FOUNDATIONS *FOR* COMMUNITY HEALTH WORKERS

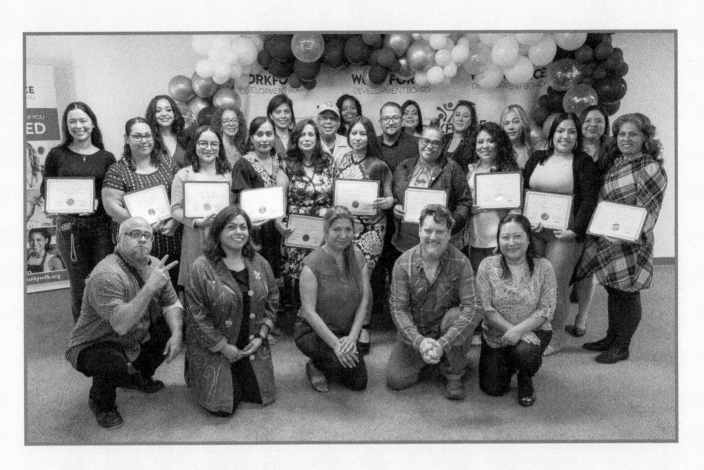

FOUNDATIONS FOR
COMMUNITY
HEALTH WORKERS

THIRD EDITION

Tim Berthold and Darouny Somsanith, Editors

JB JOSSEY-BASS™

A Wiley Brand

Library of Congress Cataloging-in-Publication Data applied for
PaperBack ISBN 9781394199785
ePDF: 9781394199839
ePub: 9781394199792

Cover design: Wiley
Cover images: Courtesy of Amy Sullivan

Set in 9/13pt Merriweather by Straive, Pondicherry, India

SKY10084566_091324

Contents

Part 1   Community Health Work: The Big Picture 1

Part 2   Core Competencies for Providing Direct Services 113

Acknowledgments

We are grateful for the dedication of our **27 authors.** Short biographical statements are provided for each author in the next section of the book.

Thank you to everyone who contributed a **CHW Profile**: Cristina Arellano, Joe Calderon, Estela Munoz de Cardenas, Lorena Carmona, Dante Casuga, Mattie Clark, Faith Fabiani, Durrell Fox, Abdul'Hafeedh bin 'Abdullah, Fadumo Jama, Michelle James, Pennie Jewell, Floribella Martinez-Redondo, Francis Julian Montgomery, Avery Nguyen, Silvia Ortega, Nilda Palacios, Monica Rico, Tahrio Sanford, Sengthong Sithounnolat, Porshay Taylor, Kim Lien Tran, and David Valentine.

We honor the other CHWs who contributed to the book through their **quotes, photographs, and participation in educational videos**, including Veronica Aburto, Victoria Adewumi, Juanita Alvarado, Leticia Olvera Arechar, Jill Armour, Kathleen Banks, Precious Beddell, Maha Begum, Lidia Benitez, Ramona Benson, John Boler, Anthony Brooks, Tomasa Bulux, Jessica Calderon-Mitchell, Rene Celiz, Esther Chavez, Andrew Ciscel, Dorel Clayton, Phuong An Doan-Billings, Cameron Dunkley, Rosaicela Estrada, Jaenia Fernandez, Felipe Flores, Ariann Harrison, Toni Hunt Hines, Alexander Fajardo, Darnell Farr, Tracy Reed Foster, Thomas Ganger, Jason Gee, Kayla Green, Lee Jackson, Sandra Johnson, Yemisrach Kibret, Yudith Larez, Rose Letulle, Michael Levato, Celeste Sanchez-Lloyd, Chelene Lopez, Inez Love, Sabrina Lozandieu, Phyllis Lui, Galen Maloney, Sergio Matos, Jermila McCoy, Richard Medina, Paul Mendez, Hugo Rengifo Ochoa, Olivia Ortiz, Sophia Simon-Ortiz, Jade Rivera, Kent Rodriguez, Keara Rodela, Romelia Rodriguez, LaTonya Rogers, Ron Sanders, Martha Shearer, Jerry Smart, Denise Octavia Smith, Abby Titter, Michelle Vail, Alma Vasquez, and Emory Wilson.

Photographs for the third edition were taken by Amy Sullivan, Francis Julian Montgomery, Susan Mayfield-Johnson, and Darouny Somsanith. Both Amy and Francis Julian are graduates of the CCSF CHW Certificate Program.

Many of the **graphics** for the new edition were designed by Blanca Goodman, a CHW and visual designer.

We thank the organizations and professionals who contributed **Case Studies** highlighting better practice standards: Dr. Marilyn Jones of Because Black is Still Beautiful; Sandy Singh with HOPE SF; Morgan Gliedman with the Transitions Clinic Project; Gayle Tang with City College of San Francisco's Health Care Interpreter Program; Cristy Dieterich with the San Francisco Department of Public Health; Ashley Kissinger with the California Department of Public health; Susan Mayfield-Johnson with the University of Southern Mississippi; Mattie Clark with the G.A. Carmichael Family Health Center; Michelle James of Friendship House; and Randi Tanksley with the Homeless Prenatal Project.

The **educational videos** linked throughout the book were codirected by Tim Berthold and Jill Tregor. Matt Luotto and Amy Hill served as videographers. The digital stories featured in Chapters 1 and 15 were produced by the Center for Digital Storytelling (with the leadership of Amy Hill and Matt Luotto).

We are grateful to the **members of the C3 and C1 teams** who consulted with the editors of the *Foundations* book and helped ensure that the content was reflective of emerging national standards for the CHW profession. Thank you to J. Nell Brownstein, Durrell Fox, Lily K. Lee, Floribella Martinez-Redondo, Paige Menking, E. Lee Rosenthal, and Julie St-John.

Pamela DeCarlo, Terri Massin, and Mike Kometani supported the development of the *Foundations* textbook by interviewing CHWs to develop profiles, by writing the Case Studies that appear throughout the book, and by reviewing early drafts of chapters.

We acknowledge and thank the faculty who have taught in the CCSF CHW Certificate Program and collaborated with students and community-based organizations to develop the curriculum that informs this book. We also thank the thousands of CCSF CHW graduates who are working with communities to promote health equity. We are grateful for the lessons you have taught us that inform the content and approach of the *Foundations* book.

We dedicate this book to community health workers: past, present, and future. We also dedicate this book to our beloved colleague and author, **Lorena Carmona**, who passed away just a few months before its publication. Lorena was a gifted and dedicated CHW leader. She will be missed and remembered by everyone who knew her.

Contributors

Cristina Arellano, CHW, BA.   Cristina is a Case Manager at LifeLong Medical Care in Oakland, California. She has served as a trainer and mentor for the Monterey County CHW Training Project.

Tim Berthold, MPH.   Tim Berthold has worked closely with community health workers for over 35 years. He supervised CHWs in public health settings in the United States and internationally. Tim develops and facilitates CHW trainings as part of a consulting group. He previously served as a faculty member and program coordinator for the CHW certificate program at City College of San Francisco.

J. Nell Brownstein, PhD.   During Nell Brownstein's 26 years at CDC, she focused on increasing recognition of the valuable roles played by CHWs as members of the public health workforce and health care teams, especially in diverse communities. She did this through CHW research and evaluation projects, written policy and scientific papers, educational products, and closely working with the CHW Special Interest Group of APHA and many other CHW allies.

Joe Calderon, AS, CHW.   Joe Calderon is dedicated to working with diverse and marginalized communities. He spent a decade leading the training and mentoring of Community Health Workers (CHWs) for the Transitions Clinic Network on a national scale. Joe continues to contribute to CHW training through the Foundations for Community Health Workers Consulting Group. Currently serving as a Program Manager at Urban Alchemy, he oversees and trains Employee Care Coordinators (CHWs) for the REAP (Reentry Employment and Prosperity) program. In this role, Joe supports individuals reentering society from state prisons, addressing the complex challenges of reentry and the collateral consequences of incarceration.

Lorena Carmona, BA, CHW.   Lorena Carmona is a Community Health Worker and Program Manager with Alameda County Care Connect at Roots Community Health Center in Oakland. Lorena trains and supervises CHWs and provides case management, health education, chronic condition management, and advocacy services. She serves on the Community Advisory Board for the CCSF CHW Certificate Program.

Mattie Clark, CHW.   Mattie Clark is a Clinical Community Health Worker with the G. A. Carmichael Family Health Center (FQHC). She has conducted many trainings and events for the community addressing health issues such as hypertension, diabetes, and COVID-19 and is a co-author of a study on cardiovascular disease among African Americans. Mattie is a member of the National Association of CHWs and Secretary of the Mississippi Community Health Workers Association.

Pau I. Crego, MPH. Pau I.   Crego is an advocate, educator, and author with a passion for advancing equity for transgender, LGBTQI+ and immigrant communities. Over the past two decades, his social justice work has spanned direct services, training and education, program design and implementation, as well as policy research and analysis. Most recently, Pau served as the Executive Director of the San Francisco Office of Transgender Initiatives. He is also part-time faculty in the CHW certificate program at City College of San Francisco, and a published author and translator in the fields of public health and trans equity.

James Figueiredo, Ed.M.   James Figueiredo is grateful for joining and remaining in the CHW field since 1991, when he served as an HIV outreach worker and case manager for over a decade on an integrated clinical team at the Cambridge Health Alliance. He later served as a longtime CHW supervisor and training facilitator across the United States and throughout sub-Saharan Africa. James is the CEO and Founder of Community Workforce Institute, where he leads a diverse team of trainers and CHW allies dedicated to supporting CHWs and supervisors.

Amie Fishman, MPH.   Amie Fishman has worked at the intersections of public health, education, and antiracist organizing for over 25 years. Much of her work has been in support of people affected by incarceration, including training CHWs to assist clients returning home. Amie currently works as a director of equity and culture for the San Francisco Department of Public Health.

Marilyn Gardner, RN, BS.   Marilyn Gardner is a writer and public health nurse living in Boston, Massachusetts. Her work with CHWs and CHW supervisors began internationally and has included four countries and several states. She is passionate about working alongside CHWs and CHW supervisors to find creative solutions for community resources and care. Marilyn is the Director of Clinical and Cross-Cultural Training at Community Workforce Institute in Cambridge, MA.

Lisa Renee Holderby-Fox, AS.   Lisa Renee is a proud member of the CHW workforce with over 30 years of experience. She is the Director of CHW Leadership Development and Envision Co-Director at the Center for Community Health Alignment, Arnold School of Public Health, University of South Carolina. Lisa Renee is a co-founder of the National Association of Community Health Workers, the New England CHW Coalition, and the Southeast CHW Network.

Pennie Jewell, CHW, AS.   Pennie has been a Community Health Worker for over 30 years. She is a member of the Michigan Community Health Worker Alliance, the National Association of Community Health Workers, and a member of the CHW Common Indicators Project Leadership Team.

Rama Ali Kased, EdD.   Rama Ali Kased is an Assistant Professor of race and resistance studies at SF State University. She has over 20 years of experience in community organizing and teaching. Her work and research center on social justice, public health, and education equity. She has an extensive background in campaign and leadership development and K-12 and higher education curriculum development.

Jimmy Ly, MA.   Jimmy Ly is a career counselor and instructor at City College of San Francisco (CCSF) with nearly 10 years of counseling experience in the areas of mental health, careers, and academics. In addition to counseling, he teaches a course on job search techniques and leads career workshops for students in various Health Education programs at CCSF including CHW, Healthcare Interpretation, and Addiction and Recovery Counseling.

Thelma Gamboa-Maldonado, DrPH, MPH.   Thelma is a community-based public health researcher, academician, and practitioner with extensive experience in non-profit, local, and state governmental public health practice. CHW inclusion and workforce development have been central to Thelma's work both internationally and in California. Thelma is a former Director of the Loma Linda University San Manuel Gateway College CHW (Promotores) Academy and is currently on faculty in the CHW Certificate Program at City College of San Francisco.

Susan Mayfield-Johnson, PhD, MCHES.   Susan Mayfield-Johnson has been a CHW ally for over 25 years. She is an Associate Professor at The University of Southern Mississippi, a member of the Leadership Team of the Community Health Worker Common Indicators Project, and a founding board member of the National Association of Community Health Workers.

Lily K. Lee, DrPH, MPH. Lily K.   Lee is a multicultural and multilingual public health professional with over 20 years of experience in program design and implementation, research and evaluation, and organizational change management. Lily developed strategic approaches to operationalize CHW/P Core Competencies in various settings and the Organizational Readiness Training program for employers familiar with or new to the CHWs/Ps roles and competencies. Lily is the founder of the KTE Strategies consulting firm, which provides Knowledge Transfer and Exchange strategies to public health and healthcare initiatives for greater impact on population health outcomes.

Savita Malik, EdD, MPH.   Savita Malik has been at the intersection of public health and education for more than 20 years. She is faculty at San Francisco State University and a co-founder and current curriculum and faculty developer for the Metro College Success Program.

Floribella Redondo-Martinez, BS.   Floribella Redondo-Martinez has been working in the scope of a CHW/ Promotora for more than 30 years. She is the co-founder and chief executive officer of the Arizona Community

Health Workers Association. Floribella is a co-founder and board member of the National Association of Community Health Workers, a member of C3 Core Team, CHW Council for Envision, and a Lead Faculty for the CHW Certificate Program at Arizona Western College.

Paige Menking, MPA. Paige Menking is a CHW ally whose over a decade of work in the field has centered around CHW training, supervision, research, and workforce development on local and national levels. She is the principal and founder of Ponderosa Public Health Consulting and lives in Albuquerque, New Mexico. She serves on the board of the National Association of CHWs and as a leader in the APHA CHW section and is on the core team of the CHW Core Consensus (C3) Project.

Francis Julian Montgomery. Francis Julian Montgomery works as a Street Crisis Response Specialist with the San Francisco Homeless Outreach Team (SF HOT). He works with the San Francisco Fire Department Community Paramedics Division, connecting unhoused people to shelter/housing, mental, medical health programs, treatment, resources, and social service support systems. Francis Julian is certified as an Addictions Treatment Counselor and is a graduate of City College of San Francisco Community Health Worker Certificate Program and the Drug and Alcohol Certificate Program.

Alberta Rincón, MPH. Alberta Rincón has served as an advocate, community organizer, change agent, health educator, trainer, and university administrator in the public health field for over 40 years. Since 2005, she has taught core community health worker coursework at City College of San Francisco.

E. Lee Rosenthal, PhD, MPH E. Lee Rosenthal has worked to support the growth and development of the Community Health Worker (CHW) workforce through collaborative research and advocacy with CHWs since the late 1980s. Lee has led the national Community Health Worker Core Consensus (C3) Project team since it began in 2014. Based at Texas Tech University Health Sciences Center El Paso, she teaches public health to medical and dental students. As of 2023, she serves as co-editor of the *Journal of Ambulatory Care Management*, which has a focus on CHW practice and research and that emphasizes CHWs roles as authors and reviewers.

Larry Salomon, PhD. Larry Salomon has been teaching in the College of Ethnic Studies at San Francisco State University for nearly 30 years. He teaches courses on social movements and community organizing, racial politics, critical thinking, and even courses focusing on the intersections between race and both sports and comedy. Larry is the author of the book *Roots of Justice: Stories of Organizing in Communities of Color*.

Darouny Somsanith, MPH. Darouny Somsanith is the coordinator of the Community Health Worker (CHW) Program and a faculty member within the Health Education Department at City College of San Francisco. She started her public health career as a CHW and has over 20 years of experience working on issues of workforce development and supporting the diverse training needs of community health workers.

Julie Ann St. John, DrPH, MPH, MA, CHWI. Julie St. John is a public health practitioner and researcher who has worked with CHWs locally, nationally, and globally for over 20 years. She is a Texas-certified Community Health Worker Instructor, served on the Texas CHW Advisory Committee for 10 years, a member of the APHA CHW Section Council, and was a founding board member of the Texas Association of Promotores/Community Health Workers. Her research and practice interests include engaging CHWs in community-based participatory research and community health development approaches; improving health status and quality of life among diverse and rural populations; addressing human trafficking through community capacity building; and equipping future public health professionals through teaching, service, research, and practice.

Jill R. Tregor, MPH. Jill Tregor is an adjunct instructor with the Community Health Worker and Alcohol and Drug Counselor certificate programs at City College of San Francisco. She has many years of experience working with community-based organizations addressing hate-motivated violence, women's health, and domestic violence.

About the Companion Website

This book is accompanied by a companion website.

http://www.wiley.com/go/communityhealthworkers3E

The website includes:

- Training guides and Video index

Introduction

Foundations for Community Health Workers is a resource for training, teaching, and credentialing CHWs. It is inspired by the curriculum for the CHW Certificate Program at City College of San Francisco (CCSF). The CCSF program (CCSF CHW Program, 2023) was established in 1992 and is still going strong.

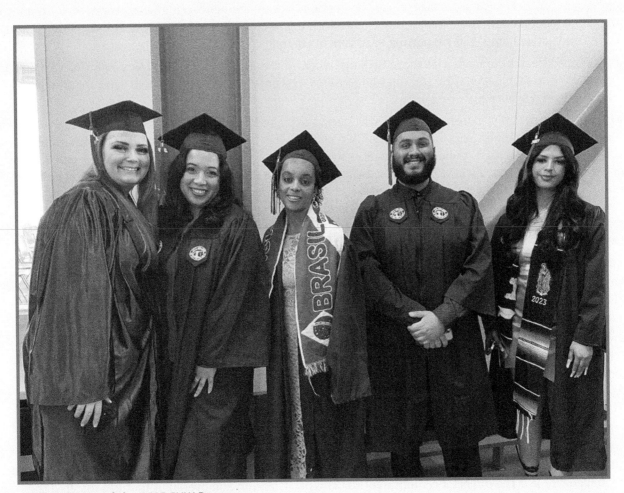

2023 graduates of the CCSF CHW Program.

Guiding principles that inform this book include a commitment to health equity and social justice, cultural humility, and person- and community-centered practice that respects the experience, wisdom, and autonomy of CHWs and the communities they serve.

The book is designed for CHWs in training and is divided into five sections:

- <u>Part One</u> provides information about the broad context that informs the work of CHWs. It includes an introduction to the role and history of CHWs, the discipline of public health, and the principles of health equity.

- <u>Part Two</u> addresses the core competencies or skills that most CHWs rely on day-to-day. This section includes chapters on ethics, person-centered practice, cultural humility, motivational interviewing, case management, action planning, and home visiting.

- <u>Part Three</u> addresses key professional skills for career success including stress management, conflict resolution, code switching, providing and receiving constructive feedback, and how to develop a resume and interview for a job.

- <u>Part Four</u> applies key competencies to specific health topics including working with people who are returning home from incarceration, supporting clients with the management of chronic health conditions, healthy eating and active living, and supporting survivors of trauma.

- <u>Part Five</u> addresses competencies that CHWs use when working at the group and community levels, including health outreach, facilitating trainings and groups, research and evaluation skills, and community organizing and advocacy.

One book cannot possibly address all the knowledge and skills required of CHWs. Our intention is to provide an introduction to the competencies most commonly required when working with clients and communities. This textbook does not attempt to provide information about all the specific health issues that CHWs will address in the field (such as type two diabetes, pediatric asthma, substance use, depression and other mental health conditions, and the challenges of being unhoused). Health knowledge changes rapidly as new research findings are released, and many reputable health organizations provide regularly updated information online. Our approach is to cover the key skills that CHWs provide in the field and to let employers take the lead in providing additional training on specific health topics and issues that they will address on the job.

The Community Health Worker Core Consensus (C3) Project (The C3 Project, 2023) has partnered with the *Foundations* textbook in its third edition to help readers understand how the skills that are featured within each textbook chapter map to the skills identified by the C3 Project.

Why the C3 Project?

- The C3 Project (2014–2018) built and now works to maintain a national consensus about CHW core roles and competencies (qualities and skills). The Project's goal is to expand cohesion in the CHW field and contribute to the visibility and greater understanding of the full potential of CHWs to improve health, community development, and access to systems of care.

- The C3 Project findings reflect a consensus-driven process that emphasized the input of CHW leaders working at the local, state, and national levels about CHW roles and competencies. CHW guidance was prioritized as a first step before Project findings were released to a wider national audience. The C3 Project team believes it is the Project's commitment to CHW participation and oversight that has fostered the wide use and support of the C3 Project core roles and competencies.

- The C3 Project core roles and competencies originated from a national study in the 1990s led by the same leadership team. In order to carry out the C3 Project, the research team used the 1994–1998 National Community Health Advisor Study (NCHAS) recommended core roles and competencies as a baseline and compared them to emerging CHW roles and competencies identified in selected policy and training sources—including *just one curriculum—the Foundations textbook itself*. The focus of the C3 Project comparison, or "crosswalk" as it is known, was to identify what new roles and skills had emerged (or disappeared) in the two decades since the original NCHAS.

From that research and supporting consensus-driven review, the C3 Project identified:

- **CHW roles or scope of practice:** Ten (10) core roles that CHWs play; together these roles form the CHW "scope of practice." The *Foundations* textbook is intended to build CHW's capacity to play these many roles in service to individuals, families, and communities.

- **CHW qualities:** Qualities are the natural and nurtured inner passion and motivation that CHWs possess—a core element of qualities is CHWs' connection to the community served. The C3 Project endorsed qualities identified in the NCHAS that were reaffirmed in consensus-driven work in New York. In the future, the C3 Project will assess these qualities more fully.

- **CHW skills:** Eleven (11) core skills range from communication to capacity-building skills. These eleven (11) skills combined give CHWs a strong foundation for their work and service.

The following table shows where each of the C3 Project's Core CHW Skills is covered in the Foundations book.

ALIGNING THE C3 PROJECT AND THE *FOUNDATIONS FOR CHWs* TEXTBOOK	
C3 CHW COMPETENCIES: CORE SKILLS	***FOUNDATIONS* CHAPTER(S)**
1. Communication Skills	Chapters 6, 7, 9, 13, 20, and 21
2. Interpersonal and Relationship-building Skills	Chapters 5, 6, 7, 9, 13, and 18
3. Service Coordination and Navigation Skills	Chapters 8, 10, 11, 16, 17, and 18
4. Capacity-building Skills	Chapters 1, 9, 15, 21, 22, and 23
5. Advocacy Skills	Chapters 2, 4, 10, and 23
6. Education and Facilitation Skills	Chapters 19, 20, and 21
7. Individual and Community Assessment Skills	Chapters 3, 8, 9, 11, 16, 17, 22, and 23
8. Outreach Skills	Chapters 19 and 23
9. Professional Skills and Conduct	Chapters 5, 7, 12, 13, and 14
10. Evaluation and Research Skills	Chapters 2, 3, and 22
11. Knowledge Base	Chapters 1, 2, 3, 4, 5, 6, 15, 16, 17, and 18

Each chapter in the *Foundations* textbook displays a brief chart at the start to allow you to make a crosswalk to the C3 Project Skills that most align with the content in the Foundation textbook chapter.

In addition to the C3 skills crosswalk in each chapter, to learn more about the C3 Project, see Chapter 1 on the role of CHWs and Chapter 2 on the history of the CHW field. We have included the C3 Project Review Checklist of CHW Roles and Competencies at the end of the book. You can use this resource to assess your progress in learning essential professional skills; you can reach the C3 Project team at: info@c3project.org

The new edition of *Foundations* includes **23 Profiles of working CHWs**—one in each chapter. Each profile captures the motivations and contributions of a CHW along with their tips and suggestions for those starting out in the profession.

The book includes **short educational videos** (QR codes are provided in the hard copy edition of the book and direct links in the e-book version) highlighting key CHW concepts and skills. These videos feature interviews with CHWs and public health experts, as well as role-plays that show CHWs working with clients. The role plays are designed to demonstrate key CHWs skills. We have also included "counter" role plays that highlight common mistakes or approaches that we wouldn't recommend for CHWs. We use these videos to generate discussion in our classrooms and to engage students in applying key concepts for working effectively with clients. All videos are posted to the Foundations for CHWs YouTube Channel at https://www.youtube.com/@foundationsforcommunityhea6889/search

Please watch the following two videos that were created by students who graduated from the City College CHW Certificate Program. These are called "digital stories," and they briefly describe what motivated each video maker to become a CHW.

A companion *Training Guide to Foundations for Community Health Workers* is available for free at Wiley (Wiley, 2023). The Training Guide presents step-by-step training plans and assessment resources corresponding to each chapter of the *Foundations* textbook. Additional educational videos are also provided.

This book is rooted in a deep hope for a world characterized by social justice and equitable access to the basic resources—including education, employment, food, housing, safety, health care, and human rights—that everyone needs in order to be healthy. CHWs play a vital role in helping to create such a world. They partner with clients and communities and support them to take action to bring this hope closer to reality.

CHW DIGITAL STORY: ROBERT'S STORY
(*Source:* Foundations for Community Health Workers/http://youtu.be/Acaf7cKFGy0/last accessed 21 September 2023.)

CHW DIGITAL STORY: LUCIANA'S STORY
(*Source:* Foundations for Community Health Workers/http://youtu.be/FS9leOmwACk/last accessed 21 September 2023.)

Tim Berthold and Darouny Somsanith

Co-editors

References

City College of San Francisco. (2023). Community Health Worker Certificate Program. https://www.ccsf.edu/degrees-certificates/community-health-worker (accessed 6 June 2023).

The Community Health Worker Core Consensus Project (C3). (2023). The Community Health Worker Core Consensus Project (C3). https://www.c3project.org/ (accessed 6 June 2023).

Wiley. (2023). Foundations for Community Health Workers Training Guide. https://bcs.wiley.com/he-bcs/Books?action=index&bcsId=10183&itemId=1119060818 (accessed 6 June 2023).

COMMUNITY HEALTH WORK: THE BIG PICTURE

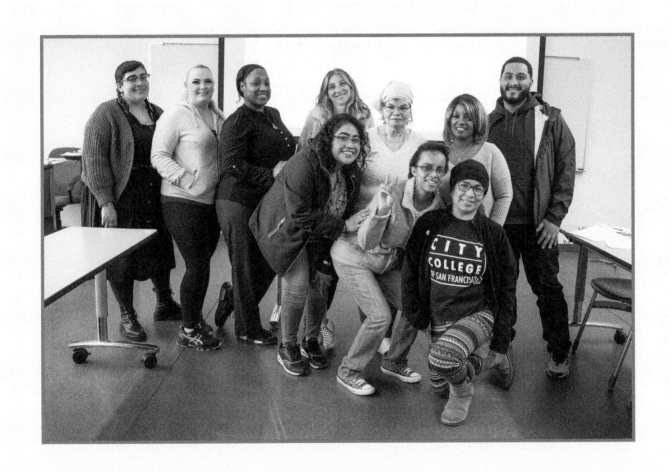

The Role of Community Health Workers—Serving with Skills and Compassion

Darouny Somsanith and Susan Mayfield-Johnson

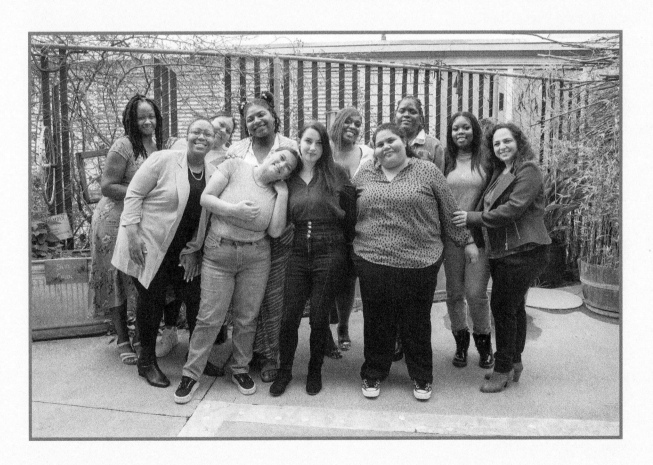

Foundations for Community Health Workers, Third Edition. Edited by Tim Berthold and Darouny Somsanith.
© 2024 John Wiley & Sons, Inc. Published 2024 by John Wiley & Sons, Inc.
Companion website: http://www.wiley.com/go/communityhealthworkers3E

Introduction

Welcome to our book! In this first chapter, you will be introduced to the key roles and competencies of Community Health Workers (CHWs) and the common qualities and values shared by successful CHWs.

You may already possess some of the qualities, knowledge, and skills common among CHWs.

- Are you a trusted member of your community?
- Have you ever assisted a family member or friend to obtain health care services?
- Are you passionate about changing the factors that are harming your community's health?
- Have you participated in efforts to advocate for social change?
- Do you hope that, in your work, you can work with your community members to become healthy, strong, and in charge of their lives?

If you answered yes to any of these questions, you have some of the qualities and characteristics of a successful CHW.

WHAT YOU WILL LEARN

By studying the information in this chapter, you will be able to:

- Describe CHWs and what they do
- Identify where CHWs work, the communities they work with, and the health issues they address
- Explain the core roles that CHWs play in the fields of public health, healthcare, and social services
- Discuss the core competencies that CHWs use to assist individuals and communities
- Describe personal qualities and attributes that are common among successful CHWs
- Discuss emerging models of healthcare and opportunities for CHWs
- Discuss the importance of language access for clients and communities with limited English language skills

C3 Roles and Skills Addressed in Chapter 1

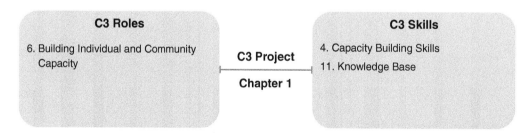

WORDS TO KNOW

Advocate (noun and verb)

Affordable Care Act (ACA)

Core Roles and Competencies

Credentialing, Health Inequities

Mortality, Social Determinants of Health

Scope of Practice

Social Justice

1.1 Who Are CHWS and What Do They Do?

CHWs help individuals, families, groups, and communities to improve their health, increase their access to health and social services, and reduce health inequities. CHWs generally come from the communities they serve and are uniquely prepared to provide culturally and linguistically appropriate services. They work with diverse and often disadvantaged communities at high risk of illness, disability, and death.

CHWs provide a wide range of services, including outreach, home visits, health education, and person-centered counseling and care management. They support clients in accessing high-quality health and social services programs. They facilitate support groups and workshops and support communities to organize and advocate (to actively speak up and support a client, community, or policy change) for social change to advance the community's health and welfare. CHWs also work with public health, healthcare, and social services agencies to enhance their capacity to provide culturally sensitive services that truly respect the diverse identities, strengths, and needs of the clients and communities they serve.

As a result of the contributions of CHWs, clients and communities learn new information and skills, increase their confidence, and enhance their ability to manage health conditions and advocate for themselves. Most importantly, the work that CHWs do reduces persistent **health inequities** or differences in the rates of illness, disability, and death (**mortality**) among different communities (Hurtado et al., 2014).

The term community health worker describes both volunteers who contribute informally to improve their community's health and those who are paid for providing these services. Regardless of compensation, CHWs serve as "frontline" health and social service workers and are often the first contact a community member has with a health or social service agency. Typically, CHWs are trusted members of the community they serve, having deep knowledge of the resources, relationships, and needs of that community.

As helping professionals, CHWs are motivated by compassion and the desire to assist those in need. Their core professional duties are to work for equity and **social justice**, a belief that all people deserve to be valued equally and provided with equitable access to essential health resources such as housing, food, education, employment, health care, and civil rights. Many CHWs take on this work because they have experienced discrimination and poverty themselves. Others simply see a need and want to improve conditions in their communities. Regardless of how the CHW comes to the work, every CHW is an **advocate**—someone who speaks up for a cause or policy or on someone else's behalf—working to promote health and better the conditions that support wellness in local communities.

The American Public Health Association adopted an official definition for CHWs in 2009, developed by CHWs, researchers and advocates:

> *A Community Health Worker (CHW) is a frontline public health worker who is a trusted member of and/or has an unusually close understanding of the community served. This trusting relationship enables the CHW to serve as a liaison/link/intermediary between health/social services and the community to facilitate access to services and improve the quality and cultural competence of service delivery. A CHW also builds individual and community capacity by increasing health knowledge and self-sufficiency through a range of activities such as outreach, community education, informal counseling, social support, and advocacy. (American Public Health Association, 2009).*

In 2010, U.S. Department of Labor, Bureau of Labor Statistics, approved a standard occupational code—SOC 21-1094—and further defined CHWs as professionals who:

> *Assist individuals and communities to adopt healthy behaviors. Conduct outreach for medical personnel or health organizations to implement programs in the community that promote, maintain, and improve individual and community health. May provide information on available resources, provide social support and informal counseling, advocate for individuals and community health needs, and provide services such as first aid and blood pressure screening. May collect data to help identify community health needs. (Bureau of Labor Statistics, 2023).*

Having a standard occupational code allowed for CHW positions to be reported as part of employment statistics. Prior to this, CHWs were included in the broad category of "social and human service assistants," which undercounted their total numbers in the U.S. workforce, as many were not counted at all in official statistics. Complicating this further is the estimated 250 job titles that are associated with the CHW profession, which made it hard to truly capture this classification of worker.

Denise Octavia Smith: How are we unique? At the heart of being a CHW—and I know a lot of CHWs that did not work with this title for many years or maybe even decades doing this work—what has always set us (CHWs) apart is this sort of Venn diagram of our lived experience, our commitment to community well-being, both individual and the larger community of families, and ecosystems that sort of supported this burden. I would say we build both the capacity for people to find what they need to achieve health and well-being, and we advocate to change those things that prevent health and well-being. Right? It's like when these things all come together, you would call it a community health worker.

You may know a CHW already. You might be one. Health departments, community-based organizations, hospitals and clinics, faith-based organizations, foundations, and researchers value the important contributions of CHWs to promoting the health and well-being of low-income and at-risk communities. CHWs work under a wide range of professional titles. Some of the most popular are listed in Table 1.1.

Table 1.1 Common Titles for CHWs

Case manager/Case worker	Health ambassador
Community health advocate	Health educator
Community health outreach worker	Health worker
Community health worker	Lay health advisor
Community health representative	Public health aide
Community outreach worker	Patient navigator
Community liaison	Peer counselor
Community organizer	Peer educator
Enrollment specialist	Promotor/a *de salud*

- *Can you think of other titles for CHWs?*

What Do
YOU?
Think

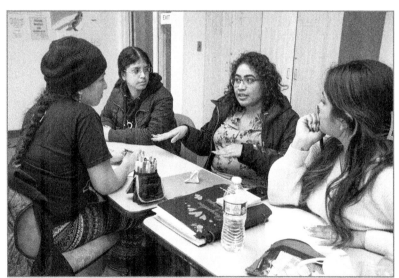

A team of CHWs planning their work

Please watch this video interview about *Becoming a CHW*.

(*Source:* Foundations for Community Health Workers/http://youtu.be/BASkvuq1epw)

Lisa Renee Holderby-Fox: My first job as a CHW was doing home visiting with high-risk pregnant women and teens. I was living in an area of Massachusetts that had the highest infant mortality rate for Black women and Latinas. They were looking to hire individuals who had common experiences. I had been a teen parent and had needed the same services as many of those I'd be working with. Many times, I did not know what was out there or what was available for additional support. It was a lot of trial and error for me. I thought that if I could help someone else and help them get the services and support they needed, it would be a really interesting job. I applied and was hired.

The first person I worked with was referred by her primary care provider. She was diabetic and pregnant, and he (the provider) called her "noncompliant." He said that she wasn't eating well; she wasn't taking her insulin the way she should take it, and that put her at higher risk during pregnancy and delivery. That's why he referred her to our program.

She was in the hospital because of her diabetes when I met her. She had a really tough exterior, but I don't know, there was something interesting about her. I wanted to get to know more, get to know her a little better, and maybe I could offer some assistance. When I did my first home visit, she had no electricity. Without electricity, she couldn't keep food in the fridge or store her insulin. I was able to get her electricity back on, and we got a second-hand fridge from a local agency (they just gave it to us).

Over time, I saw that she was taking her insulin, eating better, and had a successful delivery. After giving birth, she disclosed partner abuse. I knew I could not tell her to leave because that is not what women want to hear in that moment. That's not what I wanted to hear when I was in an abusive relationship, so I just worked with her over time, gave her resources, and let her know gradually that there was something better for her out there, that she deserved more, and she finally left him. She was a great mom, and I was able to see all of that happen. That's when I knew I had a purpose and a place in this work. As I got to work with more women who had a variety of different needs, it just became apparent to me that I had something to give.

It has been difficult to determine how many CHWs are working in the United States due to the wide variety of CHW job titles and duties. In the last 15 years, several national studies have attempted to take inventory of CHWs, most notably the 2007 study by the U.S. Department of Health and Human Services and the University of Texas in San Antonio (USDHHS, 2007) and the two National Community Health Worker Advocacy Surveys (Arizona Prevention Research Center, 2014) completed in 2010 and 2014. The following data comes from the U.S. Bureau of Labor Statistics data from 2022 to get an overview of the profession (Bureau of Labor Statistics, 2023):

- The growth rate for CHWs over the 10-year period from 2021 to 2031 is forecasted to be 16%. This growth rate is faster than average, when compared to other occupations.

- In May 2021, there were an estimated 61,000 CHWs working in the United States. However, this number is likely to be an undercount of CHWs in the United States due to the diverse job titles that CHWs hold, as well as the undercounting of Promotores de Salud or others working in a volunteer or contract capacity. In 2014, the Center for Disease Control (CDC) estimated the workforce to be closer to 100,000 (Centers for Disease Control and Prevention, 2014), and there has been substantial growth in the profession since then.

- CHWs earn an average wage of $22.97/hour and $47,780/year. Note that wages vary considerably across the United States.

- The top ten industries with the highest employment of CHWs were: local government (excluding schools), individuals and family services, outpatient care centers, general medical and surgical hospitals, insurance carriers, social advocacy organizations, community food housing and emergency services, grantmaking and giving services, home health care services, and skilled nursing facilities.

From the 2007 HRSA study, we find that most CHWs work within the field of public health (see Chapter 3) and primarily with low-income communities. They address a wide range of health issues, including homelessness, violence, environmental health, mental health, recovery, and civil and human rights issues, as well as more traditional health issues (cancer prevention, asthma, and HIV disease). They work with children, youth and their families, adults and seniors, men and women, and people of all sexual orientations and gender identities. CHWs are flexible and can work with individual clients and families, with groups, and at the community level. More about the history of Community Health Work will be shared in Chapter 2.

MODELS OF CARE

The CHW National Workforce Study identified five "models of care" that incorporate CHWs. These models are common in both healthcare and community settings:

1. **Member of a care delivery team:** CHWs work with other providers (e.g., doctors, nurses, and social workers) to care for individual patients.

2. **Navigator:** CHWs are called upon to use their extensive knowledge of the complex health care system to assist individuals and patients in accessing the services they need and gain greater confidence in interacting with their providers.

3. **Screening and health education provider:** CHWs administer basic health screening (e.g., pregnancy tests, blood pressure checks, and rapid HIV antibody tests) and provide prevention education on basic health topics.

4. **Outreach/enrolling/informing agent:** CHWs go into the community to reach and inform people about the services they qualify for and encourage them to enroll in these programs and benefits.

5. **Organizer:** CHWs work with other community members to advocate for change on a specific issue or cause. Often their work aids community members to become stronger advocates for themselves.

- *When did you first become aware of CHWs?*

- *Are CHWs working in your community?*

- *Do some or all of the five models of care resonate with your understanding of the CHW profession?*

1.2 CHWs and Public Health

CHWs often work within the field of public health. Unlike medicine, public health works to promote the health of entire communities or large populations, and to prevent the further impact of disease and illness within the community (see Chapter 3). Public health understands the primary causes of illness and health to be more than just access to health care, but also whether or not people have access to basic resources and rights, including food, housing, education, employment with safe working conditions and a living wage, transportation, clean air and water, and civil rights. Collectively, the broad range of factors and conditions that influence and contribute to health are called the "**social determinants of health**."

Across the world, CHWs are working to promote the health of local communities. Due to their close understanding of the unique needs of the communities they serve, it is no surprise that during the COVID-19 pandemic, CHWs became expert public health professionals that people turned to for information, support, and assistance.

The field of public health not only provides services to prevent illness and improve care, but it also influences the social determinants of health by advocating for policies to assure basic resources and rights for all people. CHWs share in this advocacy work. For example, one of the core values listed on the website of the Community Health Worker Network of New York City states, "Community health workers are agents of change who pursue social justice through work with individuals and communities to improve social conditions" (CHW Network of New York City, 2023).

To achieve the goal of eliminating health inequities, attention must shift to address the social determinants of health that contribute to disease. Included in the list of social determinants of health are social support, social cohesion, and universal access to medical care. Social support refers to support on the individual level when resources are provided by others, and social cohesion refers to support on a community level when the trust and respect between different sections of society result in cherishing people and their health. CHWs impact these social determinants of health as they build supportive relationships with community members and community groups to promote access to resources and health care (Hispanic Health Council, 2018).

1.3 Roles and Competencies of CHWs

The roles that CHWs take on, and the competencies that CHWs need to fulfill those roles, continue to evolve in response to changing public health strategies and healthcare delivery models. CHWs have proven to be effective in promoting improved patient health outcomes and reducing health care costs in programs focused on prevention, chronic conditions management, healthy maternity, and health care access or enrollment (Crespo, Christiansen, Tieman & Wittberg, 2020). CHWs help to ensure that services are culturally and linguistically appropriate, especially when they are involved in designing those services. As more CHWs are employed in healthcare and public health, and as new mechanisms for funding and institutionalizing CHW positions emerge, the demand for greater clarity in defining CHW roles and competencies has also increased.

The **Community Health Worker Core Consensus Project (C3 Project)** has taken on the task of convening a national consensus of these roles and skill sets through their collaborative work with CHWs, allies, and employer partners (C3 Project, 2023). The C3 Project built upon the work of the landmark 1998 Community Health Advisor Study (Rosenthal, Wiggins, Brownstein, Rael & Johnson, 1998). One of the first major studies of the CHW profession, it documented the duties that CHWs perform, identified core CHW roles and skill sets, and discussed the values or personal characteristics that many CHWs share (see Chapter 2 for more details of this study). A summary of the C3 Roles and Competencies or Skills can be found in Table 1.2.

It should be noted that defining what CHW does is not without controversy. Other health professionals may raise concerns when they see an overlap between their profession and that of CHWs in areas such as health education, counseling, systems navigation, and case management. Some CHWs, as they serve in so many different capacities and models of care, worry that too tight a definition of the CHW role could leave out some valuable CHW practices. Yet CHWs and others who work with them advocate for a clearer definition of the CHW role to better define a CHW's scope of practice. A **scope of practice** refers to the range of services and duties that a specific category of worker, such as CHWs, is competent to provide. While many CHWs express mixed feelings about how far the field should be formalized, all agree that the work they do deserves more recognition from government and other professionals, and increased funding.

The official classification of CHWs by the U.S. Department of Labor, Bureau of Labor Statistics, in 2010 was a significant step toward national recognition of the CHW occupation. This recognition has facilitated mechanisms for reimbursements of CHW services from state and federal programs such as Medicaid and Medicare. Reimbursement of CHW services under Medicaid was formally allowed under the **Affordable Care Act** of 2010 (the ACA), and each state has the option to establish policies to do this. Even before the ACA passed, states could seek a Medicaid waiver to allow "fee for service" reimbursement for certain CHW services. As this textbook goes to print, 20 state Medicaid programs now reimburse for CHW services (with an additional 3 states allowing reimbursement on a narrower scope of services). Reimbursement for CHW services through large public insurance programs like Medicaid establishes a more sustained and stable funding stream for CHWs jobs, instead of a reliance on grants that come and go. Formal recognition of the occupation also makes other avenues of financing CHW jobs more feasible.

Table 1.2 CHW Core Consensus (C3) Project Roles and Competencies

C3 ROLES	C3 COMPETENCIES/SKILLS
1. Cultural Mediation Among Individuals, Communities, and Health and Social Services Systems 2. Providing Culturally Appropriate Health Education and Information 3. Care Coordination, Case Management, and System Navigation 4. Providing Coaching and Social Support 5. Advocating for Individuals and Communities 6. Building Individuals and Community Capacity 7. Providing Direct Services 8. Implementing Individual and Community Assessments 9. Conducting Outreach 10. Participating in Evaluation and Research	1. Communication Skills 2. Interpersonal and Relationship-Building Skills 3. Service Coordination and Navigation Skills 4. Capacity Building Skills 5. Advocacy Skills 6. Education and Facilitation Skills 7. Individual and Community Assessment Skills 8. Outreach Skills 9. Professional Skills and Conduct 10. Evaluation and Research Skills 11. Knowledge Base

The C3 Project is an important reference for the CHW profession. As CHW coalitions and public health advocates have worked to develop mechanisms for greater employment of CHWs and reimbursement of CHW services under the ACA, states have defined CHW roles differently. While there has been substantial overlap with the roles and competencies identified in the 1998 study, some roles have been added or defined in more detail (such as outreach and participatory research). New terminologies such as system navigation and care coordination have emerged—these concepts were present in the 1998 study, but not articulated as such, and more sophisticated methods of providing these services have been developed together by CHWs and other health professionals in the last ten years. The C3 Project works collaboratively with CHWs and allies throughout the nation to provide a unifying national reference on CHWs roles and skills. Identifying CHW competencies allows trainers and employers to better support CHWs in their work.

Below we present the 10 core roles and 11 core competencies identified by the C3 Project. We address each of these roles and competencies in this book. The Introduction includes a chart that shows which C3 Roles and Competencies are addressed in each chapter of the book.

What are Core Roles and Competencies?

Core roles are the major functions a person performs on the job. For example, the core roles of a farmer include clearing fields, planting, and harvesting crops. The core roles of CHWs include providing outreach, health education, person-centered counseling, case management, community organizing, and advocacy.

Core competencies are the knowledge and skills a person needs in order to perform a job well. Again, a farmer must be able to operate equipment, assess timing for planting, and prepare the soil. Core competencies for CHWs include knowledge of public health, behavior change, ethics, and community resources and the ability to provide health information, facilitate groups, resolve conflicts, and conduct an initial client interview or assessment. CHW educational programs seek to strengthen CHW competencies or skills.

10 CORE CHW ROLES

1. **Cultural mediation among individuals, communities, and health and social services systems.** Intimate knowledge of the communities they work with permits CHWs to serve as cultural brokers between their clients and health and social services systems. As a bridge that links community members to essential services, CHWs ensure that the clients receive quality care.

> **Avery Nguyen:** As a non-binary CHW working exclusively with female clients, I do not disclose my transgender identity to all but one of my clients. The one client who knows I'm trans, I disclosed to because she is also trans, and it is a major part of how she sees herself and how she navigates the world. While from different class backgrounds, regional upbringing and generations, I feel so grateful that I have the opportunity to connect with this client and advocate/represent her. Knowing from personal experience and witnessing it with her, I am very protective of my client against transphobia, overt or otherwise. Overall, working with clients who have chronic illness, I help them navigate the various medical systems they need to go through to get the care they need. This can be so exhausting, and people can get burnt out. I'm thankful when I can reduce the burden on my clients.

2. **Providing culturally appropriate health education and information.** Because CHWs usually come from the communities they serve, they are familiar with the cultural identities of the clients they work with (e.g., language, values, customs, sexual orientation, and so on) and are better prepared to provide health information in ways that the community will understand and accept. Health education can be provided one-on-one, in small groups, or through large presentations.

Abby Titter: Having the ability to give real, valuable, and individualized education to members of my community on topics that matter to them not only helps positively change the lives of each member, but the community as a whole. Education is a huge priority in what we do here. I am not just going to say, "here's a few facts about diabetes." I am not going to tell you "Just to eat right." We are going to look at the issue and figure out what needs to be done together. For example, I had a community member who had had gastric bypass surgery. Of course, he could not have certain foods, but he was doing what he needed to do and constantly getting sick. We sat and down and analyzed his diet; we looked at everything he was eating. We realized that the issue was aspartame. In an effort to try to eat a healthier diet, he was consuming sugar free foods and beverages that has aspartame as a substitute. I provided the education that he needed, explained what was going on, and worked with him to make substitutions that did not make him sick. He said that this was an "eye opening thing for him." It changed his quality of life, and he tells everyone about it.

3. **Care coordination, case management, and system navigation.** CHWs provide support to clients by coordinating care from multiple service providers and by helping them navigate complex health and social services organizations and programs. Navigating systems and accessing services is often confusing or overwhelming for clients, especially if they are unhoused, living with pain or chronic health conditions, have limited English Proficiency skills, or a past history of discriminatory treatment from service providers.

Cristina Arellano: I provide services to the unhoused and previously unhoused populations in my role as a CHW Case Manager. Once they are housed, clients share that they are noticing aches and pains they couldn't pay attention to before. That's my signal to step in and offer to connect them to a primary care doctor. Because I'm connected to a Community Health Center, I can access client's medical insurance information. I sit and call the doctor's office with a client to make an appointment. I note it in my calendar and will remind the client the day before or morning of their appointment. If I sense a client is nervous about the appointment or has a history of missing appointments, I offer to attend the first appointment under the pretense of "going to help with paperwork." It's a good opportunity for me to get to know the Client, and review with them what they'd like to share with the primary care doctor. The supportive housing program I work for allows us to schedule transportation to and from medical or social service appointments for Clients. Providing transportation removes a barrier for many clients that have serious chronic and health conditions.

4. **Providing coaching and social support.** CHWs provide person-centered care through informal counseling or coaching to support clients to live healthier lives. A CHW may help clients set health-related goals and may use techniques such as motivational interviewing (see Chapters 9 and 10) to support clients in reducing health-related risk behaviors. CHWs support clients in identifying their internal and external resources, as well as affirm their positive qualities, intentions, and accomplishments. These strengths are often the most important resources to support a client in making changes that will promote their health.

Pennie Jewell: One of my greatest joys as a CHW is when a client shows obvious signs of improvement in their physical and/or mental health and overall well-being as a direct result of our relationship. Social support is especially important when a client lives alone and does not have family or friends nearby. I have provided support in a variety of ways; all of which are beneficial. I have facilitated group activities, such as outings to local events/venues, encouraged clients to obtain care when needed, supported them to create and reach their goals, helped them feel confident to self-manage their chronic conditions, and coached them through challenges they encountered. In my experience, however, I've found that listening is by far the most important skill and service you can provide within this role - active listening with no judgement. Most clients just need someone to talk to and to feel that someone truly cares. All of the other activities you do when providing social support and coaching are simply an added bonus.

5. **Advocating for individuals and communities.** CHWs speak out with and on behalf of clients and communities. They advocate—with the community whenever possible—to make sure that clients are treated respectfully and given access to the basic resources that they need in order to live healthy lives.

Celeste Sanchez-Lloyd: For me, advocacy starts with being a CHW, but it does not just end with me. We speak out for our community members to their providers, to referral organizations, and to policy makers. My role as a CHW has been centered around how "we" can influence a continuum of change for our communities. We acknowledge and elevate our communities as the key for solutions because they (the community) know what they need, and we can help find solutions. As CHWs, we are working with communities to reclaim our power.

6. **Building individual and community capacity.** CHWs support clients and community members to develop the skills and the confidence to promote and advocate for their own health and well-being. This work is done with individual clients, or clients and their family members. CHWs also work with groups and community networks to build the capacity to speak out and take action in their own lives and communities. Finally, CHWs also build their own skills and confidence and support the capacity building of the CHW profession.

Veronica Barragan: When I think of capacity building, it happens at many levels, both personal and with health systems. In the over 20 years of working for my health center, I've worked in many roles and capacity as a CHW—doing outreach, referrals, health education, care coordination, and patient advocacy—to build my community's capacity to live healthier lives and help my health center better serve them. With so many years of doing work around chronic disease management, I am now helping to build a CHW unit that will embed CHWs as part of our medical team at the clinic, they are now part of the care team! My role is to build the capacity of our clinic to better respond to the social determinants of health of our patients. For the CHWs that I now supervise, we do regular training on motivational interviewing, harm reduction, resource navigating, so that they build up their skills to help our diverse clients. Our providers are now understanding that CHWs sometimes make the biggest difference in the health outcomes of our clients because clients disclose more to us and trust us to understand them culturally.

7. **Providing direct services.** Some CHWs provide direct care to clients through the services they are trained and qualified to provide, such as blood pressure monitoring, reproductive health counseling, or HIV antibody test counseling. They may also provide case management or chronic conditions management services or otherwise link clients to services by knowing what services exist and referring clients appropriately.

Felipe Flores: Like many CHWs, I began my career by noticing a gap of services in my community. For me, it was being able to provide HIV test counseling services to Spanish speaking communities. My role in providing culturally sensitive, bias and stigma free information around HIV and sexual health was empowering. The reflection of supporting my peers and community, sharing information, and demystifying often taboo topics paved the way for what would become my career. We could talk about anything and everything because we understood each other, our backgrounds, and challenged values in a way that was respectful to the lived experience and upbringings that were similar in our stories.

8. **Implementing individual and community assessments.** CHWs work with individuals, families, groups, and communities to assist them in assessing their outstanding concerns, priorities, and resources. Advocacy cannot be done without a true understanding of the needs of the community, the gaps in services, and the effectiveness of the services that are being provided. CHWs are a key part in doing these assessments because they work the closest to the communities being served.

Victoria Adewumi: One of the first things I did after being hired as a Health Department Community Liaison was to go door to door, talking with people in their neighborhoods. We would stand on people's porches and talk to them about what they liked about their neighborhood, if they knew their neighbors and what health concerns mattered to them. The stories and experiences generously given to us would ultimately create the foundation for future place-based health interventions, but for me it was a powerful experience in connecting with people in their context to understand the historical and environmental factors that shaped their lives.

9. **Conducting outreach.** CHWs conduct outreach to link community members to information, resources, and services. A CHW often is the first person many clients interact with, whether through an outreach encounter, or when a client arrives at an agency or clinic.

Chelene Lopez: I have over 30 years of experience of conducting outreach in Sonoma County with a specialty for working with Farmworkers and Day Labor Workers. It is really important when conducting outreach at a health fair, or event to not be on your phone or talking to others at your booth or table. You need to be looking at the people that are passing by the booth asking them questions or inviting them to come see the information that you have available for them.

10. **Participating in evaluation and research.** Some CHWs participate in efforts to evaluate health programs and services or to conduct research about community health priorities. Evaluation and research efforts are most effective when they incorporate the participation and leadership of the communities affected by the issues and programs they seek to investigate.

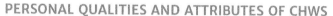

Abdul Hafeedh Bin Abdullah: As CHWs, we partnered with Youth Leaders to implement a mix method approach, including a block-by-block assessment and photo voice project that provided great insights into what young people identified as supports or barriers to their health and well-being. CHWs offer authentic voice, perspective, and facilitate increased access within communities they support. They know and are a part of these communities. These unique qualities enhance the value of evaluation and research projects they participate in.

- *Have you ever taken on any of these CHWs' roles?*
- *What were some of the challenges that you faced in performing the role?*
- *Can you think of other roles that a CHW might play?*

What Do YOU Think?

PERSONAL QUALITIES AND ATTRIBUTES OF CHWS

The CHW profession depends upon building positive interpersonal relationships with people of diverse backgrounds and identities. Without the capacity to build relationships based on trust, CHWs cannot do their job effectively. The qualities that enable this capacity can be strengthened through practice and self-reflection.

We highlight several desirable personal qualities and attributes in Table 1.3, developed by CHWs in Zimbabwe (International Training and Education Center on HIV, unpublished curriculum). With these qualities and attributes, CHWs inspire confidence and trust and build positive professional relationships with clients and communities. They also allow CHWs to more effectively perform the core CHW

Table 1.3 Personal Qualities of Successful CHWs

PERSONAL QUALITIES	DEFINITIONS
1. Interpersonal warmth	The ability to listen, care, and respond to clients and communities with compassion and kindness
2. Trustworthiness	Being honest, allowing others to confide in you, maintaining confidentiality, and upholding professional ethics
3. Open-mindedness	The willingness to embrace others' differences and the ability to be nonjudgmental in your interactions with them
4. Objectivity	Striving to work with and view clients and their circumstances without the influence of personal prejudice or bias
5. Sensitivity	To be aware of and truly respect the experience, culture, feelings, and opinions of others
6. Competence	Developing the knowledge and skills required to provide quality services to all the clients and communities you work with
7. Commitment to social justice	The commitment to fight injustice and to advocate for social changes that promote the health and well-being of clients and communities
8. Self-care and wellness	Investing in your self-care and wellness so that you have the mental and emotional capacity to perform your work professionally, without doing harm to clients, colleagues, or yourself
9. Self-awareness and understanding	Being willing and able to reflect upon and analyze your work with clients, including mistakes you may make, and your own values and biases to ensure that they do not negatively affect your interactions with clients and colleagues

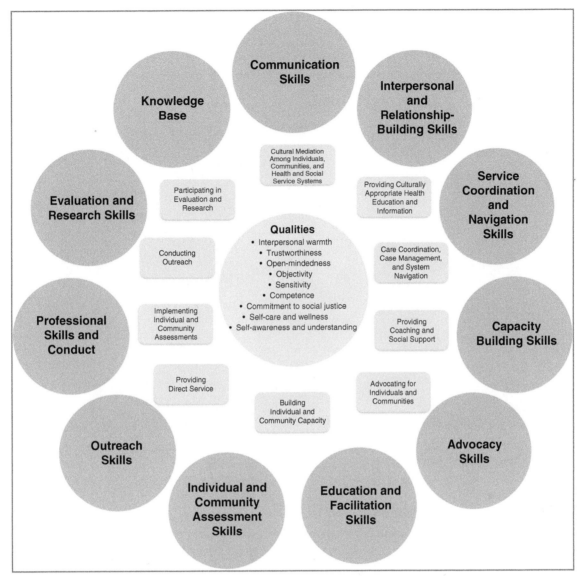

Figure 1.1 The Relationship Between CHW Qualities, Roles, and Core Competencies

competencies, within their various roles. The interconnectedness of Personal Qualities and its relation to the C3 Roles and Skills are illustrated in Figure 1.1.

- *What other personal qualities and values should CHWs have?*

- *What personal qualities and values do you bring to this work?*

- *What qualities do you want to build and enhance?*

The last quality in the list above has special importance: self-awareness serves as a foundation that assists CHWs to cultivate other key qualities and skills. For example, developing awareness of our own personal biases helps to ensure that you won't harm a client by judging them based on your own values and beliefs. This is an ethical obligation for all CHWs and is essential for three key principles of CHW practice: person-centered practice, community-centered practice, and cultural humility.

Throughout this book, you will find questions directed to you as a CHW. Some of the questions invite you to take time to reflect and to cultivate self-awareness. The questions also invite you to bring your own experience, insights, ideas, and wisdom into the conversation. Your life experience, whatever it may be, is an important foundation for the work you will do as a CHW.

The challenges of developing self-awareness and using it to inform your work as a CHW is a theme that runs throughout this book. It is addressed in greater detail in Chapters 5, 7, and 9.

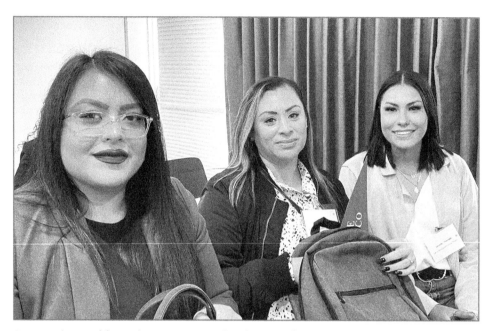

Community Health Workers support each other to reflect and enhance their knowledge and skills

11 CORE COMPETENCIES FOR CHWS

Core competencies are the skills and knowledge that enable CHWs to carry out their roles. There are some core competencies that all CHWs use—communication skills, interpersonal skills, organizational skills, and a knowledge base relevant to the clients and communities served and the types of services provided. Other core competencies are commonly used by many CHWs, but the extent to which they are used depends upon the roles that the CHW fulfills and the organizations they work for. These include teaching skills, service coordination skills, capacity-building skills, and advocacy skills.

The 11 core competencies that are highlighted below also come from the C3 Project. These are a partial list of CHW competencies based on a national consensus process. For example, CHW tasks and skills include family engagement, problem solving, treatment adherence promotion, harm reduction, translation and interpretation, leading support groups, and documentation, among others. Many of these duties fit within the eight broad competencies discussed in this chapter (e.g., documentation can be considered an organizational skill).

The 11 broad competencies, as well as many more specific duties and tasks, are addressed in subsequent sections and chapters of this book.

1. **Communication skills:** CHWs must be good listeners to learn about their clients' experiences, behaviors, strengths, and needs, and to provide health information and person-centered counseling or coaching. Communication skills are also essential for facilitating group- and community-level interventions such as facilitating trainings or support groups or participating in community organizing and advocacy efforts.

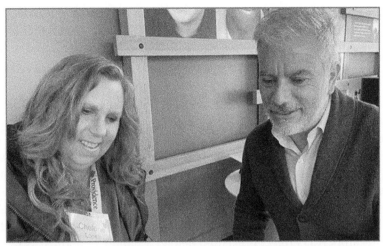

CHWs working collaboratively through active listening and good communication skills

2. **Interpersonal and relationship-building skills:** CHWs work with diverse groups of people and must be able to develop positive relationships with clients, community members, colleagues, and policymakers. This includes the ability to provide and receive constructive feedback and to resolve conflict.

3. **Service coordination and navigation skills:** The health care and social service systems are complex, not very well integrated, and sometimes difficult to access. CHWs sometimes work as case managers and frequently support clients to access available services and to create and follow realistic plans to improve their health, despite the complexity of the systems.

4. **Capacity-building skills:** CHWs don't want clients and communities to become dependent upon them or other service providers. They teach and support clients and communities to develop new skills and increase their own confidence to promote their own health, including communication skills, risk reduction behaviors, chronic disease management, and community organizing and advocacy skills.

5. **Advocacy skills:** CHWs sometimes speak up on behalf of their clients and their communities within their own agencies, with other service providers, and to support changes in public policies. More importantly, CHWs support clients and communities in raising their own voices to create meaningful changes—including changes in public policies—that influence their health and well-being.

6. **Education and facilitation skills:** CHWs educate clients about how to prevent and manage health conditions. CHWs teach about healthy behaviors and support clients in developing healthier habits. They also facilitate groups and workshops designed to teach or enhance knowledge, skills, and support.

7. **Individual and community assessment skills:** CHWs frequently assist in assessing a client's needs, risks, and priorities. They also play an important role in program and community assessments to determine whether services are accessible and working effectively, as well as identify emerging needs for the community. With their close connection to the communities they serve, they can collect the necessary data and bring it back to inform program improvements.

8. **Outreach skills:** CHWs perform outreach to share program information and public health education with local communities in-person and via social media. Performing outreach—to potential new clients, other programs, and organizations—allows CHWs to stay connected to what is happening on the ground, to learn about emerging needs within the community, to advertise their organization's services, and to network and learn about essential programs/resources.

9. **Professional skills and conduct:** CHWs work with colleagues at their own agencies, with helping professionals at other health and social services agencies, and with the community at large. It is essential for CHWs to conduct themselves professionally and within their scope of practice (more on Ethics and Scope of

Practice will be discussed in Chapter 5). Additionally, as CHWs are tasked with supporting individuals, families, and communities in getting the services they need, the work is demanding, with many things to keep track of and document. Learning the skills to prioritize, stay organized, and properly document services provided is critical in ensuring they can appropriately follow up with clients and accurately document data for their employers.

10. **Evaluation and research skills:** CHWs are key members of the public health workforce. They assist in gathering and sharing health data and information to improve the quality of health programs. As more work is done to address the social determinants of health and the complex challenge of promoting health equity, CHWs are tasked with learning how to evaluate the quality and effectiveness of health programs and policies. CHWs are also key members of research initiatives that seek to better understand complex health issues, risk factors, and promotion strategies. CHWs help to ensure that research and evaluation efforts partner with community members and investigate questions designed to benefit local communities. This means there are many opportunities for CHWs to provide input on the growth of the profession [see the CHW Common Indicators (CI) Project presented below]. Chapter 23 addresses the role of CHWs in research and evaluation.

11. **Knowledge base:** CHWs need to commit to being a lifelong learner and spend time getting to know the communities they work with and the range of health and related services that may be available to clients. CHWs must also be knowledgeable about the health issues they address on the job such as diabetes, domestic violence, depression, or infectious diseases.

- *What other competencies or skills are important for CHWs to have?*

- *Which of the 11 core CHW competencies have you already developed?*

- *Which competencies do you want to learn or improve?*

THE COMMON INDICATOR (CI) PROJECT – CHW CENTERED EVALUATIONS

"The folks who started the Common Indicators project noticed there was a lack of standardized ways of measuring CHW practice. There was nothing that was commonly used across all CHW programs at the state and national level. You can't aggregate data when everyone's measuring things differently. Measurement drives practice and as an epidemiologist colleague of mine says, "if you don't measure it, it doesn't exist." Keara Rodela, Community Health Worker Leadership Team Member, Community Health Worker Common Indicators Project, Portland, Oregon (K. Rodela, personal communication).

The purpose of the CHW Common Indicators (CI) Project is to contribute to the integrity, sustainability, and viability of CHW programs through the collaborative development and adoption of a set of common process and outcome concepts and indicators for CHW practice. The CI Project began in 2015 when 16 CHWs, researcher, evaluators, and program administrator allies from five states across the country met in Portland, Oregon, to identify an initial set of concepts and indicators for CHW program evaluation. Over the past seven years, the project has built a national constituency of over 300 CHWs, CHW program staff, CHW researcher/evaluators, and others committed to project objectives. The Leadership Team has expanded to four CHWs and three CHW allies, and the project included a CHW Council, a Researcher Council, and an Advisory Group. In order to develop a set of 12 measures that are important to CHWs and their allies, project staff conducted focus groups, workshops at conferences, and national summits. They are currently piloting the indicators with community-based organizations, state health departments, and other agencies.

Three core values and four beliefs make the CI Project different from other CHW research projects. The CI Project values a participatory process and bases all its work on the philosophy and methodology of popular education, also referred to as "people's education." Popular education (see Chapter 21 for more information about popular education) creates settings in which people most affected by inequities can share what they know, learn from others in their community, and use their knowledge to create a more just and equitable society. Popular education and the CHW model grew out of many of the same historical roots and share key principles, such as the ideas that people most affected by inequity are the experts about their own lives, and that experiential knowledge is just as important as academic knowledge. The philosophy of popular education is also present in another essential value for the CI Project, which is CHW self-determination. Leadership of and involvement in research and evaluation about their own profession is essential to CHW identity. Finally, CI values combine quantitative and qualitative methods to fully understand the conditions CHWs need in order to be successful and the outcomes of their work.

The four beliefs are (Northwest Regional Primary Care Association, 2023):

1. Evaluation reflects the point of view of those who design and conduct it.

2. Consistent data will promote sustainable funding of the CHW field.

3. Indicators will contribute to the viability of grassroots CHW programs.

4. Measurement drives practice. Carefully chosen process and outcome measures will support CHWs to play a wide range of roles.

While the intent of the CI Project is to identify common process and outcome indicators and promote the uptake of those indicators, the scope of the project has expanded to include a focus on modeling how to support CHWs to become the researchers and evaluators of their own profession. Although CHWs have been involved in various stages of data collection, they have seldom been engaged as full partners in all stages of evaluation and research, from conceptualization to analysis to publication. As one of the cofounders of the CI Project, Dr. Noelle Wiggins notes:

> *"I think evaluation and research are like the last hold-out in not involving community health workers integrally in both participation and leadership. That may be because of how we think about evaluation and research. To some degree, research and evaluation has its own unique language and jargon, and research and evaluation is thought of as something that is only done by "experts," and usually experts with a PHD, or at least a master's degree. Because most CHWs don't have a PhD or a master's degree, they've been pretty systematically excluded from knowledge production about their own profession. I think that the way that the CI Project attempts to change this thought process is by breaking down this final barrier. The CI Project asserts that you do not have to have a master's degree or PhD to be involved in research and evaluation. In fact, to produce valid and reliable findings, you **must** have the insight of those who are closest to the work, in this case, CHWs. Some CHWs will want to continue their formal education and obtain to a masters or doctoral degree, and we want to and will support them to do that. For CHWs who, for whatever reasons, don't want to or can't go get a masters or doctoral degree, they still have incredibly valuable input into research and evaluation about their own field. The CI Project is attempting to provide capacity building and access to these initiatives so that CHWs can lead their own profession." (N. Wiggins, personal communication).*

The CHW Common Indicator Project hopes to build the foundation for an ongoing process through which CHWs (some of whom are researchers and evaluators), researchers and evaluators, and community members can engage together. The CI Project also promotes CHW research and evaluation centered on CHW leadership and utilizes popular or people's education to embody the values and principles of community-based participatory research and produces research that leads to a full acknowledgment and awareness of the unique role that CHWs play in addressing health inequities. The CI Project has been supported by the Centers for Disease Control and Prevention and the National Association of Chronic Disease Directors through a cooperative agreement. Funding has supported piloting and testing current indicators, expanding constructs to cultivate additional indicators, and for development in scope and breadth. For more information about the CI Project, please see the Resources at the end of the chapter.

1.4 The Role of CHWs in the Management of Chronic Conditions

Increasingly, CHWs are hired by healthcare organizations to assist patients with the management of chronic health conditions (Chapter 16 addresses the role of CHWs in Chronic Conditions Management in greater detail).

Chronic health conditions—also known as chronic diseases—include diabetes, high blood pressure and other forms of heart disease, cancer, asthma and other chronic respiratory diseases, arthritis, depression, bipolar condition, Alzheimer's disease, HIV, and other mental health and disabling conditions that last for at least one year. Chronic conditions are the leading cause of illness, hospitalization, and death in the United States (National Center for Chronic Disease Prevention and Health Promotion, 2022).

Traditional medical models for the treatment of chronic conditions have not worked well, especially for low-income, aging, and other vulnerable patients who are often living with more than one chronic disease. New models for the management of chronic conditions feature patient-centered care, a team-based approach, and supporting patients with the self-management of their conditions. These emerging models often address the social determinants of health such as the lack of access to safe housing and healthy and affordable food. CHWs are particularly knowledgeable and skillful in talking with patients about the social determinants of health and in assisting them to access key services and resources. Hiring CHWs and integrating them into these team-based approaches has been shown to be effective in improving patient health outcomes and in reducing healthcare costs (Centers for Disease Control and Prevention, 2014; Kangovi, 2020).

Federal policies and some state policies support hiring CHWs to work in primary healthcare environments, particularly in settings that serve Medicaid populations. As a result, healthcare organizations across the United States are recruiting and hiring CHWs for a variety of positions, including general primary care clinics and specialty clinics addressing specific health conditions such as pediatric asthma or cancer clinics. Most of these positions assign CHWs to assist patients with the management of chronic health conditions.

The roles and scope of practice of CHWs who work in the field of chronic conditions can vary widely depending upon the policies and protocols of their employers. These roles and tasks include providing health education about chronic conditions and topics such as physical activity and healthy nutrition; facilitating patient education or support groups; providing case management and referrals to local resources; assistance with health system navigation and accompaniment; supporting patients to develop and implement realistic action plans for the management of their chronic conditions; medications counseling; supporting patients with advocacy when appropriate; and providing home visits.

For further information about chronic conditions management and the role of CHWs, please see Chapter 16: Chronic Conditions Management and Chapter 17: Healthy Eating and Active Living.

1.5 The Role of CHWs in Promoting Language Access Justice

The demographics of the U.S. population are changing. The United States is one of the most diverse countries in the world and continues to become increasingly multicultural and multilingual. Immigrant, refugee, limited English proficient, as well as non-English proficient populations, continue to grow. According to the 2020 U.S. Census, the Hispanic/Latino population in the United States has surpassed 62 million (18.7 percent of the total U.S. population), making it the largest minority group in the country (Jones, Marks, Ramirez & Rios-Vargas, 2021). Communities of color are expected to reach 50% of the U.S. population by 2044 (Ibid).

More than half of the Hispanic/Latino population in the United States speak Spanish at home, making it the country's most common non-English language, and many in this group may be limited in English proficiency. Other significant limited-English-speaking groups include speakers of Asian, African, and other European languages and dialects.

The Importance of Trained Healthcare Interpreters

GAYLE TANG, COORDINATOR OF THE HEALTHCARE INTERPRETER CERTIFICATE PROGRAM AT
CITY COLLEGE OF SAN FRANCISCO

There are key benefits for health organizations and patients when trained healthcare interpreters are employed to provide language services.

Research indicates that the lack of language access or having a qualified healthcare interpreter to assist with communication between patients and providers can be harmful to patient health (Allen, Johnson, McClave & Alvarado-Little 2020; Dahima, Luo & Dhongrade, 2023; Labaf, Shahvaraninasab, Baradaran, Seyedhosseini & Jahanshir, 2019). One study revealed an average of 31 interpreting errors made on each doctor visit by people who were not trained interpreters. Although some mistakes were small, such as leaving out a word that didn't change the meaning of what the doctor was saying, 63% were considered serious errors that affected diagnoses and understanding of treatment regimens (Flores, 2005). Such errors included omitting medication dosage instructions and/or the provider's questions about drug allergies and instructing a patient not to answer personal questions (Ibid).

Linguistic and cultural training helps to minimize these medical errors. When patients and providers are able to communicate through a trained interpreter, providers receive accurate information from the patients to make diagnoses and recommend treatments. Patients provided with quality interpreting services can better understand their treatment plan, leading to greater adherence, fewer hospital visits, and increased satisfaction (Centers for Medicare and Medicaid Services, 2022).

Providing language services also benefits health organizations financially. When patients and providers can communicate more effectively, the amount of staff time needed for the patient is reduced, misdiagnosis and medical errors that the hospital may be liable for are less likely, and the number of emergency room visits decreases.

In addition to the direct benefits for health consumers and providers, there are also legal and regulatory requirements that health organizations and providers must comply with. To ensure equal access and quality health services, there are federal and state laws that require healthcare organizations and social service facilities to provide culturally and linguistically appropriate care and services for their clients, and health consumers.

The changing demographics of the United States present unique challenges to healthcare organizations. Studies indicate that language is a major determinant in accessing health care (Healthy People 2030, 2023). Further studies aimed at the investigation of patient adherence issues and medical errors point to the use of untrained interpreters and the lack of effective communication as the underlying cause. Consequently, the demand for trained healthcare interpreters has increased dramatically.

THE ROLE OF MULTILINGUAL COMMUNITY HEALTH WORKERS

Multilingual CHWs who speak more than one language very well are invaluable in serving clients who speak different languages. Multilingual CHWs may be called upon to provide language services, such as speaking to a client in a non-English language or providing interpretation services between people who speak different languages or providing translation of written documents. Multilingual CHWs may or may not have received additional training or certification in healthcare interpreting.

Multilingual CHWs are often asked to accompany clients to medical visits or are employed within a healthcare organization where they provide health education, help with service navigation, and connect clients to other medical providers (such as mental health provider or any other type of specialist). While many healthcare organizations understand the role of a medical interpreter, it is not uncommon for these organizations to ask multilingual CHWs to do basic interpreting. Many multilingual CHWs are being asked to interpret, develop in-language material, and/or translate written documents from one language to another (interpretation refers to verbal communication skills and translation to written communication skills). *However, when does simple interpreting become too complex for a multilingual CHW to manage?*

If you are a multilingual CHW, it is important to understand and clearly communicate the limits of your language and interpretation skills. Carefully consider each language service request. Is it beyond your scope of knowledge? Do you have sufficient time to provide quality service? Are your language skills strong enough that you can interpret every word that patients and providers speak in both languages? Are you familiar with medical terminology in both languages?

When in doubt of your language or interpretation skills, the most honorable thing to do is to graciously say "no" and to request a trained interpret for your patients. Explain that you are not trained in healthcare interpretation and encourage your colleagues to request a professional language service provider, such as a professional interpreter or translator. We all have responsibility to ensure quality services that promote patient safety. As Mark Twain famously once said, "The difference between the almost right word and the right word is really a large matter – 'tis the difference between the lightning bug and the lightning" (Fatout, 1976).

Bridging linguistic and cultural gaps requires a specific skill set and knowledge base. This knowledge base needs to continue to expand through continuous learning and ongoing practice. Unless the CHW has received specialized training and meets the qualifications of health care interpreter or translator, they should not be providing those services.

Potential errors can negatively impact the health and safety of the client or patient. Also, performing outside of one's role without the necessary training and qualifications is against the established laws and regulations related to the importance of providing culturally and linguistically competent care and services. We encourage you to talk to your supervisor about your concerns and ask for clarification if you are in doubt of your role and skills as a multilingual CHW.

For more information about healthcare interpretation, please see the resources listed at the end of this chapter.

1.6 Professionalizing the Work

The CHW field is rapidly growing and transforming. You will learn more about this in Chapter 2. There are disagreements among CHWs, researchers, educators, employers, and other health professionals about how best to professionalize the field. Some people advocate for **credentialing** (CHWs would need certification from an educational institution, professional association, or employer in order to work) and greater integration into the healthcare field. Many states have developed credentialing policies. Others worry that CHWs may lose their connection to the community and their commitment to social justice. Everyone, however, seems to agree that the field deserves greater recognition, respect, and funding.

THE NATIONAL ASSOCIATION OF COMMUNITY HEALTH WORKERS

The National Association of Community Health Workers (NACHW) is a voice for the CHW profession. It was founded in April 2019 after several years of planning and organizing by CHWs and allies across the United States (see Chapter 2). The organization is currently led by Denise Octavia Smith, its first executive director, who is also a CHW. NACHW is governed by a national board of directors consisting of CHWs and CHW allies with decades of research and expertise in CHW training and workforce development, community organizing and engagement, intervention design, equity and social justice advocacy, research, and policy leadership.

> *"We are a young organization that has grown up, and, I think, solidified our value and necessity in the midst of a global pandemic when the voice of community and when the requirement for racial equity became paramount to protect people's lives. What this has done is that it has allowed us to test our values and our vision that a unified CHW workforce would be able to come together across geography, ethnicity, sector, race, gender, and lived experience to support communities, to achieve health, equity, and social justice" (Octavia Smith, personal communication).*

NACHW is a 501(c)(3) nonprofit membership-driven organization with a mission to unify CHWs across geography; ethnicity; sector; and experience to support communities to achieve health, equity, and social justice. Their work is guided by values that include self-determination and self-empowerment of the CHW workforce; emphasizing integrity of character; dignity and respect for every human being; social justice; and equity to ensure fair treatment, access, opportunity, and outcomes for all individuals and communities.

> *"We have tested these values in our Johnson and Johnson 2021 National CHW Survey. Among 867 CHWs from 859 zip codes, speaking 28 different languages, with over 190 working titles out of 26 options for what are the values that describe community health workers, EVERY single one of these individuals who participated identified as a CHW and regardless of their title, and they identified the 6 values that NACHW was founded on as fundamental to their identity." (Octavia Smith, personal communication.)*

NACHW seeks to engage CHWs, allies, supporters, sponsors, and key professional influencers; educate stakeholders on the impact of CHWs; expand membership, recognition, opportunities, and collective action; establish a national voice and sustainable strategies on issues related to CHW workforce; and enhance CHW leadership skills and opportunities. For more information about NACHW, please see the references provided at the end of the chapter.

LOCAL CHW NETWORKS AND STRATEGIES

Advancing the mission of NACHW on a national level also requires local and state strategies for advancing the CHW profession. These include:

- Conducting research about the field to further clarify what CHWs do and how effective they are
- Establishing state and regional CHW organizations as a way for CHWs to have a collective voice in determining the development of their profession and to advocate on behalf of the communities they serve
- Developing appropriate ways to credential or certify the work of CHWs
- Developing training programs and materials that teach the core competencies required for success as a CHWs
- Advocating for policy changes that will result in more stable and continuous funding for CHWs
- Developing regulations and procedures to take advantage of the funding opportunities in the Affordable Care Act

- *What are some key opportunities and challenges for the CHW profession?*

- *Does your state have a CHW Association?*

- *What are some of the potential benefits of joining a CHW Association?*

1.7 Introducing 23 CHWS

Throughout this book, you will find quotes from CHWs who have firsthand knowledge, experience, and information to share. The book also includes 23 Profiles of experienced CHWs, one in each chapter of the book. We hope that you enjoy reading about their contributions to the profession, their motivation for becoming CHWs, and their tips or suggestions for people who are just starting their careers.

The CHWs who have generously contributed Profiles highlighting their work are **Cristina Arellano, Joe Calderon, Lorena Carmona, Dante Casuga, Mattie Clark, Faith Fabiani, Durrell Fox, Fadumo Jama, Michelle James, Pennie Jewell, Abdul' Hafeedh bin 'Abdullah, Floribella Martinez-Redondo, Francis Julian Montgomery, Estela Munoz de Cardenas, Avery Nguyen, Silvia Ortega, Sengthong Sithounnolat, Nilda Palacios, Monica Rico, Tahrio Sanford, Porshay Taylor, Kim Lien Tran, and David Valentine.**

CHW Profile

Estela Munoz De Cardenas, She/Her

Community Outreach Worker

Alameda County, CA. Center for Healthy Schools & Communities

Low-income and Immigrant families

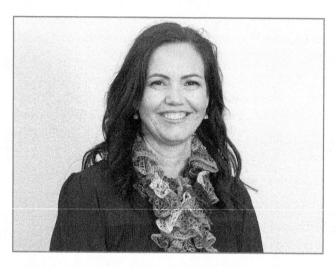

When I arrived in the United States in 1991, I didn't speak English. The language and cultural barriers made basic activities like shopping or doctor's appointments difficult, and I couldn't always find help when advocating for myself and others. As immigrants, we struggle to adjust to a new country and to communicate when we don't speak the language. My determination and commitment come from my mother, who always helps in any way she can. Mom always said to me, "be humble and kind to others. Don't be a bystander—when you see someone struggling, help them." For me, it is just human kindness. We all need to feel that we are part of our community.

Today, I work for the School Health Division of Alameda County's Health Care Services Agency, providing services in various districts guided by a school-linked family engagement model. I get referrals from school nurses, counselors, and social workers. I serve clients from immigrant communities (newcomers, immigrant workers, and refugees/asylees) and other marginalized populations. I meet with clients at schools, Starbucks, or other places in the community that they suggest. I provide family resource navigation and community health care coordination, specifically focusing on current or eligible Medi-Cal (Medicaid) clients. I support clients to access medical and dental care and other basic needs. My clients have a hard time connecting with services because they don't speak English. I work in partnership with local school districts to follow up on particularly complex and urgent cases.

I'd like to share a story from one of my previous jobs: I got a referral for a client who arrived in the United States and needed services like housing, health insurance for her family, and help enrolling her kids in school. The client's main concern was to meet with a lawyer about her immigration status. I accompanied her to the immigration office for the first time to help with interpretation. I found an organization that supports families free of charge. After her second interview, the lawyer agreed to represent her for free. The client walked out smiling, hugged me, and said, "Thank you, Estela. You don't understand. Nobody does this—brings me in your car, calls the lawyer, brings me the second time." Months later, the client called me to let me know her immigration was approved, and she got her work permit and social security. She was so happy because she could support her family to have a better life.

(continues)

CHW Profile
(continued)

As a CHW, I want to support all clients' needs. I'm good at my job and I have the resources to help people. But sometimes I meet a client in crisis or who is difficult to communicate with, and I want to improve, to do better. When a client tells me—"I know it was difficult at first. I was anxious and angry, but you've been so patient and kind, you helped me"—it reminds me that I need to keep going one client at a time. I just need to listen to them. I need to respond to all of my clients with compassion and kindness, and to embrace people of different cultures and backgrounds with love and respect. It is really a blessing for me to have a career as a CHW.

One tip I would share with new CHWs is not to assume you have all the answers for your clients. People come to you for support, not for knowledge. They already have the knowledge. They might be more knowledgeable than you are! People know what they need. Listen to your clients is the most important part of your job.

Chapter Review

1. Which communities or populations do CHWs most commonly work with? What experiences (if any) have you had with CHWs in your own community?

2. What health issues do CHWs commonly address in their work? Which health issues most motivate you as you train to work as a CHW?

3. How would you explain the relationship between CHW roles and competencies?

4. Which of the 10 core CHW roles are you most comfortable fulfilling? Which do you know the least about?

5. Explain the 11 core competencies of CHWs and provide an example of each. Have you had the opportunity to develop and practice any of these skills? Which of these skills are you currently least prepared to put into practice?

6. Describe personal qualities and attributes that are common among successful CHWs. Which of these qualities will you bring to the work? What additional qualities, attributes, or values will you bring?

7. Think about a chronic condition that you or a family member lives with. How could you as a CHW working as part of a clinical team, support you or your family in managing this chronic condition?

8. Why is it important for patients with limited or no English language proficiency who are meeting with English-speaking health care providers to have access to a well-trained health care interpreter?

9. What are some guidelines for multilingual CHWs who are asked to provide health care interpretation?

10. What are some of the key contributions and resources of the National CHW Association?

11. Why is CHW leadership important for the continued advancement of the CHW profession?

12. As the profession grows, what are some of the challenges that CHWs face? What new opportunities or recognition would you like to see CHWs gain?

References

Allen, M., Johnson, R., McClave, E., & Alvarado-Little, W. (2020). *Language, interpretation, and translation: A clarification and reference checklist in service of health literacy and cultural respect.* National Academy of Medicine. https://nam.edu/language-interpretation-and-translation-a-clarification-and-reference-checklist-in-service-of-health-literacy-and-cultural-respect/ (accessed 12 June 2023).

American Public Health Association [APHA]. (2009). Policy statement 20091. http://www.apha.org/policies-and-advocacy/public-health-policy-statements/policy-database/2014/07/09/14/19/support-for-community-health-workers-to-increase-health-access-and-to-reduce-health-inequities (accessed 10 June 2023).

Arizona Prevention Research Center. (2014). *National Community Health Worker Advocacy Survey (NCHWAS)*. University of Arizona. http://www.institutephi.org/wp-content/uploads/2014/08/survey-of-Community-Health-Workers.pdf (accessed 10 June 2023).

Bureau of Labor Statistics [BLS]. (2023). Occupational employment and wage statistics: 21-1094 Community Health Workers. https://www.bls.gov/oes/current/oes211094.htm (accessed 10 June 2023).

Centers for Disease Control and Prevention. (2014). Technical assistance guide: States implementing community health worker strategies. Retrieved from https://www.cdc.gov/dhdsp/programs/spha/docs/1305_ta_guide_chws.pdf.

Centers for Medicare and Medicaid Services (CMS). (2022). Guide to developing a language access plan. Retrieved from https://www.cms.gov/About-CMS/Agency-Information/OMH/Downloads/Language-Access-Plan.pdf

CHW Core Consensus Project (2023). https://www.c3project.org/ (accessed 12 June 2023).

Community Health Worker Network of New York City. (2023). Core values. https://www.chwnetwork.org/ (accessed 10 June 2023)

Crespo, R., Christiansen, M., Tieman, K., & Wittberg, R. (2020). An emerging model for community health worker–based chronic care management for patients with high health care costs in rural Appalachia. *Preventing Chronic Disease*, 17, 190316. http://dx.doi.org/10.5888/pcd17.190316.

Dahima, R. Luo, M., & Dhongrade, V. (2023). *Medical interpretation in the U.S. is inadequate and harming patients. Hastings bioethics forum*. The Hastings Center. https://www.thehastingscenter.org/medical-interpretation-in-the-u-s-is-inadequate-and-harming-patients/ (accessed 12 June 2023).

Fatout, P. (1976). *Mark Twain speaking*. Iowa City, IA: University of Iowa Press.

Flores, G. (2005). The impact of medical interpreter services on the quality of health care: A systematic review. *Medical Care Research and Review* 62(3), 255–299. http://doi.org/10.1177/1077558705275416.

Healthy People 2030. (2023). Language and Literacy. https://health.gov/healthypeople/priority-areas/social-determinants-health/literature-summaries/language-and-literacy (accessed 10 June 2023).

Hispanic Health Council. (2018). Policy brief – addressing social determinants of health through community health workers: A call to action. Retrieved from https://www.cthealth.org/wp-content/uploads/2018/01/HHC-CHW-SDOH-Policy-Briefi-1.30.18.pdf.

Hurtado, M., Spinner, J. R., Yang, M., Evensen, C., Windham, A., Ortiz, G., & Ivy, E. D. (2014). Knowledge and behavioral effects in cardiovascular health: Community health worker health disparities initiative, 2007–2010. *Preventing Chronic Disease*, 11, 130250. http://dx.doi.org/10.5888/pcd11.130250.

Jones, N., Marks, R., Ramirez, R., & Rios-Vargas. (2021). *Improved race and ethnicity measures reveal U.S. Population is much more multiracial – 2020 Census illuminates racial and ethnic composition of the country*. United States Census Bureau. https://www.census.gov/library/stories/2021/08/improved-race-ethnicity-measures-reveal-united-states-population-much-more-multiracial.html (accessed 12 June 2023).

Kangovi, S. (2020). Evidence-based community health worker program addresses unmet social needs and generates positive return on investment. *Health Affairs* 39(2), 207–213. https://doi.org/10.1377/hlthaff.2019.00981.

Labaf A., Shahvaraninasab A., Baradaran H., Seyedhosseini J., & Jahanshir A. (2019). The effect of language barrier and non-professional interpreters on the accuracy of patient-physician communication in emergency department. *Advanced Journal of Emergency Medicine*. https://doi.org/10.22114/ajem.v0i0.123.

Northwest Regional Primary Care Association. (2023). CHW Common Indicators Project. https://www.nwrpca.org/page/CHWCommonIndicators (accessed 11 June 2023)

Rosenthal, E. L., Wiggins, N., Brownstein, J. N., Rael, R., & Johnson, S. (1998). *The final report of the national community health advisor study: Weaving the future.* Tucson, Arizona: University of Arizona. Retrieved from http://crh.arizona.edu/publications/studies-reports.

U.S. Department of Health and Human Services. (2007). *Community Health Worker National Workforce Study.* Health Resources and Services Administration, Bureau of Health Professions. https://bhw.hrsa.gov/data-research/review-health-workforce-research/archive (accessed 27 December 2023).

Additional Resources

American Public Health Association. (n.d.). Community health workers section. https://www.apha.org/apha-communities/member-sections/community-health-workers.

California Healthcare Interpreting Association. (n.d.). https://www.chiaonline.org/.

Certification Commission for Healthcare Interpreters. (n.d.). https://cchicertification.org/certifications/.

City College of San Francisco Health Education Department. (n.d.). Community Health Worker Certificate Program. https://www.ccsf.edu/degrees-certificates/community-health-worker.

Community Health Workers Health Disparities Initiative of the National Institutes of Health. (n.d.). Medicaid will allow reimbursement for community health worker preventative services. http://www.abcardio.org/articles/cms:rule.html (accessed 10 June 2023)

Community Health Worker Network of New York City. (n.d.). http://www.chwnetwork.org/.

Community Health Worker Project of the Urban Institute. (n.d.). http://www.urban.org/careworks/.

Massachusetts Association of Community Health Workers. (n.d.). http://www.machw.org/.

National Association of CHWs. (2023). www.nachw.org (accessed 10 June 2023).

National Board of Certification for Medical Interpreters. (n.d.). https://www.certifiedmedicalinterpreters.org/.

University of Southern Mississippi Center for Sustainable Health Outreach. (n.d.). http://www.usm.edu/health/center-sustainable-health-outreach.

The Evolution of the CHW Field in the United States

The Path We Walk—The Mountains We Climbed

E. Lee Rosenthal, Paige Menking, Floribella Redondo-Martinez, and J. Nell Brownstein

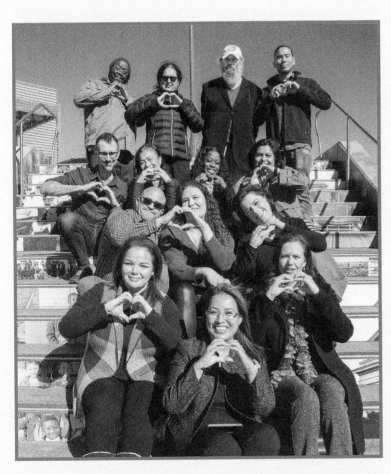

Foundations for Community Health Workers, Third Edition. Edited by Tim Berthold and Darouny Somsanith.
© 2024 John Wiley & Sons, Inc. Published 2024 by John Wiley & Sons, Inc.
Companion website: http://www.wiley.com/go/communityhealthworkers3E

A great river always begins somewhere. Often it starts as a tiny spring bubbling up from a crack in the soil, just like the little stream in my family's land (in Ihithe), which starts where the roots of the fig tree broke though the rocks beneath the ground. But for the stream to grow into a river, it must meet other tributaries and join them as it heads for a lake or the sea . . .

—*Wangari Maathai, Unbowed (2007).*

Introduction

The focus of this chapter is the growth and development of Community Health Workers in the United States, including ongoing efforts to define CHW roles or "scope of practice" (what CHWs do). We will look at the early origins of the field in the United States and various trends that affect the CHW field, including developments in both evaluation and research, as well as in approaches to education, training, and capacity building. We also look at the development of policies aimed at sustaining CHW services and programs and an overview of CHW local and national network building in the United States. You will find stories of CHWs and allies working to build the field. In addition to our focus on CHWs in the United States, be sure to learn to look at the podcast script about CHWs around the world and other supplemental materials regarding the CHW field that are posted on the publisher's website (Berthold, 2024).

The history of the CHW field in the United States includes the contributions of many individuals and organizations working together to establish culturally tailored and community-specific ways to promote the health of our most vulnerable communities. CHWs and their allies understand that CHWs support families and communities by enabling them to take greater control over their own lives and health and to better access and use formal health care systems.

A Note on Writing Down Histories

When people met my mother, Betty Clark Rosenthal, she would tell them about her life and the work she did, and they would say, "You should write down your story." Betty would say, "I am too busy living my life and doing my work to stop and write it down."

Just because something is published in a book or article does not mean that it is the only story or the best story. Research can only tell us about what has been documented in some way, especially in the articles published in scientific journals. These research articles are a valuable source of history. Yet our experiences are also valuable sources of information. As someone who has played a role in the US CHW field for many years, I have been honored to contribute to its history. I am pleased to have a chance to share some of what I have witnessed and learned. I also understand that, even with the literature to help me, I am only able to shed light on a small piece of the much bigger and richer CHW story.

As we begin this review of the CHW journey in the US, take a moment to ask yourself, "Where have I made my contributions?" If you are new to CHW work, ask yourself, "Where will I fit into this history?" Think about your role in assisting people – your neighbors and friends – and any role you have played in making your community healthier. You already have, or one day will have, an important story to tell about your contributions as a CHW.

–E. Lee Rosenthal, original edition author.

MEET COMMUNITY HEALTH WORKERS: PAST AND PRESENT

There are many Community Health Workers (CHWs) throughout the United States and the world. In all communities, we see natural helping and aid-giving networks that may include CHWs. Formal CHW programs and services, however, including both paid and volunteer CHWs, are not universally found. In the United States, CHWs are not yet a routine part of health and human service systems, but they are becoming increasingly common. CHWs are seen by many as invaluable members of the safety net and as important contributors to protecting and improving the health of individuals, families, and communities.

The COVID-19 Pandemic that started in late 2019 and that lasted several years helped to change the visibility of CHWs today. Increasingly, CHWs became recognized for their important work in reaching marginalized (so-called hard-to-reach) populations. During this period, CHWs gained much overdue value as they were acknowledged in the United States and abroad as First Responders who played a pivotal role in emergency response (Mayfield-Johnson et al., 2020; Rahman, Ross, & Pinto, 2021; Rodriguez et al., 2023).

With this as our backdrop, let's explore the history of the CHW field.

WHAT YOU WILL LEARN

By studying the material presented in this chapter, you will be able to:

- Describe the contributions and the role of CHWs in promoting the health of individuals and communities in the United States and around the world
- Identify and discuss major trends and policy debates that have impacted the development of the CHW field in the United States
- Discuss the role that CHWs have played in advocating for greater recognition and respect for their field
- Explain the history and role of professional organizations in the field and in workforce development

C3 Roles & Skills Addressed in Chapter 2

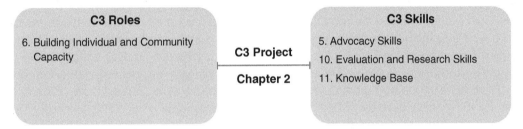

C3 Roles		C3 Skills
6. Building Individual and Community Capacity	C3 Project Chapter 2	5. Advocacy Skills 10. Evaluation and Research Skills 11. Knowledge Base

WORDS TO KNOW

Natural Helping System

Self-Determination

Why Study History?

Some say the past predicts the future or creates the present, so looking at history helps us to understand the world we live in today. As you study and work as a CHW, you are becoming part of something bigger—a world shared with your peers—other CHWs known by many names including *promotores*, Community Health Representatives, and peer health educators. At times, people working as CHWs and their allies would describe this field as part of a movement—one dedicated to health equity, social justice, and the economic development for those served by CHWs and for the CHWs themselves. Learning about how the CHW field has grown in the United States since the 1950s can give you insights about your work today, the people you serve, and the relationships CHWs have with others also working in community and clinical settings throughout the nation to promote health and deliver medical care.

Please reflect on your own story as a CHW and the story of the communities you come from:

What Do YOU Think?

- *When did you start identifying with the role of being a CHW? Were others in your family history a part of a healer or advocacy tradition?*

- *If you work formally as a CHW, either paid or volunteer, when and how did that begin?*

- *How has your work impacted you?*

- *How has your work as a CHW impacted clients, families, and communities?*

- *How have you helped to build the CHW field (or how would you like to help develop the CHW field)?*

2.1 Neighbor Assisting Neighbor

The history of CHWs began when neighbors first aided each other to take care of their health. Over time, those seeking to promote wellness saw the promise of building on these **natural helping systems and formal** approaches to CHW work evolve. The many programs and CHW services we see today include both paid CHWs and volunteer "lay" aid programs and networks. The informal assistance-giving tradition continues today; CHWs extend that tradition.

What is a "Natural Helping System"?

A natural helping system is a naturally occurring community network through which family, friends, neighbors, and others, connected by shared experience (in the same geographic setting or shared experience) watch out for one another and reach out with assistance on a regular basis and in times of crisis.

- *What natural helping networks do you rely on?*

2.2 CHW Names, Definitions, and Competencies

As the CHW field has evolved, no one definition for a CHW has been adopted. In this textbook, we use the term *community health worker* to include the volunteer and paid health practitioners known nationally and internationally by many different names or titles. The National Community Health Advisor Study (NCHAS) identified more than sixty titles for CHWs, including lay health advocate, *promotor,* outreach educator, Community Health Representative, peer health promoter, and of course, CHW (Rosenthal, 1998); according to sources today more than 100 names for CHWs have been identified (CHW Initiative of Sonoma, 2015). The Center for Disease Control series on community health workers refers to more than 20 popular names (Centers for Disease Control and Prevention, 2023). The name CHW is used by the World Health Organization and is the title most commonly used in international settings. It is also used by the American Public Health Association CHW Section.

Having many titles reflects the diversity of the field, but it can make it hard for CHWs to identify one another and find the support they need for training, improving practice, and their own professional development.

> **Durrell Fox:** During a series of meetings in the mid '90s of diverse leaders in the CHW movement in the United States, it was decided that we needed a unifying, umbrella term for the many titles under which CHWs fall. CHW was the agreed-upon, common, unifying term to help the movement for sustainability of our CHW workforce to progress, especially to help inform policy development.
>
> —Durrell Fox, served on the Executive Board of the American Public Health Association from 2011 to 2015 and was a founding member of the National Association of CHWs in 2019

DEFINING CHWs

Because CHWs work in so many communities, under a wide variety of titles, and provide such a wide variety of services, the field and the occupation were not well defined for many years.

As part of a movement for greater recognition and respect for the work that CHWs do, several groups have been advocating for a formal CHW definition. In the early 2000s, a newly formed Policy Committee for the American Public Health Association (APHA) CHW Special Interest Group (SPIG, later a Section of APHA) took the lead in developing such a definition (APHA, 2001). As a part of this effort, the Center for Sustainable Health Outreach (CSHO) collected definitions from CHWs and CHW networks across the United States and from other sources.

In 2006, the APHA CHW SPIG submitted a definition of CHWs to the U.S. Department of Labor (DOL) for consideration. Other groups also submitted definitions for consideration. In March 2009, the U.S. Department of Labor (DOL) approved a separate occupational (work-related) category—21-1094—for CHWs (U.S. Bureau of Labor Statistics, 2009). The Department of Labor's new definition was used in collecting U.S. Census data in 2010 for the first time and that continues through today.

In 2014, CHWs and their supporters, with leadership once again from the Policy Committee of the CHW Section of APHA, advocated for an updated definition that better reflects the community-based nature of CHWs. Many local and state CHW networks have adopted the APHA CHW definition as a part of a campaign to create greater unity in the field. CHW Lisa Renee Holderby-Fox played a pivotal role on behalf of the APHA CHW Section in getting feedback from CHW network leaders across the United States to confirm the CHW definition during this time. The updated (2014) definition is presented in Chapter 1 of this book.

CHW COMPETENCIES AND ROLES

Chapter 1 provides an overview of the Community Health Worker Core Consensus (C3) Project recommended core competencies and roles (The Community Health Worker Core Consensus Project, 2023). The C3 Project is important because just as there was no formal definition of CHWs as discussed above, there was no formal agreement about CHW roles or scope of practice in the United States. In the absence of official roles and competencies, many looked to the National Community Health Advisor Study (NCHAS) conducted from 1994–1998. Notably, roles and competencies identified in the Study (Wiggins & Borbon, 1998) were not formally endorsed by the field, but they were adopted in 2000 by the American Public Health Association. Though not formally identified as standards, the NCHAS roles and competencies influenced many CHW job descriptions, training curricula, and state-level guidance on roles and scope of practice and training standards (Rosenthal et al. 1998).

Given the continual use of the NCHAS roles and competencies and the absence of national standards, a team came together in 2014 to carry out the C3 Project and revisit and update the core roles and competencies from the NCHAS (Rosenthal et al., 2014). The focus of the C3 Project looked at the 1994–1998 roles and competencies and compared them with more current role and competency documents that reflected the current scope of practice and CHW competencies. The C3 Project's original review was completed in 2016. Before the release of the review, the C3 Project team, including all authors of this chapter, released the findings to U.S. CHW network leaders (Rosenthal et al., 2018; Rodela et al., 2021). These networks were invited to review the findings and provide input to confirm a field-driven list of roles and competencies. Following the network review, the C3 Project team released the list of competencies and roles for general use.

The short-term goal of the project was achieved: developing an updated list of competencies and roles and a national awareness of CHWs competencies and scope of practice. The longer-term goal was the use and endorsement of the identified roles and competencies by local, state, and national organizations. Through the field-driven review process, many came to know and trust the C3 Project findings and many programs and states utilize the C3 Project roles and competencies to organize trainings, programs and services, and to guide policies.

CHW Competencies and Roles: CHW Competencies Support CHW Roles or "Scope of Practice"

Competencies

In talking about the uniqueness of different professions, it is important to understand the skills individuals need to do their job. In the CHW field, we recognize that in addition to skills, CHWs bring valuable life experience to their work, and they are connected to the community they serve. These elements and others, often called qualities or attributes, are critical to the competence of CHWs.

- As defined in the Community Health Worker Core Consensus (C3) Project (2018), CHW Competencies include many Qualities and 11 core Skills.

(continues)

CHW Competencies and Roles: CHW Competencies Support CHW Roles or "Scope of Practice"

(continued)

- **Qualities**: Qualities, also known as traits or attributes, are an important part of the competence that CHWs bring to their service. One of the most important qualities often cited is "connection to the community served." Identifying Qualities in those who would like to formally serve as CHWs can be a valuable tool in selecting CHWs.
- **Skills**: Skills learned through life experience, on-the-job, and in formal training and educational programs, are key to CHW success in their service. Strong skills in a wide range of areas support CHW work in their many potential roles.

Roles or Scope of Practice

Scope of practice is defined as the "Definition of the rules, the regulations, and the boundaries within which a fully qualified practitioner with substantial and appropriate training, knowledge, and experience may practice in a defined field. Such practice is also governed by requirements for continuing education and professional accountability" (Federation of State Medical Boards, 2005).

Within the CHW field, we use the term scope of practice more broadly to talk about the breadth and depth of CHW roles or functions that allow you to do your work. A scope of practice for CHWs may be found in various places, including CHW job descriptions or within State legislation.

- The C3 Project identified 10 core CHW roles by looking at their early work in the field (Wiggins & Borbon, 1998) on this topic and contrasting with current policies and selected training content that support CHW work today. Together, the 10 CHW Roles form a CHW's Scope of Practice. This Scope allows CHWs to function in a wide range of roles in both clinical and community settings. Having a broad scope of practice allows CHWs to do direct work in promoting the health and well-being of individuals, families, and communities as well as advocating for access to care and community development overall.

- In some instances, CHW funding and policies only support a narrow set of roles for CHWs, allowing them only to focus on select approaches or issues. The C3 Project recommended that CHWs be prepared for all their identified roles allowing them to functio n at their fullest potential.

To learn more about the Community Health Worker Core Consensus Project and CHW Competencies and Roles, see the resources posted at the end of this chapter (C3 Project, 2023).

THE CHW WORKFORCE—A FORCE FOR HEALTH AND COMMUNITY DEVELOPMENT

In general, health professions have become recognized by defining themselves and helping others to understand what they do to improve health. At times, health professionals have faced conflicts with other professions and have had to struggle for respect and legitimacy. This has been true for many health professions groups such as nurse practitioners, midwives, home health aides, and CHWs (Rosenthal, 2003). In the past several decades, U.S. CHWs have organized at the local, state, and national levels to ensure that their knowledge, skills, and contributions are valued, respected, and integrated into health and public health systems. CHWs have also worked to understand basic characteristics that best help CHWs and others understand CHWs in the landscape of the many health professions.

The History of the National Association of CHWs' Six Pillars Describing the CHW Workforce

Another way of defining the CHW workforce is to describe the characteristics of the workforce overall. NACHW identified a gap in the breadth of information describing the CHW workforce and developed another cornerstone piece that helps to define and describe the CHW workforce. Having spent several years collecting data and working with CHWs and CHW networks and associations throughout the United States, in early 2023 NACHW released "The 6 Pillars of CHWs." The six pillars include descriptions of the diversity and strength of CHWs but also the fragility of the workforce. These 6 pillars state the following: 1) CHWs are a unique workforce, 2) CHWs are a community-based workforce, 3) CHWs are a historic and diverse workforce, 4) CHWs are a cross-sector workforce, 5) CHWs are a proven workforce, and 6) CHWs are a precarious workforce. To learn more about the 6 Pillars of CHWs, visit the NACHW website (National Association of CHWs, 2023).

Additional Readings About CHW History and Leaders

There is simply not enough space in this chapter for all we want to share with you about the history of the CHW profession. To read more about the global history of CHWs, the founding of the National CHW Association, and the contributions of Yvonne Lacey, an influential leader in the CHW field, please see the Additional Resources posted at the end of this chapter and on the Wiley website.

CHW Profile

Durrell Fox (He/Him)

CHW Consultant—JSI Research and Training

Founding Board of Directors

National Association of Community Health Workers (NACHW)

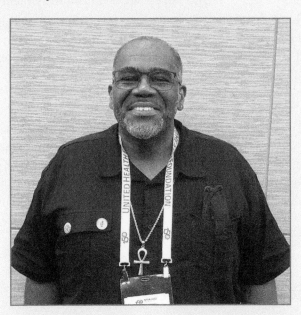

One of the major driving forces for being a CHW was my mom, a single mother living in a housing development in the Roxbury section of Boston. She began receiving services from anti-poverty agencies. That led her to working for and becoming the Executive Director of one of the agencies before serving as a state legislator. I spent most of my life seeing community service in action providing services like childcare, food, housing support, and gifts during the holiday seasons. Community service was in my blood.

I began my journey as a CHW in 1991 providing direct services, outreach, policy, and advocacy support for HIV+ adolescents and their families. One lesson I learned from my mom was that you can help one client at a time, but if you change a policy related to housing, food insecurity, etc., you can help the whole community.

(continues)

CHW Profile

(continued)

Currently, I provide technical assistance and advocacy support for CHWs on several JSI projects and in my role in state, regional, and national CHW networks and associations including the National Association of CHWs (NACHW). I continue to volunteer as a CHW for programs serving young adults of color. In recent years, I've been supporting young men's health, fatherhood, youth violence, and COVID-19 prevention programs. The main crux of my work is about addressing the social determinants of health (SDOH). SDOH like housing, education, and jobs play a larger role in community health outcomes than healthcare. I've spent more time at client graduations, job interviews, and court appearances than in clinic with them, which has led to improved health and wellness outcomes. Some common activities include proving supported referrals, informal counseling, motivational interviewing, and system navigation.

Since the early 90s, I've been engaged in many local and state regional initiatives, including being honored to serve as a founding board member of a statewide CHW Association in Massachusetts. I'm currently helping to build a CHW network in Georgia.

I am most proud of my role as a founding member of NACHW. It took over four years of organizing by the founding members, building on a decade of past efforts, to develop a truly diverse, truly CHW-led national CHW association. We launched NACHW in 2019, and less than a year after launching, the COVID-19 pandemic began. Suddenly hundreds of millions of dollars became available for healthcare overnight including for CHWs. Within a year of our NACHW launch, this funding provided the opportunity to exponentially grow and expand. This period, 2020–2022, is a major milestone and historic moment in the CHW movement.

I was born into community service, and after becoming a CHW and receiving training, my CHW-health equity lens and view shaped and guided me. In my early years as a man of color, I was never in touch with my feelings--my father and other male role models rarely showed emotions. Part of my journey as a CHW included getting in touch with and tapping into feelings and emotions. CHWs' values, qualities, attributes, and practice include keeping a close connection to the heart—this has served CHW and community wellness efforts well!

I encourage new CHWs to get and stay connected with other CHWs and CHW allies locally, statewide, regionally, and nationally. That connection to and support from CHWs across the country has been paramount to my journey and trajectory to CHW leadership roles. I also urge CHWs to always be engaged in advocacy and policy development to support our workforce and communities. CHWs use the same advocacy skills assisting a family in addressing their SDOH needs as we use to develop policies that can help the entire community address SDOH needs!

2.3 CHWs' Evolution in the United States

The important role of CHWs in the United States is increasingly being recognized. In many settings, from clinics to community-based organizations, CHWs work in partnerships with community members and organizations, other CHWs, and with those in health and human services with the goal of improving health and access to systems of care. CHWs carry out many or all the roles described in the previous chapter to do this work. For example, in their role of cultural mediator, they can help make health and social service systems more culturally competent. Often the communities they represent have traditional healing systems that were developed long before their introduction to Western medicine. CHWs help these two systems to co-exist, with individuals and families integrating what they consider the best from both systems to maintain or improve their health. For example, in American Indian communities, traditional healers such as medicine men were and are an important part of health networks (Mohatt & Elk, 2002). In Latino communities, *curanderos* assist in promoting health in the community (Brown & Fee, 2002; Gonzalez & Ortiz, 2004; Reyes-Ortiz, Rodriguez, & Markides, 2009; Rothpletz-Puglia, 2013). CHWs help to bridge these worlds and to increase the two-way flow of information so that both providers and those they serve can identify ways to promote health and use formal medical and social prevention and treatment services. CHWs also work to enhance understanding of other social, political, and economic issues. This bridging role of CHWs is just one of the many ways CHWs help those they serve and ultimately promote improved health and health equity (APHA, 2009).

Many different groups recognize the potential and importance of CHWs in health promotion and disease prevention. Public health and other health professionals recruit and partner with individuals who are connected to the natural helping networks in their communities (Eng & Young, 1992; Gilkey, Garcia, & Rush, 2011) supporting them to develop skills as a formal CHW. CHWs address many health and social issues, sometimes prioritized by community members themselves, as well as issues identified by organizations that serve the community. Health care systems and community-based agencies are increasingly hiring and integrating CHWs to serve within teams in public health departments, hospitals, community clinics, or other sites (Martinez, Ro, Villa, Powell, & Knickman, 2011). Other CHWs contribute on a volunteer basis in these settings and in community centers and social and faith-based organizations. In these cases, programs often provide incentives such as educational credits or modest financial stipends to CHWs to support their participation.

CHWs' FORMAL EARLY HISTORY IN THE UNITED STATES: 1950–2000

In the 1950 and 1960s, the first documented formal volunteer and paid CHW programs were established in the United States. During this period, Native American tribes and migrant farm workers were the best-known programs (Giblin, 1989; Gould & Lomax, 1993; Hoff, 1969; Meister, Warrick, de Zapién, & Wood, 1992). Strong CHW programs still serve these communities today.

The Federal Migrant Act of 1962 required federally qualified migrant clinics to conduct outreach in migrant labor camps. CHWs were hired to provide this outreach, a move that established many CHW programs. This outreach was built on the *promotor(a)* tradition common in Mexico and Latin America, where many farm workers were raised or have family ties (Mahler, 1978).

The largest program of this period got its official start in the late 1960s: the Community Health Representative (CHR) Program. It was established by the Indian Health Service (IHS) with support from the Office of Economic Opportunity (OEO) and in collaboration with American Indian tribes (Indian Health Service, 2023; Satterfield, Burd, Valdez, Hosey, & Shield, 2002). The OEO ran the original program unit and IHS took the reins in 1972. In 1975, the Indian Self-Determination and Education Assistance Act, P.L. 93-638, facilitated Tribal authorities to contract with the Federal government to operate programs and health systems serving tribal members. Today, approximately 95% of Tribal CHR programs are tribally governed, representing 264 Tribes. The CHR program has stood the test of time and today CHRs work in nearly all tribal communities in the United States.

As CHR programs manage and oversee both community-based and community-specific health services critical to improving health and health outcomes, they are a poised, highly trained, and well-established standardized workforce serving the medical and social needs of American Indian communities. The CHR scope of practice includes outreach and communication, advocacy, social support, basic health education, referrals to community clinics, and hospitals and providing social and primary preventive services reflecting underserved populations in rural and hard-to-reach Tribal communities. CHR core roles and competencies affirm CHR training and "lived experience" as a valuable member of the public health and health care system offering cultural, linguistic, and traditional knowledge central to care coordination and case management. The primary purpose of the CHR program is unique and in line with broader CHW workforce roles and competencies recognized by several federal entities, including (1) relationship and trust-building—to identify specific needs of clients, (2) communication—especially continuity and clarity, between provider and patient, and traditional knowledge and language, and (3) focus on social determinants of health—conditions in which people are born, grow, work, live, and age, including social connectedness, traditional knowledge, and spirituality, relationship to the environment and a shared history.

CHRs played pivotal roles during the COVID-19 pandemic, leading efforts around contact tracing and meeting basic health and social needs during lockdown. Many rural reservation communities cover large areas and CHRs often assist families with transportation to health care providers. CHR programs across the country have developed best practices for addressing social determinants of health and cultural competency and are national leaders in the CHW field. Many tribal entities and organizations have recently received federal funds to build CHR capacity in their communities and contribute to the CHW profession overall. The IHS continues to play a large role in the national CHW landscape and is working to progress the CHR program alongside the CHW field in areas like CHR integration within systems and teams, sustainability, certification, and standardization.

In the 1960s and 1970s, new CHW programs continued to develop throughout rural and urban communities. CHW programs addressed important public health issues and were often credited with creating valuable employment opportunities for people who had a hard time entering the paid workforce (Domke, 1966). The Office of Economic Opportunity invested in CHWs in many urban areas (Meister, 1997). CHWs and other community-based workers were seen as critical to the reorganization of the human services system (Pearl & Riessmann, 1965). CHWs were recognized for their connection to the community and their unique insight into the individuals they served (Withorn, 1984).

In this period, opportunities for paid and volunteer CHWs and *promotores* increased and were hailed as contributing to the reorganization of health and human services delivery systems (Pynoos, Hade-Kaplan, & Fleisher, 1984; Service, 1977). CHWs were paid to work across a range of health projects and programs targeting different issues and populations (Hoff, 1969; Potts & Miller, 1964; Wilkinson, 1992). In this era, groups like the Black Panther Party and the Young Lords advocated for the government to provide free healthcare, including prevention services, and accessible services to treat drug addiction for African American, Latino, and all oppressed peoples. Though their more controversial activities received public attention, the Black Panthers also created free breakfast programs for school children and free medical clinics for their communities (Stanford University, 2023).

Beginning in the mid-1960s, CHWs were an important part of Community Health Centers (CHC), helping to establish these clinics and tie them to communities (Northwest Regional Primary Care Association, 2015). Today, many CHCs integrate CHWs into health promotion and other community programming where they help to ensure that CHCs achieve their mission of delivering culturally competent and community-centered services (National Association of Community Health Centers, 2010; Spiro et al., 2012).

In the 1970s, Service et al., (1977) started to use the term "lay health advisors" (LHAs) and called attention to the important community roles of LHAs, such as health promotion, social support, mediation (helping two sides reach an agreement), and community empowerment (Salber, 1979).

In the 1980s, funding for job creation programs slowed, and the number of paid CHWs participating in forums such as the American Public Health Association declined. At the same time, a number of CHW programs expanded their roles. Programs for migrants grew with funding from private and government sources (Booker, Grube-Robinson, Kay, Najjera, & Stewart, 2004; Harlan, Eng, & Watkins, 1992; Meister, Warrick, de Zapién, & Wood, 1992). The number of CHWs making home visits to aid mothers and infants increased (Julnes, Konefal, Pindur, & Kim, 1994; Larson, McGuire, Watkins, & Mountain, 1992; McFarlane & Fehir, 1994; Poland, Giblin, Waller, & Hankin, 1992). The federal Healthy Start program began to rely on outreach workers to address inequalities in infant mortality rates, especially in cities among African Americans mothers and infants. CHWs also started supporting community members at risk for chronic conditions or diseases (e.g., high blood pressure, cancer, and diabetes) to maintain better control, keep appointments with and talk to their doctors, check their blood pressure, and blood sugar levels, and know the signs of serious illness (Brandeis University, 2003; Brownstein, Bone, Dennison, Hill, Kim, & Levine, 2005; Norris et al., 2006).

In this same period, the emergency of HIV/AIDS challenged and motivated activists to organize and advocate for civil rights protections and investment in community health outreach, education and testing programs, research into treatments, and access to quality health care. Perhaps the best-known activist organization was the AIDS Coalition to Unleash Power (ACT UP), founded in 1987. ACT UP built on the protest traditions that came out of the civil rights movement and opposition to the Vietnam War (Klitzman, 1997). Activists were successful in building strategic alliances with health and public health professionals, in drawing public attention to HIV/AIDS, in advocating for changes to public policies and the creation of new public health programs and research on treatments for HIV disease. As a result, local health departments and community-based organizations began to hire CHWs to conduct outreach and provide client-centered education, counseling, and HIV antibody testing services. CHWs conducted home and hospital visits, facilitated support groups, trained physicians and other providers in providing culturally competent care, initiated syringe exchange programs, and much more. With the development of the AIDS epidemic in the United States, "a disease [became] the basis of a political movement" (Klitzman, 1997). The success of CHWs in aiding to address the HIV epidemic in turn influenced the development of the CHW field.

In the 1990s, CHWs gained increased recognition for their important contributions to health and job creation (Rosenthal, 1998; Witmer, Seifer, Finocchio, Leslie, & O'Neil, 1995). Job creation was pushed by Welfare Reform, which brought renewed federal attention and resources. Welfare-to-work programs explored CHW jobs as an important option for individuals newly entering or reentering the paid workforce. CHW program coordinators reminded all involved of the importance of looking for individuals who were already known to be natural aides in their communities when recruiting CHWs (Aguirre, 1997).

From 2000 to 2019, workforce studies, articles, and reports about CHWs became more common (Love et al., 2004; Matos, Findley, Hicks, Legendre, & Do Canto, 2011; Proulx, 2000a, b). At the same time, public and private grant funding for CHW programs continued to grow, focusing on assisting individuals in managing health conditions such as HIV, diabetes (Norris et al., 2006; Tang et al., 2014), high blood pressure (Allen, Dennison Himmelfarb, Szanton, & Frick, 2014; Brownstein et al., 2007; CDC, 2015, 2018), cancer, and asthma (Margellos-Anast, Gutierrez, & Whitman, 2012; Prezio, Pagán, Shuval, & Culica, 2014) and other health areas (CDC, 2015). During this period, we learned more about the work of CHWs and the evidence base grew. A colorectal cancer navigation program designed for Hispanic men showed an increase in life expectancy by six months for participant as compared to non-participants with a health care savings of $1,148 per program participant (Wilson, Villarreal, Stimpson, & Pagán, 2014). Interventions incorporating CHWs were found to be effective in improving knowledge about cancer screening, as well as screening outcomes for both cervical and breast cancer (Viswanathan et al., 2009). Integrating CHWs into multidisciplinary health teams emerged as an effective strategy for improving the control of asthma, diabetes, and high blood pressure among high-risk populations, along with cost savings (CDC, 2015). With this growing evidence base showing the impact that CHWs make, interest in developing the CHW workforce continued to grow.

As discussed in Chapter 1, the National Association of CHWs (NACHW) was officially launched in Spring of 2019, after years of work by its founding board to build consensus and formalize its charter. The emergence of NACHW and the COVID-19 pandemic which followed less than a year later, mark important moments in the development of the CHW workforce on a national level.

2020 to today: The impact of the COVID-19 pandemic on the CHW workforce in the United States cannot be overstated. CHWs gained increasing recognition as a frontline, essential workforce during the initial response to the pandemic, the roll-out of vaccinations, and the ongoing work of addressing misinformation, vaccine hesitancy, and persistent COVID-related health inequities (Kangovi, 2020; Peretz, Islam, & Matiz, 2020; Smith & Wennerstrom, 2020).

During the pandemic, many CHWs were recruited to help with contact tracing efforts and efforts to curb spread of COVID-19 through public education campaigns, resource referrals, and helping community members meet basic needs without risking infection (Rosenthal, Menking, & Begay, 2020). CHWs working in clinical settings often helped with COVID screenings, vaccine administration, and other frontline activities related to the pandemic (Moir et al., 2021; Nawaz et al., 2023).

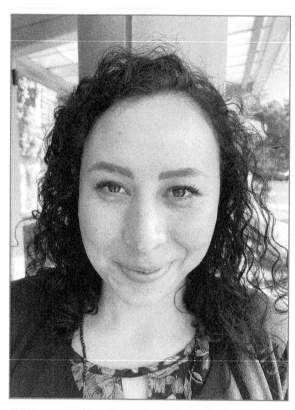

CHWs are working throughout the United States.

This time period saw a dramatic increase in the workforce, policies supporting CHW infrastructure, and federal funding aimed directly at CHW programs. The Centers for Disease Control and Prevention, Health Resources and Services Administration, and the National Institutes of Health all offered multimillion-dollar grants specifically to support building and supporting the CHW workforce. Some leaders of the CHW field, including NACHW, raised concerns about some of these funding opportunities, which were structured to favor large institutions and government entities over community-based organizations (Smith, 2022). Still, it is worthwhile to note the importance of these groundbreaking federal investments in the CHW workforce as the first of their kind.

While much of this federal funding was specifically written for COVID-19 response, CHW work has always been firmly rooted in addressing social determinants of health and the prevention and management of chronic disease. Given the focus on infectious disease funding, CHWs across the United States have been tasked with balancing addressing COVID-19 and other infectious diseases with their foundational work addressing health disparities (American Diabetes Association, 2020). CHW programs have had to continue to be nimble, rising to the ever-changing nature of the pandemic while also meeting the pre-existing social and physical and mental health needs of patients and community members.

In 2020, with the death of George Floyd at the hands of the Minneapolis police, we saw an increase in conversations in the public health field about the effect of racism on health and the role CHWs can play in addressing systemic racism and state violence. The CHW Section of the American Public Health Association wrote *Policy 20227: A Strategy to Address Systemic Racism and Violence as Public Health Priorities: Training and Supporting Community Health Workers to Advance Equity and Violence Prevention* with the support of more than 30 CHW leaders and allies (APHA, 2022). The policy was passed with overwhelming support from the APHA voting delegates at the 2022 APHA Annual Meeting in Boston, MA.

This time period has also seen increased numbers of devastating natural disasters due to the changing climate. More and more, CHWs are being regarded as essential allies in disaster response and preparedness given their strong connection to communities disproportionately affected by the effects of climate change across the United States, be they hurricanes, winter storms, wildfires, or flooding (Nicholls, Picou, & McCord, 2017; Springgate, Wennerstrom, & Carriere, 2011).

As the urgency of the COVID-19 pandemic eases, CHWs are dealing with the inevitable mental health effects and burnout that come after years of emergency response and high-stress work environments. CHW organizations across the country have responded to the increased stress of CHW work during the pandemic and other community emergencies with CHW-specific mental health and self-care offerings, a focus that will surely continue into the future (Byrd-Williams et al., 2021; Powell & Yuma-Guerrero, 2016).

2.4 Trends in the CHW Field

The CHW field has been increasingly recognized in the United States as evidenced by the development of public policy related to CHWs in numerous states (NASHP, 2021) and activities in federal agencies in support of CHWs and attention to CHWs in peer review literature, in the press, and on social media (Goldfield et al., 2020). With the focus in health care on the often cited "**triple aim**" of improved health outcomes, improved experience of care, and efficiency related to costs, interest in CHWs is not surprising. CHW services have sought to address all three aim areas with promising impacts documented (Findley, Matos, Hicks, Chang, & Reich, 2014). The Patient Protection and Affordable Care Act passed in 2010 also increased attention to CHWs and the roles they have in improving access to care and in prevention services delivery. Related regulations opened up more opportunities for the sustainability of CHW services (Widget, Kinsler, Dolatshahi, & Hess, 2014).

With this promising horizon in place for CHWs, let's explore what trends are influencing development in the field today.

CAPACITY BUILDING AND EDUCATION

CHW training programs have increased in the 21st century and vary widely in terms of the competencies addressed, curriculum requirements, quality and type of instruction, and other factors. Many states closely monitor or certify the curriculum used for CHW training and/or certification, some have just one officially approved curriculum that all training sites must use, and others are fully decentralized, allowing each training site to develop their own capacity-building programs with full autonomy. **Capacity building** refers to strengthening the knowledge, skills, and confidence of individuals—like CHWs—or communities. CHWs learn from many sources and in many settings and these keep changing over time.

You are likely participating in a CHW capacity-building activity right now since you are reading this textbook! You might be participating in a virtual CHW training course or attending classes in person. You may be receiving instruction through a community college, a community or faith-based organization, a health department, a clinical provider, or your employer. Your instructor could be a CHW or may have a different connection to the CHW field. Your training might be 60 or 160 hours long. Many trainings include skill building and practicums or internships in a practice-driven curriculum (George et al., 2021; Lee et al., 2021). Some training programs even begin as early as high school (Williams-Livingston et al., 2020; Zheng, Williams-Livingston, Danavall, Ervin, & McCray, 2021). CHW training and the types of people that facilitate the trainings vary across region, state, community, and setting, which is part of what allows the CHW field to nimbly respond to an ever-changing public health landscape.

While training techniques vary, there is little clear evidence in the CHW literature about which training characteristics lead to the best outcomes in CHW programs and interventions (Adams et al., 2021). There is wide variability in the way CHW trainings are evaluated and how those results are reported, leading to a lack of clear peer-reviewed guidance around how to structure and deliver CHW training, especially for CHWs from particular racial or ethnic backgrounds (Lee et al., 2021; Ramalingam, Strayer, Breig, & Harden, 2019).

CHW TRAINING GUIDES AND CURRICULA

Many training guides and educational curricula have been developed for CHWs. Some educational resources are shared freely, while other training materials are proprietary and are not made available by the individuals and organizations that developed them. Public and privately developed curricula address specific health issues, such as diabetes, heart health, cancer, HIV/AIDS, and prenatal health. In the early 1990s, the National Commission for Infant Mortality developed a curriculum for maternal and child CHW programs that included a training manual, a CHW pocket manual, and even a community guide to starting CHW programs. Though issue-specific curricula are still very common, there appears to be a shift to curriculum that develops core or foundational CHWs skills. In Minnesota, a core curriculum on CHWs was developed collaboratively by educators, employers, and CHWs in that state (Willaert, 2005); that curriculum was designated as a required curriculum for CHWs seeking reimbursement. As states have begun to formalize regulations for CHWs, some have considered the option of a single curriculum, but more have chosen to identify core competencies and play a role in approving a range of curricula (Miller, Bates, & Katzen, 2014) to address these areas. As of 2015, no single CHW curriculum, book, or textbook for CHWs has been adopted throughout the United States, but some resources have been widely used. *Helping Health Workers Learn*, developed by the Hesperian Foundation, has been popular, especially in international settings (Werner & Bower, 2012). The City College of San Francisco developed the textbook you are now using. This is the first textbook specifically developed for use by CHWs in classroom settings. It was first released in 2009, revised in 2015, and now this third edition is being updated in 2023. ***The book itself is of historic significance, especially for the U.S. CHW field.***

ON-THE-JOB LEARNING

On-the-job learning (also known as on-the-job training) has been a mainstay of CHW education (HRSA, 2007). In the early days of the field in the United States, CHW program coordinators often developed CHW training in their own organizations (Rosenthal, 1998). It was helpful to CHWs to access trainings and to have employers cover the costs of education. It meant that CHWs could be selected from communities directly due to the qualities that make them good CHWs versus their prior formal learning (Jennings, 1990). This meant high access to the field for CHW candidates. At the same time, training on the job requires significant resources from each employer. CHWs also reported that on-the-job training was a barrier to career development because it was not recognized when they moved from one job to another (Rosenthal, 1998). Additionally, some CHWs and administrators reported that on-the-job training was too limited and even off-base (Love et al., 2004).

Today, it is increasingly common for CHWs to come into a paid CHW position with their core training already behind them (Rosenthal & Macinko, 2011). In this way, employers are largely freed from covering CHW educational costs. In some cases, however, employers sponsor CHWs to participate in educational programs. Also, many employers take responsibility for CHW continuing education needs, scheduling training, and covering the time and costs associated with participation for their staff or volunteers. In the state of Massachusetts, organizations receiving public funds for CHW services are required to support ongoing training and CHW networking opportunities.

APPRENTICESHIPS FOR CHWs—IN THE CLASSROOM AND ON THE JOB

On the job learning is closely related to the skills development approach that is found in professions whose training is based on an apprenticeship model where a mentor professional called a journeyman or journeywoman mentors an apprentice. In the United States, the Department of Labor runs a formal system of Registered Apprenticeships (Department of Labor, 2023). Their model has certain standards and blends a required classroom learning with a significant on the job learning. It also requires that apprentices be paid and gives an incentive for increased pay during the apprenticeship training period. Due to collaborative efforts in the state of Texas, in 2011, the Department of Labor officially accepted the CHWs workforce as eligible for apprenticeship opportunities.

In 2022, HRSA released a grant opportunity specifically to fund CHW training and apprenticeship programs. Ultimately, HRSA awarded $255 million to 83 organizations around the country (HRSA, 2022).

The Homeless Prenatal Program (HPP), CHW Apprenticeship Program

The reasons for family poverty and homelessness are as diverse as the families that experience them. However, persistent unemployment and/or underemployment and a lack of sufficient income can not only initiate but set a trend of poverty and homelessness that becomes increasingly difficult for families to escape. After 33 years of experience working with low-income and homeless families, the Homeless Prenatal Program (HPP) in San Francisco, CA knows that sustainable employment and economic security are key to creating and maintaining long-term family stability.

(continues)

The Homeless Prenatal Program (HPP), CHW Apprenticeship Program

(continued)

HPP provides housing assistance, a transitional housing shelter for pregnant and post-partum women, and wellness services including mental health and parenting, childcare and prenatal services, and family counseling. Another service is the Community Health Worker (CHW) Apprenticeship program, which is an accredited, 16-month, paid workforce development program (with an education component) that prepares low-income members of the community for professionally rewarding and economically self-sustaining careers in the nonprofit and healthcare sectors.

The CHW Apprenticeship hires members of the community who face barriers to employment. HPP recruits apprentices from the agency's client population. Most applicants are former clients or are referred by former clients. Prior to hire, these individuals are typically unemployed and/or on public assistance. Most are mothers, and most are single parents. Most apprentices have been homeless or at-risk of homelessness and many are survivors of domestic violence and/or child abuse. Some of these participants are formerly incarcerated adults. Some have also struggled with substance abuse and/or have been involved with child welfare/foster care. All apprentices are recovering from trauma and living with a tremendous amount of stress. For many, the CHW Apprenticeship is their first paid job. The CHW Apprenticeship effectively disrupts cycles of poverty and homelessness for the individuals who participate in the program and their families, setting the stage for long-term stability.

HPP has offered highly successful CHW training alongside its broader continuum of supportive services since 1995. Of the 206 individuals who have participated in the program, 85% graduated, and 92% of graduates secured a job (living wage plus benefits) within 30 days of graduation.

Juanita Wortham participated in the CHW Apprenticeship and now works as a Wellness Counselor for HPP. "It was definitely a game changer, not only in my career path but with my personal relationships with others," said Juanita. "I learned a lot about myself and how I can be perceived by others that need my services. My highlight was cultural humility because HPP works with families from all walks of life and having cultural humility is critical to helping our clients. The improvement in my personal life from learning about vicarious trauma helps me overall with others and being able to make space for others' trauma without taking it with me and holding it."

To learn more about the Homeless Prenatal Program, go to https://homelessprenatal.org/.

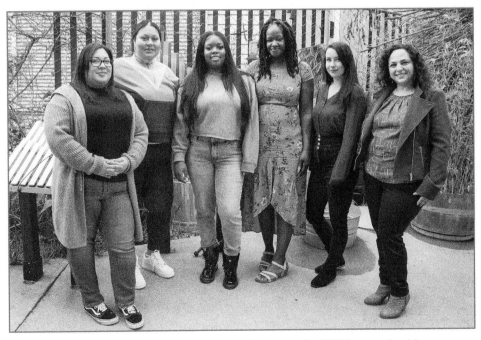

Recent Graduates from the Homeless Prenatal Program's CHW Apprenticeship Certification Program.

CENTER-BASED AND COLLEGE-BASED CHW EDUCATIONAL APPROACHES

In the 1990s, there was a move toward center-based training (rather than on-the-job training), as well as college-supported educational programs for CHWs. An early example of center-based training comes from Boston's Community Health Education Center, developed by the City of Boston to respond to a citywide need for CHW capacity building. Since the 1990s, the center has provided core initial training to CHWs. It has also been a resource center for training and other materials and has served as a gathering place for CHWs, with activities like job-sharing luncheons.

Early in their history, efforts were made in some areas to assist CHWs to gain access to academic pathways and credit within college programs. Early reports of CHWs in academic settings showed that there were challenges in the college setting; some CHWs felt their competence gained through life experience and experience on the job were undervalued (Sainer, Ruiz, & Wilder, 1975).

City College of San Francisco started a CHW Certificate Program in the early 1990s. The program, designed to address some of these challenges and barriers, offered the first full-scale college credit-bearing educational opportunity for CHWs (Love et al., 2004). Building on this model and other emerging programs, Project Jump Start at the University of Arizona (1998–2002) focused on creating credit-bearing training for CHWs through four Arizona community colleges predominately serving rural communities (Proulx, 2000b). During 2004–2008, CHWs, allies, and representatives of twenty-two CHW college-based educational programs formed the CHW National Education Collaborative (CHW NEC) to advise college-based CHW programs about best practices for such programs (Proulx, Rosenthal, Fox, Lacey, & Community Health Worker National Education Collaborative Contributors, 2008). The Project saw CHW leadership as vital, and its majority CHW Advisory Council and co-chairs Lacey and Fox were important to the Project; the Project was lead Don Proulx, Lee Rosenthal, and anchor coordinator Nancy Collyer. In 2008, as the CHW NEC project came to an end, we produced a guidebook for the field, looking at ways colleges and other institutions can start and strengthen CHW educational and capacity-building programs.

Today, CHW training centers can be found in many types of organizations. Community Colleges continue to play a large role in the instruction of CHWs, but other community-based organizations, public health entities, and educational or job training organizations also provide CHW instruction and certification courses.

HOW DOES THE ORGANIZATION OF CHW TRAINING AND EDUCATION IMPACT THE FIELD?

Many of the skills and personal qualities needed to excel as a CHW can be learned on the job and through life experience. The skills that lead to success in higher education do not, in themselves, translate into job effectiveness as a CHW. Veteran CHWs have often been suspicious of college-based training programs: the typical college classroom is not open to all community members. In addition, it is common in the health workforce that higher education credentials are set as a requirement for employment. This can limit access to employment for CHWs who are highly skilled but lack formal education. Specifically, requirements for college-based programs may present barriers to and negatively affect the very communities with the greatest potential to be outstanding CHWs, including low-income communities, communities of color, undocumented immigrant communities, and English language learners. At the same time, college credit and education are closely linked to employment outcomes, career advancement, and higher income. Well-designed educational programs that are accessible and that offer college credit to CHWs can provide these students with valuable opportunities for professional growth and advancement.

Many in the CHW field believe it is important to maintain multiple approaches to CHW education and training and to develop ways to recognize and credit the value of life and job experience. To the extent that college-based training becomes more widespread, it is important to ensure that these programs are accessible to CHWs financially and in their preferred teaching approaches. It is also important to make sure that employers continue to support and fund CHW training and education, which historically has been an important ingredient for success in the field maintaining access to many CHWs who are and become increasingly outstanding CHWs.

THE USE OF TECHNOLOGY AND ONLINE EDUCATION

Many CHW training programs offer online education, both in real time and self-paced. Online training became more common during the COVID-19 pandemic, and many have continued to offer online options or hybrid educational events. Online resources come from both public and private sources. Some are offered at no cost, while others have associated fees and, in some cases, credits. No matter what the cost, online or distance education training means that there are more resources available for CHW learning that may be especially valuable for CHWs in geographically isolated communities. In using online training curricula, it is important to consider how this approach may impact what we could call the "high touch" role of CHWs. Generating a hybrid plan for face-to-face learning time and online education still seems the best fit for CHWs.

RESEARCH: BUILDING THE EVIDENCE BASE ABOUT THE WORK OF CHWs

Through the 1990s, researchers conducted a number of regional and national studies of CHWs. Together, these studies demonstrated the power, value, and importance of the work that CHWs have been doing in the United States in a form that could be understood by the fields of public health and medicine.

The National Community Health Advisor Study was a participatory research project, meaning the group being studied participated in designing the study and analyzing, and interpreting findings (Rosenthal, et al. 1998). The majority of the NCHAS advisory council were CHWs, and the council alone was responsible for making recommendations based on the data for the field. Many of the actions recommended by the 36 council members are now being implemented throughout the United States. These include increased access to CHW educational programs that offer college credit and the then controversial recommendation to credential CHWs.

In addition to identifying the core roles and competencies of CHWs, the NCHAS documented the many community and clinical settings where CHWs work, including homes, schools, clinics, and hospitals. The settings in which CHWs work clearly influence the activities of CHWs. According to the California Workforce Initiative, CHWs working in clinics are more likely to perform duties focused on traditional patient care, whereas CHWs working door-to-door act more in the roles associated with social workers and community organizers (Keane, Nielsen, & Dower, 2004).

In 1995, a commentary entitled "*Community Health Workers: Integral Members of the Health Care Work Force*" appeared in the *American Journal of Public Health* (Witmer, Seifer, Finocchio, Leslie, & O'Neill, 1995). The article's title alone stimulated attention to the field. The Institute of Medicine's landmark book, *Unequal Treatment: Confronting Racial and Ethnic Disparities in Health Care*, addressed the importance of CHWs in reducing health inequalities (Institute of Medicine, 2003). A study funded by the Centers for Medicare and Medicaid Services (CMS) on approaches to cancer prevention among elders of color found that CHWs were the "primary mechanism for cultural tailoring" (Brandeis University, 2003).

Early workforce studies in the San Francisco Bay Area (Love, Gardner, & Legion, 1997) inspired other regions and states to conduct similar assessments to determine the extent and roles of CHWs in local labor markets. The Annie E. Casey Foundation funded another study of the CHW workforce, looking at the potential of worker-owned CHW cooperatives (Rico, 1997). In 2007, the federal government funded and coordinated the CHW National Workforce Study (HRSA, 2007). The study explored the roles and functions of CHWs in different settings and estimated that there were 120,000 CHWs throughout the United States in 2005.

Over the years, research has continued to document the evidence of the effectiveness of CHWs in promoting health outcomes (Giblin, 1989; HRSA, 2007; Nemcek & Sabatier, 2003; Swider, 2002; Rosenthal et al., 2011; Smedley et al. 2003). In 2007, CHWs, researchers, and other stakeholders met to develop a CHW Research Agenda by and for the field (Rosenthal, de Heer, Rush, & Holderby, 2008). At this two-day conference led by Carl Rush, conference participants identified the most important areas for additional research:

- CHW cost-effectiveness or return on investment
- CHW impact on health status
- Building CHW capacity and sustaining CHWs on the job
- Funding options
- CHWs as capacity builders
- CHWs promoting real access to care

The Massachusetts Department of Public Health released an influential report in 2009 entitled "*Community Health Workers in Massachusetts: Improving Health Care and Public Health*" (Massachusetts Department of Public

Health, 2009). The report presented strong evidence that the state's nearly 3,000 CHWs have improved access to health care and the quality of that care. It suggested state policy changes—including workforce development and training, occupational regulation, guidelines for research and evaluation, and sustainable financing—are needed to promote and sustain CHWs services.

States and organizations (e.g., CHW Network of New York, California, Virginia, Community Health Foundations, Foundations for Health Generations, and American Association of Diabetes Educators) have developed reports on a variety of CHW issues such as scope of practice, training, financing, and cost effectiveness. These and other states continue to explore options for supporting CHW integration and sustainability. New research studies on workforce issues help inform those who are trying to integrate CHWs into healthcare teams and sustain their employment (Obrien, Squires, Bixby, & Larson, 2009; Volkman & Castañares, 2011; Nielson et al., 2023; Massachusetts Department of Public Health, Community Health Worker Advisory Council, 2009).

The Centers for Medicare and Medicaid Services Innovation Center (CMMI) funded projects from 2013 to 2016 to work on models that reduce costs, improve care for populations with special needs, test approaches to transform clinic models, and improve the health of populations by focusing, for example, on diabetes or hypertension prevention programs that go beyond clinics. Many of the funded projects centered on CHWs. For example, Oregon was given a grant to test the effects of its Coordinated Care Organizations (CCOs) and new payment model on health outcomes and costs. All of the CCOs integrated CHWs into their care teams (Foundation for Health Generation, 2013).

Over the years, research has continued to document evidence of the effectiveness of CHWs in preventing and managing various diseases and health conditions including asthma, cancer, diabetes, hypertension, immunizations, HIV/AIDS, maternal and child health, nutrition, and tuberculosis (Brownstein et al., 2005, 2007, 2011; Giblin, 1989; Guide to Community Preventive Services, 2015; HRSA, 2007; Kangovi et al., 2018; Nemcek & Sabatier, 2003; Swider, 2002). More recent studies show a continuation of this trend, for example, in cancer, diabetes, social work and rural studies, HIV/AIDs, and COVID-19.

Cancer: The scope of work for CHWs and patient navigators (PNs) includes addressing various cancers and covers prevention, detection, diagnosis, treatment, and survivorship. CHWs and PNs educate, address barriers to care, and advocate, link, and navigate patients through healthcare systems and to community resources (Roland et al., 2017).

Diabetes: In 2017, the Community Preventive Services Task Force (CPSTF) recommended interventions that engage CHWs to help community members manage their diabetes. CHW interventions improve patients' blood glucose and cholesterol control and reduce their healthcare use. Economic evidence indicates these interventions are cost-effective (The Community Guide, 2015, 2022). The use of digital health devices such as mobile phones and wearable technology for glucose monitoring and management, along with CHW support, can result in better daily self-monitoring of blood glucose (Whitehouse et al., 2022).

Social workers and CHWs: A small number of studies report successful collaborations between CHWs and social workers in chronic disease prevention and care and mental health outcomes, with significant improvements in at least one health outcome (Noel et al., 2022).

Rural health: Studies of CHW interventions in rural populations of the United States show that the interventions focused on chronic conditions, women's health, health education, and links to community resources had positive outcome improvements. Fully one-third of the interventions integrated CHWs into health care teams. The studies showed that CHWs can improve access to care in rural areas and may be a cost-effective investment (Berini, Bonilha, & Simpson, 2022).

HIV/AIDS: CHWs provide valuable links to community resources and services and have successfully helped people get easier access to HIV/AIDS prevention and treatment (Hammack, Bickam, Gilliard, & Robinson, 2021). The stigma and fear associated with HIV infection and mistrust of the healthcare system are reduced by CHWs, who themselves are often members of priority populations. The CDC offers various funding opportunities for "Ending the HIV Epidemic." The initiative is funding innovative activities unique to local communities including peer-to-peer learning and support (CDC, 2019).

COVID-19: The COVID-19 pandemic disproportionately affected communities with social and health inequities. Since 2020, CHWs efforts include identifying and educating high-risk (elderly, immunocompromised, with underlying conditions such as diabetes and asthma) community members, combating fear and distrust, and supporting the use of COVID-19 preventive behavioral practices such as the use of face masks, social distancing, testing, and vaccinations to reduce their exposure to COVID-19. CHWs played an important role in advocating for their communities and linking individuals to public and volunteer networks to address socioeconomic barriers such as food and housing insecurity and mental health issues (Valeriani et al., 2022). Follow-up services provided by CHWs ensured that community members had access to services (St. John, Mayfield-Johnson, & Hernandez-Gordon, 2021).

Practitioners, policy makers, and researchers continue to examine the workforce to help us understand the changing landscape of the CHW world. Research on the work of CHWs is key to making the case for bringing more resources to the field. CHWs continue to play pivotal roles in community health research, exercising a core role of participating in conducting research, for, with, and about the communities they serve. You will learn more about the CHW's role and the skills you need to play a role in conducting research within your community and other communities in which you work in Chapter 23. Durrell Fox observes that CHWs have an important role to play in conducting research; he observed that CHWs have already informed research and public health theories and science for decades (Rosenthal, de Heer, Rush, & Holderby, 2008) and will continue to do so.

How Research Can Influence Policy: CHWs Helping People Control High Blood Pressure. Testimonial from J. Nell Brownstein.

During my work at the Centers for Disease Control and Prevention (CDC), I learned of several research studies focused on CHWs efforts in helping people control high blood pressure (also called hypertension). Uncontrolled high blood pressure is a major risk factor for stroke, heart, and kidney disease. Most of the existing studies were carried out by researchers at Johns Hopkins University. I invited those researchers to join me in writing a paper (Brownstein et al., 2005) in which we summarized the research involving CHW work and made recommendations for future research and practice.

We recommended that CHWs be included in healthcare teams and in community-based research to allow CHWs to play an important role in helping to reduce disparities in heart disease and stroke. We noted that what was needed was sustainable funding and reimbursement for CHW services, better use of CHW skills, improved CHW supervision, training and career development, policy changes, ongoing education, and a reporting of CHW program costs. Since then, other researchers, agencies, program developers, evaluators, practitioners, and other CHW stakeholders have addressed these issues through meetings, reports, and new studies. The CDC provides a variety of CHW policy resources as part of its CHW Toolkit (CDC, 2023).

In 2007, I was the lead author of a team that conducted a systematic literature review of the effectiveness of CHWs in the care of persons with high blood pressure. Our review showed that most of the studies had significant improvements in blood pressure because CHWs helped people keep medical appointments and stay on their prescribed medicines.

This paper influenced the 2010 Institute of the Medicine Report (A Population-Based Approach to Prevent and Control Hypertension) that recommended that the CDC work with state partners to bring about policy and systems changes that result in trained CHWs ". . . deployed in high-risk communities to help support health living strategies that include a focus on hypertension."

(continues)

How Research Can Influence Policy: CHWs Helping People Control High Blood Pressure. Testimonial from J. Nell Brownstein.

(continued)

In 2013, the CDC gave states the opportunity to work on (1) integrating CHWs into health care teams to support self-management and ongoing support for adults with high blood pressure diabetes, (2) having CHWs lead or support diabetes self-management classes, and (3) having CHWs promote linkages between health systems and community resources for adults with high blood pressure and diabetes.

In 2015, the CDC's Community Preventive Task Force released the results of its systematic review of 23 CHW hypertension studies (Centers for Disease Control and Prevention, 2015). It recommends "interventions that engage community health workers to prevent cardiovascular disease (CVD). There is strong evidence of effectiveness for interventions that engage community health workers in a team-based care model to improve blood pressure and cholesterol in patients at increased risk for CVD. There is sufficient evidence of effectiveness for interventions that engage community health workers for health education, and as outreach, enrollment, and information agents to increase self-reported health behaviors (physical activity, healthy eating habits, smoking cessation) in patients at increased risk for CVD."

I developed and supported others to develop resources for CHWs including technical assistance, a heart disease and stroke prevention training, and *fotonovelas* about blood pressure and sodium and cholesterol in English and Spanish.

2.5 CHW Workforce Policy

Since the early 1990s, there have been movements around the nation to build respect, recognition, and a sustainable path for the CHW profession. Many states are developing movements around CHW advocacy, policy, and systems change processes in efforts to develop a vital and sustainable workforce. To better understand these movements, CHW advocate Carl Rush has divided the history of CHW policy into five phases. You can see more about the five phases in our online supplement and an updated version of Phase 5 below provided by Carl H. Rush (Berthold, 2023).

STATE AND FEDERAL INTEREST IN THE CHW PROFESSION (PHASE 5: 2007–PRESENT)

The publication by the U.S. Health Resources and Services Administration (HRSA) of the CHW National Workforce Study launched a period of rapid growth in policy activity in the CHW field. Several trends helped to stimulate interest in policies favorable to CHWs including a new emphasis on health equity, an appreciation of the importance of "social determinants of health," and renewed efforts for health care reform or transformation at the national level, including the establishment of the Patient Protection and Affordable Care Act (ACA). This period also has seen more concerted efforts to integrate CHW positions into ongoing financing of public health and health care, to move away from short term grants and contracts to finance paid CHW positions.

- In 2007, the State of Minnesota submitted a Medicaid State Plan Amendment (SPA) to authorize reimbursement for CHW "self-management education" services to Medicaid recipients. The State specified completion of a standard training curriculum as a requirement for CHWs to be Medicaid "providers." Since that time, nine additional states (as of 2022) have approved SPAs, the most recent covering an increasing range of CHW activities. A number of these took advantage of a 2014 change in Medicaid regulations allowing greater flexibility in paying for preventive services provided by "nonlicensed" individuals (Rush, Higgins, & Wilkniss, 2022).

- In 2009, the Office of Management and Budget published a series of changes to the Standard Occupational Classification, used to classify employment data from employers and the Census. Effective in 2010, the system now includes "community health worker" as a distinct occupation (SOC 21-1094).

- Licensing was ruled out in three states as a means of credentialing CHWs. Licensing boards in New York, Massachusetts, and Virginia all declined to consider licensing of CHWs, finding that there is minimal risk of harm to the public from the work of CHWs.

- During this period, the Centers for Disease Control and Prevention (CDC) dramatically increased their emphasis on the role of CHWs in chronic disease prevention and treatment, funding numerous demonstration projects and the creation of specialty training curricula for CHWs in fields like diabetes and heart disease. The CDC's National Center for Chronic Disease Prevention and Health Promotion included in their strategic priorities encouraging policy and system change to increase employment of CHWs and published several policy briefs and reports related to evidence-based policy. The CDC modified its state chronic disease grants program to create competitive "resilience" grants specifically focused on CHW services, and health disparities grants, which have also been used by states to create infrastructure to support the CHW workforce.

- State legislation calling for task forces to recommend CHW policies was passed in Massachusetts in 2010 (creating a CHW Board of Certification), and rapidly passed in 2014 in New Mexico, Illinois, and Maryland. Many other states created CHW policy initiatives during the period, most of these with active sponsorship and/or participation by state government officials. By mid-2015, almost all states had some form of CHW policy initiative underway.

- Several states have created new policy initiatives involving CHWs, such as Oregon's "Coordinated Care Organizations" and a pilot of Medicaid funding of CHWs in South Carolina (2021–2024). Rhode Island created "Health Equity Zones" and "Community Health Teams" built around CHWs.

- Experience with the COVID-19 pandemic (2020–2022) led more state and federal officials to realize the unique capabilities of CHWs in addressing the needs of low-income and disenfranchised communities. In 2022, the Health Resources and Services Administration (HRSA) awarded $225 million in CHW training grants to 83 organizations.

- Federal interest in CHWs led to the development of numerous committees and work groups:

  - The CDC created an internal CHW Work Group in 2011, which is still active (CDC, 2022).

  - The Office of Minority Health in USDHHS convened a department wide work group in 2022 to develop national strategies for sustainability of the CHW workforce.

  - In 2021, the Office of the Assistant Secretary of Health (OASH) tasked all federal Regional OASH offices to work with states and CHW networks within their region to advance policies for CHWs.

SELF-DETERMINATION BY CHWs

With the recognition CHWs gained in the aftermath of the COVID-19 pandemic, the CHW profession is better positioned to define their own roles and scope of practice. The importance of CHW self-determination continues to be voiced by the CHW workforce and the CHW allies that support CHW practice and policies.

In 2014, the APHA passed a resolution entitled "Support for Community Health Worker Leadership in Determining Workforce Standards for Training and Credentialing" that called for CHWs to be 50 % of participants in all efforts aimed at defining or regulating CHWs (APHA, 2014). Two of the four action steps directly reference this important topic:

- State governments and other entities creating policies regarding CHW training standards and credentialing are urged to engage in collaborative CHW-led efforts with local CHWs and/or CHW professional groups. If CHWs and other entities partner in order to pursue policy development on these topics, a working group of at least 50% self-identified CHWs should be established.

- State governments and any other entity drafting new policy regarding CHW training standards and credentialing are encouraged to establish a governing board composed of at least 50% CHWs. This board should, to the extent possible, minimize barriers to participation and ensure a representation of CHWs that is diverse in terms of language preference, disability status, volunteer vs. paid status, past source of training received, and CHW roles.

CHW CREDENTIALING AND CERTIFICATION

Many health occupations use credentialing in some form, including certification and licensure, in an effort to assure that workers have the knowledge and skills necessary to do their jobs. Credentials may be administered by a public entity, such as a state health department, or by a free-standing organization led by members of the occupation itself, or by another interested organization. Credentialing may directly certify individuals (nurses, social workers, or CHWs) or may credential programs (agencies, clinics, training curriculum, and training institutions). Trainers may also be certified. In some cases, all of these strategies are used.

Credentialing has been a controversial issue in the CHW field (Keane, Nielsen, & Dower, 2004; National Human Services Assembly, 2006; Rosenthal, 1998). Some feel that credentialing will support the ongoing effort to increase recognition and respect for CHWs and to create stable sources of funding for CHW positions. Others question or oppose credentialing because they feel that it may make the field too bureaucratic and weaken the strong ties and allegiance that CHWs have to the community. Others are concerned that it may keep people from being CHWs who otherwise have the necessary commitment, knowledge, and skills. For example, many CHWs have had an experience, such as felony drug convictions, that would disqualify them from receiving a credential if the process is modeled after those of other professions. At the same time, individuals with this background may be the best fit for working with marginalized communities that could fall through the cracks without CHWs who share aspects of their identity and life experience. There are also concerns that credentialing is driven by the norms of other health care professionals rather than a genuine understanding of CHW work and a desire to strengthen the field.

Despite these concerns, it is increasingly common for states to pursue approaches to formally certify CHWs and/or the agencies where they work. Texas was the first state to formally establish a CHW credentialing program in 2001. The credential is coordinated by the Department of Health Services with a committee that includes certified CHWs (Nichols, Berrios, & Samar, 2005). In 2003, Ohio adopted a credentialing program regulated by the state Board of Nursing. Since then, many other states have adopted credentialing programs and others are considering credentialing at various levels, including credentialing individual CHWs, their trainers and/or curricula, and CHW programs.

Many states have started or begun planning for ways to monitor CHWs. In some states, like Florida, a network of CHWs has taken the lead in creating and administering CHW certification, diminishing the role of the state in this process. Other states like Massachusetts are choosing voluntary certification in recognition that certification, in some cases, may prevent qualified people from serving as CHWs. To learn more about what states are doing to establish credentialing and related processes, see the interactive maps from the National Academy for State Health Policy (NASHP, 2021).

FINANCING

A 2014 ruling by the Center for Medicare & Medicaid Services (CMS) allows states to develop payment systems for preventive services by unlicensed individuals, such as CHWs. The ruling improves people's access to preventive services, aids the partnerships between health care providers and CHWs, increases access to CHWs, reduces program costs, and has the potential for CHWs to be reimbursed under Medicaid. States must include a summary of the qualifications of CHWs, their required training, education, experience, and credentialing or registration. Credentialing of CHWs is not required by CMS (CDC, 2015).

The certification, credentialing, and or licensure that many states have pursued has opened the door to this payment stream for CHW services. Many states have authorized reimbursement of CHW services through Medicaid or are in the process of doing so. This reimbursement is done under a State Plan Amendment (SPA) or Section 1115 demonstration authority. According to the National Association of State Health Policymakers (NASHP, 2021), as of 2022, 10 states have reported payment being authorized under the Medicaid state plan and six more or are in the process (NASHP, 2021; Rush, Higgins, & Wilkniss, 2022). Among the most recent to take this step are California, Louisiana, Nevada, and Rhode Island, which implemented their coverage in 2022. Also, according to NASHP, an additional 10 states allow managed care organizations to reimburse for services or hire CHWs directly. The remaining 27 states do not yet reimburse CHW services through Medicaid.

Many other states have been moving toward a reimbursement option and are working to add CHW reimbursement processes in 2023 (Wennerstrom et al., 2023). In Arizona, Medicaid reimbursement is in the process via a State Plan Amendment. The CHW Coalition and AzCHOW have been working with the Arizona Health Care Cost

Containment System (AHCCCS) to ensure input from the CHW workforce. Advancing the process for CHW reimbursement was only possible after the Arizona CHW Voluntary Certification application was opened in late 2022. This policy change was a result of the years of advocacy work that the Arizona CHW Coalition and the Arizona CHW Association continue to conduct.

Since Medicaid is controlled by the states, each state has a different structure to its reimbursement process, based on the advocacy and policy work that CHWs and CHW allies conduct in their states/regions. One state may reimburse for a service that other state may not. Training and certification requirements for CHWs also vary across states; for those states with related policies, CHW certification may be voluntary or mandatory.

2.6 Convening CHWs: Nothing About Us Without Us

ORGANIZATIONS

As the landscape of the CHW profession continues to expand, national organizations are learning how to support and promote the growth and recognition of CHWs. Some of the key national organizations that have been supporting the development of the CHW workforce are listed below. To learn about their work and how they might contribute to your work as a CHW, see the Additional Resources posted at the end of the chapter.

- Centers for Disease Control and Prevention
- Indian Health Service
- National Association of County and City Health Officials
- NASHP: National Academy for State Health Policy
- ASTHO: Association of State and Territorial Health Officials
- Families USA the Voice for Health Care Consumers
- Office of Minority Health

At the state level, the number of dedicated departments and offices to support CHW work is beginning to grow. This is especially common as states establish training and certification requirements. Texas and Massachusetts were among the first to take this step. Find out what resources your state dedicates to supporting CHWs. Reach out locally to find out more; the national organizations noted above can also be a source of inventories of state-level activity, a roadmap for what is happening in your state.

CONFERENCES

Many states and regional associations organize gatherings for the CHW workforce. Some hold regular conferences, meetings, and trainings. For example, the Center for Community Health Alliance in South Carolina organized several states in the southeastern United States and held their first regional Southeast Community Health Worker Network Summit in 2022. In Texas, local CHW networks, coalitions, and alliances have come together to hold the Texas CHW Association Conference, and in Arizona, the Arizona Community Health Workers Association hosts an annual conference. Check with your local CHW association or network to see what conferences are being held in your area.

Beginning in 2000, CHWs from around the United States began meeting under the auspices of the National Center for Sustainable Health Outreach (CSHO), a partnership between Southern Mississippi University ("CSHO south"), and Georgetown University Law School in Washington, D.C. ("CSHO north"). After nearly a decade of collaboration, the CSHO partnership ended, but Dr. Susan Mayfield Johnson continued to coordinate the Unity Conference, bringing together CHWs every one to two years in various cities across the United States. In 2019, the Unity conference was handed over to NACHW and after three virtual conferences during the COVID-19 pandemic, the first in-person, NACHW-organized Unity Conference was held in Austin, Texas, in August 2023.

NETWORKS

CHWs have organized local, state, and national networks out of the belief that they must have a strong voice in shaping the field as it evolves and to provide mutual support, mentoring, and peer learning.

Durrell Fox: In 2001 there was a crisis in public health funding in my state [Massachusetts] that deeply impacted CHWs. We had emergency budget cuts. Our state had new and long-standing outreach and prevention programs with evidence of effectiveness. Some programs that had a full year of funding were notified that funding was cut in half. Some programs were notified on a Wednesday that by Friday they would have no more funding. They had to close and lay off staff, including CHWs. We began to see a pattern where CHWs were the first to go and last to know.

Since some CHWs were already connected through training and networking we got together and said, "We've got to do something" We created the Massachusetts Association of CHWs (MACHW) to build strength, support, independence, and sustainability for CHWs. At the time, CHWs were not paid well, were disenfranchised, and disconnected. We had maternal child health outreach workers, HIV outreach workers Convening CHWs: Networks and Conferences funded by different agencies and not communicating with each other. You could be in a housing development stepping over other outreach workers who might be dealing with some of the same families but had no communication or coordination. This was crazy and inefficient. We didn't have enough resources to have six CHWs serving one family. So MACHW brought CHWs together to learn about what each other was doing and what communities they serve. We began to do strategic planning to help CHWs be more efficient and effective.

MACHW linked up with a couple of training programs, one in Boston (CHEC) and in Worcester (Outreach Worker Training Institute – OWTI in Worcester), and that's where we developed a way to have CHWs coming together from across the state to network, support, and learn from each other.

NATIONAL AND REGIONAL NETWORKS

There are many national groups in the United States that assist in regularly convening CHWs. The names of the groups and their size and capacity have varied with funding and other support over the years, but each group works to provide leadership and opportunities for CHW networking and sharing.

The APHA CHW Section

In 1970, five hundred CHWs and their supporters joined together within the American Public Health Association (APHA) in what was then called the New Professionals Special Primary Interest Group (SPIG). The "new professionals" name was chosen in protest to the many terms used to describe them, including nonprofessional, subprofessional, aide, auxiliary, and paraprofessional (Bellin, Killeen, & Mazeika, 1967; D'Onofrio, 1970; Murphy, 1972). In the year of their formation, the New Professionals wrote:

> For too long, non-degreed health workers have been left out of the mainstream of planning for the delivery of health services and [have] gone without recognition and reward . . . . It is our hope that the National New Professional Health Workers will be able to change the status of workers across the country and thereby improve the health of the nation. (American Public Health Association, 1970)

In the 1980s, membership and activity in the SPIG declined. In the 1990s, the SPIG membership was small, and was held together by longtime CHW member and SPIG leader Ruth Scarborough. At that stage, those working in the field were looking for a way to stay connected and in the early 1990s, we began to rebuild the SPIG. Many CHWs and allies played a role in this effort, and the group grew strong once again. We created a visible niche within APHA for CHWs. Many CHW allies (including the authors of this chapter) and CHWs worked together to build the SPIG. One CHW SPIG leader in the late 1990s Yvonne Lacey pushed for the New Professional SPIG to become the CHW SPIG. A few years later, with another push under the leadership of Sergio Matos and Lisa Renee Holderby-Fox, the CHW SPIG became the CHW Section, which meant we now had a greater number of members and were a bigger part of APHA.

The CHW Section continues to grow and in 2022, the Section once again saw overflowing rooms at its annual APHA meeting. This steady attendance followed several years of virtual and hybrid meetings during the COVID-19 pandemic. With growth of the Section, its committees have become stronger and taken on important tasks of working on issues impacting CHWs both inside and outside APHA.

The National Association of Community Health Representatives

The National Association of Community Health Representatives (NACHR and pronounced "nature") is a network of CHRs and CHR coordinators. It was founded in the 1970s to be the voice of CHRs serving their tribal communities across the United States. The association has twelve service areas and leadership includes representatives from each of these twelve health service regions. They coordinate the activities of NACHR in collaboration with the Indian Health Service (Indian Health Service, 2023; The National Association of Community Health Representatives, 2023). For many years, NACHR held national meetings every three years, when more than 1,000 CHRs gathered to learn about health issues and programs as well as to honor leadership and longevity in the CHR program. Currently, meetings are less frequent, but NACHR regional leaders work together to connect CHRs across the country and some of the twelve regional CHR networks meet regularly to explore issues in their area. CHRs continue to play pivotal leadership roles in many regional and national CHW organizations, serving as board members in state CHW associations and the National Association of CHWs.

The National Association of Hispanic CHWs

The National Association of Hispanic CHWs grew out of the CHW National Network Association, based in Yuma, Arizona, at the regional Western Area Health Education Center. The Association was established in 1992 in Arizona to serve southwestern states; it grew to include people from other regions, including the Midwest and New England, eventually becoming a national network. The annual conference was held primarily in Spanish along with simultaneous translation of selected sessions. In 2007, the organization announced that it would officially focus on Hispanic promotores while maintaining its interest in all CHWs. The association no longer convenes, but its legacy lives on with many promotores now actively networking at the state level and participating in national meetings on behalf of CHWs.

The American Association of CHWs

CHWs and allies came together in 2006 to explore development of a national CHW leadership organization or association. The CSHO (noted above) staff played an important role in supporting this strategic network development meeting and Unity meetings provided an important networking forum before and after this key meeting. The meeting led to the development of the American Association of Community Health Workers (AACHWs). Though the Network's efforts were not sustained in the long term, many important lessons can be learned to inform future efforts to develop or restart other regional and national networks. The group left the legacy of a Code of Ethics that it established (see Chapter 5). Over its few years of collaboration, the association focused on organizing issues generally and around providing support for regional and national efforts to promote CHW sustainability.

To learn more about AACHW, read the thoughts of two CHWs, Durrell Fox and Sergio Matos, posted to the Wiley website and referenced in Additional Resources at the end of the chapter.

The National Association of CHWs

A much-anticipated organization for the CHW field was finally formally announced in 2019. Many efforts to build a national CHW network served as the foundation for the National Association of Community Health Workers (NACHW) through which CHW leaders can now collaborate to develop the field. It has become an important convening organization for CHW networks, large and small, across the country, and provides a welcome place for the development of CHW workforce policy. It also provides a resource for CHWs to influence policies that impact the many communities they serve. See more about NACHW in Chapter 1 and be sure to visit their website (NACHW, 2023) to learn more and consider becoming an individual and/or network member.

- Forming this vital organization took several years of planning and organizing by national CHW leaders and allies from across the United States. Founding board members of NACHW include Mae-Gilene Begay, Durrell Fox, Floribella Redondo-Martinez, Lisa Renee Holderby-Fox, Wandy Hernandez-Gordon, Catherine Haywood, Julie Smithwick, Naomi Cottoms, Maria Lemus, Ashley Wennerstrom, Gail Hirsh, Geoffrey Wilkinson, Susan Johnson, Carl Rush, Napualani Spock, Sergio Matos, and Anita McDonnell.
- The mission-vision of the national CHW association is *to unify the voices of the community health workers and strengthen the profession's capacity to promote healthy communities.*

Regional and State Networks

By joining together in regional, state, and national networks and associations, CHWs are taking leadership in the development of the field, defining their roles, establishing new standards, research priorities, educational and training models, and advocating for greater recognition and increased funding to support the valuable contributions of CHWs. Visit the NACHW website to help you find local, regional, and national networks and associations (NACHW, 2023).

If you cannot find a regional or state CHW association on the NACHW website, reach out to other colleagues to be sure there is not a newly forming one or a longstanding one in need of your energy and input.

If you identify that there is a gap and that there is no network of CHWs in your area, think of it as an opportunity for you, and your colleagues to start one!

Chapter Review

Review your understanding of the key information and concepts addressed in Chapter 2 by answering the following questions:

1. Why is it so hard to develop a common definition of CHWs and CHW roles and competencies? How could a common definition of roles and competencies benefit the CHW field?

2. What has been the role of CHW leaders in defining and developing the CHW field?

3. Why is academic research about CHWs important to developing the CHW field? What are the research priorities for the CHW field?

4. How are developments in CHW training, education, reimbursement, and credentialing shaping the CHW field? Why are these developments controversial?

5. What does the phrase "Nothing about us without us" mean to the CHW profession, and why is it so significant?

6. How do CHW networks develop and why are they important to the future of CHWs in the United States?

7. Are there CHW networks in your city, county, or state? How can you get involved?

References

Adams, L. B., Richmond, J., Watson, S. N., Cené, C. W., Urrutia, R., Ataga, O., Dunlap, P., & Corbie-Smith, G. (2021). Community health worker training curricula and intervention outcomes in african american and latinx communities: a systematic review. *Health Education & Behavior*, 48(4), 516–531. https://doi.org/10.1177/1090198120959326.

Aguirre, A. (Director). (1997). El Rio Colorado Border Vision.

Allen, J. K., Dennison Himmelfarb, C. R., Szanton, S. L., & Frick, K. D. (2014). Cost-effectiveness of nurse practitioner/community health worker care to reduce cardiovascular health . *The Journal of Cardiovascular Nursing*, 29(4), 308–314. https://doi.org/10.1097/JCN.0b013e3182945243.

American Diabetes Association. (2020, May 9). Diabetes Core Update: COVID-19—The Role of Community Health Workers as First Responders|American Diabetes Association. American Diabetes Association. https://professional.diabetes.org/podcast/diabetes-core-update-covid-19-role-community-health-workers-first-responders.

American Public Health Association. (1970). *Meeting minutes: New professionals special primary interest group.* American Public Health Association.

American Public Health Association. (2001). *Recognition and support for community health workers' contributions to meeting our nation's health care needs*. American Public Health Association. https://www.apha.org/policies-and-advocacy/public-health-policy-statements/policy-database/2014/07/15/13/24/recognition-and-support-community-health-workers-contrib-to-meeting-our-nations-health-care-needs.

American Public Health Association. (2009, November 10). *Support for community health workers to increase health access and to reduce health inequities*. American Public Health Association. https://www.apha.org/policies-and-advocacy/public-health-policy-statements/policy-database/2014/07/09/14/19/support-for-community-health-workers-to-increase-health-access-and-to-reduce-health-inequities.

American Public Health Association. (2014, November 18). *Support for Community Health Worker Leadership in Determining Workforce Standards for Training and Credentialing*. American Public Health Association. https://www.apha.org/policies-and-advocacy/public-health-policy-statements/policy-database/2015/01/28/14/15/support-for-community-health-worker-leadership.

American Public Health Association. (2022). *A Strategy to Address Systemic Racism and Violence as Public Health Priorities: Training and Supporting Community Health Workers to Advance Equity and Violence Prevention 20227*. American Public Health Association. https://www.apha.org/Policies-and-Advocacy/Public-Health-Policy-Statements/Policy-Database/2023/01/18/Address-Systemic-Racism-and-Violence

Bellin, L. E., Killeen, M., & Mazeika, J. J. (1967). Preparing public health subprofessionals recruited from the poverty group—Lessons from an OEO work-study program. *American Journal of Public Health and the Nations Health*, 57(2), 242–252. https://doi.org/10.2105/AJPH.57.2.242.

Berini, C. R., Bonilha, H. S., & Simpson, A. N. (2022). Impact of community health workers on access to care for rural populations in the United States: A systematic review. *Journal of Community Health*, 47(3), 539–553. https://doi.org/10.1007/s10900-021-01052-6.

Berthold, T. (2024). *Foundations for community health workers. Supplemental resources*. Wiley.

Booker, V., Grube-Robinson, J., Kay, B., Najjera, L. G., & Stewart, G. (2004). *Camp Health Aide Program Overview*. Migrant Health Promotion.

Brandeis University. (2003). Evidence Report and Evidence-Based Recommendations: Cancer Prevention and Treatment Demonstration for Ethnic and Racial Minorities. https://www.cms.gov/files/document/cptdbrandeisreportpdf (accessed 29 December 2023).

Brown, T. M. & Fee, E. (2002). Sidney Kark and John Cassel: Social Medicine Pioneers and South African Emigrés. *American Journal of Public Health*, 92(11), 1744–1745. https://doi.org/10.2105/AJPH.92.11.1744.

Brownstein, J. N., Bone, L. R., Dennison, C. R., Hill, M. N., Kim, M. T., & Levine, D. M. (2005). Community health workers as interventionists in the prevention and control of heart disease and stroke. *American Journal of Preventive Medicine*, 29(5 Suppl 1), 128–133. https://doi.org/10.1016/j.amepre.2005.07.024.

Brownstein, J. N., Chowdhury, F. M., Norris, S. L., Horsley, T., Jack, L., Zhang, X., & Satterfield, D. (2007). Effectiveness of community health workers in the care of people with hypertension. *American Journal of Preventive Medicine*, 32(5), 435–447. https://doi.org/10.1016/j.amepre.2007.01.011.

Brownstein, J. N., Hirsch, G. R., Rosenthal, E. L., & Rush, C. H. (2011). Community health workers "101" for primary care providers and other stakeholders in health care systems. *The Journal of Ambulatory Care Management*, 34(3), 210–220. https://doi.org/10.1097/JAC.0b013e31821c645d.

Byrd-Williams, C., Ewing, M., Rosenthal, E. L., St. John, J. A., Menking, P., Redondo, F., & Sieswerda, S. (2021). Training needs of community health workers facing the COVID-19 pandemic in Texas: a cross-sectional study. *Frontiers in Public Health*, 9, 689946. https://doi.org/10.3389/fpubh.2021.689946.

Centers for Disease Control and Prevention. (2015). *Addressing chronic disease through community health workers: A policy and systems-level approach*. Centers for Disease Control and Prevention. https://www.cdc.gov/dhdsp/docs/chw_brief.pdf.

Centers for Disease Control and Prevention. (2018). *How the Centers for Disease Control and Prevention (CDC) supports community health workers in chronic disease prevention and health promotion*. Centers for Disease Control and Prevention. https://www.cdc.gov/dhdsp/programs/spha/docs/chw_summary.pdf.

Centers for Disease Control and Prevention. (2019). Strengthening the Nation's HIV Prevention Workforce: Capacity Building Assistance for High-Impact HIV Prevention. https://www.cdc.gov/hiv/funding/announcements/ps19-1904/executive-summary.html.

Centers for Disease Control and Prevention. (2022). The Role of Community Health Workers in Addressing Food and Nutrition Security and Social Support During the COVID-19 Pandemic. https://stacks.cdc.gov/view/cdc/122282.

Centers for Disease Control and Prevention. (2023). *Community Health Worker (CHW) Toolkit*. Centers for Disease Control and Prevention. https://www.cdc.gov/dhdsp/pubs/toolkits/chw-toolkit.htm.

CHW Initiatives of Sonoma County. (2015). CHW job titles. CHW Initiative of Sonoma County. Retrieved from https://chwisc.org/job-titles (accessed 30 April 2023).

Community Health Worker Core Consensus (C3) Project (2018). https://www.c3project.org/

D'Onofrio, C. N. (1970). Aides—Pain or panacea? *Public Health Reports*, 85(9), 788–801. https://www.ncbi.nlm.nih.gov/pmc/articles/PMC2031769/.

Domke, H. R. (1966). Project planning and development by official health agencies. 3. The neighborhood-based public health worker: Additional manpower for community health services. *American Journal of Public Health and the Nations Health*, 56(4), 603–608. https://doi.org/10.2105/AJPH.56.4.603.

Eng, E. & Young, R. (1992). Lay health advisors as community change agents. *Family & Community Health: The Journal of Health Promotion & Maintenance*, 15, 24–40. https://doi.org/10.1097/00003727-199204000-00005.

Federation of State Medical Boards. (2005). Assessing Scope of Practice in Health Care Delivry: Critical Questions in Assuring Public Access and Safety. https://www.fsmb.org/ (accessed 26 December 2023).

Findley, S., Matos, S., Hicks, A., Chang, J., & Reich, D. (2014). Community health worker integration into the health care team accomplishes the triple aim in a patient-centered medical home: A Bronx tale. *The Journal of Ambulatory Care Management*, 37(1), 82–91. https://doi.org/10.1097/JAC.0000000000000011.

Foundation for Health Generation. (2013). *Community health white paper: Report and recommendations*. Foundation for Health Generation.

George, S., Silva, L., Llamas, M., Ramos, I., Joe, J., Mendez, J., . . ., Balcazar, H. (2021). The development of a novel, standards-based core curriculum for community facing, clinic-based community health workers. *Frontiers in Public Health*, 9. https://www.frontiersin.org/articles/10.3389/fpubh.2021.663492.

Giblin, P. T. (1989). Effective utilization and evaluation of indigenous health care workers. *Public Health Reports*, 104(4), 361–368. https://www.ncbi.nlm.nih.gov/pmc/articles/PMC1579943/.

Gilkey, M., Garcia, C. C., & Rush, C. (2011). Professionalization and the experience-based expert: Strengthening partnerships between health educators and community health workers. *Health Promotion Practice*, 12(2), 178–182. https://doi.org/10.1177/1524839910394175.

Goldfield, N. I., Crittenden, R., Fox, D., McDonough, J., Nichols, L., & Lee Rosenthal, E. (2020). COVID-19 crisis creates opportunities for community-centered population health: Community health workers at the center. *Journal of Ambulatory Care Management*, 43(3), 184–190. https://doi.org/10.1097/JAC.0000000000000337.

Gonzalez A. L., Ortiz, L.(2004). Neighborhood and Community Organizing in Colonias: A Case Study in the Development and Use of Promotoras. *Journal of Community Practice* 12(1/2): 23–35. https://doi.org/10.1300/J125v12n01_03

Gould, J. M. & Lomax, A. R. (1993). The evolution of peer education: Where do we go from here? *Journal of American College Health: J of ACH*, 41(6), 235–240. https://doi.org/10.1080/07448481.1993.9936333.

Hammack, A. Y., Bickham, J. N., Gilliard, I., & Robinson, W. T. (2021). A community health worker approach for ending the HIV epidemic. *American Journal of Preventive Medicine*, 61(5), S26–S31. https://doi.org/10.1016/j.amepre.2021.06.008.

Harlan, C., Eng, E., & Watkins, E. (1992, May 10). Migrant lay health advisors: A strategy for health promotion. Third International Symposium: Issues in Health, Safety and Agriculture, Saskatchewan, Canada.

Hoff, W. (1969). Role of the community health aide in public health programs. *Public Health Reports*, 84(11), 998–1002. https://www.ncbi.nlm.nih.gov/pmc/articles/PMC2031701/.

HRSA. (2007). *Community Health Worker National Workforce Study.* U.S. Department of Health and Human Services Health Resources and Services Administration Bureau of Health Professions. https://bhw.hrsa.gov/sites/default/files/bureau-health-workforce/data-research/community-health-workforce.pdf.

HRSA. (2022). FY 2022 community health worker training awards|Bureau of Health Workforce. HRSA. https://bhw.hrsa.gov/funding/community-health-worker-training-fy2022-awards.

Indian Health Services. (2023). Community Health Representative|Indian Health Service (IHS). Community Health Representative. Retrieved from https://www.ihs.gov/chr/ (accessed April 28, 2023).

Institute of Medicine (US) Committee on Understanding and Eliminating Racial and Ethnic Disparities in Health Care. (2003). *Unequal treatment: Confronting racial and ethnic disparities in health care.* . In B. D. Smedley, A. Y. Stith, & A. R. Nelson (Eds.), https://nap.nationalacademies.org/catalog/12875/unequal-treatment-confronting-racial-and-ethnic-disparities-in-health-care. (accessed 29 December 2023).

Jennings, W. (1990, October). *Barriers to employment for public health assistance recipients.* New York: American Public Health Association.

Julnes, G., Konefal, M., Pindur, W., & Kim, P. (1994). Community-based perinatal care for disadvantaged adolescents: Evaluation of The Resource Mothers Program. *Journal of Community Health,* 19(1), 41–53. https://doi.org/10.1007/BF02260520.

Kangovi, S. (2020). *Want to help battle COVID-19? Bring in more community health workers.* AAMC. https://www.aamc.org/news-insights/want-help-battle-covid-19-bring-more-community-health-workers.

Kangovi, S., Mitra, N., Norton, L., Harte, R., Zhao, X., Carter, T., Grande, D., & Long, J. A. (2018). Effect of community health worker support on clinical outcomes of low-income patients across primary care facilities: A randomized clinical trial. *JAMA Internal Medicine,* 178(12), 1635–1643. https://doi.org/10.1001/jamainternmed.2018.4630.

Keane, D., Nielsen, C., & Dower, C. (2004). *Community health workers and promotores in California.* San Francisco: The Center for the Health Professions; University of California. https://healthforce.ucsf.edu/sites/healthforce.ucsf.edu/files/publication-pdf/3.1%20%28issue%20brief%29%202004-09_Community_Health_Workers_and_Promotores_in_California.pdf.

Klitzman, R. (1997). *Being positive: The lives of men and women with HIV* (1st edition). Ivan R. Dee.

Larson, K., McGuire, J., Watkins, E., & Mountain, K. (1992). Maternal care coordination for migrant farmworker women: Program structure and evaluation of effects on use of prenatal care and birth outcome. *The Journal of Rural Health: Official Journal of the American Rural Health Association and the National Rural Health Care Association,* 8(2), 128–133. https://doi.org/10.1111/j.1748-0361.1992.tb00338.x.

Lee, L. K., Ruano, E., Fernández, P., Ortega, S., Lucas, C., & Joachim-Célestin, M. (2021). Workforce readiness training: A comprehensive training model that equips community health workers to work at the top of their practice and profession. *Frontiers in Public Health,* 9, 673208. https://doi.org/10.3389/fpubh.2021.673208.

Love, M. B., Gardner, K., & Legion, V. (1997). Community health workers: Who they are and what they do. *Health Education & Behavior: The Official Publication of the Society for Public Health Education,* 24(4), 510–522. https://doi.org/10.1177/109019819702400409.

Love, M. B., Legion, V., Shim, J. K., Tsai, C., Quijano, V., & Davis, C. (2004). CHWs get credit: A 10-year history of the first college-credit certificate for community health workers in the United States. *Health Promotion Practice,* 5(4), 418–428. https://doi.org/10.1177/1524839903260142.

Maathai, W. (2007). *Unbowed: A Memoir* (Reprint edition). Anchor.

Mahler, H. (1978). Promotion of primary health care in member countries of WHO. *Public Health Reports,* 93(2), 107–113. https://www.ncbi.nlm.nih.gov/pmc/articles/PMC1431881/.

Margellos-Anast, H., Gutierrez, M. A., & Whitman, S. (2012). Improving asthma management among African-American children via a community health worker model: Findings from a Chicago-based pilot intervention. *The Journal of Asthma: Official Journal of the Association for the Care of Asthma,* 49(4), 380–389. https://doi.org/10.3109/02770903.2012.660295.

Martinez, J., Ro, M., Villa, N.W., Powell, W., & Knickman, J.R. (2011). Transforming the delivery of care in the post-health reform era: what role will community health workers play? *American Journal of Public Health*, 101(12), e1–5. https://doi.org/10.2105/AJPH.2011.300335. Epub 2011 Oct 20. PMID: 22021289; PMCID: PMC3222444.

Massachusetts Department of Public Health. (2009). *Community health workers in Massachusetts: Improving health care and public health: report*. Massachusetts Department of Public Health. https://archives.lib.state.ma.us/handle/2452/49271.

Massachusetts Department of Public Health, Community Health Worker Advisory Council. (2009). Community Health Workers in Massachusetts: Improving Health Care and Public Health. https://www.mass.gov/community-health-workers (accessed 29 December 2023).

Matos, S., Findley, S., Hicks, A., Legendre, Y., & Do Canto, L. (2011). *Paving a path to advance the community health worker workforce in New York State: A new summary report and recommendations*. The New York State Community Health Worker Initiative.

Mayfield-Johnson, S., Smith, D. O., Crosby, S. A., Haywood, C. G., Castillo, J., Bryant-Williams, D., . . ., Wennerstrom, A. (2020). Insights on COVID-19 from community health worker state leaders. *The Journal of Ambulatory Care Management*, 43(4), 268–277. https://doi.org/10.1097/JAC.0000000000000351.

McFarlane, J. & Fehir, J. (1994). De Madres a Madres: A community, primary health care program based on empowerment. *Health Education Quarterly*, 21(3), 381–394. https://doi.org/10.1177/109019819402100309.

Meister, J. S. (1997). Community outreach and community mobilization: Options for health at the U.S.-Mexico border. *Journal of Border Health*, 2(4), 32–38.

Meister, J. S., Warrick, L. H., de Zapién, J. G., & Wood, A. H. (1992). Using lay health workers: Case study of a community-based prenatal intervention. *Journal of Community Health*, 17(1), 37–51. https://doi.org/10.1007/BF01321723.

Miller, P., Bates, T., & Katzen, A. (2014). *Community health worker credentialing: state approaches*. Center for Health Law and Policy Innovation, Harvard Law School. https://chlpi.org/wp-content/uploads/2014/06/CHW-Credentialing-Paper.pdf (accessed 29 December 2023).

Mohatt, G. & Elk, J. E. (2002). *The price of a gift: A Lakota Healer's story*. U of Nebraska Press.

Moir, S., Yamauchi, J., Hartz, C., Kuhaulua, R., Kelen, M., Allison, A., Kishaba, G., & Vocalan, C. (2021). The critical role Hawai'i's community health workers are playing in COVID-19 response efforts. *Hawai'i Journal of Health & Social Welfare*, 80(10 Suppl 2), 46–49. https://www.ncbi.nlm.nih.gov/pmc/articles/PMC8538113/.

Murphy, M. A. (1972). Improvement of community health services through the support of indigenous nonprofessional. *New York State Nurses Association*, 3, 29–33.

NACHC. (2010). *Community health centers lead the primary care revolution*. National Association of Community Health Centers. http://www.nachc.org/wp-content/uploads/2015/06/Primary_Care_Revolution_Final_8_16.pdf.

NACHW. (2023). *The six pillars of community health workers*. National Association of Community Health Workers. https://nachw.org/the-six-pillars-of-community-health-workers/.

NASHP. (2021, December 11). State Community Health Worker Models. https://nashp.org/state-community-health-worker-models/.

National Human Services Assembly. (2006). *Community health workers: Closing the gap on family's health resources*. Family Strengthening Policy Center.

Nawaz, S., Moon, K. J., Vazquez, R., Navarrete, J. R., Trinh, A., Escobedo, L., & Montiel, G. I. (2023). Evaluation of the community health worker model for COVID-19 response and recovery. *Journal of Community Health*. https://doi.org/10.1007/s10900-022-01183-4.

Nemcek, M. A. & Sabatier, R. (2003). State of evaluation: Community health workers. *Public Health Nursing (Boston, Mass.)*, 20(4), 260–270. https://doi.org/10.1046/j.1525-1446.2003.20403.x.

Nicholls, K., Picou, S. J., & McCord, S. C. (2017). Training community health workers to enhance disaster resilience. *Journal of Public Health Management and Practice*, 23, S78–S84. https://www.jstor.org/stable/48516966.

Nichols, D., Berrios, C., & Samar, H. (2005). Texas' community health workforce: From state health promotion policy to community-level practice. *Preventing Chronic Disease*. https://www.cdc.gov/pcd/issues/2005/nov/05_0059.htm.

Nielsen, V. M., Ursprung, W. W. S., Song, G., Hirsch, G., Mason, T., Santarelli, C., . . ., Behl-Chadha, B. (2023). Evaluating the impact of community health worker certification in Massachusetts: Design, methods, and anticipated results of the Massachusetts community health worker workforce survey. *Frontiers in Public Health*, 10. https://www.frontiersin.org/articles/10.3389/fpubh.2022.1043668.

Noel, L., Chen, Q., Petruzzi, L. J., Phillips, F., Garay, R., Valdez, C., Aranda, M. P., & Jones, B. (2022). Interprofessional collaboration between social workers and community health workers to address health and mental health in the United States: A systematised review. *Health & Social Care in the Community*, 30(6), e6240–e6254. https://doi.org/10.1111/hsc.14061.

Norris, S. L., Chowdhury, F. M., Van Le, K., Horsley, T., Brownstein, J. N., Zhang, X., Jack, L., & Satterfield, D. W. (2006). Effectiveness of community health workers in the care of persons with diabetes. *Diabetic Medicine: A Journal of the British Diabetic Association*, 23(5), 544–556. https://doi.org/10.1111/j.1464-5491.2006.01845.x.

Northwest Regional Primary Care Association. (2015). *Celebrating 50+ years in the American Community Health Center Movement—Northwest Regional Primary Care Association*. Northwest Regional Primary Care Association. https://www.nwrpca.org/page/chc50th_anniversary.

O'Brien, M. J., Squires, A. P., Bixby, R. A., & Larson, S. C. (2009). Role development of community health workers: An examination of selection and training processes in the intervention literature. *American Journal of Preventive Medicine*, 37(6 Suppl 1), S262–S269. https://doi.org/10.1016/j.amepre.2009.08.011.

Pearl, A., & Riessmann, F. (1965). *New careers for the poor: Nonprofessionals in human service*. New York, NY: Free Press.

Peretz, P. J., Islam, N., & Matiz, L. A. (2020). Community health workers and Covid-19—Addressing social determinants of health in times of crisis and beyond. *New England Journal of Medicine*, 383(19), e108. https://doi.org/10.1056/NEJMp2022641.

Poland, M. L., Giblin, P. T., Waller, J. B., & Hankin, J. (1992). Effects of a home visiting program on prenatal care and birthweight: A case comparison study. *Journal of Community Health*, 17(4), 221–229. https://doi.org/10.1007/BF01321654.

Potts, D. & Miller, C. (1964). The community health aide. *Nursing Outlook*. https://oa.mg/work/2397314022

Powell, T. & Yuma-Guerrero, P. (2016). Supporting community health workers after a disaster: Findings from a mixed-methods pilot evaluation study of a psychoeducational intervention. *Disaster Medicine and Public Health Preparedness*, 10(5), 754–761. https://doi.org/10.1017/dmp.2016.40.

Prezio, E. A., Pagán, J. A., Shuval, K., & Culica, D. (2014). The Community Diabetes Education (CoDE) program: Cost-effectiveness and health outcomes. *American Journal of Preventive Medicine*, 47(6), 771–779. https://doi.org/10.1016/j.amepre.2014.08.016.

Proulx, D. E. (2000a). Arizona's project jump start: A community college/AHEC Partnership. *National AHEC Bulletin*, 17.

Proulx, D. E. (2000b). Project jump start: A community college and AHEC partnership initiative for community health worker education. *Texas Journal of Rural Health*, 18(3), 6–16.

Proulx, D. E., Rosenthal, E. L., Fox, D., Lacey, Y., & Community Health Worker National Education Collaborative Contributors. (2008). *Key considerations for opening doors: Developing community health worker educational programs*. University of Arizona.

Pynoos, J., Hade-Kaplan, B., & Fleisher, D. (1984). Intergenerational neighborhood networks: A basis for aiding the frail elderly. *The Gerontologist*, 24, 233–237. https://doi.org/10.1093/geront/24.3.233.

Rahman, R., Ross, A., & Pinto, R. (2021). The critical importance of community health workers as first responders to COVID-19 in USA. *Health Promotion International*, 36(5), 1498–1507. https://doi.org/10.1093/heapro/daab008.

Ramalingam, N. S., Strayer, T. E. I., Breig, S. A., & Harden, S. M. (2019). How are community health workers trained to deliver physical activity to adults? A scoping review *Translational Journal of the ACSM*. https://journals.lww.com/acsm-tj/Fulltext/2019/03150/How_Are_Community_Health_Workers_Trained_to.1.aspx.

Responses to Comments on 2010 SOC: U.S. Bureau of Labor Statistics. (2009). U.S. Bureau of Labor Statistics. April 28, 2023. Retrieved from https://www.bls.gov/soc/soc2010responses.htm.

Reyes-Ortiz, C. A., Rodriguez, M., & Markides, K. S. (2009). The role of spirituality healing with perceptions of the medical encounter among Latinos. *Journal of General Internal Medicine*, 24(Suppl 3), 542–547. https://doi.org/10.1007/s11606-009-1067-9.

Rico, C. (1997). *Community health advisors: Emerging opportunities in managed care.* Annie E. Casey Foundation and Seedco—Partnerships for Community Development.

Rodela, K., Wiggins, N., Maes, K., Campos-Dominguez, T., Adewumi, V., Jewell, P., & Mayfield-Johnson, S. (2021). The community health worker (CHW) common indicators project: Engaging CHWs in measurement to sustain the profession. *Frontiers in Public Health*, 9. https://www.frontiersin.org/articles/10.3389/fpubh.2021.674858.

Rodriguez, B., Saunders, M., Octavia-Smith, D., Moeti, R., Ballard, A., Pellechia, K., Fragueiro, D., & Salinger, S. (2023). Community health workers during COVID-19: supporting their role in current and future public health responses. *Journal of Ambulatory Care Management*, 203–209. https://doi.org/10.1097/JAC.0000000000000466.

Roland, K. B., Milliken, E. L., Rohan, E. A., DeGroff, A., White, S., Melillo, S., . . ., Young, P. A. (2017). Use of community health workers and patient navigators to improve cancer outcomes among patients served by federally qualified health centers: A systematic literature review. *Health Equity*, 1(1), 61–76. https://doi.org/10.1089/heq.2017.0001.

Rosenthal, E. L. (1998). *A Summary of the National Community Health Advisor Study.* University of Arizona and Annie E Casey Foundation. https://crh.arizona.edu/sites/default/files/2022-04/CAHsummaryALL.pdf.

Rosenthal, E. L. (2003). The sustainability dance: Lessons to learn for an emerging force in community health [Doctoral Dissertation].

Rosenthal, E. L. & Macinko, J. (2011). JACM special issue on community health workers and community health worker practice. *The Journal of Ambulatory Care Management*, 34(3), 208–209. https://doi.org/10.1097/JAC.0b013e31821c6438.

Rosenthal, E. L., Wiggins, N., Brownstein, J. N., Johnson, S., Borbon, A., Rael, R., . . ., Blondet, L. (1998). *The final report of the national community health advisor study: Weaving the future.* University of Arizona and Annie E. Casey Foundation.

Rosenthal, E. L., de Heer, H., Rush, C. H., & Holderby, L.-R. (2008). Focus on the future: A community health worker research agenda by and for the field. *Progress in Community Health Partnerships: Research, Education, and Action*, 2(3), 183–184, 225–235. https://doi.org/10.1353/cpr.0.0025.

Rosenthal, E. L., Wiggins, N., Ingram, M., Mayfield-Johnson, S., & De Zapien, J. G. (2011). Community health workers then and now: An overview of national studies aimed at defining the field. *The Journal of Ambulatory Care Management*, 34(3), 247–259. https://doi.org/10.1097/JAC.0b013e31821c64d7.

Rosenthal, E. L., Menking, P., St. John, J., Fox, D., Holderby-Fox, L.-R., Redondo, F., . . ., Rush, C. (2014, 2023). CHW Core Consensus Project. https://www.c3project.org.

Rosenthal, E. L., Menking, P., & St. John, J. (2018). The Community Health Worker Core Consensus (C3) Project: A Report of the C3 Project Phase 1 and 2, Together Leaning Toward the Sky, A National Project to Inform CHW Policy and Practice. Texas Tech University Health Sciences Center. www.c3project.org

Rosenthal, E. L., Menking, P., & Begay, M.-G. (2020). Fighting the COVID-19 merciless monster: Lives on the line—Community health representatives' roles in the pandemic battle on the Navajo Nation. *Journal of Ambulatory Care Management*, 43(4), 301–305. https://doi.org/10.1097/JAC.0000000000000354.

Rothpletz-Puglia, P. (2013). Building social networks for health promotion: Shout-out health, New Jersey, 2011. *Preventing Chronic Disease*, 10. https://doi.org/10.5888/pcd10.130018.

Rush, C., Higgins, E., & Wilkniss, S. (2022, December 8). *State approaches to community health worker financing through Medicaid State Plan Amendments*. NASHP. https://nashp.org/state-approaches-to-community-health-worker-financing-through-medicaid-state-plan-amendments/.

Sainer, E. A., Ruiz, P., & Wilder, J. F. (1975). Career escalation training. Five-year follow-up. *American Journal of Public Health*, 65(11), 1208–1211. https://doi.org/10.2105/AJPH.65.11.1208.

Salber, E. J. (1979). The lay advisor as a community health resource. *Journal of Health Politics, Policy and Law*, 3(4), 469–478. https://doi.org/10.1215/03616878-3-4-469.

Satterfield, D., Burd, C., Valdez, L., Hosey, G., & Shield, J. E. (2002). The "in-between people": Participation of community health representatives in diabetes prevention and care in American Indian and Alaska Native Communities. *Health Promotion Practice*, 3(2), 166–175. https://doi.org/10.1177/152483990200300212.

Service, C., Salber, E. J., & Duke University Community Health Education Program. (1977). *Community health education: The lay advisor approach*. In Connie Service and E. J. Salber (Eds.), *Community Health Education Program*, Dept. of Community and Family Medicine, Duke University Medical Center.

Smedley, B., Stith, A., & Nelson, A. (2003). *Unequal treatment: What healthcare providers need to know about racial and ethnic disparities in healthcare*. Washington, DC: Institute of Medicine, Committee on Understanding and Eliminating Racial and Ethnic Disparities in Health Care.

Smith, D. (2022, May 24). NACHW Letter to HRSA Regarding, pp. 22–124. https://nachw.org/wp-content/uploads/2022/05/NACHW-Letter-to-HRSA-Regarding-22-124-May-24-2022.pdf.

Smith, D. O. & Wennerstrom, A. (2020). To Strengthen the Public Health Response to COVID-19, We Need Community Health Workers. *Health Affairs Forefront*. https://doi.org/10.1377/forefront.20200504.336184.

Spiro, A., Oo, S. A., Marable, D., & Collins, J. P. (2012). A unique model of the community health worker: The MGH Chelsea Community Health Improvement team. *Family & Community Health*, 35(2), 147–160. https://doi.org/10.1097/FCH.0b013e3182465187.

Springgate, B., Wennerstrom, A., & Carriere, C. (2011). Capacity building for post-disaster mental health since Katrina: The role of community health workers. *The Review of Black Political Economy*, 38(4), 363–368. https://doi.org/10.1007/s12114-010-9083-x.

St. John, J. A., Mayfield-Johnson, S. L., & Hernandez-Gordon, W. D. (Eds.). (2021). Promoting the Health of the Community. https://link.springer.com/book/10.1007/978-3-030-56375-2.

Stanford University. (2023). Black Panther Party Research Project. Stanford University. https://www.bpp55stanford.com/ (accessed 29 December 2023).

Swider, S. M. (2002). Outcome effectiveness of community health workers: An integrative literature review. *Public Health Nursing (Boston, Mass.)*, 19(1), 11–20. https://doi.org/10.1046/j.1525-1446.2002.19003.x.

Tang, T. S., Funnell, M. Sinco, B., Platt, G., Palmisano, G., Spencer, M. S., Kieffer, E. C., & Heisler, M. (2014). Comparative effectiveness of peer leaders and community health workers in diabetes self-management support: results of a randomized controlled trial. *Diabetes Care*, 1525–1534. https://doi.org/10.2337/dc13-2161.

The Community Guide. (2015). HDSP: Community Health Workers|The Community Guide. The Community Guide. https://www.thecommunityguide.org/findings/heart-disease-stroke-prevention-interventions-engaging-community-health-workers.html.

The Community Guide. (2022, October 18). Engaging Community Health Workers Recommended to Prevent Cardiovascular Disease|The Community Guide. The Community Guide. https://www.thecommunityguide.org/news/engaging-community-health-workers-recommended-prevent-cardiovascular-disease.html.

The Community Health Worker Core Consensus Project. (2023). C3 Project Findings: Roles & Competencies. https://www.c3project.org/roles-competencies. (accessed 26 December 2023).

The Guide to Community Preventive Services. (2015). Cardiovascular Disease Prevention and Control: Evidence-Based Interventions for Your Community. The Centers for Disease Control and Prevention. https://www.cdc.gov/dhdsp/pubs/docs/cpstf-what-works-factsheet.pdf (accessed 29 December 2023).

The National Association of Community Health Representatives. (2023).

U.S. Department of Labor: Apprenticeship. (2023, April 30). DOL. Retrieved from http://www.dol.gov/agencies/eta/apprenticeship.

Valeriani, G., Sarajlic Vukovic, I., Bersani, F. S., Sadeghzadeh Diman, A., Ghorbani, A., & Mollica, R. (2022). Tackling ethnic health disparities through community health worker programs: A scoping review on their utilization during the COVID-19 outbreak. *Population Health Management*, 25(4), 517–526. https://doi.org/10.1089/pop.2021.0364.

Viswanathan, M., Kraschnewski, J., Nishikawa, B., Morgan, L. C., Thieda, P., Honeycutt, A., . . ., RTI International-University of North Carolina Evidence-based Practice Center. (2009). Outcomes of community health worker interventions. *Evidence Report/Technology Assessment*, 181, 1–144. A1-2, B1-14, passim.

Volkmann, K. & Castañares, T. (2011). Clinical community health workers: Linchpin of the medical home. *The Journal of Ambulatory Care Management*, 34(3), 221–233. https://doi.org/10.1097/JAC.0b013e31821cb559.

Wennerstrom, A., Haywood, C. G., Smith, D. O., Jindal, D., Rush, C., & Wilkinson, G. W. (2023). Community health worker team integration in Medicaid managed care: Insights from a national study. *Frontiers in Public Health*, 10, 1042750. https://doi.org/10.3389/fpubh.2022.1042750.

Werner, D. & Bower, B. (2012). Helping Health Workers Learn: A Book of Methods, Aids, and Ideas for Instructors at the Village Level (First Edition). Hesperian Health Guides.

Whitehouse, C., Knowles, M., Long, J., Mitra, N., Volpp, K., Xu, C., . . ., Kangovi, S. (2022). Digital health and community health worker support for diabetes management: A randomized controlled trial. *Journal of General Internal Medicine*, 38. https://doi.org/10.1007/s11606-022-07639-6.

Wiggins, N. & Borbon, A. (1998). Chapter 3: Core roles and competencies of community health advisors. In The Final Report of the National Community Health Advisor Study: Weaving the Future, pp. 15–49. https://www.orchwa.org/resources/Documents/Chapter-3-from-CH-Advisor-Report-Wiggins0001.pdf.

Wilkinson, D. Y. (1992). Indigenous community health workers in the 1960s and beyond. In R. L. Braithwaite & S. E. Taylor (Eds.), *Health issues in the black community* (pp. 255–266). Jossey-Bass.

Willaert, A. (2005). *Minnesota community health worker workforce analysis: Summary of findings for Minneapolis and St. Paul.* Mankato, MN. Healthcare Education Industry Partnership.

Williams-Livingston, A. D., Ervin, C., & McCray, G. (2020). Bridge builders to health equity: The High School Community Health Worker Training Program. *Journal of the Georgia Public Health Association*, 8(1). https://doi.org/10.20429/jgpha.2020.080114.

Wilson, F., Villarreal, R., Stimpson, J., & Pagán, J. (2014). Cost-effectiveness analysis of a colonoscopy screening navigator program designed for Hispanic men. *Journal of Cancer Education : The Official Journal of the American Association for Cancer Education*, 30. https://doi.org/10.1007/s13187-014-0718-7.

Witgert, K. E., Kinsler, S., Dolatshahi, J., & Hess, C. (2014). *Strategies for supporting expanded roles for non-clinicians on primary care teams.* National Academy of State Health Policy. https://ciswh.org/resources/strategies-supporting-expanded-roles-non-clinicians-primary-care-teams/.

Withorn, A. (1984). *Serving the People: Social Services and Social Change.* Columbia University Press.

Witmer, A., Seifer, S. D., Finocchio, L., Leslie, J., & O'Neil, E. H. (1995). Community health workers: Integral members of the health care work force. *American Journal of Public Health*, 85(8 Pt 1), 1055–1058. https://www.ncbi.nlm.nih.gov/pmc/articles/PMC1615805/.

Zheng, J., Williams-Livingston, A., Danavall, N., Ervin, C., & McCray, G. (2021). Online high school community health worker curriculum: Key strategies of transforming, engagement, and implementation. *Frontiers in Public Health*, 9. https://www.frontiersin.org/articles/10.3389/fpubh.2021.667840.

Additional Resources

Association of State and Territorial Health Officials. (2022, January 24). Community Health Workers. https://www.astho.org/topic/population-health-prevention/healthcare-access/community-health-workers/.

Barbero, C., Mason, T., Rush, C., Sugarman, M., Bhuiya, A. R., Fulmer, E. B., . . ., Wennerstrom, A. (2021). Processes for implementing community health worker workforce development initiatives. *Frontiers in Public Health*, 9. https://www.frontiersin.org/articles/10.3389/fpubh.2021.659017

Centers for Disease Control and Prevention. (2023, March 1). Community Health Worker Resources|CDC. https://www.cdc.gov/chronicdisease/center/community-health-worker-resources.html.

Community Health Worker Resources | CDC. (2023, March 1). https://www.cdc.gov/chronicdisease/center/community-health-worker-resources.html.

Community Health Worker Resources from Families USA. (2023). https://familiesusa.org/community-health-worker-resources-from-families-usa/.

Community Health Worker Workgroup—The Office of Minority Health. (2021). https://minorityhealth.hhs.gov/omh/browse.aspx?lvl=3&lvlid=125.

Lee, C. N., Matthew, R. A., & Orpinas, P. (2023). Design, implementation, and evaluation of community health worker training programs in Latinx communities: A scoping review. *Journal of Community Psychology*, 51(1), 382–405. https://doi.org/10.1002/jcop.22910.

National Academy for State Health Policy: Community Health Workers. (n.d.). NASHP. Retrieved from https://nashp.org/policy/health-care-workforce/community-health-workers/ (accessed 1 May 2023).

National Association of County and City Health Officials. (2023). https://www.naccho.org/.

An Introduction to Public Health

Rama Ali Kased and Savita Malik

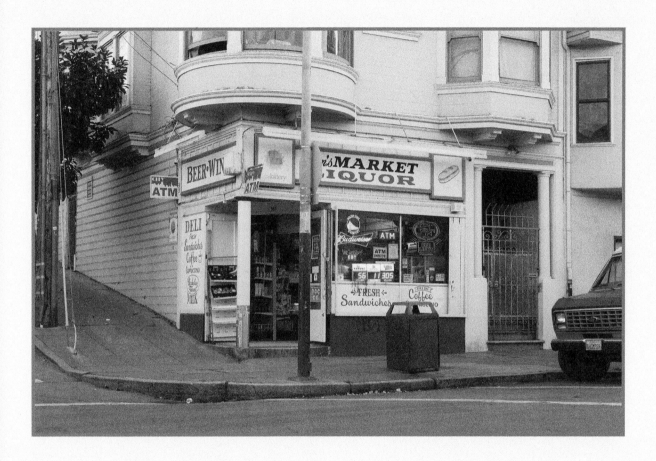

Foundations for Community Health Workers, Third Edition. Edited by Tim Berthold and Darouny Somsanith.
© 2024 John Wiley & Sons, Inc. Published 2024 by John Wiley & Sons, Inc.
Companion website: http://www.wiley.com/go/communityhealthworkers3E

My passion and purpose found their ideal field in public health, a discipline which, by its very nature, strives to improve lives, reduce inequalities and make real, practical changes in the service of people and communities. It ties together all other disciplines and is a powerful tool in the fight for social justice.

—*Leana S. Wen, President of Planned Parenthood, 2021, page 314*

Introduction

This chapter provides an introduction to the interdisciplinary field of public health. We focus on the concepts we believe are most essential to guiding your work as a community health worker.

WHAT YOU WILL LEARN

By studying the information in this chapter, you will be able to:

- Define public health and explain how the field of public health is different from the field of health care
- Explain how public health analyzes the causes of illness and health of populations and emphasizes the social determinants of health
- Explain why public health is concerned with health inequities
- Discuss the relationship between promoting social justice and promoting public health
- Describe the ecological model of public health and apply it to specific public health issues
- Discuss public health's emphasis on prevention
- Explain the spectrum of prevention and provide examples for each of the six levels

C3 Roles and Skills Addressed in Chapter 3

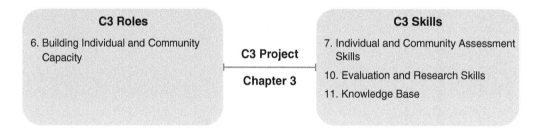

WORDS TO KNOW

Ecological Model	Prevalence
Epidemiology	Primary Prevention
Infant Mortality	Secondary Prevention
Interdisciplinary	Social Determinants
Life Expectancy	Spectrum of Prevention
Population	Tertiary Prevention

3.1 Defining Health

Sophia Simon-Ortiz: The practice of public health is about understanding all the components of our lives that impact our health—and going beyond health care and genetics, which are important factors but not the whole picture. The conditions in which we live, work, experience connection or marginalization in our communities, and more, all also impact our health significantly. The practice of public health centers on prevention instead of treatment only: preventing harms to health before they happen and changing conditions to support thriving.

Public health promotes the health and well-being of all people. There are many definitions of health. The World Health Organization (WHO) defines health as "the complete state of physical, mental, and social well-being, not just the absence of disease" (World Health Organization, 2023). This widely used definition encourages us to think about health broadly and in positive terms. By including "social well-being," it suggests that an individual's health is linked to the health of his or her family and community. Other definitions of health emphasize additional dimensions, such as emotional, intellectual, occupational, environmental, political, and spiritual health as depicted in Figure 3.1 below. The WHO further defines public health as

> *all organized measures (ether public or private) to prevent disease, promote health, and prolong life among the population as a whole. Its activities aim to provide conditions in which people can be healthy and focus on entire populations, not on individual patients or diseases. Thus, public health is concerned with the total system and not only the eradication of a particular disease* (World Health Organization, 2015).

- *How do you define health?*

What Do YOU Think?

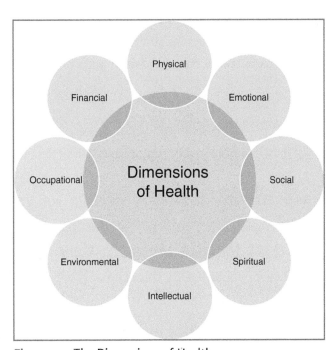

Figure 3.1 The Dimensions of Health

PUBLIC HEALTH VERSUS HEALTH CARE

Public health has long been confused with health care. While these two concepts are partners, there are distinct differences between them. Health care and public health have been described as trains on parallel tracks—with windows facing opposite directions, looking out on the same landscape. Those on the medical train see the individual trees: the subtle differences in size, color, age, and health. Those aboard the public health train see the forest: populations of similar trees, growing together and weathering the same storms. This analogy gives clarity to the distinctions. Public health sees health from a population perspective. Health care treats the individual.

PUBLIC HEALTH	HEALTH CARE
Focus is on supporting the health of entire populations	Focus is on diagnosing and treating individual patients
Driven by the goal of public well being	Promoting the health of individuals. Often driven by profit and revenue generation
The responsibility of local, state and federal government in partnership with private agencies	The responsibility of employers, private providers and local, state, and federal government

The field of public health embraces the broadest definition of health. The discipline addresses a broad range of issues that influence human health including illness, accidents, and disability, as well as challenges such as homelessness, hunger and access to sufficient food, violence, and civil and human rights issues.

To increase health for all, the United States sets national health goals and objectives every ten years. Healthy People 2030 (U.S. Department of Health and Human Services, 2023) establishes five overarching goals and dozens of focus areas. The goals are to:

1. Create healthy, thriving lives and well-being
2. Achieve health equity by eliminating health disparities
3. Create social and physical environments that promote health
4. Promote quality of life and healthy behaviors across all life stages.
5. Engage leadership and communities to take action and design policies that improve the health and well-being of all

- *What do you think of the Healthy People 2030 goals?*

- *What do you consider to be the most important public health issues facing the communities you live in and work with?*

- *How would you explain the difference between public health and health care?*

3.2 Defining the Field of Public Health: Key Concepts

To further define and describe the field of public health, this chapter discusses several key concepts.

PUBLIC HEALTH IS POPULATION BASED

While health care focuses on the health of individual patients, public health is concerned with the health of large groups of people or **populations**. These populations are usually defined by one or more factors, such as:

- Geographic and political boundaries (ZIP code, city, county, and nation)
- Demographic characteristics such as ethnicity, gender, age, and immigration status
- Health-related data on groups with similar patterns of risk factors, illness, injury, disability, or mortality

For example, a population could be defined as women in the United States, Latina women in California, or college-educated Latina women under the age of twenty-five in the city of Oakland, California.

- *What populations do you belong to?*

- *Which populations are you most interested in working with as a CHW?*

PUBLIC HEALTH EMPHASIZES PREVENTION

Public health goes beyond treatment. It attempts to prevent illness or injury before it starts, or as soon as possible when illness is diagnosed, or injury occurs. This emphasis on prevention distinguishes public health from health care, which typically treats a health condition after it is identified or diagnosed.

The "upstream story" is frequently used to illustrate this point.

The Upstream Story of Prevention

Four hikers walking beside a river heard cries for help and saw a person struggling against the current, trying to reach the shore. They managed to rescue the person in the river, but just as they were pulling them to safety, along came a small child slamming against the boulders. Before they pulled the child out, two more people passed by in the current: the hikers barely rescued them. Exhausted, they treated the victims. Then they heard another cry for help. One of the hikers said, "That's it—I'm going upstream to investigate!" The others said, "You can't! More people will need to be rescued, and we can't do it without you. If you leave, someone might drown." The hiker replied, "I want to find out why they are falling in the river, so we can find a way to stop it."

Just as the hiker moved upstream to see what could be done to prevent people from falling into the river, public health tries to intervene "upstream" to prevent illness or epidemics from developing in the first place. Money spent on upstream programs and policies that promote equity and access to basic resources not only saves lives but also helps to prevent the expense of caring for people who may become ill. If we apply this to the example of depression, public health emphasizes the importance of investing "upstream" in programs and policies that help to prevent new cases of depression.

Primary, Secondary, and Tertiary Prevention

Public health emphasizes three different types of prevention.

Primary prevention prevents the development of a health condition before it starts. An example of primary prevention as applied to depression is programs and policies designed to address social determinants that are associated with a higher risk of promotion. This includes policies that promote equity (such as access to housing, food, health care, and education) and prevent discrimination and violence (implementation of civil rights protection and community-based violence prevention programs).

Secondary prevention involves the early diagnosis and treatment of illnesses or conditions before they become symptomatic or turn into something worse. Targeted prevention programs aimed at high-risk populations (those with serious risk factors or precursors of disease) are considered secondary prevention, too. Secondary prevention might include educational and social media campaigns to heighten awareness about depression, and the widespread use of depression screening in schools, clinics and hospitals, jails and prisons, and other social services settings.

Tertiary prevention involves services for those already living with illness or injury to delay further progression of disease, alleviate symptoms, prevent complications, and delay death. Tertiary prevention often involves treatment, and in this way, it overlaps with the role of clinical medicine. Tertiary prevention might include access to culturally relevant, free, and low-cost mental health services and treatments that are easily accessible for those living with depression.

- *What role can CHWs play at each level of prevention?*

- *At which level of prevention do you want to work?*

PUBLIC HEALTH IS ROOTED IN SCIENCE

Public health is an **interdisciplinary** field. This means that it taps into a wide range of science, social science, and professional disciplines, including biology, anatomy, economics, demography, statistics, business, urban planning, law, anthropology, sociology, medicine, psychology, and political science.

Public health has also developed its own science of **epidemiology**, the study of the health and illness of populations.

Dr. John Snow is often called the father of modern epidemiology. He worked to stop a cholera epidemic in London in 1854. Cholera is a terrifying disease that causes extreme vomiting and diarrhea and can result in death from dehydration in a matter of hours. Today we know that disease can be spread from person to person by invisible microorganisms, such as the bacteria that cause cholera and viruses that cause the flu. Before the twentieth century, people were unsure what caused diseases like cholera, smallpox, or measles (known as communicable diseases). Many people believed that disease was spread by *miasma* or foul air identified with the conditions of poverty.

Snow thought that cholera was spread by contaminated water. He interviewed cholera patients and their surviving family members and studied death records. He plotted deaths from cholera on a map of London and saw that the death rate was much higher among families who got their water from the Broad Street Pump. Snow convinced local leaders to turn off the Broad Street Pump. Once the handle to the pump was removed, there was a sudden and dramatic decline in the number of local residents infected with and dying from cholera (Tulchinsky, 2018).

The methods that John Snow used to investigate the cholera epidemic are still used today. They are used to study epidemics as varied as COVID-19, HIV/AIDS, tuberculosis, automobile accidents, and child malnutrition.

Today, public health applies a range of scientific methods, including epidemiology, to:

- Identify patterns of illness, injury, disability, and death within populations
- Compare disease rates between different populations to identify those with the highest rates of illness and death
- Guide the development of public health programs and policies designed to promote the health of populations
- Address health disparities and ensure health and wellness for marginalized communities.
- Evaluate the effectiveness of public health programs and policies

Public health analyzes existing government data and gathers new information to examine patterns of disease and death. The National Center for Health Statistics, of the Centers for Disease Control and Prevention (Murphy, Kochanek, Xu, & Arias, 2020), lists the leading causes of death in the United States for 2020 as follows:

1. Heart disease: 696,962
2. Cancer: 602,350
3. COVID-19: 350,831
4. Accidents (unintentional injuries): 200,955
5. Stroke (cerebrovascular diseases): 160,264
6. Chronic lower respiratory diseases (such as emphysema): 152,657
7. Alzheimer's disease: 134,242

8. Diabetes: 102,188

9. Influenza and Pneumonia: 53,544

10. Kidney disease (nephritis, nephrotic syndrome, and nephrosis): 52,547

The year 2020 marked a shift in the way we think of the leading causes of death. For previous years, **chronic diseases** remained at the top of the list, such as heart disease, cancer, stroke, chronic lung diseases, and diabetes. A century ago, in 1900, the leading causes of death were **infectious diseases** such as tuberculosis, the flu, pneumonia, and diarrheal diseases. In 2020, the globe endured the COVID-19 pandemic, pushing COVID-19 into the number 3 spot of the leading causes of death. This changed the landscape to include both chronic and infectious diseases in the top ten leading causes of death in the United States.

A baby born in 1900 was expected to live only to age 47, while by the year 2020, that life expectancy had grown to age 77. People often assume that the dramatic change in the leading causes of death during the twentieth century must have been due to innovations in medicine; however, public health research shows the change was mainly a result of new public policies and public health actions. While reductions in infectious disease came about in through the development of vaccines and antibiotics, changing social conditions had an even bigger impact. These changes include shifts such as universal schooling, safer worksites, improvements in sanitation, more access to clean water, the establishment of a minimum wage, and improved nutrition.

Records of births and deaths are generally available, but it is not as easy to document the number of people living with a specific illness or disability, such as COVID-19 or HIV disease.

Epidemiology gathers information from a sample (a smaller, but representative number) of the population. Based on the sample, it then estimates how many people have a particular illness and how it might be increasing within a population. Researchers use statistics to figure out how to gather this information, whom to gather it from, and how many people must be sampled in order to provide a reliable estimate of the number or percentage of the population who are affected.

For example, the field of public health uses statistical methods to estimate the **prevalence** (percentage of a population with a specific health condition) of depression among people in the United States in 2020, during the global COVID-19 pandemic. A study conducted by Columbia University in 2020 estimated that 9% of Americans ages 12 and older experienced a major depressive episode, and the rate among youth ages 12–17 was 17% (Columbia University, 2022). Mental Health America conducted over 2.6 million surveys to determine that the prevalence of anxiety or depression for Asian or Pacific Islanders increased 7% between 2019 and 2020. In contrast, the prevalence of anxiety or depression among the white (non-Latino) population dropped by 7% during that same time frame (Mental Health America, 2020).

Epidemiologists use basic health indicators to describe the health of a population. These indicators are also used to compare the health status of different populations. The most widely used health indicators are infant mortality and life expectancy. **Infant mortality** is the estimated number of children, out of every 1,000 children born alive, who die before the age of one. In 2020, the infant mortality rate in the United States was 5.42 deaths for every 1000 live births (Centers for Disease Control and Prevention, 2020b). In stark contrast, the infant mortality rate in 2020 for Zimbabwe was 36.5 deaths for every 1,000 live births (UNICEF, 2023).

Life expectancy is the estimated number of years that people will live. In 2021, life expectancy in the United States was estimated at 73 years for males and 79 years for females. In comparison, life expectancy in Zimbabwe was estimated at 58 years for males and 64 years for females (United Nations, 2020a, United Nations, 2020b). As a discipline, public health often starts with the statistical information in health indicators to raise new questions about what shapes our health, and what we can do about it.

What Do
YOU?
Think

- *Are you surprised by the large difference in infant mortality and life expectancy rates between the United States and Zimbabwe?*

- *What do these life expectancy and infant mortality rates tell you about the relative health of each nation?*

- *What questions do you have about the infant mortality and life expectancy rates in your area?*

While CHWs are not expected to have an in-depth knowledge of epidemiology or statistics, the more you know, the better prepared you will be to participate in decisions about public health research, programs, and policies. Look up the website for your county or state's health department and select a report to read or skim. Identify language or information that you do not fully understand and talk about it with a colleague.

- *What type of health statistics do you most want to learn about?*

- *How can health data guide and support your work as a CHW?*

What Do
YOU?
Think

CASE STUDY   COVID-19

The COVID-19 pandemic provides a unique look at epidemiology in action as well as how science and politics can impact a public health response. In the early phases of the pandemic, public health experts agreed that a unified national strategy based on scientific evidence was critical. However, the response that followed was political in nature and science was often ignored or undermined. In a Pew Research Study conducted in June 2020, 73% of Democrats said that ordinary Americans could impact the spread of COVID-19, compared to 44% of Republicans (Jurkowitz & Mitchell, 2020).

Public health experts used scientific methods to recommend ways that individuals could help stop the spread of the virus. By April 2020, nearly all states had coronavirus restrictions in place, such as stay-at-home orders, school closures, mask wearing, and social distancing. Yet the partisan nature of the United States government meant the messages that reached the American people were confusing, at best. The Brookings Institution found that the political party people aligned with was a more influential role in people's behavior around the coronavirus than age, health status, or even local infection rates published by health departments. (Rothwell & Makridis, 2020). By November 2020, the United States was recording COVID-19 infection rates of over 1,000,000 per day and neared 10 million total cases as well as 250,000 deaths. Concern for the coronavirus remained, and states chose to handle their response independently of what the federal government was recommending. The Centers for Disease Control as well as local public health departments continued to

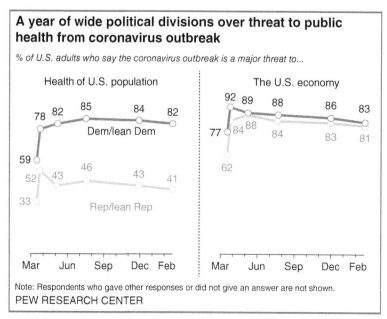

A year of wide political divisions over threat to public health from coronavirus outbreak

% of U.S. adults who say the coronavirus outbreak is a major threat to...

Health of U.S. population
78 82 85 84 82
Dem/lean Dem
59
52 43 46 43 41
33
Rep/lean Rep

Mar Jun Sep Dec Feb

The U.S. economy
92 89 88 86 83
77 84 88 84 83 81
62

Mar Jun Sep Dec Feb

Note: Respondents who gave other responses or did not give an answer are not shown.
PEW RESEARCH CENTER

(*Source*: Pew Research, 2023.)

(continues)

(continued)

publish data, giving governments as much information as they could. This is a clear example of the impact data can have on epidemiology, as well as the role that politics plays in listening to the data.

Leana Wen, the President of Planned Parenthood states that "[Public health] is based on science, but relies on winning over hearts and minds to follow evidence-based guidelines. Public health needs to balance diverging interests. It's messy and complicated, but the stakes are too high for us to get it wrong" (Wen, 2021, pp. 298).

CHW Profile

Tahrio Sanford (she, her)
Community Wellness, Test, and Vaccination Site Lead
Rafiki Coalition for Health and Wellness
Low-Income Communities of Color

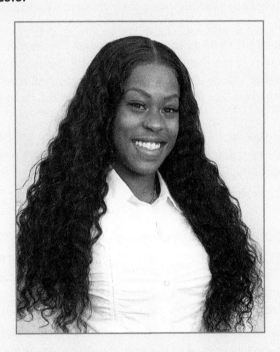

I've worked in my community since I was 14 years old. My family was on government assistance, and I learned how they treat the community. I was working at the Bayview Hunters Point YMCA in the financial department and a co-worker came in and said she had just graduated from the CHW program. I got really interested because I always wanted to work with my community, be a case manager or therapist. So I applied and got in!

I am the Site Lead at the COVID-19 testing and vaccination sites in the Bayview/Hunters Point area, a diverse low-income community. We collaborate with the Department of Public Health (DPH). I explain about COVID-19 tests and vaccinations and help register folks in the community. For anyone who tests positive for COVID-19, we send out food boxes and clean supplies. Anyone who comes to our sites, we give PPE (personal protective equipment) bags with hand sanitizer, gloves, face masks, face shields, and home tests for COVID-19. We also have extra goodies such as coloring books, crayons, and snacks when we get donations.

(continues)

CHW Profile
(continued)

At first, nobody wanted to come and get tested. People were scared to get vaccinated. One day two young ladies walked past the site and I asked if they wanted a test or a vaccine. One lady was like: I don't need a test; I don't want a shot; I don't want anybody shooting anything in me. So I'm like, it's okay, all right, well, if you know anybody who wants one, let me know.

Then her friend asked why she couldn't get more of the PPE bags; she was upset that we didn't have enough supplies. She wanted us to tell the DPH that they need to do more for our community. The community wants to know about this stuff; it's important to them.

I try to do my best to get services to the community, no matter what they may want, or how they come at me. You gotta be prepared to code switch and make sure you stay professional at all times. That's why I just love working in the community; you get so many different atmospheres, so many different personalities.

Now our community actually comes out and gets tested a lot, and we've had more people get vaccinations. Now people are comfortable walking from their house to our site to get tested or driving through and getting tested from the car. They bring their families, bring their cousins, or whoever. It makes us feel good that they're happy to see us there.

Working as a CHW has changed me to being more open minded. I've learned to speak up and ask questions. We hear the voices and concerns of the people we're working for. So you've gotta speak up and promote your services and make sure that you do what you say you're gonna do. Now I want to go back to school and get my degree in public health. It makes my son happy to see that his mom likes to work to create a better community.

For a CHW just starting their training I would say, don't give up! There will be very hard times where you want to give up or quit, but keep going. Use your voice. You have a lot to offer, a lot of knowledge, so don't let anyone make you come out of your character. And keep your pride. You're gonna need it!

PUBLIC HEALTH EMPHASIZES THE SOCIAL DETERMINANTS OF HEALTH

The field of public health understands the factors that cause illness and death differently than the field of medicine does. Traditionally, medicine focuses on the causes of disease located within the individual patient. If a patient goes to their doctor with symptoms of depression, often the physician will ask questions about their overall mental state and refer them to a licensed mental health provider for medication and/or therapy.

In contrast, public health looks at the factors that cause and contribute to patterns of illness and death in populations. This is, of course, closely related to the public health commitment to social justice. Public health research has demonstrated that the most significant of these factors are located at the societal level. These **social determinants of health** include economic, social, and political policies and dynamics that influence whether people have access to resources and opportunities essential to good health. In general, populations with less access to resources experience higher rates of illness and death. These resources, rights, and opportunities include:

- Safe housing and public transportation
- Proper and sufficient nutrition
- Personal safety (from domestic violence, police brutality and war, for example)
- Civil rights and protection from discrimination
- Employment, safe working conditions, and a living wage
- Clean water, air, and soil
- Quality education

- Recreational facilities and green space
- Cultural resources
- Affordable health care

All these factors affect health. For this reason, working to ensure that all people have access to these resources and opportunities *is* public health work.

- *What resources and opportunities do you consider to be essential for the health and wellness of the communities you belong to or work with?*

Jade Rivera: Public Health frameworks align with community self-determination and calls from grassroots movements to reimagine public safety and redistribute public resources away from state violence and into life-affirming social investments including education, housing, and health services.

3.3 The Practice of Public Health

PUBLIC HEALTH IS PRACTICED BY MANY PEOPLE, GROUPS AND ORGANIZATIONS

Public health is not a coordinated system, and is practiced by a large and diverse group of public (government) and private sector agencies, groups, and individuals, including:

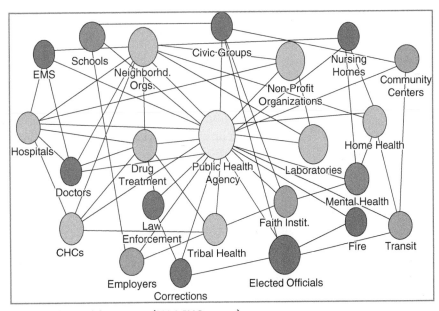

The Public Health System (NAACHO, 2013).

International and intergovernmental organizations such as the World Health Organization and the United Nations Children's Fund (UNICEF).

Local, state, tribal, and national government agencies, such as the department of public health in your city or county, and national organizations such as the Department of Health and Human Services, the Centers for Disease Control and Prevention, and the Office of Minority Health.

- *Which government agencies in your area are involved in the community's health?*

Public and private clinics and hospitals, particularly those that provide health care services to low-income and uninsured patients.

- *Which clinic or hospital, if any, provides services to low-income patients in your community?*

Colleges and universities with departments or schools of public health, health education, medicine, public policy, and social work that educate professionals and conduct research and advocacy related to public health.

- *Is there a college or university close to where you live? Does it provide education and training or conduct research or advocacy related to public health?*

Many small and large private or nongovernmental organizations provide health and social services to promote the health of low-income and at-risk communities (communities with increased risks for illness, disability, injury, or premature death). These may include agencies that work with youths or seniors and address issues such as domestic violence, homelessness, or drug and alcohol use.

- *Which agencies provide services in your community?*

Individuals, groups, and associations work to promote the health and welfare of low-income and otherwise vulnerable communities. Individual activists lobby local governments to develop policies or fund programs to improve health. Informal groups of people come together to advocate on behalf of shared issues. For example, public housing residents might advocate for the repair of hazardous living conditions. More formal associations are also active in public health and social justice. Labor unions, for example, have taken leadership in promoting occupational health.

- *Can you identify individual activists, groups, or associations that are working to promote public health in your community?*

Though the practice of public health is largely invisible and not often publicized, our lives are affected by public health programs and policies every day. When you turn on the tap, do you drink clean water? Are you or your children immunized against infectious disease? Do you ride in a vehicle that has seatbelts and airbags? Each of these measures represents a very concrete gain in quality of life, achieved through public health efforts. *Can you think of other examples?*

Public health agencies in the United States have been historically underfunded. Funding remains inadequate, despite increased public concern about re-emerging infectious diseases and new threats to health, like terrorism, global pandemics, and climate change. The vast majority of health-related funding is spent on expensive and relatively inefficient health care services. Public health professionals seek to change the balance of these investments and to increase government spending on effective public health programs and policies.

Policies that affect the public's health are largely determined by the decisions that our governments make, including the level of investment in essential resources such as education, housing, transportation, food, safe working conditions, and access to comprehensive health care. Every time your government makes a decision about where to invest public dollars, it has an impact on public health (Please note that everyone, regardless of citizenship status, pays taxes, including sales taxes, automobile, gasoline, and tobacco taxes). When governments enforce civil rights, raise the minimum wage or build affordable housing, they are promoting public health. When international bodies negotiate a cease-fire or treaty, or fail to, they are taking action that affects public health.

What Do
YOU?
Think:

- *What decisions has your local government made in the past year that affect the health of the communities you work with?*

- *How can you—and the communities you work with—influence such decisions to improve the community's health?*

THREE CORE FUNCTIONS OF PUBLIC HEALTH

There are three core functions that help distinguish public health from other related fields, and 10 essential public health services that fall under these three broad categories. At the foundation of these functions is a commitment to health equity, connecting public health to social justice in a real and meaningful way. Every public health department carries out these three functions, in one way or another, to improve population health:

- Assessment
- Policy Development
- Assurance

THE PUBLIC HEALTH SYSTEM AND THE TEN ESSENTIAL PUBLIC HEALTH SERVICES

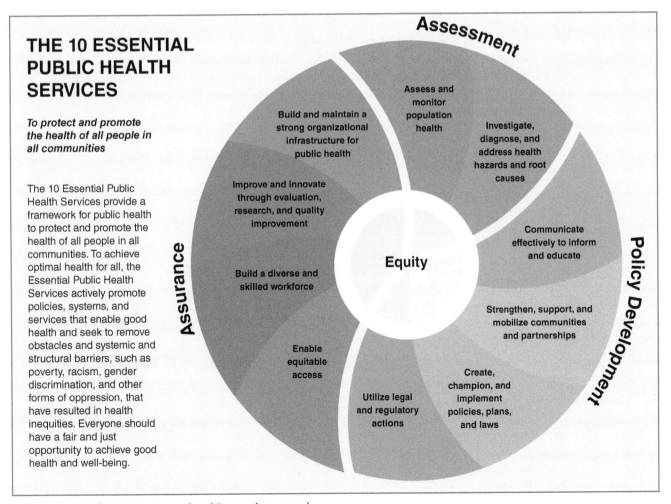

(*Source*: Centers for Disease Control and Prevention, 2023.)

Assessment helps public health professionals understand a health issue before taking action. Examples of assessment include:

- Monitoring health through regular reporting of the community's health status, such as the number of births, deaths, diabetes, or flu cases.

Policy Development is what public health professionals do to address a problem and promote a better health outcome. It means taking actions such as:

- Mobilizing community partnerships to change the conditions of health in the neighborhood, city, or county. For example, a community task force on children's health might bring together schools, service providers, parents, and youth to take action to reduce health risks for children.

Assurance means making sure that a policy, program, or service is implemented properly. Assurance includes actions such as:

- Enforcing the laws that protect our health—for example, inspecting restaurants for cleanliness, or making sure that the drinking water supply is kept clean.
- Ensuring that the workforce is highly skilled by providing training and education for people who work in public health, including CHWs.

To carry out these functions, every public health department organizes itself into specialized units. For example, a health department might have units for infectious disease, chronic disease, maternal and child health, environmental health, public health nursing, nutrition, and epidemiology.

PUBLIC HEALTH USES ECOLOGICAL MODELS TO UNDERSTAND AND PROMOTE HEALTH

The factors that have the greatest influence on health are the social determinants of health. **Ecological models** are frequently used in public health to examine risk factors that lead to disease and to develop policies and programs to address them. Ecological models help us to better understand how smaller and larger environments influence health.

- *What do you see in your community that contributes to illness or injuries? What do you see that contributes to good health and well-being?*

- *Have you witnessed a community's health improve because a root cause or a risk factor was eliminated or reduced? For example, a source of pollution was cleaned up, or a dangerous traffic or pedestrian street became safer.*

Because **ecological models** emphasize the social and physical environment, they draw attention to the social determinants of health. These models guide CHWs and other public health practitioners to view individual clients in the context of their families, neighborhoods, and the broader society in which they live. While there are many different ecological models used in the field of public health, we refer throughout this book to the model presented as Figure 3.2.

Figure 3.2 shows interconnected circles representing the individual; relationships with family and friends; the neighborhood or community in which people live, work, and go to school; and the broader society.

The individual: The innermost circle represents the individual. A person's health status is influenced by their genes/biology, values, beliefs, knowledge, and behaviors. In reference to depression, this includes how people think and feel about themselves (self-esteem) and their interpretation of stigma in accessing support for mental health concerns. In addition, individuals' acceptance of and comfort with therapy, medication for depressive symptoms, and a willingness to discuss depression openly, all contribute to people's decisions around seeking support.

- *Can you think of other ways that individuals influence their own health?*

- *How do you influence your own individual health?*

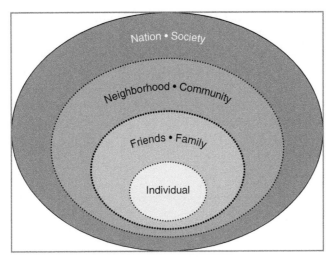

Figure 3.2 Ecological Model of Health

Family and friends: The next circle represents family and friends, who may influence health in many ways. Family and peer dynamics, including the presence of harassment or abuse, can increase the risks for depression. Families have varied responses when loved ones tell them they are depressed. Some families have judged, alienated, and even disowned relatives who suffer from depression. Other families are supportive, regardless of the identities and behaviors of their relatives. While friends sometimes encourage healthy behaviors, they may also promote behaviors such as the use of drugs and alcohol that may increase risks for depression. Familial and cultural stigma around depression also contributes to individuals choosing not to pursue medication or therapy.

- *Can you think of other ways in which family and friends influence health status?*

- *How do your family and friends influence your health?*

The community: The next circle represents the neighborhood or community we live in. Our health—including our mental health status—is strongly influenced by whether or not we have a safe home to live in, safe working conditions, a living wage, or exposure to environmental hazards and violence. Neighborhoods and communities also influence whether people have access to recreational and cultural activities, public transportation to get back and forth from their homes to school, work, or grocery stores and to visit with family and friends. In reference to depression, some neighborhoods have free or low-cost mental health services that provide culturally appropriate individual therapy, support groups, and access to medications. Other neighborhoods do not have access to these services. Some communities have safe places for youths to congregate and openly talk about their feelings, while others do not. Some communities experience high rates of prejudice and discrimination; others do not. Some communities have good schools and job training, with easy access to jobs and social services; others do not. Living in neighborhoods that lack these basic resources results in chronic stress and increased risks for illness and premature death (please see Chapter 4).

- *Can you think of other ways in which a community may contribute to the risks of disease?*

- *How does the neighborhood and community you live in and belong to influence your health?*

The nation or society: The outermost circle in Figure 3.2 represents the nation or society we live in, and the social, cultural, economic, and political factors that influence our health status. The decisions that our governments make about where and how to invest public funds largely determine which populations have greater access to resources such as safe housing, loans, transportation, recreational facilities, quality schools, social services, and employment opportunities. The media, including television and social media, may encourage risky behavior or healthy choices. Economic dynamics influence access to jobs that provide safe working conditions and a living wage. Prejudice and discrimination that target certain communities also have a profound impact on health (see Chapters 4 and 12).

In reference to depression, some communities face ongoing prejudice, harassment, and other forms of discrimination, which increase their risks for depression (Alvarez-Galvez & Rojas-Garcia, 2019; Hudson, Collins-Anderson, & Hutson, 2023; Lee et al., 2022). Poverty and income inequality also contribute to the risks of depression (Zare, Fugai, Azadi, & Gaskin, 2022). Appropriate mental health services are not accessible to everyone who needs it. The most vulnerable populations (unhoused, incarcerated, undocumented, and communities of color) are at greater risk of not receiving appropriate or timely care to manage their depression. Not all people in the United States have health coverage, and the high cost of services can be a barrier to access.

Whether CHWs work with individuals, families, or communities, an ecological perspective is essential to guide their efforts.

- *What would you add to the ecological model presented above?*

- *Can you think of other ways that our society and our government influence our health?*

DEVELOPING PROGRAMS AND POLICIES FOR PREVENTION

The Spectrum of Prevention provides a framework for understanding different "levels" of prevention activities. It has proven to be a useful resource for guiding the development of public health programs in areas such as injury prevention, violence prevention, nutrition, HIV/AIDS, and fitness for over twenty years (Prevention Institute, 2023).

Below, we provide an example of how CHWs can work at each level of the spectrum of prevention. An intervention is a public health program or activity aimed at producing a change. The examples provided in Table 3.1 address depression and mental health. In the Chapter Review, you will have a chance to apply the spectrum of prevention to a different public health issue.

- *Have you participated in programs that represented one or more levels of the Spectrum of Prevention?*

- *Which levels of the Spectrum of Prevention have you worked at?*

- *Which levels do you hope to work at over the course of your career as a CHW?*

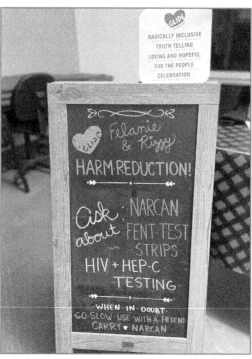

Public health supports harm reduction policies and programs.

Table 3.1 The Spectrum of Prevention

LEVEL OF PREVENTION	DEFINITION	EXAMPLE
1. Strengthening individual knowledge and skills	Enhancing an individual's ability to prevent injury or illness and promote safety	CHWs work in a clinic and provide person-centered education about mental health, symptoms of depression, and ways to seek support.
2. Promoting community education	Reaching groups of people with information and resources to promote health and safety	CHWs visit local high schools and give educational presentations designed to assist youths in accessing mental health services.
3. Educating providers	Informing health providers who will transmit skills and knowledge to others	CHWs facilitate trainings for the staff at a youth-serving organization on signs to watch for, resources around supporting youth with depression, and how to combat stigma around accessing services.
4. Fostering coalitions and networks	Bringing individuals and groups together to work for common goals with a greater impact	CHWs facilitate the formation and planning process of a coalition of youths and youth-serving organizations interested in supporting young people around their mental health.
5. Changing organizational practices	Adopting regulations and shaping norms within organizations to improve health and safety	CHWs work with local youth networks and youth leaders to advocate with local schools or school districts to provide comprehensive mental health support, free of charge to youth. This could lesbian, gay, bisexual, and transgender students, students who have history with incarceration, undocumented students, and students who are unhoused.
6. Influencing policy and legislation	Developing strategies to change laws and policies in order to influence health outcomes	CHWs advocate with state policymakers on behalf of new policies such as funding more mental health professionals in youth organizations and schools, services like job training and living wages and expansion of mental health covered by Medicaid.

PUBLIC HEALTH PRACTICE RELIES ON EVIDENCE

The field of public health gathers data to identify the populations at greatest risk for illness and premature death, and to evaluate the effectiveness of public health programs and policies. Using epidemiology and research evidence to assess effective programs is another example of how science informs the practice of public health. This information is then used to guide planning and programming for subsequent public health interventions. This data-driven approach helps support programs that have already proven to be successful. While using data is important, we must also remember that if a program or policy works for one community, that is no guarantee that it will work in another community with a different population. We must be mindful to examine the feasibility of replicating public health programs before assuming they will work in another community or setting.

At the same time, it is important to acknowledge that political beliefs and goals sometimes undermine this process, and scientific evidence may be disregarded in the development of policies. For example, state and federal governments have favored incarceration over mental health and drug treatment and defunded mental health supports within school systems despite overwhelming evidence that kids are more likely to access mental health services when they are available at school (Panchal, Cox, & Rudowitz, 2022).

As a CHW, you can benefit from keeping up-to-date with public health research about the issues you address in your work. You can learn from both successful and unsuccessful public health programs to find more effective ways to serve your clients and communities. The most useful research evidence will be drawn from program models and strategies that are very similar to your own, and with populations that are very similar to those you work with. For example, just because a diabetes management program was effective with Native American women in Arizona, a similar program may not be equally successful serving white men in New Hampshire. As we have tried to emphasize, the environment in which people live and the identities and culture of the community you serve need to be taken into consideration. Public health departments, research universities and the CDC are all good sources for evidence about model programs that have been demonstrated to work, at least in some settings. A few of these are listed in the Resources section at the end of this chapter.

Finally, as a CHW you may have opportunities to participate in public health research and will certainly have opportunities to participate in the evaluation of the programs and services you provide. We encourage you to talk with your colleagues about the programs you work with. How were they developed? Are they guided by existing research? Have they been evaluated? If so, what are the findings? If they haven't been evaluated, ask to participate in developing an evaluation method to learn if and how the programs are making a positive difference. It is also helpful to ask questions about whose voices are being heard in the research process. Is community input being gathered and listened to? Do community members benefit from being involved in writing the questions? Even if you are unfamiliar with research or evaluation methods, your experience as a CHW may be vital in identifying what information to gather from the community and how to gather it. Please refer to information provided in Chapter 23 for an introduction to evaluation and research.

HOPE SF

HOPE SF is developing vibrant, mixed-income communities at four public housing communities in San Francisco, CA without mass displacement of original residents. Through a holistic approach that incorporates social services and environment-friendly building practices, they will replace all 1,900 public housing units one-for-one and add affordable and market-rate units, nearly tripling the total number of homes to 5,300. As the nation's first large scale, explicitly anti-racist community development initiative, HOPE SF will center resident voice, build community wealth, and support healthy communities.

The four community housing sites (Alice Griffith, Potrero Terrace and Annex, Hunters View, and Sunnydale) are home to a mix of cultures, including African American, Hispanic, Pacific Islander, and Asian communities. Residents are at the center of HOPE SF and drive the priorities and vision of the project. One of the ways this is done is through the Community Health Ambassador Program (CHAMP), based in the Urban Services YMCA in San Francisco. CHAMP hires community residents who are compassionate, resilient, and committed to promoting resident-driven health initiatives, supporting resident empowerment, and leadership. CHAMPs are enrolled in the Community Health Worker (CHW) Certificate Program at City College of San Francisco (CCSF).

The Ambassadors work at each of the four sites at the community wellness center, where the YMCA partners with the Department of Public Health (DPH) to provide clinicians, nurses, and case managers. The CHAMP team supports the DPH team to provide extra support to residents who are seen by the nurses and clinicians. This can include getting them rides to medical appointments or providing extra resources for residents.

The Ambassadors live in the community and often grew up there, and can respond to issues as they arise, such as holding a memorial service when someone is killed, working with the family and survivors of violence. Because of occasional turf issues between the sites, they strive to honor the person who passed in a safe way. During the COVID-19 pandemic, CHAMPs handed out PPE (masks, gloves, and hand sanitizer) and informed residents of best practices for avoiding COVID-19.

CHAMP offers individual outreach and weekly programming such as Zumba and yoga classes, mental health promotion, a women's group, and harm reduction education. They facilitate monthly family fun programs and celebrate *Dia de los Muertos*, Lunar New Year, Black History Month, and Asian and Pacific Islander Month.

(continues)

HOPE SF

(continued)

Priscilla Wilson started as an Ambassador four years ago. Priscilla earned her CHW Certificate from CCSF and now works for HOPE SF as a site manager. She started the popular Wellness Wednesdays in the community, where she makes smoothies for kids, explaining what's in them and why they're beneficial.

CHAMP is committed to creating health and wellness programs within the Hope SF communities, in addition to empowering Ambassadors as they become experienced CHWs. For more information about HOPE SF, please visit https://www.hope-sf.org/

3.4 Public Health and Social Justice

Public health is directly linked to a social justice framework. CHWs who engage in any level of the ecological model, will often need to consider the other levels when designing programs and interventions for their communities. To make the most impact on health equity for a community, a CHW must work to address the factors upstream that are impacting the health of the individuals they work with. The American Public Health Association explains social justice as the view that everyone deserves equal rights and opportunities and that includes the right to good health. There are inequities in health that are avoidable, unnecessary, and unjust (American Public Health Association, 2022). A public health perspective that is characterized by social justice argues that public health problems are primarily socially generated (Wallack, 2019).

PUBLIC HEALTH IS CONCERNED WITH SOCIAL JUSTICE AND HEALTH INEQUITIES

One of the most important public health issues of our time is the growing inequity in health among different populations. Health inequities, also referred to as *disparities*, occur when one group of people experience significantly higher rates of illness and death than others. As you will read in Chapter 4, epidemiological data documents these differences in health status between nations and between different communities within the United States.

An example of the health inequities that strip away the opportunity of some populations or communities to live and die in conditions of dignity is the dramatic inequity in HIV prevalence between the populations of the United States and Zimbabwe presented earlier. The data underscore the critical need facing the people of Zimbabwe, where about 12% percent of the population lives with HIV disease. Dr. Paul Farmer points out that the HIV epidemic follows patterns of class, race, and gender inequities in which the health care needs of the poor are too often ignored (Gupta & Koenig, 2022). In Zimbabwe, colonialism, unequal distribution of basic economic resources, political oppression, poverty, famine, and rigid gender roles set the stage for HIV/AIDS. Health cannot be separated from the social and economic conditions that shape human lives.

HIV disease is also unequally distributed among populations within the United States. For example, the chance of a woman being diagnosed with HIV in her lifetime is more than 15 times higher for African American women compared to white women (Centers for Disease Control and Prevention, 2020a). While African Americans make up 14 percent of the total population in the United States, they account for 44 percent of estimated AIDS cases. Although women are still disproportionately affected by HIV/AIDS, there was a promising 5% decrease in new infections among women between 2015 and 2019, yet another indication that health inequities *can* be reduced with concerted effort (Ibid)

Health inequities are not inevitable. They are the consequence of the way a society structures access to the basic resources, rights, and opportunities that all people require in order to live long and healthy lives. Eliminating health inequities requires changing social policies that determine access to resources that all people need to be healthy such as housing, food, education, employment, health care, safety, and human rights.

Leading institutions in the United States and internationally—including the National Association of County and City Health Officials (NACCHO), Centers for Disease Control and Prevention, the Institutes of Medicine (IOM), the Office of Minority Health (OMH), and the World Health Organization—have recognized health inequities as a public health priority. The Healthy People 2030 goals presented earlier in this chapter emphasize both the elimination of health inequities and the creation of social and physical environments that promote health.

For many of us, working to eliminate health inequities is the central challenge facing public health today. CHWs, working directly with communities that experience disproportionately high rates of illness and death, have a significant role to play in the movement to eliminate health inequities.

PUBLIC HEALTH ADVOCATES FOR SOCIAL JUSTICE

The factors that often have the biggest impact on human health are social determinants, including political decisions about where and how to invest public resources. It follows, therefore, that the most powerful strategy for promoting public health is to advocate for changes to public policies that will provide equal access to the resources and opportunities that are essential to health (education, housing, nutrition, safety, civil rights, and so on). If everyone, regardless of their educational background, income, ethnicity, immigration status, or other demographic characteristics, had access to these resources and opportunities, our society would not experience such high rates of infectious or chronic disease, or such pronounced inequities in illness, disability, and death between different populations.

We define *social justice* as the equal access to these basic human resources, rights, and opportunities. Leading public health researchers and institutions such as the American Public Health Association, schools of public health at many universities, the National Association of County and City Health Officials, and the World Health Organization have articulated the connections between social justice and public health and committed themselves to advocating for social justice as a best practice for promoting public health.

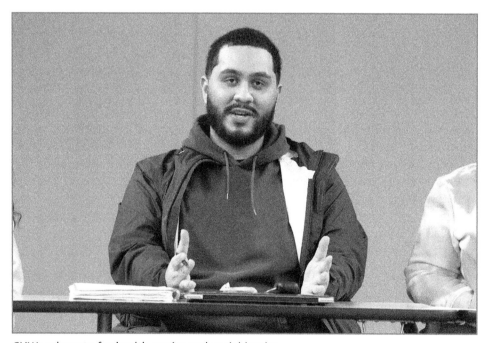

CHWs advocate for health equity and social justice.

Anthony Iton, former Medical Officer for the Alameda County Health Department in Oakland, California, stated:

> In virtually every public health area ... be it immunizations, chronic disease, HIV/AIDS ... or even disaster prepar-
> edness, local public health departments are confronted with the consequences of structural poverty, institutional
> racism and other forms of systemic injustice. By designing approaches that are specifically designed to identify

existing assets and build social, political and economic power among residents of afflicted neighborhoods, local public health departments can begin to sustainability reduce and move towards eliminating health inequities in low-income communities of color. Additionally, local public health agencies must simultaneously seek opportunities to strategically partner with advocates for affordable housing, labor rights, education equity, environmental justice, transportation equity, prison reform. ... Without such a focus, local health departments will most likely only succeed in tinkering around the edges of health disparities at a cost too great to justify. (Iton, 2006, p. 135)

One of the primary roles of all public health practitioners, including CHWs, is to advocate for social justice on behalf of and in partnership with the clients and communities you serve. Only by doing so can we change and improve the conditions that have the biggest impact on health status.

Galen Maloney: What I love about public health is that it provides a lens and a toolkit in order to obtain social justice goals. It's not quite a back door to address important social justice issues and achieving equity, but it's kind of a side door that hasn't been used too frequently and not enough. It's like the house is being renovated right now to allow for better Feng shui and the public health door is a key component. I got into public health because I saw an amazing organizing effort to characterize the impacts of police violence more comprehensively, so that it is not only a matter of civil rights but also a public health crisis..... And I think the same could be said for a multitude of issues including housing, education, systemic, racism, mental health, substance use, public space, and on and on and on. Public health has its roots in a dressing social ills and it's time to return to those roots. Not only time for that, but it is essential that we use public health to do that, or our society and planet will suffer for our lack of action sand letting our most powerful tools rust in the tool shed.

Public Health Has Not Always Promoted Justice

Unfortunately, public health is sometimes practiced from the top down: professional "experts" develop and implement programs and policies they think will promote the health of a vulnerable community. This approach has sometimes resulted in significant harm to the community. For example, the Tuskegee Syphilis Trials, an infamous public health research project, withheld treatment from African American men who were being studied to learn more about syphilis. As a result, men enrolled in the study were disabled and died (For more information about Tuskegee, see Chapter 7).

The eugenics movement in the 20th century is another devastating example of state-sponsored harm in the name of public health. The premise was that only white elites should determine who is "fit" and "unfit" to breed and this led to forced sterilizations of Black, Mexican, and Indigenous women from 1950 to as recently as 2010 (Nelson, 2003). Unfortunately, public health history has many such examples.

- *Have your communities been harmed by public health programs or policies in the past?*

- *How do the communities you belong to view the government?*

What Do YOU? Think

PUBLIC HEALTH WORKS IN PARTNERSHIP WITH COMMUNITIES

At its best, public health works in collaboration with the communities that have the most to gain or lose. One of the key roles of CHWs is to assist in flipping the top-down strategy just described and to partner with communities to develop public health programs and policies that represent and benefit from the wisdom, creativity, skills, and leadership of affected communities. This is important for many reasons, including:

- *It is the right thing to do*: Communities with the most to gain or lose from a public health program or policy should be consulted regarding its design, management, and evaluation. The right of a community to self-determination, and a voice in the decisions that affect them, is rooted in our most fundamental beliefs in democracy.

- *Long-term effectiveness*: Public health programs and policies come and go. Programs developed with leadership from the community are much more likely to be culturally relevant and to result in significant and lasting changes.

- *Capacity building*: You may have heard the expression, "Give a person a fish and they will eat well for a day. Teach a person to fish, and they will eat well forever." A key dimension to enhancing the health of communities is to foster community leadership and skills that they may use to address other health concerns in the future.

The quality of your work as a CHW can be judged to a great extent by the degree to which you establish and maintain respectful partnerships with the communities you work with and your ability to facilitate and support their leadership. (For more information about community-centered practice and the role of the CHW, please see Part Five of this textbook.)

PUBLIC HEALTH PROMOTES THE HEALTH OF THE NATURAL ENVIRONMENT

Our ancestors understood that human health was dependent upon the health of the planet. Modern societies have largely forsaken this knowledge and often operate in ways that harm our planet, the air and atmosphere, our oceans, groundwater, soil, plants, and animal species. The health of the planet and the health of human populations are integrally connected and mutually dependent, and increasingly, public health is beginning to promote both goals.

Modern society has concentrated its industrial pollution in certain areas where often poorer people and people of color live. The branch of public health known as Environmental Health works to decrease exposures to pollution in communities and worksites. CHWs often serve as an invaluable bridge between researchers and communities in public health efforts to clean up pollution and protect health. Campaigns that address the inequities that result from concentrating pollution in certain areas are part of the broader environmental justice movement.

Increasingly, public health has turned its attention to global climate change. Public health practitioners have an important role in developing policies both to mitigate (slow down or reverse) climate change and to adapt to a changing world. Public health leaders in California, for example, have been key supporters of the response to climate change (California Department of Public Health, 2023). They have supported laws to reduce the amount of carbon that goes into the atmosphere, while at the same time preparing for the worst (heat waves, fires, floods, etc.).

One creative contribution that public health makes to the policy discussions around climate change is an emphasis on the health co-benefits. A **health co-benefit** is like a positive side effect; it's something that, in addressing climate change, also improves the health of the population—for example, building bike paths so that people can around cities on a bicycle improves cardiovascular health, at the same time as it burns less gasoline. When addressing climate change, just like any other major health threat, particular attention must be paid to health equity. While climate change affects all populations, the poorest and most marginalized are often at greatest risk and have the least resources to adapt. A strong public health infrastructure is essential to handling the ongoing effects of climate change, including heat waves, floods and natural disasters, food shortages, and changes in patterns of infectious disease.

Chapter Review

To review, answer the following questions and apply the ecological model and the spectrum of prevention to the public health issue of gun violence.

POLICE VIOLENCE IN THE UNITED STATES

Recent social movements have re-centered police violence as a public health issue. Marginalized communities are disproportionately affected (e.g., people of color, immigrants, individuals experiencing homelessness, people with disabilities, the lesbian, gay, bisexual, transgender and queer community, individuals with mental illness, and people who use drugs and sex workers) by police practices including searches, arrests, assaults, and deaths. On average, 1,000 people are killed by police each year. Racial inequities in deaths by police are stark. Black and Indigenous people are two to three times more likely to be killed by police than their white counterparts and disproportionately suffer anxiety, depression, and post-traumatic stress disorder as a result (Human Impact Partners, 2020).

Policies that protect law enforcement have not held police accountable for this violence (American Public Health Association, 2018). While these statistics provide an overview of the problem and the populations most affected, the public health framework requires us to dig deeper to understand what actually causes police violence and what we can do about it.

1. Apply your understanding of the ecological model to the public health issue of police violence. What types of factors contribute to police violence and inequities in police violence among different communities?

2. Why is police violence considered to be a public health issue?

3. How might the three functions of public health—assessment, policy development, and assurance—be used to help prevent police violence?

4. Imagine that you are going to work with a public health program focused on preventing police violence in a large city. What type of public health statistics would you want to study?

5. How would promoting social justice help to prevent police violence in the United States?

6. Using the spectrum of prevention framework shown in Table **3.2**, provide examples of public health strategies that CHWs can participate in, to assist in preventing police violence, or gun violence in general.

Table 3.2 The Spectrum of Prevention Applied to Police Violence in the United States

SPECTRUM	STRATEGY
1. Influencing policy and legislation	CHWs will
2. Changing organizational practices	CHWs will
3. Fostering coalitions and networks	CHWs will
4. Educating providers	CHWs will
5. Promoting community education	CHWs will
6. Strengthening individuals' knowledge and skills	CHWs will

References

Alvarez-Galvez, J. & Rojas-Garcia, A. (2019). Measuring the impact of multiple discrimination on depression in Europe. BMC Public Health. https://bmcpublichealth.biomedcentral.com/articles/10.1186/s12889-019-6714-4 (accessed 10 March 2023).

American Public Health Association. (2018). Addressing Law Enforcement as a Public Health Issue. Retrieved from https://www.apha.org/policies-and-advocacy/public-health-policy-statements/policy-database/2019/01/29/law-enforcement-violence (accessed 10 March 2023).

American Public Health Association. (2022). Social Justice and Health. https://www.apha.org/what-is-public-health/generation-public-health/our-work/social-justice (accessed 6 February 2023).

California Department of Public Health (2023). Climate Change and Health Equity. https://www.cdph.ca.gov/Programs/OHE/pages/CCHEP.aspx (accessed 3 March 2023).

Centers for Disease Control and Prevention. (2023). 10 Essential Public Health Services. https://www.cdc.gov/publichealthgateway/publichealthservices/essentialhealthservices.html (accessed 10 March 2023).

Centers for Disease Control and Prevention (CDC). (2020a) Reproductive Health. https://www.cdc.gov/reproductivehealth/maternalinfanthealth/infantmortality.htm (accessed 6 February 2023).

Centers for Disease Control and Prevention, National Center for Health Statistics. (2020b). Deaths: Final Data for 2020. National Vital Statistics Reports, No. 427, December 2021. https://www.cdc.gov/nchs/data/data-briefs/db427.pdf

Columbia University. (2022). Nearly One in Ten Americans Reports Having Depression. Mailman School of Public Health. https://www.publichealth.columbia.edu/public-health-now/news/nearly-one-ten-americans-reports-having-depression (accessed 9 March 2023).

Gupta, R. & Koenig, S. P. (2022). The power of one—in memoriam of Paul E. Farmer. *Journal of the International AIDS Society*. https://doi.org/10.1002/jia2.25903.

Hudson, D., Collins-Anderson, A., & Hutson, W. (2023). Understanding the impact of contemporary racism on the mental health of middle class Black Americans. *International Journal of Environmental Research and Public Health*. https://doi.org/10.3390/ijerph20031660.

Human Impact Partners. (2020). How Health Departments Can Address Police Violence as a Public Health Issue. https://humanimpact.org/hipprojects/how-health-departments-can-address-police-violence-as-a-public-health-issue/ (accessed 10 March 2023).

Iton, A. (2006). Tackling the root causes of health disparities through community capacity building. In R. Hofrichter (Ed.), *Tackling health inequities through public health practice: A handbook for action* (pp. 115–136). Washington, D.C.: National Association of County and City Health Officials.

Jurkowitz, M & Mitchell, A. (2020). "Cable TV and COVID-19" Pew Research Center. https://journalism.org/2020/04/01/cable-tv-and-covid-19-how-americans-perceive-the-outbreak-and-view-media-coverage-differ-by-main-news-source (accessed 10 March 2023).

Lee, Y. H., Liu, Z., Fatori, D., Bauermeister, J. R., Luh, R. A., Clark, C. R., ..., Smoller, J. W. (2022). Association of everyday discrimination with depressive symptoms and suicidal ideation during the COVID-19 pandemic in the all of US Research Program. *JAMA Psychiatry* https://doi.org/10.1001/jamapsychiatry.2022.1973.

Mental Health America. (2020). How Race Matters: What We Can Learn from Mental Health America's Screening in 2020. mhanational.org/mental-health-data-2020 (accessed 10 March 2023).

Murphy, S. L., Kochanek, K. D., Xu, J. Q., & Arias, E. (2020). *Mortality in the United States. NCHS Data Brief, no 427.* Hyattsville, MD: National Center for Health Statistics. https://dx.doi.org/10.15620/cdc:112079external icon.

National Association of County & City Health Officials. (2013). National Public Health Performance Standards: Local Implementaion Guide. https://www.naccho.org/uploads/card-images/public-health-infrastructure-and-systems/2013_1209_NPHPS_LocalImplementationGuide.pdf (accessed 26 February 2024).

Nelson, J. (2003). *Women of color and the reproductive rights movement.* New York, New York: NYU Press.

Panchal, N., Cox, C., & Rudowitz, R. (2022). The Landscape of School-Based Mental Health Services. https://www.kff.org/other/issue-brief/the-landscape-of-school-based-mental-health-services/ (accessed 10 March 2023)

Pew Research Institute. (2023). A Year of U.S. Public Opinion on the Coronavirus Pandemic. https://www.pewresearch.org/2021/03/05/a-year-of-u-s-public-opinion-on-the-coronavirus-pandemic/ (accessed 26 December 2023).

Prevention Institute. (2023). The Spectrum of Prevention. http://www.preventioninstitute.org/tools/spectrum-prevention-0 (accessed 10 March 2023).

Rothwell, J. & Makridis, C. (2020). Politics is Wrecking America's Pandemic Response. Brookings Institution. https://www.brookings.edu/blog/up-front/2020/09/17/politics-is-wrecking-americas-pandemic-response/ (accessed 10 March 2023).

Tulchinsky, T. H. (2018). John Snow, cholera, the broad street pump; waterborne diseases then and now. *Case Studies in Public Health.* https://doi.org/10.1016/B978-0-12-804571-8.00017-2.

U.S. Department of Health and Human Services. (2023). About Healthy People. https://health.gov/healthypeople (accessed 10 March 2023).

United Nations. (2020a). UN Data Country Profile: United States. https://data.un.org/CountryProfile.aspx?crName=United%20States%20of%20America#Social (accessed 10 March 2023).

United Nations. (2020b). UN Data Country Profile: Zimbabwe. https://data.un.org/CountryProfile.aspx?crName=ZIMBABWE#Social (accessed 10 March 2023).

United Nations Children's Fund (UNICEF). (2023). Country Profiles: Zimbabwe. https://data.unicef.org/country/zwe/ (accessed 11 March 2023).

Wallack L. (2019). Building a social justice narrative for public health. *Health Education & Behavior: The Official Publication of the Society for Public Health Education.* https://doi.org/10.1177/1090198119867123.

Wen, L. (2021). *Lifelines: a doctor's journey in the fight for public health.* New York, NY: Metropolitan Books.

World Health Organization. (2015b). WHO Definition of Public Health. http://www.who.int/trade/glossary/story076/en/# (accessed 10 March 2023).

World Health Organization. (2023). Constitution. https://www.who.int/about/governance/constitution (accessed 10 March 2023).

World Health Organization (WHO). (2015). Social Determinants of Health. Retrieved from http://www.who.int/social_determinants/en/.

Zare, H., Fugai, A., Azadi, M., & Gaskin, D. J. (2022). How income inequality and race concentrate depression in low-income women in the US; 2005–2016. *Healthcare (Basel).* https://doi.org/10.3390/healthcare10081424.

Additional Resources

American Public Health Association. https://www.apha.org/.

Centers for Disease Control and Prevention. https://www.cdc.gov/.

Health Impact Partners. https://humanimpact.org

Just Cause/Causa Justa. https://cjjc.org/.

Office of Minority Health. https://www.minorityhealth.hhs.gov/.

Partners in Health. https://www.pih.org.

PolicyLink. https://www.policylink.org.

Prevention Institute. https://www.preventioninstitute.org/.

Public Health Awakened. https://publichealthawakened.org/.

United States Department of Health and Human Services. (2020). Healthy People 2030. https://health.gov/healthypeople (accessed 9 March 2023).

World Health Organization. https://www.who.int/.

Promoting Health Equity

4

Amie Fishman and Pau I. Crego

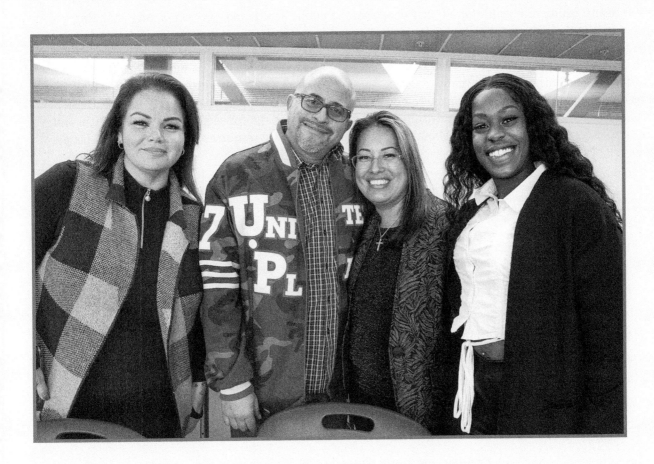

Foundations for Community Health Workers, Third Edition. Edited by Tim Berthold and Darouny Somsanith.
© 2024 John Wiley & Sons, Inc. Published 2024 by John Wiley & Sons, Inc.
Companion website: http://www.wiley.com/go/communityhealthworkers3E

Health inequities are differences in health status or in the distribution of health resources between different population groups, arising from the social conditions in which people are born, grow, live, work and age. Health inequities are unfair and could be reduced by the right mix of government policies.

(World Health Organization, 2018).

Introduction

The idea of health equity or "health for all" has deep roots in public health and has been a long-standing goal and aspiration. Yet throughout the United States and the world, people continue to experience dramatic health inequities. This means that some communities, and especially low-income communities of color, get sick more often and die much earlier than others. These inequities do not happen by chance, by merit, or as the result of genetic differences. Contrary to what many of us are taught to believe, health inequities are not the result of poor choices—people do not generally *choose* to be without resources to support their health. Rather, these inequities are socially, politically, and historically constructed: they are the consequences of the political and economic decisions we make as societies about the allocation of the basic resources and rights that all people require to live healthy lives.

It is within our power and our responsibility to prevent health inequity, and CHWs play an important role in these efforts.

WHAT YOU WILL LEARN

By studying the information in this chapter, you will be able to:

- Define health inequities
- Discuss and analyze the data that show health inequities among populations
- Describe the differences between sex assigned at birth, gender identity, and sexual orientation
- Explain how social inequities result in health inequities
- Discuss how health inequities are harmful to our society
- Describe and analyze how health inequities are preventable
- Examine the role of CHWs in overcoming health inequities and promoting social justice
- Connect the ideas from this chapter to issues of health equity in your own community

C3 Roles and Skills Addressed in Chapter 4

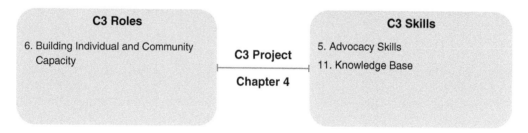

WORDS TO KNOW

Birthing Parent Mortality

Child Mortality

Cisgender

Gender Binary

Gender Identity

Pronouns

Redlining

Sex Assigned at Birth

Social Gradient

Transgender

Targeted Universalism

4.1 Defining Health Equity

Health equity means that everyone, regardless of their age, race/ethnicity, income, sexual orientation, documentation status, or any other aspect of their identity or experience, has a fair and just opportunity to be as healthy as they can possibly be. On the other hand, health inequities (also referred to as "health disparities") are differences in health status between communities that are avoidable and preventable, and therefore unfair and unjust.

What is the difference between equity and equality? Equality means giving everyone the same and expecting the same result. For example, a health equality approach was demonstrated during the COVID-19 pandemic, when the federal government initially provided four free COVID tests to every household. People living alone each got four tests, but for families with more than four people in a household, four tests were not enough to promote their health or achieve the outcome of people having access to free tests. Even further, for people who were unhoused or who had no permanent address, or those who used a P.O. box, no tests were made available. While attempting to provide "equal" access to health, the federal government actually contributed to health inequity. Why? Because they tried to give everyone *the same thing* rather than accounting for what people actually needed.

In contrast, health equity aims to give everyone what they need in order to achieve their highest level of health and wellness. This example from the Robert Wood Johnson Foundation helps us understand the difference. On the top of the image is "equality," where everyone gets the same bike (Robert Wood Johnson Foundation, 2017). We can see right away that the same bike does not work for everyone—some people need a bigger or smaller bike, or a bike they can operate with their arms. The bottom portion demonstrates equity, where people are given the same access—in this case, the ability to ride a bike—but that access looks different depending on each person's needs (Figure 4.1).

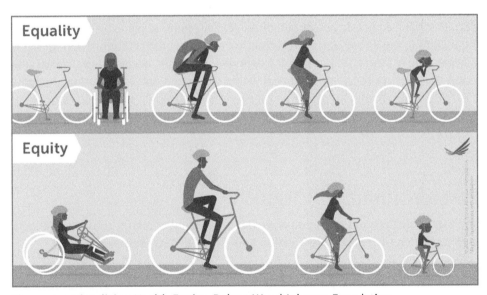

Figure 4.1 Visualizing Health Equity, Robert Wood Johnson Foundation

Here's another image that demonstrates the concept in relationship to communities (Figure 4.2):

The second image, created by artist Matt Kinshella, looks at how community resources are distributed (Kinshella, 2006). On the left side, we see two very different communities—one has broken windows, no trees, and few resources. The other is thriving. If we were to give "equal" amounts of resources to each of these communities, what would we expect to see in terms of outcomes? The community on the left would continue to struggle, while the one on the right would continue to thrive. Attempts to achieve health equality do not account for people's differing and diverse needs, nor the differential access to health that people are afforded based on political and economic policies.

On the right side of this graphic, we see a demonstration of equity, where each community is given the amount of resources it needs in order to thrive. This means that the community on the left side, which has been systematically under-resourced and under-supported, will need *more* resources, not the same, in order to achieve

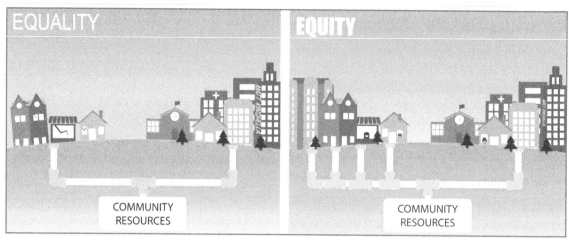

Figure 4.2 Equity Compared to Equality, Kinshella

the level of wellness and health that the community on the right enjoys. That is health equity in action, in practice, and in community.

Addressing the root causes of health inequities is an essential "upstream" approach for transforming the conditions of health everywhere and is especially critical in communities that experience the worst health outcomes due to disparities.

Public health researchers have long highlighted the connections between social conditions, democracy, and health. The national plan for health in the United States—Healthy People 2030—includes a goal to "Eliminate health disparities, achieve health equity, and attain health literacy to improve the health and well-being of all" (Healthy People, 2030, 2023a). Fostering equitable health outcomes is also a guiding principle for many international entities and efforts, including the World Health Organization and the United Nations (UN). In 1948, the UN ratified the International Declaration of Human Rights, which included Article 25, declaring that "Everyone has the right to a standard of living adequate for the health and well-being of himself and of his family, including food, clothing, housing and medical care and necessary social services..." (United Nations, 2023).

- *What resources do the communities where you live and work require access to in order to achieve health equity?*

What Do YOU? Think

4.2 Social Determinants of Health

Health is shaped by the conditions and the context we live in. In public health, these are called the social determinants of health, which the Centers for Disease and Control (CDC) defines as:

> *the nonmedical factors that influence health outcomes. They are the conditions in which people are born, grow, work, live, and age, and the wider set of forces and systems shaping the conditions of daily life. These forces and systems include economic policies and systems, development agendas, social norms, social policies, racism, climate change, and political systems.* (Centers for Disease Control, 2022a)

The field of public health focuses on the factors that cause and contribute to patterns of illness and death in populations, and the social determinants of health are the single most influential factor in the health of communities. Out of five overarching goals, Healthy People 2030 notes that it is crucial to "create social, physical, and economic environments that promote attaining the full potential for health and well-being for all" (Healthy People, 2030, 2023b).

In order to further understand this important public health concept, take a few moments to consider how the social determinants of health may have influenced your own life and that of your communities.

- What were the conditions in which you were born and grew up?
- Consider factors such as you and your family's access to food, stable housing, education, jobs at a living wage, affordable and culturally responsive health care, and civil rights protections.

Upon reflection, many of us are likely to conclude that the social conditions we just mentioned affect our lives and health to some extent. The social determinants also interact with one another. For example, a person's experiences in education, and access (or lack of access) to higher education will often determine what type of jobs they are able to secure. The type of employment they have (as well as how much money they earn in that job) will dictate the choices they can afford with regard to housing, food, and health coverage, among other things.

ECONOMIC STATUS, EMPLOYMENT, AND EDUCATION

Economic inequity has grown dramatically in the United States and in many other countries in the Global North, though income inequity is higher in the United States than in other wealthy nations (Horowitz, Igielnik, & Kochhar, 2020). Since the 1970s, the richest 1% of the U.S. population has experienced the fastest rate of income growth (Inequality.org, 2023). As of 2019, the richest 1% of people in the United States make 84 times as much as the bottom 20% (Inequality.org, 2023). As income and wealth gaps have increased between the richest and the poorest residents, poverty rates have essentially remained the same. In the United States, one of the wealthiest countries in the world, 1 in 10 people live in poverty (Semega, Kollar, Creamer, & Mohanty, 2019).

Income (the amount of money a person or household makes during a year) and wealth (the total value of a person's property, possessions, and money) are closely connected to health. Think about how someone's health may be impacted if they have enough resources to live comfortably, compared to someone who is constantly struggling to make ends meet. A person with economic opportunity and stability will likely have more access to nutritious food, physical activity, lower stress levels, better mental health, and easier access to health care. In contrast, a person who is struggling financially will generally rely on cheaper (and often less nutritious) food, may not have time to engage in physical activity, will have higher stress levels and consequently worse mental health, and may not have high-quality health care. However, it is not just our individual economic status that influences our health; economic inequity in and of itself can lead to worse health outcomes for a population. How income is distributed, and the stress caused by having low status in a hierarchical society, negatively impacts everyone's health. Since wealth is accrued over generations, homeownership is a primary way that people in the United States gain wealth because property values tend to rise over time. But some communities—particularly people of color—have been systematically excluded from homeownership in this country, which has resulted in serious wealth inequities at the population level (see the example of "redlining" below, for an example of how anti-Black policies have created unjust differences in homeownership and wealth).

Education, and the opportunities it opens up in terms of employment, are associated with better health overall (Zajacova & Lawrence, 2018). Some examples of how educational advancement can improve health include:

- Higher education often leads to jobs that pay better and offer more choices of what type of job to pursue. As we discussed earlier, economic stability opens the door to better nutrition, physical activity, and other health behaviors that reduce the likelihood of developing health conditions.

- Better compensation, and more comprehensive benefits, can improve our relationship to work and stress. Higher-paying jobs tend to be less stressful, less reliant on physical labor (which can lead to injuries), and more manageable when there is access to time off through vacation and personal time. Sick leave and comprehensive health coverage make it easier to take good care of one's own health and the health of family members.

- People with higher levels of education have more health knowledge and health literacy and can better use that information to improve their health habits.

- People with higher levels of education tend to have a larger and more diverse social network, along with higher economic status and greater agency to control or influence what happens to them. These aspects are associated with better stress management and healthy behaviors.

Nevertheless, serious inequities exist in access to high-quality education, from childhood education through college. The amount of money invested in education per child—and therefore, the quality of education each child receives—varies significantly by state, and even more by locality. This, coupled with the disparate treatment in schools of Black, disabled, Lesbian, Gay, Bisexual, Transgender, Queer and/or Questioning, Intersex, Asexual, and other identities (LGBTQIA+), and children of color, leads to consequential inequities due to geography, race, immigration status, income, and other identities. Furthermore, our early childhood experiences in school strongly impact our ability and desire to pursue higher education as adults, and since higher education is extremely costly, with much of the cost even at public institutions being charged to students directly, high levels of student loan debt have become increasingly common. These all constitute major barriers to education, which as noted earlier, is a crucial avenue for economic advancement and improved health.

- *How does the quality of education vary across different areas of the city or county where you live?*

- *What role does education play in promoting the health and well-being of the communities you serve?*

- *How accessible and affordable is a college education to low-income students in the city, county, or state where you live?*

NEIGHBORHOOD QUALITY AND ENVIRONMENTAL HEALTH

The physical environment we live in can pose health hazards, like pollution or radiation. It can influence our health behaviors including eating, physical movement, social connection, or isolation. The physical environment can expose us to chronic stress, which results in serious consequences for our mental and physical health (such as impacts on our cardiovascular and immune systems—see Chapter 12 for more discussion of the effects of chronic stress).

In recent decades, public health efforts have taken a comprehensive look at the places people live, to try to improve their chances of a long, healthy life by improving neighborhoods.

Although nutritious and affordable food is essential for good health, low-income neighborhoods frequently lack grocery stores and have to rely instead on fast-food restaurants and liquor stores, which mostly sell processed foods, tobacco, and alcohol. Low-income neighborhoods also tend to have less green spaces and fewer parks for people to exercise.

Other aspects of the physical environment, such as transportation and violence, also strongly influence health. Living in a neighborhood without adequate transportation can affect the likelihood of getting a good job or pursuing higher education, or even reaching a health clinic, while also requiring a lot of time that could otherwise be used for health-promoting activities. Limited access to health care facilities in some neighborhoods affects preventative care, timely diagnosis of life-threatening illness, and management of chronic conditions. The rate of violence in a community not only causes injury and death to those it impacts directly; it also discourages people from engaging in outdoor physical activity and from establishing social connections with their neighbors and community members. The combination of less physical activity, feelings of isolation, and more stress leads to higher rates of chronic illness (see Chapter 16).

HEALTH CARE ACCESS AND QUALITY

Access to health care is not universal in the United States, and the lack of access contributes to health inequities between populations. When health care is not available or affordable, many people miss out on preventative care (screening tests, health advising, and vaccinations), chronic conditions are less likely to be well-managed, and diseases like cancer may be diagnosed later in their development.

Since the passage of the Affordable Care Act (ACA) in 2010, the rate of uninsured people in the United States has been reduced by almost half. The Commonwealth Fund reports that in 2013 (shortly before the implementation of the main parts of the ACA) 20.4% of people in the United States were uninsured, and the differences between racial groups were significant: while 14.5% of white people were uninsured, the rates of uninsured Black residents (24.4%) and Latine/a/o residents (40.2%) were much higher. Cost was a barrier to care for many people, but again impacted mostly Latine/a/o and Black people: 27.8% and 23.2%, respectively, avoided care within the previous year because of cost, compared with 15.1% of whites (Commonwealth Fund, 2023). Between 2013 and 2021, insurance coverage rates improved for all groups (12.1% uninsured), and the coverage gap between racial groups got smaller: in 2021, 8.2% white people, 13.5% Black people, and 24.5% Latine/a/o people were uninsured (Commonwealth Fund, 2023).

In addition to insurance barriers, differences in the quality of health care also contribute to serious inequities. These differences in the quality of care can be due to prejudice and bias of medical professionals, as well as bias within the institutions and practices of health care delivery themselves (more on health inequities later in this chapter). An example of this is the alarmingly high rates of transgender and gender nonconforming people who are denied care and mistreated by medical providers. Fifty-five percent (55%) of those who sought coverage for gender-affirming surgeries and 25% of those seeking hormone treatment (both established medically necessary treatments for some transgender people) were denied health care, and 33% of all transgender people who saw a health care provider in a one-year period had one or more negative experiences related to transphobia such as being refused treatment, verbally harassed, or physically or sexually assaulted, or having to teach the provider about transgender people in order to get appropriate care (James et al., 2016). In addition, these experiences cause transgender and gender nonconforming people to avoid health care encounters with 23% of transgender people in the United States not visiting a doctor when they need to due to fear of being mistreated (James et al., 2016).

Given these challenges of inequitable access to quality health care, CHWs have an important role to play in helping to ensure that all patients are treated with dignity and respect.

Defining Sex, Gender, and Gender Identity

To talk about gender and gender identity, it is important to first define some terms.

While often used interchangeably, gender and sex are actually two distinct aspects of human identity and experience. **Sex assigned at birth** refers to the category given to a child when they are born, generally based on their distinctive sexual organs or genitalia. While most of us have been taught to believe that there are only two distinct sexes, male or female, in reality there are also intersex people, meaning those that are born with ambiguous or a combination of sexual organs. Gender or **gender identity** is different from sex—it refers to behavioral, cultural, and psychological traits through which one expresses their gender (Merriam Webster, 2023).

Dominant notions of gender tend to fall into an either/or framework (meaning either masculine or feminine)—this is also known as the **gender binary**. It asserts that people are either men who are masculine, or women who are feminine. We learn this from the very beginning of our lives, when we are told that girls like pink and are "emotional," whereas boys like blue, and "don't cry," or that they are "strong." These ideas shape our lives, what we believe is possible for us, and how we see ourselves in the world.

People whose gender identity corresponds with gender expectations based on their sex assigned at birth are known as **cisgender**. Alternately, **transgender** refers to people whose gender identity differs from the expectations associated with the sex they were assigned at birth. While we are referencing sex assigned at birth, people who identify as transgender exist on a spectrum in which some have "transitioned," which may include some combination of hormone treatments and/or gender-affirming surgeries or not.

Pronouns is another term that often comes up when talking about gender identity. In this context, pronouns are the words we use to refer to someone when speaking about them, without using their name, usually she/her, he/him, or they/them. We use pronouns all the time to avoid repeating the person's name over and over again. Often, people assume a person's pronouns based on their perceptions about that individual's gender identity, but this may lead to using incorrect pronouns.

SOCIAL AND COMMUNITY CONTEXT

Social and community support (or lack thereof) affect our physical, emotional, and psychological health. For example, the stress of being perceived and/or treated as "less than" on the basis of race, ethnicity, gender identity, sexual orientation, educational level, immigration status, national origin, age, disability status, or for any other reason, causes physiological reactions in the human body that contribute to chronic disease.

These high levels of chronic stress from racism and other forms of discrimination result in higher rates of physical and mental health conditions, premature aging, and death (Greenberg, 2020; Guidi, Lucente, Sonino, & Fava, 2021; Sandoiu, 2021). Exposure to chronic stress over a lifetime helps explain why a person whose social status changes over time—for example, someone who grew up low-income and later moved into a middle-class economic status—may still have higher levels of chronic disease than those who experienced higher status all their lives—even when both groups have similar health habits as adults.

What Matters Most: Individual or Social Factors?

While in recent decades, the field of public health has relied on the framework of the social determinants of health to better understand and address health inequities, historically (and sometimes, to this day) health professionals mistakenly assumed that health inequities were mainly affected by genetics and personal health behaviors.

Genes certainly influence our health. Some illnesses tend to run in families, and some of those illnesses are influenced by genes that are passed down, biologically, from parent to child. Some genes, or combinations of genes, give people a certain weakness or predisposition toward an illness. However, while genes can explain the differences in health between one family and another, they do very little to explain health inequities among different populations.

Health behaviors are often presented as the leading cause of illness, especially those that are sexually transmitted (such as HIV) or strongly affected by nutrition and physical activity (such as diabetes and hypertension). But health behaviors are strongly influenced by the social determinants of health. While personal behaviors do influence health—many CHWs work specifically on helping clients adopt healthier behaviors—efforts to improve health behaviors are generally more effective if they take into account the social environment. Likewise, changes in the community or in public policy can make it easier for people to change health-related behaviors (such as policies that promote easier access to affordable and healthy foods).

It is now well-established that health is mainly influenced by social and political factors, while still being somewhat impacted by genetics and personal health behaviors. This understanding of the social determinants of health guides CHWs and other public health professionals in promoting health equity.

THE INFLUENCE OF POLITICAL, ECONOMIC, AND SOCIAL FORCES

There are dramatic differences in how essential resources—access to food, housing, health care, education, civil rights, etc.—are distributed between and within nations. These inequities are not random. To a large extent, they are created by political, economic, environmental, and social forces, which are often translated into policies.

The CDC's Office of Policy, Performance, and Evaluation defines policy as "a law, regulation, procedure, administrative action, incentive, or voluntary practice of governments and other institutions" (Center for Disease Control and Prevention, 2022b). Institutions design and implement policies to create guidelines or rules for how resources should be distributed, how processes should be organized, and how people should behave. Generally, the policies that influence the social determinants of health are those put in place by government entities; these are also called public policies.

An example of how policies have influenced the social determinants of health, and consequently had grave impacts on the health of entire communities, is the practice of "**redlining**." In the United States, between the 1930s and the 1960s, the percentage of people who owned their homes skyrocketed, but Black communities and other communities of color were *intentionally* locked out of the opportunity to build wealth through homeownership. Neighborhoods where Black people and other communities of color lived were "redlined" on city maps. City maps were color-coded based on how desirable the neighborhood was—according to the Home Owners' Loan Corporation and other government agencies—ranging from green (which were predominantly white neighborhoods) to red (which were majority Black areas). Simply because Black people lived in those neighborhoods, properties in those areas were considered less desirable, and therefore property values were expected to go down. To learn more about redlining, visit the *Mapping Inequality* website listed in Additional Resources at the end of the chapter.

Black families were also denied bank loans due to widespread racism, under the excuse that homes in traditionally Black neighborhoods would lose value over time. Between 1934 and 1962, the Federal Housing Administration and the Veterans Administration financed over $120 billion in new housing; however, less than 2% of this was available to communities of color, and it was mostly located in segregated areas (Lipsitz, 2009). Speculators exploited these anti-Black policies to make more money at the expense of Black communities. For example, they would use scare tactics to get white homeowners to sell at low prices, and then turn around and sell those same properties to Black families at higher prices. Since most Black Americans could not get bank loans, speculators would loan money to Black families so they could afford a home but would do so at high interest rates; speculators would also loan money on a "contract" system that turned over full ownership of the house to the speculator if the family was even slightly late with a payment (Coates, 2014). As a result of these anti-Black federal housing and lending policies, fewer Black people and communities of color were and are homeowners, compared to whites. Since homeownership is a key avenue to building wealth, redlining policies have had a lasting impact on economic inequities in this country.

When we examine any aspect of life where stark inequities are present, we find that public policies have played a large role in creating and maintaining those inequities. As a key avenue through which political, social, and economic forces are put into practice, policies can significantly influence the social determinants of health, and in turn, materially affect the health of individuals and communities. *The good news is that policies are not set in stone, and CHWs and public health professionals have an important role in advocating for change to improve the health of communities* (see Section 4.4 on Public Health and Social Justice).

Anti-Trans Legislation and Population Health

Policies and laws are sometimes created with the intent to harm specific communities. This happens when people who have the power to draft and implement policies are motivated by prejudice and fear.

In recent years, the United States has seen a rise in anti-transgender sentiment that has motivated an increasing number of bills introduced to state legislatures with the explicit goal of harming transgender people. The sudden surge in legislative hate in the past few years is alarming: in 2020 66 anti-trans bills were introduced, and every year since the number of anti-trans bills has increased (144 in 2021 and 174 in 2022). As of May 2023, 549 anti-trans bills had been introduced to state legislatures and this number increases every week (Trans Legislation Tracker, 2023).

These bills—many of which are becoming state laws—intentionally create additional barriers to health care and other key aspects of health for transgender people. They do so by limiting access to public restrooms, sports, and medically necessary gender-affirming health care for adults and children. Furthermore, these laws encourage schools, families, and individuals to report transgender people entering public restrooms in accordance with their gender identity, to deny transgender children the opportunity to participate in school sports, and to access transition-related treatments considered safe and medically necessary for some transgender people. Some of these laws ban using correct names or pronouns and providing gender-affirming care to transgender children, and encourage reporting trans-affirming schools, families, and medical providers.

The rise of anti-trans legislation is a striking example of how political forces can seriously influence the social determinants of health, and in turn, worsen health outcomes for a community. These laws will undoubtedly have long-lasting negative effects on the health and mental health of transgender and gender nonconforming adults and children in this country, at a time when this community already experiences grave inequities.

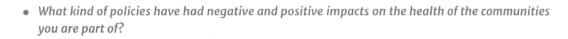 *What kind of policies have had negative and positive impacts on the health of the communities you are part of?*

 What Do YOU Think?

4.3 Health Inequities Between Communities

The reality that inequity exists is not surprising; however, the large-scale and enduring quality of many health inequities—and the impact they have on human lives—represents an urgent public health and human rights crisis. Health inequities are neither natural nor unchangeable. In reality, they have been created and perpetuated throughout history, codified and enforced through laws and policies, and justified through dominant beliefs often rooted in prejudice and discrimination. The fact that these inequities are often accepted as "just the way things are" or viewed as reflective of innate deficiencies within marginalized communities—a belief that is itself inherently racist and biased—further limits our collective outrage and determination to address this societal harm.

Rather than being the result of "bad choices," "bad fortune," or genetic predisposition, most of the poor health outcomes that communities experience are the result of decades and generations of cumulative harm from the lack of access to essential resources. CHWs often work with clients experiencing the mounting negative health effects that generations of poverty, discrimination, and other social and economic exclusion create. Many CHWs have been affected by these same barriers in their own lives. Yet it can still be surprising, and even shocking, to learn of the range of health inequities that persist today.

HEALTH INEQUITIES BETWEEN NATIONS

There is no shortage of data about health inequities. It is important to remember that these data represent real people and their lived experiences. Behind the data are the stories, lessons, struggles, and resilience of communities experiencing the highest rates of illness and premature death.

Life expectancy or the number of years people live on average, is one of the most common measures and comparisons of health. While life expectancy has increased dramatically all over the world in the last 150 years, there are dramatic differences in life expectancy between different populations. For example, in 2020 life expectancy was estimated at 61 in Zimbabwe, 69 in Iraq, and 85 in Japan. In other words, people in Japan live, on average, 16 years longer than people in Iraq and 24 years longer than people in Zimbabwe (World Bank, 2023).

Child mortality or the estimated number of children who die before the age of five out of every 100,000 live births, and **Birthing parent mortality**, or the estimated number of people who die as a result of pregnancy or childbirth per 100,000 live births, are other commonly used measures of comparative health. Recent data show that in 2021, children born in Somalia were 38 times more likely to die before the age of five than children born in Sweden (112 deaths per 100,000 compared to 3 per 100,000). People giving birth in Afghanistan in 2020 were 124 times more likely to die from complications related to pregnancy and childbirth than those giving birth in Sweden (620 deaths per 100,000 compared to 5 per 100,000) (World Bank, 2023). These are not small or trivial differences or inequities in health: they represent devastating losses for families, communities, and nations.

Learning About Health Inequities

When we present data on health inequities at City College of San Francisco, CHW students often experience anger, frustration, sorrow, and other powerful emotions. The authors of this book share these responses. We usually pair the evidence of deep inequities in health with evidence that inequities can be changed for the better, by advocating for and improving public policies that shape health. Our hope is that a growing awareness of health inequities will inspire us to advocate for a more just world.

- *What are your reactions as you study the topic of health inequities?*

HEALTH STATUS IN THE UNITED STATES COMPARED TO OTHER WEALTHY NATIONS

The United States spends significantly more money on health care than other wealthy nations yet ranks near the bottom in most leading health indicators. While the United States spends more money on health care than any other country, it ranks 70th among nations in terms of life expectancy (2021 data), lower than Australia, Greece, or China.

A study of 11 wealthy nations including Canada, France, Australia, Sweden, and the United States showed that the United States ranked last in almost all key health indicators. "U.S. performance is lowest among the countries, including having the highest infant mortality rate (5.7 deaths per 1,000 live births) and lowest life expectancy at age 60 (23.1 years)" (Commonwealth Fund, 2021).

> The Commonwealth Fund concludes: "Four features distinguish top performing countries from the United States: (1) they provide for universal coverage and remove cost barriers; (2) they invest in primary care systems to ensure that high-value services are equitably available in all communities to all people; (3) they reduce administrative burdens that divert time, efforts, and spending from health improvement efforts; and (4) they invest in social services, especially for children and working-age adults" (Commonwealth Fund, 2021).

HEALTH INEQUITIES WITHIN THE UNITED STATES

In general, people in the United States experience a steady and direct relationship between social advantage and health, sometimes referred to as a **social gradient**. This means that for each step one goes up or down in social advantage (e.g., going up in income), there is a corresponding change in health. The same is true for educational level—people with college degrees tend to be healthier than high school graduates, and high school graduates tend to be healthier than those who do not finish high school.

The social gradient does not only apply to income and health but can also be used to understand the ways that intersecting experiences of social advantage work together to determine health. A study released in 2022 reviewed 2 million births in California and found that while wealthy people had the highest number of at-risk births, they and their newborns were most likely to survive the year after childbirth, unless the family was Black. The richest Black people giving birth and their babies are *twice as likely to die* as the richest white people giving birth and their babies (Kennedy-Moulton et al., 2022).

This trend suggests that if we want to improve health across the population, it is not enough to get everyone over some threshold, like the Federal Poverty Level. Instead, we need to address the many ways inequity affects the nation as a whole. One way of thinking about this is what is known as the *"curb-cut effect."* The idea is simple: curb cuts, or sloped areas that connect sidewalks to streets, were a hard-fought victory for the disability rights community in the 1970s, a necessary modification to allow accessibility onto sidewalks and into buildings for wheelchair users, people with walkers and canes, and others with limited mobility. But who uses curb cuts today? People pushing strollers, people delivering supplies, people carrying luggage, and more. In fact, we all benefit from the curb cut.

Angela Glover Blackwell explains how curb-cut thinking animates the idea of equity in her article "The Curb-cut Effect":

> There's an ingrained societal suspicion that intentionally supporting one group hurts another. That equity is a zero sum game. In fact, when the nation targets support where it is needed most—when we create the circumstances that allow those who have been left behind to participate and contribute fully—everyone wins. The corollary is also true: When we ignore the challenges faced by the most vulnerable among us, those challenges, magnified many times over, become a drag on economic growth, prosperity, and national well-being. (Blackwell, 2017)

Pervasive social and economic inequities in the United States due to differential and discriminatory treatment and access based on race, class, education level, gender, gender identity, ability, immigration status, sexual orientation, geographic location, and more, are at the root of health inequities. These characteristics and experiences have undoubtedly affected your clients' lives and experiences and are important to understand.

Of these, inequities based on income and race have received the most attention and focused research. We discuss several of these inequities in more detail below.

RACE, ETHNICITY, AND HEALTH INEQUITY

Health inequities based on race or ethnicity are significant and increasing in the United States, despite our federal government's policy to eliminate health disparities. The CDC recognizes racism as a "serious threat to the Public's health" (Centers for Disease Control and Prevention, 2021).

We must make the distinction that it is not someone's race or ethnicity that causes health inequities, but rather the discriminatory or preferential treatment that person or group may receive *because of their race*.

As we discuss racial inequities in health, it is also important to understand that race is a social and historical construct rather than a truly biological one. There is much more genetic variation among people of any given race, than between different races. While individuals who share a specific place of origin (say Greek Americans or Laotian Americans) have certain genetic traits in common, the Greek American who is "white" may have no more genes in common with an Irish American as they do with a Japanese American. Likewise, Laotian Americans, Japanese Americans, and Pakistani Americans may all be considered "Asian/Pacific Islander," but their genes are tremendously varied. Also many people identify with more than one race or ethnicity. Our racial categories have been constructed socially and often do not accurately reflect people's experience or identity.

Who is considered to be "white" in the United States has changed over time and is deeply connected to this country's history of slavery and genocide of indigenous communities. The Pew Research Center has an interactive website dedicated to this history, looking at how the Census categories changed over time to reflect dominant political, economic, and social beliefs and practices (Pew Research Center, 2020).

While not a biological fact, race remains a deeply meaningful term historically, socially, economically, and politically. Many people identify strongly as being a member of a particular race, and even if they do not, others may treat them in a certain way based on assumptions about their race. In a race-conscious (and racially stratified) country like the United States, there are some similarities in experience within any given race. For CHWs, your clients' racial identities and experiences will shape their needs, priorities, and interactions with you. For all of these reasons, it is meaningful to discuss racial and ethnic inequities in health.

While great variation in health exists within any racial or ethnic group, the overall picture is one of higher rates of illness and premature death among non-white populations in the United States. This has remained true even with the increase in access to health care due to policies such as the Affordable Care Act, which reduced the percentage of uninsured people across all racial and ethnic groups in the United States.

Another reason for these disparities is the ways that racism and bias exist within health care institutions themselves and are perpetuated by health care providers, who "are less likely to deliver effective treatments to people of color when compared to their white counterparts - even after controlling for characteristics like class, health behaviors, comorbidities, and access to health insurance and health care services" (American Bar Association, 2023).

Health inequities between Black and white people in the United States have been most studied because they have been the most extreme and pervasive. Chapter 15 goes deeper into the historical roots of this inequity. Black Americans of all ages die at higher rates than whites. The data presented in Table 4.1 show that Black infants are more than two times as likely to die before the age of one than white infants born in the United States. Black people are two and half times more likely to die due to complications of pregnancy or childbirth than whites in the United States. Finally, white people are expected to live almost 6 years longer than Black people.

It is important to note that the health inequities between Black and white people are not static. Like the curb-cut effect, change and improvement happen when targeted interventions occur. But in order for these changes to be sustained, we must also address the social determinants and institutional or structural barriers to equity.

- *What is the gap or inequity between life expectancy for Black and white people in your city? Have they narrowed or grown over the last few years?*

What Do
YOU ?
Think :

- *What things might you do as a CHW to help narrow these gaps?*

Table 4.1 Health Indicators for Black and White People in the United States

POPULATION	INFANT MORTALITY (2019) PER 1,000 LIVE BIRTHS	MATERNAL MORTALITY (2020) PER 100,000 LIVE BIRTHS	LIFE EXPECTANCY (2021) LIFE SPAN EXPECTED AT BIRTH
Black residents	10.6	37.3	70.8
White residents	4.5	14.9	76.4

Source: National Institutes of Health (2021), Centers for Disease Control and Prevention (2019), and Hill, Ndugga, & Artiga, (2023).

The data regarding health inequities for Indigenous, Latine/a/o, and Asian communities in the United States are more mixed. Life expectancy for Indigenous communities in 2021 was 65.2 years, compared to 77.7 for Latine/a/os, 76.4 for whites, and 83.5 for Asians (Hill, Ndugga, & Artiga, 2023; Office of Minority Health, 2023a, b). Indigenous and Black communities saw the largest declines in life expectancy from 2019 to 2021, during the COVID-19 pandemic. That said, it is important to note that subgroups within these racial or ethnic categories are often lumped together, even though there are many significant differences between them. For example, the infant mortality rate for Puerto Ricans (5.6 per 1000 live births) is significantly higher than for whites. However, the rates for other Latino groups are similar to or lower than the rate for whites (Cuban: 3.8; Central & South American: 4.0) (Office of Minority Health, 2018). Asian American & Pacific Islander (AAPI) parents experienced an infant mortality rate of 3.39 (Ely et al., 2022). Unfortunately, it is still rare to find health data that distinguish among the many distinct AAPI populations, who trace their roots to 20 different countries within Asia. When available, the data usually indicate wide variation in rates of disease or premature death among different AAPI communities. For example, Burmese American households in 2021 had lower incomes than Asian American households overall: $44,400 vs. $85,800 (Budiman & Ruiz, 2021).

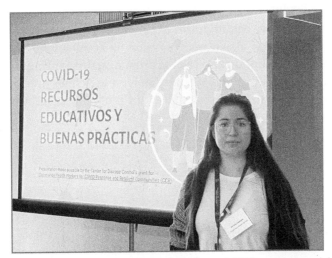

A CHW facilitates a presentation about COVID-19 in Spanish.

MIGRATION AND DOCUMENTATION STATUS

Health inequities also persist in the United States based on migration and documentation status. While migrants to the United States generally have a higher life expectancy than people born in the United States, they are much less likely to have health insurance or receive preventative health care services. Nearly half of undocumented immigrants (46%) and a quarter of documented immigrants were uninsured in 2021, compared with less than 10 percent of citizens (Kaiser Family Foundation, 2022). Interestingly, new migrants to the United States tend to have better health than those born here of the same gender, age, income, and educational level; this pattern is called the "Latino paradox" or the "immigrant paradox." However immigrants' health status declines the longer they live in the United States (Sax, 2021). Changes in diet and activity levels can contribute to this decline, along with the loss of social ties with extended family, and increased exposure to discrimination.

GENDER IDENTITY

Like race, gender is a socially constructed idea, and one that often misses much of the complexity and richness of human experience. In reality, people express their gender in all kinds of ways, and humans of all genders experience and express emotions, strength, and a combination of characteristics that have been labeled "masculine" or "feminine." In fact, many people do not self-identify within this gender binary, and instead see themselves as gender nonconforming or gender non-binary. This means that, while these gendered characteristics sometimes align with a person's sex assigned at birth, often they do not, and some people choose to express their gender in ways that do not fit neatly in either category.

This is not a new concept—people have existed and thrived outside of the gender binary throughout history and across all cultures and countries. In some places, they have been vilified, but in others, they hold important roles in society and communities. Indigenous communities in what is now called the United States for example have long recognized two-spirit members. Zapotec communities in Oaxaca, Mexico, recognize the Muxes as a third gender. Samoan communities recognize four gender roles, including fa'afafine, and fa'afatama, which are both fluid. These are just a few of the many places where people have not only recognized but celebrated gender expression outside of the gender binary.

This reality challenges dominant views and people who express themselves outside of this binary, or in ways that differ from how others think they ought to, are often targets of discrimination, harassment, violence, and even political attacks. The rise in state-wide laws banning drag queens is just one example of these political attacks. Drag queens are performers who often include exaggerated interpretations of femininity in their performances—through hair, makeup, dress, and mannerisms, that play with stereotypes of gender. These expressions of transphobia and sexism translate to health disparities for non-cisgender male communities, including women, transgender people, and gender nonconforming people.

Transgender and gender nonconforming communities experience some of the highest rates of HIV infection in the United States, as well as high rates of violence, depression, unemployment, and attempted suicide (James et al., 2016). Due to persistent discrimination and related stigma against such groups, comparably little research is available regarding the health status of transgender and gender nonconforming communities. Fortunately, this is beginning to change. For CHWs, one of the most important ways you may advocate for all of your clients is by helping ensure they receive gender-inclusive care.

Gender-Inclusive Care

HERE ARE SOME TIPS FOR PROVIDING GENDER-INCLUSIVE CARE FOR ALL CLIENTS:	
DOS	**DON'TS**
DO ask people what they like to be called, including what name and pronouns they would like you to use.	DON'T assume a person's gender or pronouns.
DO ask questions to understand the client's needs and experiences and how to best support them.	DON'T ask questions out of sheer curiosity that you don't need to know. *Questions about whether a transgender person has had gender-affirming surgery, or what their name used to be, are deeply personal questions that would be inappropriate to ask anyone in casual conversation.*
DO practice cultural humility.	DON'T expect the client to educate you on all things transgender.
DO demonstrate respect by using the person's correct name and pronouns. If it is difficult for you to understand, seek out support and practice with your colleagues.	DON'T make comments about how weird or hard or different it is to refer to the person correctly.
DO accept that you will make mistakes and be prepared to offer a sincere apology and a commitment to keep learning.	DON'T get defensive if you are corrected; simply apologize, and then move on.

While women have a higher life expectancy than men in most nations, they experience disproportionately higher rates of domestic and sexual violence, with the resulting trauma, depression, and other chronic health conditions. They also face discrimination in the diagnosis and treatment of certain health conditions, and experience more days of illness per year, higher rates of disability, and poorer health overall (Crimmins, Shim, Zhang, & Kim, 2019; National Center for Health Statistics, 2023). While some inequities in health can be directly tied to biological differences between the sexes (e.g., higher rates of breast cancer in women than men), others are largely influenced by the status and treatment of women and girls (e.g., higher rates of depression in women than men).

When the U.S. Supreme Court overturned Roe vs. Wade in 2022, effectively ending federal protection of access to abortion, the United States saw a dramatic rise in state-wide level abortion bans. These restrictions directly impact the health of people who require reproductive health care and cannot access it, or fear that their attempts to access it will result in discrimination, physical harm, or criminal prosecution for themselves or their providers.

SEXUAL ORIENTATION

Like gender identity, sexual orientation exists along a spectrum, and continues to evolve to include new orientations and expressions. As of 2022, 7.1% of the U.S. population identified as LGBTQIA+. That number is significantly higher (over 20%) for those in their 20s (Jones, 2022). The large increase in young people who identify as LGBTQIA+ may indicate increased acceptance and visibility of diverse sexual orientation and expression; however, health inequities continue to exist and persist based on sexual orientation across the lifespan (Jones, 2022).

Repealing the "Don't ask, Don't tell" policy in 2010 that barred LGBTQIA+ people from serving in the military, and the Defense of Marriage Act in 2015 that barred LGBTQIA+ people from marrying demonstrated increased acceptance for LGBTQIA+ people into mainstream society. However, that increased acceptance was met with increased backlash, resulting in the introduction of new state-level laws targeting gender identity and sexual orientation. These include Florida's "Don't Say Gay" bill, passed into law in 2023, which restricts educators from being able to discuss gender and sexual orientation in their classrooms, and restrictions on access to gender-affirming care.

Policies like these directly result in negative health outcomes, including increased stress, depression, suicidality, substance use, tobacco use, alcohol use, and other behaviors. They also result in diminished access to health care because LGBTQIA+ people may experience discrimination or the fear of discrimination from health care providers themselves, meaning they may be less likely to seek out medical care when needed. This is precisely why affirming care is so critical and why CHWs play such an important role in understanding the barriers clients may face to accessing health care and supportive services, and standing with them as they navigate through those challenging situations.

4.4 Public Health and Social Justice

Health inequities—and the social, political, and economic forces that cause them—are not fixed. Every day, health advocates, community leaders, public health departments, and other health professionals engage in organizing and advocacy to improve health conditions at the local, state, and national levels. Like other public health practitioners, CHWs have a professional responsibility to be knowledgeable about health inequities and their causes, to acknowledge their impacts on clients and communities, and to address the social determinants that lead to health inequities.

The framework of targeted universalism is an approach to advance equity. "**Targeted universalism** is based on exploring the gaps that exist between individuals, groups, and places that can benefit from a policy or program and the aspiration-establishing goal. Targeted universalism policy formulations do more than close or bridge such gaps, but ultimately clarify and reveal the barriers or impediments to achieving the universal goal for different groups of people... Targeted universalism emphasizes goals, and recenters the policy debate toward a focus on outcomes" (Powell, Menendian, & Ake, 2019).

The ecological model—first introduced in Chapter 3—is a helpful tool for identifying where to intervene to create change. By reviewing the ecological model, you will see that there are opportunities to advocate for health equity at every level: individual, family and friends, neighborhood and community, and nation and society levels. CHWs play an important role in promoting social justice and health equity, whether they are supporting individuals to manage chronic conditions, facilitating support groups, or engaging in community organizing campaigns.

In their day-to-day work, CHWs typically influence change at the individual, and friends and family, levels. For example, when CHWs help people access health care, find transportation, apply for jobs, plant a community garden, manage their asthma, or reduce tobacco use, they promote better health outcomes. Supporting change at the individual level also empowers people to influence their own health and that of their communities. The sense of accomplishment and social support that a client often feels when they work toward a health goal with a CHW can also help relieve the chronic stress that is common among communities most impacted by inequity.

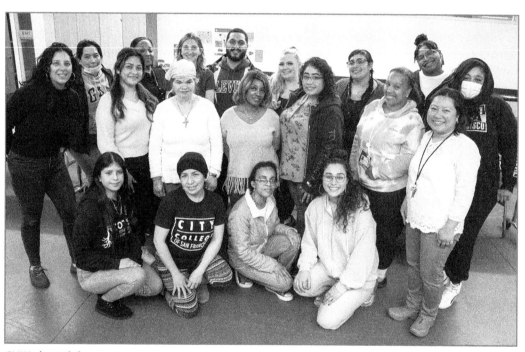
CHWs in training.

There are many opportunities for CHWs to promote health at the levels of community and society. They can do this by changing social environments, addressing equitable allocation of resources, removing physical hazards, and changing public policies. CHWs identify health inequities that impact the lives of communities they work with and belong to. This knowledge is a necessary first step to envisioning social justice and can lead to community organizing. When CHWs and the people they serve speak up at city council meetings or before state legislators, they are influencing public policy. When they mobilize community action to build more parks or close down a source of pollution, that mobilization contributes to health equity. When they partner with other organizations to confront racism, xenophobia, or any other form of oppression, helping institutions recognize and address bias in any of their practices, CHWs are changing the social determinants of health for the better. For more information about Community Organizing, see Chapter 23.

CHW Profile

Abdul Hafeedh Bin Abdullah. He/Him

Executive Director and Co-Founder of CHASM

Quality Life Blueprint/Sokoto House. Wilmington, North Carolina

Historically oppressed populations exposed to violence

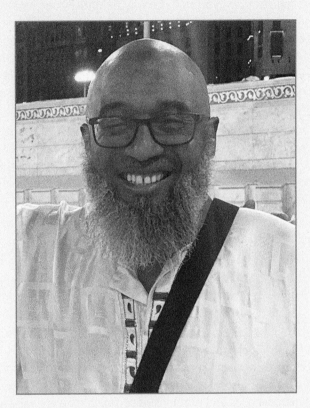

Growing up in the crack cocaine era, I was exposed to gang violence, gang activity, and mass incarceration: I was incarcerated at age seventeen and spent eight years in prison. I went through some significant transformations there, seeing people who used their gifts to build community instead of destroying it. I wanted to participate in that building process. When I came home, I engaged in community organizing around violence and gang activity. In 2010, I was introduced to a program from Portland Oregon that addressed violence from a public health lens. I realized violence needed to be prevented before it happened. Community members have a significant role to play in that, right? I engaged full throttle in being a CHW and trying to advance the field of violence prevention.

I adapted the program from Oregon for Wilmington, North Carolina as a community-based public health response to violence. Instead of the program coming down from the CDC or a health department, we built it from the community up. We serve anyone who's been exposed to violence—a perpetrator, a victim, or a witness. In our program, CHWs provide community members with wrap-around services. We connect them to housing or food resources or mental health services. As much as it's important to provide personal assistance, you also need to build community power to shift the norms of the system, right? So, we make sure the voice of the community is being heard inside rooms where decisions are being made that dictate where resources go. We train CHWs to help the community articulate their priorities.

(continues)

CHW Profile

(continued)

I worked with a young man, a middle school student, who kept finding himself in confrontations with his peers. An incident with school resource officer escalated the situation to the criminal justice system. They brought me in to connect with him. It became apparent that this was a nice kid who had a whole lot of other stuff going on. When things triggered him in school, the way he understood how to deal with it, because of all the toxic stress he was under, was to fight. The school social worker wasn't able to reach his mom, so I knocked on her door. I told her what was at stake with her son. She was single mom with severe health issues. Instead of being suspended for ten days, the young man spent that time with me. I introduced him to other professionals and people at the community center, asked him to write about it. He shared that with his school. I helped his mother connect with local resources and get back on her feet. The end result is that the young man graduated from middle school, made it to high school, became a local star for soccer.

Looking at the accomplishments of CHWs and community-based organizations, it shows something can be done, even if it can't always be done at the system level. I can mitigate the challenges of family members I'm interacting with day to day. I can organize communities to be more vocal about their needs, to address the racial inequities and other root drivers of why they are living in crisis. For me, being a CHW has cultivated a heightened sense of hope that something can be done.

It's important for CHWs to have confidence in the profession they've taken on. The CHW profession is well established in terms of its ability to address and improve the conditions of the communities that we serve. Don't get stuck in what your job description is. Build your career, enhance your skills, because as a CHW you may be called to another professional opportunity.

It is important to note that there is no one way to make change. All social changes with the goal of improving people's lives are important to the broader movement toward equity and justice. Some advocates believe in the benefits of making incremental changes, while others believe in entirely overhauling the structures that govern our lives. Similarly, some activists want to see improvements immediately, and others would rather prioritize working toward longer-term changes. All perspectives and methods of social change are valid and have an important role in the fabric of seeking broader justice for communities most impacted by health and social inequities.

Regardless of the approach, successful advocacy requires the participation and leadership of the communities most impacted by the issue at hand. It also requires building broad-based coalitions of diverse stakeholders who can work together. Fruitful partnerships can be formed among people and organizations working squarely in public health and those working in other sectors, such as affordable housing, urban planning, rural development, food security, economic justice, workers' rights, and racial justice, among others. CHWs have a crucial role to encourage communities most impacted to fully participate in these efforts, and to advocate for the changes that will truly address the needs and vision of those communities.

Improving Health Through Economic Justice

The social determinants of health influence the health status of individuals and populations. When considering avenues for social justice change, it can sometimes be overwhelming to know where to start, and how to make the most impact. It can be especially challenging to consider how to make change within the large political, social and economic forces, and structures that govern our lives. Nevertheless, it is possible to successfully make tangible changes that meaningfully improve the health of communities, by improving the social determinants of health in relatively small ways.

(continues)

Improving Health Through Economic Justice

(continued)

The Stockton Economic Empowerment Demonstration (SEED) is an example that has made a positive impact on the health of a population by addressing economic barriers: SEED was launched in 2019 by then-Mayor Tubbs to alleviate income inequities in the city of Stockton, California (Stockton Economic Empowerment Demonstration, 2021). This program gave $500/month of unconditional cash to 125 randomly selected residents, for 24 months. The SEED initiative showed that unconditional cash recipients' lives improved in various ways: a significant number of participants were able to secure full-time employment; financial stability lowered depression and anxiety and improved the well-being of participants; recipients' financial scarcity was alleviated, which increased self-determination, goal-setting, and the ability to take risks in pursuit of greater opportunities.

Due to the resounding success of this initiative, advocates and governments across the country have felt inspired to start similar pilot programs, usually called "guaranteed income" or "basic income" programs. To learn more about the SEED project, visit their website listed at the end of the chapter.

As we conclude this chapter, we want to acknowledge that many of us feel overwhelmed when confronting injustice and health inequities. As CHWs and public health practitioners, social justice values are often what motivate our work. Indeed, for many of us, social justice and health equity are extremely personal as we have experienced and/or witnessed painful examples of injustice and health inequities in our own lives and communities. As public health advocate Dr. Leana Wen has noted: "It's been said that the currency of inequality is years of life. Public health is a powerful tool to level that playing field, to bend the arc of our country away from distrust and disparities and back towards equity and justice" (Wen, 2016).

We find that, in times of hopelessness, it helps to remember that, despite the long road ahead to achieve true justice, as individuals and communities impacted by inequities, we have come a long way thanks to our resilience, hope, tenacity, and collective power. Many of us are where we are today thanks to community advocates and social justice movements that made it possible for us to have rights and access to resources that former generations would not have even dreamed of. It is our duty, and our privilege, to continue that legacy of hope, resilience, and tenacity for future generations to come.

What Do YOU Think?

- *Who inspires you to work for social justice and health equity?*

- *How do you hope to promote greater health equity?*

- *What brings you hope and energy for your work as a CHW?*

Chapter Review

To assess your understanding of the key concepts presented in this chapter, reflect on how you would answer the following questions:

1. You are talking with a friend, family member, or client about your work as a CHW. How would you explain the following concepts, *in your own words*:

   - What are health inequities?

   - What causes health inequities?

- What are the consequences of health inequities (how do they harm local communities and our society at large)?
- What can we do to reduce or eliminate health inequities?

2. Conduct research to answer the following questions about health inequities in the city, county, or state where you live:

- Where can you find reliable information and data on health inequities that impact your city, county, state, or nation?
- Which communities in your city (or county or state) experience higher rates of illness, disability, and premature death?
- What organizations are working to eliminate these inequities and to advocate for social justice?
- What policy changes are these organizations advocating for?
- What else needs to happen in your local area in order to promote health equity?
- What role can you play in these efforts?

References

American Bar Association. (2023). Racial Disparities in Health Care. www.americanbar.org/groups/crsj/publications/human_rights_magazine_home/the-state-of-healthcare-in-the-united-states/racial-disparities-in-health-care/ (accessed 2 April 2023).

Blackwell, A. (2017). The Curb-Cut Effect. www.ssir.org/articles/entry/the_curb_cut_effect (accessed 20 March 2023).

Budiman, A. & Ruiz, N. G. (2021). Key facts about Asian Americans, a diverse and growing population. Pew Research Center. Retrieved from www.pewresearch.org/short-reads/2021/04/29/key-facts-about-asian-americans/.

Centers for Disease Control and Prevention. (2019). Infant Mortality. www.cdc.gov/reproductivehealth/maternalinfanthealth/infantmortality.htm (accessed 20 March 2023).

Centers for Disease Control and Prevention. (2021). Racism and Health Disparities. www.cdc.gov/minority-health/racism-disparities/index.html (accessed 20 March 2023).

Centers for Disease Control and Prevention. (2022a). Social Determinants of Health at CDC. www.cdc.gov/about/sdoh/index.html (accessed 13 April 2023).

Centers for Disease Control and Prevention. (2022b). CDC Policy Process. www.cdc.gov/policy/paeo/process/index.html (accessed April 13, 2023).

Coates, T. N. (2014). The case for reparations. The Atlantic. Retrieved from www.theatlantic.com/features/archive/2014/05/the-case-for-reparations/361631/ (accessed 16 April 2023).

Commonwealth Fund. (2021). Mirror, Mirror 2021: Reflecting Poorly. Retrieved from www.commonwealthfund.org/publications/fund-reports/2021/aug/mirror-mirror-2021-reflecting-poorly (accessed 2 December 2022).

Commonwealth Fund. (2023). Inequities in health insurance coverage and access for Black and Hispanic adults: The impact of Medicaid expansion and the pandemic. Retrieved from www.commonwealthfund.org/publications/issue-briefs/2023/mar/inequities-coverage-access-black-hispanic-adults (accessed 16 April 2023).

Crimmins, E. M., Shim, H., Zhang, Y. S., & Kim, J. K. (2019). Differences between men and women in mortality and the health dimensions of the morbidity process. *Clinical Chemistry*, 65(1), 135–145. https://doi.org/10.1373/clinchem.2018.288332.

Ely, D. M. & Driscoll, A. K. (2022). Infant mortality among non-Hispanic Asian subgroups in the United States, 2018–2020. NCHS Health E-Stats. https://doi.org/10.15620/cdc:122451.

Greenberg, A. (2020). How the stress of racism can harm your health – and what that has to do with Covid-19. NOVA. Public Broadcasting Service. www.pbs.org/wgbh/nova/article/racism-stress-covid-allostatic-load/ (accessed 9 November 2022).

Guidi, J., Lucente, M., Sonino, N., & Fava, G. A. (2021). Allostatic load and its impact on health: A systematic review. *Psychotherapy and Psychosomatics*, 90(1), 11–27. https://doi.org/10.1159/000510696.

Healthy People 2030: Framework. (2023a). Retrieved from www.health.gov/healthypeople/about/healthy-people-2030-framework.

Healthy People 2030: Social determinants of health. (2023b). Retrieved from www.health.gov/healthypeople/objectives-and-data/social-determinants-health.

Hill, L., Ndugga, N., Artiga, S. (2023). Key data on health and health care by race and ethnicity. Kaiser Family Foundation. www.kff.org (accessed May 2023).

Horowitz, J. M., Igielnik, R., & Kochhar, R. (2020). Trends in income and wealth inequality. Pew Research Center. www.pewresearch.org/social-trends/2020/01/09/trends-in-income-and-wealth-inequality/ (accessed April 27, 2023).

Inequality.org. (2023). Income Inequality in the United States. www.inequality.org/facts/income-inequality/ (accessed 29 April 2023).

James, S. E., Herman, J. L., Rankin, S., Keisling, M., Mottet, L., & Anafi, M. (2016). The report of the 2015 U.S. transgender survey. Washington, DC: National Center for Transgender Equality. Retrieved from www.transequality.org/sites/default/files/docs/usts/USTS-Full-Report-Dec17.pdf.

Jones, J. M. (2022). LGBT Identification Ticks Up. Retrieved from www.gallup.com/poll/389792/lgbt-identification-ticks-up.aspx.

Kaiser Family Foundation. (2022). Health coverage and care of immigrants. www.kff.org/racial-equity-and-health-policy/fact-sheet/health-coverage-and-care-of-immigrants/ (accessed 24 March 2023).

Kennedy-Moulton, K., Miller, S., Persson, P., Rossin-Slater, M., Wherry, L., & Aldana, G. (2022). Maternal and infant health inequality: New evidence from linked administrative data. NBER Working Paper Series, No. 30693. Retrieved from www.nber.org/papers/w30693.

Kinshella, M. (2006) Equity Compared to Equality. Meyer Memorial Trust. https://mmt.org/news/equity-illustrated-3rd-place-equity-about-resources (accessed 29 December 2023).

Lipsitz, G. (2009). The Possessive Investment in Whiteness: How White People Profit from Identity Politics. Philadelphia, PA: Temple University Press.

Merriam-Webster. (2023). Gender. www.merriam-webster.com/dictionary/gender (accessed 4 April 2023).

National Center for Health Statistics. (2023). Life expectancy at birth, age 65, and age 75, by sex, race, and Hispanic origin: United States, selected years 1900-2019. www.cdc.gov/nchs/hus/data-finder.htm (accessed April 2, 2023).

National Institutes of Health. (2021). Life Expectancy in the U.S. Increased Between 2000 and 2019, But Widespread Gaps Among Racial and Ethnic Groups Exist. www.nih.gov/news-events/news-releases/life-expectancy-us-increased-between-2000-2019-widespread-gaps-among-racial-ethnic-groups-exist.

Office of Minority Health. (2018). Infant Mortality and Hispanic Americans. www.minorityhealth.hhs.gov (accessed 20 May 2023).

Office of Minority Health. (2023a). Profile: Hispanic/Latino Americans. www.minorityhealth.hhs.gov (accessed 20 May 2023).

Office of Minority Health. (2023b). Profile: American Indian/Alaska Native. www.minorityhealth.hhs.gov (accessed 20 May 2023).

Pew Research Center. (2020). What Census Calls Us. https://www.pewresearch.org/interactives/what-census-calls-us/ (accessed 27 April 2023).

Powell, J., Menendian, S., & Ake, W. (2019). *Targeted universalism: Policy & practice*. Berkeley: Haas Institute for a Fair and Inclusive Society, University of California. haasinstitute.berkeley.edu/targeteduniversalism (accessed May 20, 2023).

Robert Wood Johnson Foundation. (2017). Visualizing Health Equity. www.rwjf.org/en/insights/our-research/infographics/visualizing-health-equity.html#/download (accessed 10 May 2023).

Sandoiu, A. (2021). 'Weathering': What are the health effects of stress and discrimination? Medical News Today. www.medicalnewstoday.com/articles/weathering-what-are-the-health-effects-of-stress-and-discrimination (accessed 9 November 2022).

Sax, L. (2021). *The immigrant paradox: Why are children of immigrants doing better? Institute for Family Studies*. https://ifstudies.org/blog/the-immigrant-paradox-why-are-children-of-immigrants-doing-better (accessed 29 December 2023).

Semega, J., Kollar, M., Creamer, J., & Mohanty, A. (2019). Income and Poverty in the United States: 2018. U.S. Census Bureau, Current Population Reports. Retrieved from www.census.gov/content/dam/Census/library/publications/2019/demo/p60-266.pdf.

Stockton Economic Empowerment Demonstration (SEED). (2021). https://www.stocktondemonstration.org/ (accessed 16 April 2023).

Trans Legislation Tracker. (2023). 2023 Anti-Trans Bills Tracker. www.translegislation.com/ (accessed 20 May 2023).

United Nations. (2023). Universal Declaration of Human Rights. www.un.org/en/about-us/universal-declaration-of-human-rights (accessed 11 February 2023).

Wen, L. (2016). Testimony to Democratic Platform Committee: The Case for Investing in the Public's Health. HuffPost. Retrieved from www.huffpost.com/entry/testimony-to-democratic-p_b_10821932.

World Bank. (2023). www.data.worldbank.org (accessed 17 March 2023).

World Health Organization. (2018). https://www.who.int/news-room/facts-in-pictures/detail/health-inequities-and-their-causes (accessed 26 December 2023).

Zajacova, A. & Lawrence, E. M. (2018). The relationship between education and health: Reducing disparities through a contextual approach. *Annual Review of Public Health* 39, 273–289. https://doi.org/10.1146/annurev-publhealth-031816-044628

Additional Resources

Bay Area Regional Health Inequalities Initiative. (2023). Retrieved from www.barhii.org/.

California Newsreel. The Raising of America. [Video and website]. Retrieved from www.raisingofamerica.org.

California Newsreel. Unnatural Causes. [Video and website]. Retrieved from www.unnaturalcauses.org.

Economic Policy Institute. (2023). Retrieved from www.epi.org.

Gapminder. (2023). A Fact Based World View. Retrieved from www.gapminder.org/.

Government Alliance on Race and Equity. (2023). Retrieved from www.racialequityalliance.org/.

Movement Advancement Project. (2023). Retrieved from www.lgbtmap.org/.

National Association of County and City Health Officials. (2023). Roots of Health Inequity. A Web-Based Course for the Public Health Workforce. Retrieved from www.rootsofhealthinequity.org/.

PolicyLink. (2023). Retrieved from www.policylink.org/.

Race Forward. (2023). The Center for Racial Justice Innovation. Retrieved from www.raceforward.org/.

UCLA. (2023). School of Law Williams Institute. Retrieved from www.williamsinstitute.law.ucla.edu/.

University of Utah, Health Sciences. (2023). Learn Genetics: Epigenetics. Retrieved from www.learn.genetics.utah.edu/content/epigenetics/.

CORE COMPETENCIES FOR PROVIDING DIRECT SERVICES

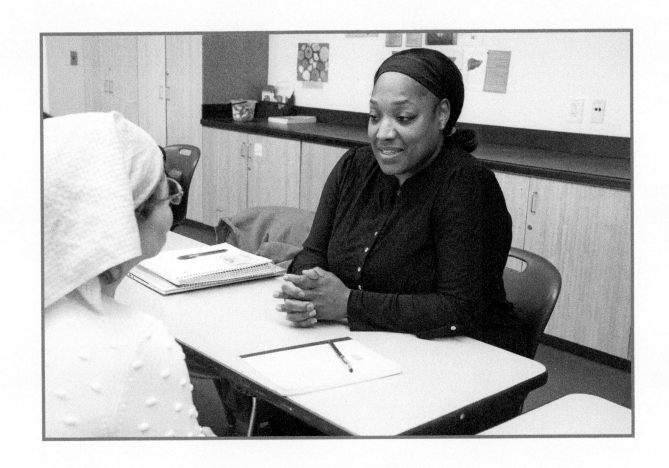

Guiding Principles: Self-Awareness, Ethics, Professional Boundaries, and Teamwork

5

James Figueiredo and Marilyn Gardner

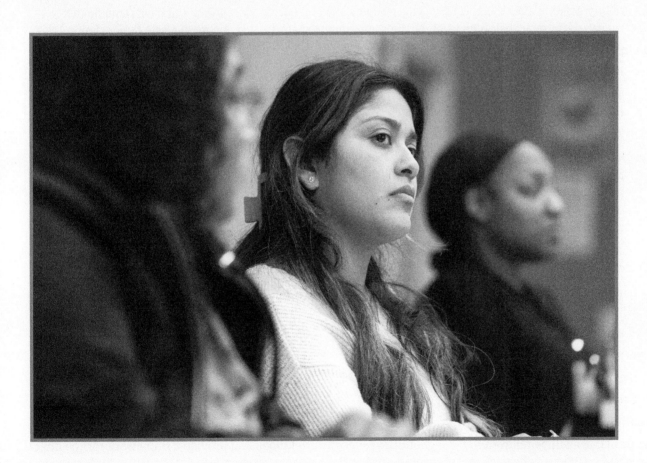

Foundations for Community Health Workers, Third Edition. Edited by Tim Berthold and Darouny Somsanith.
© 2024 John Wiley & Sons, Inc. Published 2024 by John Wiley & Sons, Inc.
Companion website: http://www.wiley.com/go/communityhealthworkers3E

CHW Scenario: Your First Job as a CHW

A month ago, you started your first paid job as a CHW. This is the first time you have worked in a health-related field. Your prior experience includes a series of customer service jobs at stores and restaurants, and as an unpaid caregiver to a family member with a chronic disability.

You are the newest member of a team that includes six CHWs, three social workers, two nurses, and two peer alcohol and drug recovery coaches. This team interacts regularly with primary care physicians, nutritionists, psychiatrists, and other health professionals. The CHWs regularly interact with community leaders and external organizations that provide services in the community. Your direct supervisor had nearly eight years of experience as a CHW before she started supervising the other CHWs on the team.

Over the last month, you went through an orientation and observed your colleagues conduct health outreach in the community, meet individually with clients, and co-facilitate health education groups for people with diabetes and cardiovascular disease.

You are impressed by how much your colleagues know and are able to accomplish. You have some doubts that you can perform at their high level. At the same time, you are excited about your new career choice.

You still have many questions about your role, including:

- *How do I protect the confidentiality of clients who are from the same tight-knit community where I live?*
- *What are the limits of confidentiality? Under what circumstances may I break confidentiality and share client information with another agency?*
- *When I am working with a client, what are the professional boundaries that I should not cross?*
- *What types of services can I provide and what services should be provided by others?*
- *How do I interact professionally and build relationships with other CHWs and health professionals on my team?*

Introduction

This chapter introduces five topics and guiding principles that will inform your work as a CHW. These guiding principles include:

- Self-awareness
- Ethics
- Scope of Practice
- Professional Boundaries
- Multidisciplinary Teamwork

These principles will be referred to throughout the *Foundations* textbook and provide a framework for the direct services that CHWs provide to clients and communities. For example, guiding principles such as Ethics, Scope of Practice (SOP), and Person-Centered Practice are critical concepts for CHWs who conduct initial client interviews or provide person-centered counseling or care management services.

WHAT YOU WILL LEARN

By studying the information in this chapter, you will be able to:

Self-awareness

- Define self-awareness
- Explain the importance of self-awareness to the work of CHWs
- Identify practical strategies for enhancing self-awareness

Ethics

- Define ethics and explain how ethics are different from laws
- Discuss key articles from the CHW Code of Ethics
- Explain ethical guidelines relating to informed consent and confidentiality

Scope of Practice

- Define Scope of Practice (SOP)
- Identify competencies that may lie within and outside the CHW SOP
- Analyze the potential consequences of working outside of the CHW SOP
- Explain how to respond when confronted with a challenge regarding your SOP as a CHW

Professional Boundaries

- Define and discuss professional boundaries and dual or multiple relationships
- Discuss how CHWs may cross professional boundaries and the potential risks of doing so
- Explain self-disclosure and analyze the potential risks and benefits for clients and CHWs

Working as Part of a Multidisciplinary Team

- Explain the key elements for successful teams
- Identify common challenges to teamwork

Discuss strategies for working successfully as part of a multidisciplinary team

C3 Roles and Skills Addressed in Chapter 5

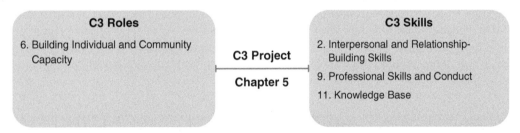

C3 Roles

6. Building Individual and Community Capacity

C3 Project

Chapter 5

C3 Skills

2. Interpersonal and Relationship-Building Skills
9. Professional Skills and Conduct
11. Knowledge Base

WORDS TO KNOW

Boundary Crossing

Confidentiality

Dual or Multiple Relationships

Ethics

Informed Consent

Professional Boundaries

Self-Awareness

Self-Disclosure

5.1 Duty of Self-awareness

"It's not about you." One of the most valuable things that CHWs and other helping professionals can learn is that the work we do with clients is not about us. It is always about the client or family, the group or community we serve.

It is counterintuitive but true that greater self-awareness makes us better able to provide person-centered care and culturally responsive services. When CHWs are unaware of their own culture, values, beliefs, and experiences, they are at greater risk of imposing these on other people without realizing they are doing so. This may harm the very people that CHWs are tasked to care for.

THE VALUE OF SELF-AWARENESS

Self-awareness can be defined as "the ability to focus on yourself and how your actions, thoughts, or emotions do or don't align with your internal standards. If you're highly self-aware, you can objectively evaluate yourself, manage your emotions, align your behavior with your values, and understand correctly how others perceive you" (Goleman, Kaplan, David, & Eurich, 2018). Self-awareness can be further defined as internal or external.

Internal self-awareness refers to how clearly we see our own values, beliefs, thoughts, feelings, behaviors, weaknesses, and strengths and their impact on others.

External self-awareness refers to how people see us based on the same factors. Research shows that when we know how others see us, we are more likely to be able to understand others' perspectives and gain empathy.

There are many ways that CHWs and other helping professionals can benefit from increasing self-awareness. Some of these benefits include:

- It frees us from being trapped by our own biases and assumptions
- It helps us to see things from multiple perspectives
- It helps us learn empathy for others
- It helps us to communicate more clearly
- It benefits not only work relationships, but also personal relationships

We do not live or work in a vacuum. When our own issues or challenges are present, powerful, and unresolved, we may not realize how they influence our ability to work with, listen to, and provide support to clients. We may unconsciously guide, direct, or pressure clients to talk about or avoid certain topics and potentially important health decisions.

For example, if you as a CHW have experiences of trauma in a refugee camp and you are meeting with a new arrival who has come from a similar situation, it may overwhelm you with memories of a difficult chapter of your life. Similarly, another CHW who has strong opinions and beliefs about reproductive rights and abortion may subconsciously impose those beliefs on a client who is pregnant. CHWs who are unaware of their own emotions of anger and defensiveness are not well prepared to deal with the anger and defensiveness of their clients.

- *Can you think of other examples of how a CHW's own issues may interfere with their ability to work effectively with clients and communities?*

- *Have you ever worked with a helping professional who seemed uncomfortable or judgmental about your identity or behavior?*

- *Can you identify past experiences or personal issues that could be re-stimulated through your work as a CHW?*

A LIFELONG TASK

Developing self-awareness is a life-long task. It involves an ongoing process of identifying and working to better understand yourself, including your:

- **Life experiences:** Such as experiences of incarceration, trauma, refugee or immigration status, chronic illness, grief and loss through death or divorce, homelessness, discrimination, and mental health challenges.

- **Values and beliefs:** Such as values and beliefs about faith and religion, reproduction and reproductive rights, sexual orientation, gender identity, substance use, the criminal justice system, and death and dying.

- **Prejudices:** We all have biases and prejudices in our background. Most of us have grown up in communities that value some people over others based on factors such as religion, education, ethnicity, immigration status, sex, gender identity, disability status, sexual orientation, and age. How we grow up and what we have been taught by others influences who we are as adults. All of us are more comfortable with certain communities—usually those that we identify with and belong to. As community health professionals, all of us have a duty to examine our assumptions, prejudices, and often hidden biases. This is an essential first step to equitable and culturally responsive services.

SELF-EVALUATION

No matter how much we know, we can still stop to self-reflect and self-evaluate. The following questions may help you to reflect on your own beliefs and values:

- What type of situations provoke your anger or judgment?
- When do you find it the most difficult to listen to others?
- What situations tempt you to want to tell someone else what to do and how to do it?
- What health and health-related topics are you least comfortable and familiar with addressing?
- What health behaviors or topics are you unprepared to address with your clients?
- What populations are you least prepared to work with? For example, are you comfortable serving people of all ages, sexual orientations, religions, and gender identities?

Maha Begum: I grew up in Bangladesh and had no idea that an LGBTQ+ community existed. When I started my job as a CHW, I was lucky to have gay and lesbian co-workers and to go to a training on addressing the health needs of transgender people. I learned a lot through conversations with my colleagues and my own research. My comfort level is so much higher now, and I know that clients are being better served because of this.

Self-Awareness Scenario

Jessica works as a CHW in a teen clinic in East Boston. She grew up bicultural and bilingual in a Brazilian neighborhood. She loves her job and her community. While the clinic serves many youth from Central and South America, many immigrant teens come from other diverse communities and backgrounds.

On a busy Wednesday afternoon, Jessica is doing an initial intake and assessment on a 16-year-old observant Muslim woman named Khadija. Khadija wears hijab and Jessica has already learned that Khadija's faith is very important to her. Jessica begins to ask questions about Khadija's sexuality and sexual activity. She does not notice that Khadija begins to turn her body away from Jessica and appears increasingly uncomfortable. She asks a question about what Khadija's sexual orientation is and Khadija abruptly gets up and says, *"I'm sorry but I must leave. I cannot answer questions like this."* Jessica is surprised and begins to defend herself when, without a backward glance, Khadija leaves the room.

Jessica is both frustrated and embarrassed about the interaction.

We are only given limited information about both Jessica and Khadija, but given what we know, how would you respond to the following questions?

- *What assumptions might you or another CHW make about Khadija, given the fact that she is a 16-year-old being raised in Boston?*
- *How might your experiences and identity affect the interaction described in the scenario?*
- *What steps could you take to better understand your own feelings about this scenario?*
- *What steps could you take to know how to interact with future patients like Khadija in order to provide the best care possible?*

The bottom line is that this interaction with Khadija is not about Jessica and her experiences. Though our experiences are important, the key point to remember is that all interactions with clients must be focused on the client's experience, beliefs, values, and priorities. In this case, the client's situation is about helping Khadija to feel safe, heard, and able to communicate about any issues, problems, questions, or concerns.

The reality is that in a clinic or other work situation, as a CHW you may have to ask questions that may seem intrusive and offensive to your client. One of the ways to handle this is by saying in advance, *"I know that some of the questions I ask you may feel uncomfortable, and you may not want to discuss them. They are standard questions, and I don't mean to offend you by asking them. If you don't want to answer or talk about a particular issue, please let me know and I'll respect your decision."*

ENHANCING SELF-AWARENESS

It is not only important to understand what self-awareness is but also to take an active approach to enhance your self-awareness. Here are some ways to do this:

- **Self-reflection:** Think about your cultural background and how you see the world. What values and beliefs are important to you? What are some of the life experiences you have that have shaped you? How do these influence the way you work with clients, families, and communities?

- **Writing and journaling:** Keep a personal journal where you write about your work experiences. Write about your successes, challenges, and feelings about your work. Writing can help you process and develop a better understanding of the ways you react to people and situations. As you journal you can use these questions as a guide: What did I do well today? What challenges did I face? How did I feel when I faced these challenges? How did I respond to praise, constructive feedback, or suggestions from others? What strengths and skills did I use to stay on task?

- **Education or training:** Participating in courses on trauma-informed care, cultural humility and culturally responsive care, and self-care can all be a part of our journey to enhanced self-awareness. For example, when you understand more about your own culture and values, then you will be in a better place to learn about the cultural values and beliefs of others. It may seem counter intuitive, but the first step in developing culturally responsive skills is increased self-awareness.

- **Trusted mentors and supervisors:** A trusted mentor or supervisor is a valuable gift to help you enhance your self-awareness. They are people who want you to grow and succeed. A good supervisor and mentor knows that giving encouragement and constructive feedback is a necessary part of growth. Meeting with them and having honest conversations about developing self-awareness is an excellent way to grow.

- **Pay attention to your emotions:** Are there emotions that you are uncomfortable with? Do you struggle with anger? Reflect and talk with a trusted mentor or supervisor.

We will build on the principle of self-awareness throughout the book and particularly in Chapter 7 on Cultural Humility.

CHW Profile

Avery Nguyen (They/Them)

Intensive Case Manager

Catholic Charities

Providing support for women living with HIV

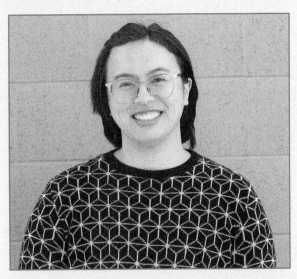

Everybody, at some point in their lives, will get sick and have to navigate the medical system: I started out in social services but began to pivot toward health when some of my loved ones started to deal with chronic illness and disabilities, and I was supporting them. It can be overwhelming and traumatizing, even in the best situations with the best doctors and the kindest providers.

I am an Intensive Case Manager at Catholic Charities, and I work with women living with HIV. HIV is still a big deal because the folks that are most vulnerable to getting HIV are the ones that are vulnerable to lots of other stressors like housing instability, trauma, financial instability, substance use. The women I work with have been living with HIV for a long time and most are now middle aged or seniors, but they still need to manage their HIV. Some are not out about their HIV status or minimize how many people know about them. So, it can get a little lonely.

For me, no two days are the same. We collaborate with clinics at the University of California, San Francisco and the General Hospital. I call to make appointments, and sometimes I'll sit in with clients and take notes. We have a van and I'll take clients to clinics, the Social Security office, and other places when transportation is an issue. I'll go to the store to buy groceries or household items for our agency to give to clients.

One client had been so disengaged from our program that they were considering closing her case. I called and told her that I was her new case manager. I met with her to complete the annual paperwork and gave her some gift cards. She smiled when we finally met. From the very beginning, it was a relationship that started off with humor, honesty, and transparency. I learned that she had a history of trauma with family members killed by gun violence. She had a partner who was very controlling about where she went and who she spent time with, so I had to figure out how to work around that. I need to be mindful of what she is going through and give her respect and space to make her own decisions. At first, she wanted me to call her to remind her of the things she needed to do. Now she is able to see it as her own responsibility; she is accountable to herself day-to-day. Building resilience and independence is a great outcome.

(continues)

CHW Profile

(continued)

When I signed up for the CHW training program, I thought: 'I'll do the training and I'm gonna learn skills and be able to help my clients check off more things on their list, and therefore be a more effective case manager.' But I learned that people are not checklists. It's about using motivational interviewing, coming up with ways to be creative and meet them where they're at, respecting their personhood, and their own agency and the choices that they make.

One thing I would tell new CHWs is to practice compassion for your clients and for yourself. Sometimes we may feel like a client has a problem to be solved and get personally frustrated when things aren't going the way we want. But I realize that my frustration is coming from me and it's because I am holding them to an expectation that comes from my understanding of my life and my personal experience. And everyone has different tools and experiences and skills. Remember that you're not here to save people; you're here to accompany them on the ride.

5.2 Ethical Guidelines for CHWs

Community Health Workers are dedicated to working with integrity at the top of their skill set. As such, it is important to recognize the importance of making ethical decisions when faced with a difficult challenge at work.

Ethics can be defined as moral principles that govern a person's behavior or activity. Ethical standards provide guidance to professionals regarding "right conduct" and what to do when faced with a workplace challenge or dilemma.

A code of ethics clarifies roles and responsibilities within a profession and provides guidance for responding to common ethical questions.

COMMON ETHICAL CHALLENGES

CHWs are motivated by a desire to help people and their communities. Often you represent the community that you are serving. This role is an honor and privilege, but it also comes with a heavy responsibility. There are times when you may face a professional challenge where the answer or isn't clear. For example, what would you do in the following situations?

- You find out that a teenager from your community is pregnant. You are friends with the family. Someone from the family comes up to you at an event and specifically asks you about the teenager.
- A former client asks you out on a date (you are single, available, and interested).
- A client asks you to attend their wedding.
- A grateful client shows up at your work with a large, expensive gift.
- One of your clients is HIV positive and is continuing to have unprotected sex with their partner without disclosing their HIV status.
- A client says that they haven't eaten and asks for some money to purchase a meal.
- You notice that one of your co-workers has the smell of alcohol on his breath during work hours. Should you confront him? Should you tell their supervisor?
- Many of your clients complain that they are treated rudely by front desk staff at your agency. Do you have a duty to report this?

All of the situations described are real-life situations and none of them has an easy answer. In fact, depending on the situation, two different CHWs might respond completely differently than each other.

A code of ethics and policies that are developed by organizations can be helpful resources for responding to workplace challenges. However, even highly experienced CHWs (and other helping professionals) will face workplace situations when they aren't sure what the "right conduct" or response is, or how to apply ethical standards. Whenever you are uncertain how to respond to a client or a workplace challenge, seek consultation and guidance from your supervisor or another senior colleague.

ETHICS AND THE LAW

Ethics and the law are integrally related, yet distinct.

Ethics is about doing what is morally right. Codes of ethics aim to standardize professional behavior and accountability. They are designed to inform clients and the public about the types of services they can expect to receive from professionals, and to ensure that clients are protected from inappropriate conduct or abuse from professionals. Typically, codes of ethics address issues such as informed consent, confidentiality, professional training, protections against discrimination, and maintaining clear professional boundaries with clients.

Laws are established by governments to prevent and punish behavior that is harmful or destructive to a society's well-being. Laws define the minimal standards that a society will tolerate and are enforced by the government. Laws include statutes, regulations, agency policies and procedures, and court decisions and may be local (city laws), state, federal (national), or international. The consequences of breaking a law tend to be more severe than a violation of a professional code of ethics. For example, the penalty for breaking the law can include imprisonment, whereas the penalty for violation of a professional code of ethics may include being fired from your job, fined, or barred from future employment in your field. Keep in mind that violations of the law and of the professional code of ethics can impact your reputation and relationship with your colleagues, community, clients, and ultimately yourself. Additionally, violations of ethical guidelines are sometimes also legal violations. For example, if you break the confidentiality of a client by disclosing her HIV-positive status to another without written consent, you are violating both your ethical guidelines and laws that protect the privacy of people with HIV disease.

THE CHW CODE OF ETHICS

The CHW Code of Ethics is based upon commonly understood principles that apply to all professionals within the health and social service fields (e.g., promotion of social justice, positive health, and dignity). It was developed by a group of CHWs and allies and is still used today to define the code of conduct and scope of practice for CHWs in the country. In total, there are four overarching "Articles" or sections of the Code of Ethics: Responsibilities in the Delivery of Care, Promotion of Equitable Relationships, Interactions with Other Service Providers, and Professional Rights and Responsibilities.

Please note that it does not address all ethical issues facing Community Health Workers and the absence of a rule does not imply that there is no ethical obligation present. As professionals, Community Health Workers are encouraged to reflect on the ethical obligations that they have to the communities that they serve and to share these reflections with others.

Article 1. Responsibility in the Delivery of Care

Community Health Workers build trust and community capacity by improving the health and social welfare of the client they serve. When a conflict arises among individuals, groups, agencies, or institutions, Community Health Workers should consider all issues and give priority to those that promote the wellness and quality of living for the individual/client. The following provisions promote the professional integrity of Community Health Workers.

1.1 Honesty

Community Health Workers are professionals who strive to ensure the best health outcomes for the communities they serve. They communicate the potential benefits and consequences of available services, including the programs they are employed under.

1.2 Confidentiality

Community Health Workers respect the confidentiality, privacy, and trust of individuals, families, and communities that they serve. They understand and abide by employer policies, as well as state and federal confidentiality laws, that are relevant to their work.

1.3 Scope of Ability and Training

Community Health Workers are truthful about qualifications, competencies, and limitations on the services they may provide, and should not misrepresent qualifications or competencies to individuals, families, communities, or employers.

1.4 Quality of Care

Community Health Workers strive to provide high-quality service to individuals, families, and communities. They do this through continued education, training, and an obligation to ensure the information they provide is up-to-date and accurate.

1.5 Referral to Appropriate Services

Community Health Workers acknowledge when client issues are outside of their Scope Of Practice (SOP) and refer clients to the appropriate health, wellness, or social support services when necessary.

1.6 Legal Obligations

Community Health Workers have an obligation to report actual or potential harm to individuals within the communities they serve to the appropriate authorities. Additionally, Community Health Workers have a responsibility to follow requirements set by states, the federal government, and/or their employing organizations. Responsibility to the larger society or specific legal obligations may supersede the loyalty owed to individual community members.

Article 2. Promotion of Equitable Relationships

Community Health Workers focus their efforts on the well-being of the whole community. They value and respect the expertise and knowledge that each community member possesses. In turn, Community Health Workers strive to create equitable partnerships with communities to address all issues of health and well-being.

2.1 Cultural Humility

Community Health Workers possess expertise in the communities in which they serve. They maintain a high degree of humility and respect for the cultural diversity within each community. As advocates for their communities, Community Health Workers have an obligation to inform employers and others when policies and procedures will offend or harm communities or are ineffective within the communities where they work.

2.2 Maintaining the Trust of the Community

Community Health Workers are often members of their communities and their effectiveness in providing services derives from the trust placed in them by members of these communities. Community Health Workers do not act in ways that could jeopardize the trust placed in them by the communities they serve.

2.3 Respect for Human Rights

Community Health Workers respect the human rights of those they serve, advance principles of self-determination, and promote equitable relationships with all communities.

2.4 Anti-Discrimination
Community Health Workers do not discriminate against any person or group on the basis of race, ethnicity, gender, sexual orientation, age, religion, social status, disability, or immigration status.

2.5 Client Relationships
Community Health Workers maintain professional relationships with clients. They establish, respect, and actively maintain personal boundaries between them and their clients.

Article 3. Interactions with Other Service Providers
Community Health Workers maintain professional partnerships with other service providers in order to serve the community effectively.

3.1 Cooperation
Community Health Workers place the well-being of those they serve above personal disagreements and work cooperatively with any other person or organization dedicated to helping provide care to those in need.

3.2 Conduct
Community Health Workers promote integrity in the delivery of health and social services. They respect the rights, dignity, and worth of all people and have an ethical obligation to report any inappropriate behavior (e.g., sexual harassment, racial discrimination, etc.) to the proper authority.

3.3 Self-Presentation
Community Health Workers are truthful and forthright in presenting their background and training to other service providers.

Article 4. Professional Rights and Responsibilities
The Community Health Worker profession is dedicated to excellence in the practice of promoting well-being in communities. Guided by common values, Community Health Workers have the responsibility to uphold the principles and integrity of the profession as they assist families to make decisions impacting their well-being. Community Health Workers embrace individual, family, and community strengths and build upon them to increase community capacity.

4.1 Continuing Education
Community Health Workers should remain up to date on any developments that substantially affect their ability to competently render services. Community Health Workers strive to expand their professional knowledge base and competencies through education and participation in professional organizations.

4.2 Advocacy for Change in Law and Policy
Community Health Workers are advocates for change and work on impacting policies that promote social justice and hold systems accountable for being responsive to communities. Policies that advance public health and well-being enable Community Health Workers to provide better care for the communities they serve.

4.3 Enhancing Community Capacity
Community Health Workers help individuals and communities move toward self-sufficiency in order to promote the creation of opportunities and resources that support their autonomy.

4.4 Wellness and Safety

Community Health Workers are sensitive to their own personal well-being (physical, mental, and spiritual health) and strive to maintain a safe environment for themselves and the communities they serve.

4.5 Loyalty to the Profession

Community Health Workers are loyal to the profession and aim to advance the efforts of other Community Health Workers worldwide.

4.6 Advocacy for the Profession

Community Health Workers are advocates for the profession. They are members, leaders, and active participants in local, state, and national professional organizations.

4.7 Recognition of Others

Community Health Workers give recognition to others for their professional contributions and achievements.

- *How do the policies at your organization compare with the CHW Code of Ethics?*

- *Does your state have its own CHW Code of Ethics? If so, how does it compare with what you read here?*

- *What are ways you can go about getting clarity on workplace policies and protocols when the rules have not been communicated?*

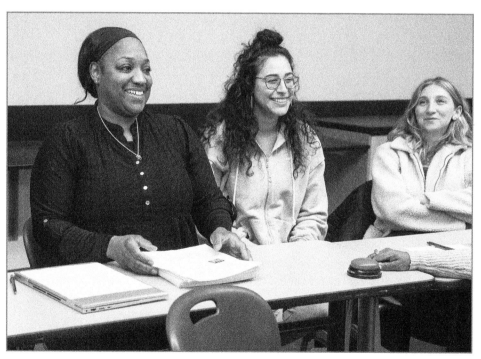

CHWs in training.

ESSENTIAL ETHICAL CONCEPTS

There are certain ethical issues and concepts that CHWs frequently encounter in the course of their work. These include informed consent and confidentiality.

Informed Consent

Informed consent is related to Article 1.1 Honesty and Article 3.3 Self-Presentation in the CHW Code of Ethics. **Informed consent** is the obligation to provide clients with the information they need in order to make a sound decision about whether to participate in a program, service, or research study. This should include information about anything that could be potentially difficult for or harmful to the client, as well as information about any costs, insurance coverage, program requirements for participation, limitations of program services, and confidentiality.

One of the reasons we highlight informed consent as an ethical issue is because organizations sometimes fail to fully inform clients about the services they are receiving. There is a history of coercing clients into services they may not be interested in. Notorious examples include the Tuskegee Syphilis Trials discussed in Chapter 7.

Informed consent is an ongoing responsibility of CHWs. We recommend that you review the informed consent policies used by the programs you work for. Is all relevant information shared with clients in order to assist them in deciding whether to participate in services? Is the information presented in a way that your clients can understand? Is the same information provided to clients who speak languages other than English? If not, the ethical principle of informed consent has been devalued.

Confidentiality

Article 1.2 of the AACHW Code of Ethics addresses confidentiality. **Confidentiality** protects a client's communication with a CHW and forms an essential component for establishing a trusting and productive professional relationship. Unless clients are confident that the CHW will not disclose their information to others, they will be reluctant to share personal information.

> ## The Health Insurance Portability and Accountability Act (HIPAA)
>
> If you work in a health care setting, every new client or patient will be asked to read and sign a Health Insurance Portability and Accountability Act (HIPAA) form and be asked to renew their understanding of this policy each yar. HIPAA is a federal law passed in 1996 that requires the protection and confidential handling of all health information. (Centers for Disease Control and Prevention, 2022)

CHWs should address issues of confidentiality and its limits with new clients before services begin and before clients have an opportunity to disclose personal and intimate information. This should include an explicit discussion of the exceptions that would cause the CHW to "break" a client's confidentiality and report private information to others, including outside agencies as a crisis response team, the police, or child protection services. It is essential for CHWs to explain confidentiality and its limits using clear and accessible language, and to make sure that clients understand the concept and policy before addressing other topics in detail.

> **Ramona Benson:** I had this big problem when I was starting out as a CHW because some of my clients would say things to other providers, things that they thought were private, and then the provider would say: "I'm a mandated reporter. I must report that to the authorities." That's the wrong way to handle things, especially with the ladies I work with. They have experienced so much racism and discrimination that it is already hard for them to trust people—and I know why! So, when I start working with a client at the Black Infant Health Program, I always tell them upfront what the rules are and what kind of information I will have to report to others. They have a right to know and it's a matter of respect.

In general, CHWs do not share private information about their clients with others, including the client's identity (such as the client's name or Social Security number), unless the client provides written consent. For example, as described in Chapter 10, clients may work with providers at more than one agency or program and may ask these providers to consult with each other. In this case, the client could ask both providers and agencies to sign a Release of Information permitting them to share information about specific issues over a specified period.

However, there are several important exceptions that limit a CHW's ability to keep a client's information private. If clients disclose information about harm or the threat of harm to themselves or others, CHWs may have an ethical and legal obligation to report to their supervisor and a third party, such as the local department of human services (such as a child protective services or elder abuse division), a local crisis response team or the police. The types of harms that could require a breach of confidentiality include suicide, and child and elder abuse (note that reporting requirements can vary by state). In such circumstances, CHWs have an ethical obligation not only to the client, but to anyone who may be harmed. This ethical obligation requires them to report the harm or threat of harm in order to protect the safety and health of the victim or potential victim.

When CHWs face a situation in which they must break the confidentiality of a client, we recommend that you consider if and how you may be able to involve the client in the reporting process. This can aid in preserving a positive working relationship between the client and the CHW. The decision about whether to participate, of course, must be left to the client. In cases of mandated reporting, it is important that the CHW fully and accurately understand the consequences of such reporting and be prepared to discuss these with the client. When necessary (or possible), the CHW may seek supervisory support in these situations.

Consider the case of a CHW working at a health clinic serving youth (see the featured example).

Client Scenario About the Limits of Confidentiality

A CHW works in a busy clinic that provides specialized services for youth. Multiple signs are clearly posted throughout the clinic—including in the waiting room, at the front desk and in meeting and exam rooms—explaining the limits of confidentiality. All clients are required to sign a HIPAA Form and update it each year. The CHW begins all client sessions by reviewing the limits of confidentiality and describing the types of information that cannot legally be kept private, including physical and sexual abuse and suicide.

After discussing the limits of confidentiality, a fourteen-year-old female client discloses that she is being sexually abused by her stepfather. Legally and ethically, the CHW (or the agency they work for) has a duty to report this information to local law enforcement authorities.

Despite having discussed the limits of confidentiality previously, the client begs the CHW not to make a report: the client is scared about what her stepfather and mother might do.

The CHW listens to the client express her fears. The CHW then explains their legal duty to report sexual abuse to the police. The CHW emphasizes concern for the client's safety and welfare. The CHW also explains why it would be wrong not to make a report: they have an obligation to do everything they can to protect clients from harm. Failing to report the abuse could send a message to the client that she shouldn't talk about what is happening to her or that the sexual abuse is acceptable or somehow doesn't matter.

The CHW calmly explains the need to call the police immediately and asks the client if she would like to help make the call, listen in on the call, or wait in another room until the call is completed. The client is also free to leave, although she and her parents will be contacted later by the police. The client decides to listen in on the call to the police. The CHW also asks the client if she would like to call the local rape crisis center and explains the type of services they offer. The client decides to call the rape crisis center after the CHW makes the call to the police. Throughout this process, it is important to assess the client's safety and make an appropriate plan to prevent further harm to her or others.

After the client leaves the clinic, the CHW documents the session and sends an email to their supervisor explaining that they called the police to provide a mandated report about the sexual assault of a minor. The next day, the CHW meets with their supervisor to review the case, complete documentation, and plan for how to check-in on the status of the client.

The client scenario described above presents a challenging situation. In the example provided, the CHW clearly explained the rules of confidentiality and its limits, and took time to listen to the client's questions, concerns, and feelings. The CHW also provided the client with several choices and supported her decisions. Ultimately, the CHW and the client acted together to report the sexual abuse to the authorities and to contact additional resources (the rape crisis center). While the situation was stressful for the client, providing her with choices also aided in giving back a measure of control. This is an important feature of person-centered practice (see Chapters 6 and 9) and working with survivors of trauma (addressed in greater detail in Chapter 18).

- *What do you think of the way in which the CHW handled this situation?*

- *Is there anything else you would want to do differently in this situation?*

What Do YOU? Think

5.3 Scope of Practice

SOP is a concept used to determine what skills, activities, and services a person in a specific job position or profession is allowed to perform based on their role and credentials. For example, doctors are trained to prescribe medications and to diagnose patients based on assessment, physical exam, and test results, but it is beyond a doctor's SOP to offer legal advice, or to do extensive electrical work in someone's house. Legal advice is within the SOP of an attorney with a license to practice law, and doing electrical work is within the SOP of a licensed electrician.

More established professions, such as medicine and social work, have a well-developed SOP guidelines that are widely recognized and accepted. Because the CHW profession is not yet as well-established, many organizations lack well-defined SOP guidelines. This presents a significant barrier to successfully integrating CHWs into care teams.

Unfortunately, questions and concerns related to the CHW SOP may not be raised until someone—usually a supervisor or colleague from another profession, such as nursing or social work—tells the CHW that they shouldn't have done something on the job. This creates stress and confusion that can lead to conflict among the team.

As discussed in Chapters 1 and 2, the CHW field is not always fully understood or respected by other professions. At times, the role of the CHW is questioned and limited so that they are not unable to work at the top of their skill set. It is important for CHW employers and colleagues to understand and appreciate the roles and contributions of CHWs.

Sabrina Lozandieu: People sometimes think that the CHW is something warm and fuzzy that feels good, but they still wonder what we really do.

Over the last several years, many state governments have developed CHW certification bodies, which has increased the professionalization and standardization of the field. In many states, the competencies legislated through the certification process are what inform the SOP for a CHW. In addition, an organization's policy will determine the SOP for CHWs employed at the organization.

FACTORS THAT INFLUENCE THE CHW SCOPE OF PRACTICE

The role of CHWs can appear to be so large and all-encompassing that it feels overwhelming. Understanding where your role begins and ends, and when to make a referral to another professional, can provide clarity and comfort to CHWs. It will also help you to avoid mistakes that may harm your clients, your agency, and your own career.

The SOP for CHWs varies considerably from one organization to another and depends on a variety of factors, such as:

- State and local laws (including employment, mandatory reporting, and Medicaid reimbursement statutes)
- The agency, program, and supervisor you work for. For example, some employers may train CHWs to co-facilitate support groups, while others do not. Some employers or unions negotiate employment contracts that specify or limit the SOP.
- The type of health issue you focus on. For example, CHWs who work in the chronic conditions management field may be trained to support patients with medication management.
- Your background, training, and skills
- Your own level of comfort and competency
- Overlapping scopes of practice of other colleagues such as nurses, medical assistants or medical evaluation assistants, senior health educators, and social workers
- Politics and perceived competition among different professions and professional associations for status, recognition, control, and pay
- The context of the work, including issues raised by clients

TASKS AND SERVICES WITHIN OR OUTSIDE OF THE CHW SCOPE OF PRACTICE

Within the CHW Scope of Practice

The following tasks and services generally lie *within* the CHW SOP:

- Outreach and recruitment of clients or study participants, including the provision of informed consent
- Supporting clients to access services
- Supporting clients in communicating their questions or concerns
- Assisting with the initial interviews or assessments for new clients
- Providing culturally and linguistically appropriate health education and information
- Facilitating health education workshops or trainings on approved topics
- Supporting clients to develop and implement a plan to reduce risks and to enhance their health
- Supporting clients in changing behaviors
- Providing informal counseling or coaching services (also referred to as peer counseling)
- Providing nonclinical care coordination (sometimes referred to as navigation or case management or community care coordination)

- *What other competencies do you think generally lie* **within** *the CHW Scope of Practice?*

OUTSIDE OF THE CHW SCOPE OF PRACTICE

The following competencies are *outside* the CHW SOP:

- Diagnosing illness and other health conditions
- Prescribing treatment or medication
- Counseling severely mentally ill clients (although CHWs will often provide outreach, peer support, health education, and case management services to clients living with severe mental illness)
- Providing therapy (rather than more limited peer/informal counseling)

- *What other competencies do you think lie outside the CHW Scope of Practice?*

SERVICES THAT MAY BE WITHIN OR OUTSIDE THE CHW SCOPE OF PRACTICE

In general, it is easier to determine competencies that lie within or outside of the CHW's SOP. However, there are several competencies that are sometimes considered to lie within, and sometimes considered to lie outside of the CHW SOP, depending on the factors identified above (state law, policies of the employer, professional politics, and training). To avoid confusion, conflict with colleagues, and harm to your clients, seek clear guidance from your supervisors regarding what you are and are not permitted to do on the job.

The following competencies may require specialized training and supervision and *sometimes lie within* and *sometimes outside* the SOP of CHWs.

Informal Counseling

While some professionals argue that CHWs shouldn't perform "counseling" and object to the use of this term, there is a strong tradition of CHWs and others providing peer-based and person-centered counseling. For example, in many agencies, CHWs are trained to use motivational interviewing techniques and practice Mental Health First Aid to appropriately support people experiencing mental health challenges. CHWs have provided risk-reduction counseling to address HIV and other infectious diseases for many decades. Many states train and certify unlicensed frontline providers as peer mental health specialists, drug and alcohol recovery counselors or specialists, and sexual assault counselors.

Clinical counseling and nonclinical counseling use different methods and have different goals. Clinical counseling, also known as mental health counseling, is a type of therapy provided by licensed clinicians with specialized training in diagnosing and treating mental health disorders using evidence-based techniques and interventions. It is generally provided in a setting such as a hospital, health center, or mental health clinic and can address complex and serious mental health conditions. The informal or nonclinical counseling offered by CHWs is focused on personal development, present-day challenges, and promoting health and wellness for people facing a wide range of health and social issues including chronic health conditions and challenges such as reentry (coming home after incarceration) and being unhoused. CHWs provide informal counseling in settings that include health clinics, homeless shelters, residential drug recovery programs, on the streets, in jails and prisons, and wherever people live.

Interpretation and Translation Services

Bilingual CHWs are frequently asked to interpret conversations between clients and providers, or to translate written documents from one language to another. Some CHWs and their employers have advocated for CHWs to provide these services. Others have advocated for all interpretation and translation services to be provided only by those with specialized training or certification because the potential consequences of mistakes made during interpretation or translation can be harmful to clients.

Home Visiting

Many CHWs visit with clients outside of the office including in their homes, in homeless shelters, on the streets, and in jail, hospitals or residential program settings. While many organizations train and support CHWs to conduct home visiting, others do not and may assign other professionals to provide these services. For more information about Home Visits, see Chapter 11.

Research Projects

CHWs may provide assistance with research projects such as by recruiting or enrolling participants. In some research projects, CHWs may work as interviewers or help facilitate focus groups. For more information, please see Chapter 22.

Determining Eligibility Status

CHWs may help in determining the client's eligibility for state benefits, federal benefits, and other forms of assistance. They may also assist clients in completing applications for these benefits.

Medications Management

Increasingly, CHWs work in partnership with clinicians and pharmacists to support clients in understanding and following medications and other treatment guidelines—sometimes referred to as medication management, medication therapy management, or treatment adherence. For example, CHWs from the Boston Public Health Commission work with families to aid them to better understand their children's asthma medications and know how to use them properly to prevent symptoms. For more information about medication management, see Chapter 16.

Accompanying Clients

CHWs may accompany clients during visits to other agencies, appointments with physicians or other professionals, or even court appearances to lend support. For example, while one client may simply need to be provided with the address and operating hours of a local food pantry, another client may benefit by being accompanied the first time they visit the food pantry.

Community Organizing

In some settings, CHWs take an active role in community organizing campaigns or movements. In other settings, these efforts are led by other professionals. For more information about community organizing, see Chapter 23.

Co-Facilitating Social or Support Groups

There are different points of view regarding the level of education or training required to facilitate groups. Some groups are facilitated by CHWs, others only licensed professionals alone or with a CHW co-facilitator. For more information, please see Chapter 21.

Crisis Intervention and Working with Survivors of Trauma

Many CHWs work as part of a team with clients who are experiencing crisis, such as a client recently exposed to sexual assault or domestic violence or other trauma, or someone who is thinking of suicide.

Some professionals argue that nonclinicians do not have sufficient training to provide these services, and the risk of inadvertently causing harm to clients is too great. These advocates believe that clients in crisis should be referred as soon as possible to licensed professionals.

On the other hand, some CHWs and professionals argue that CHWs can be trained to provide crisis intervention services and still make timely referrals to qualified licensed clinicians when needed. They argue that it is not possible for many clients in crisis to be seen by a licensed clinical provider. These advocates also point to the rape crisis and domestic violence movements as models for the provision of culturally responsive crisis intervention services by unlicensed staff.

For more information on crisis intervention and working with survivors of trauma, please see Chapter 18.

> **Anonymous:** My job is mainly about supporting older adults at a local senior center. One day I was called by the director of the senior center because an elderly woman disclosed that she was suicidal. It turned out that she only trusted me to talk with her. I called my supervisor to explain the situation, but she was not around. I drove a short distance to the center and put to practice the new skills that I learned when I became certified in Mental Health First Aid through my employer. I was able to de-escalate the situation and connect her to a clinician. When one social worker on our team found out what I did, she was very upset and vocal because she thought I went beyond my scope and that this was clinical work only. It got even more confusing because the other social worker on the same team commended me for my actions and agreed that I was working within my scope. It led to an argument between these co-workers and my supervisor did not want to take sides, which left me even more confused. How am I supposed to know my scope, if my own supervisor does not know?

- *What other competencies do you think may sometimes lie within or outside of the CHW Scope of Practice?*

> **Anonymous:** Some nurses and social workers here are suspicious that CHWs will "steal their jobs" because we earn less than they do. I think this makes them nervous and question our abilities more. I get annoyed having to deal with this. At the same time, I understand that they themselves do not fully understand what exactly it is that we do. I found it helps when I take the time to really explain my role and how the CHW Code of Ethics prohibits me from doing many things that they are allowed to do. They are shocked to find out that this code of ethics exists. Clarity is the key. As much as I don't like it, I think for a long time that I'm going to keep needing to explain what is and what's not in my scope of work.

When CHWs Work Outside Their Scope of Practice

CHWs may be tempted to work outside their SOP because of their own desire to help or pressure from their supervisor, colleagues, or the clients themselves. It can be hard to say no to these requests. It is understandable why CHWs sometimes find it hard difficult to adhere to their defined SOP.

- *Can you think of situations where you might be tempted to exceed your Scope of Practice?*

Imagine that a CHW:

- Advises a client about cancer treatment
- Gives legal advice to a client related to immigration law

- *How might this impact the client?*

- *The CHW?*

- *The organization where the CHW works?*

When CHWs step outside of their SOP, they risk doing harm to clients, themselves, and their organization. CHWs do not have the required training or licensure to diagnose or treat medical conditions, to provide legal guidance, or to provide therapy. For example, giving advice about cancer treatments could result in a client seeking inappropriate, ineffective, or harmful treatments. Under such circumstances, CHWs should refer the client to a medical provider.

Stepping outside of your SOP may negatively affect your professional reputation and could result in disciplinary action and the loss of your job. In states where CHWs are credentialed, it can lead to having your certificate revoked and negatively impact future employment opportunities. When you step outside of your SOP, you are likely taking over the role of other professionals, such as nurses or social workers, and this may damage your relationship with these colleagues.

Providing services that you are not competent or licensed to provide may also seriously damage the reputation of your program or agency. News that a CHW has done something unethical or has harmed a client will travel quickly in the community and could result in diminished support for an important agency or program.

Exceeding your SOP also breaks trust with the communities that CHWs pledge to support. Most of the communities that CHWs serve have already experienced a long history of harmful treatment by health, medical, education, law enforcement, or other government agencies or representatives. Each betrayal takes a toll on the community and makes it harder for them to establish trusting relationships with service providers.

What to Do When You Are Uncertain about Your Scope of Practice

If your SOP has not been clearly defined by the agency that employs you, or you are uncertain about the type or level of service that you should provide in a certain situation, consider the following suggestions:

- Review your job description and your agency's policies regarding your SOP.

- Examine the potential for causing harm to clients or communities.

- Be aware of your own risk factors for exceeding your SOP. For each of us, there may be types of situations or clients that may motivate our desire to go above and beyond the call of duty and may tempt us to step outside of our professional boundaries.

- Clearly explain to your client what services you can and cannot provide and stay within these professional boundaries.

- Don't let the client be your guide regarding SOP. Some clients, out of an understandable desire to meet their needs, may try to pressure you to step outside of your SOP. Hold firm to your SOP and your ethical guidelines.

- *If you are not certain that a certain duty lies within your Scope of Practice, don't do it, and consult with your supervisor.*

What to Do When you Disagree with How Your Scope of Practice is Defined

As we noted above, people sometimes disagree about which competencies are within or outside of a CHW's SOP. As a result, there may be times when you disagree with how your SOP is defined by your agency, your supervisor, or your colleagues. In such situations, you may want to advocate for your SOP to be narrowed or widened.

Sometimes, a supervisor or colleague might ask you to perform tasks that you have not been trained to do. At other times, you may find that your agency has defined a SOP that is too restrictive and that keeps you from providing services that you are truly competent to provide. In both cases, you may want to consider advocating for changes to your SOP.

Handle these challenges in a way that promotes the welfare of clients as well as your own professional reputation, and that of the program and agency you work for. Take this as an opportunity to advocate *within* your agency and with your supervisor for changes to your SOP. This might involve educating your colleagues and your supervisor about CHWs and their role and about your training, experience, and skills. It might involve finding out from your supervisor what additional training they would like you to have to provide certain services. It is likely to involve advocating for increased opportunities for professional development. In circumstances where you are being pulled away from your duties to do non-CHW work, it may involve advocating for the supervisor to come up with alternate solutions so that you can meet the demands of your role.

5.4 Upholding Professional Boundaries

Establishing and maintaining appropriate professional boundaries protects CHWs as well as the clients and communities they serve, and the programs and agencies they represent. It is an ethical duty related to Article 2 of the Code of Ethics.

Professional boundaries are the limitations or ethical guidelines that define a professional working relationship. Professional boundaries clarify what CHWs can and cannot do for the client. Your clients should know what to expect from your behavior at the outset of the relationship. The moment when a CHW deviates from their job description and professional role is known as a **boundary crossing**.

Examples of professional boundary issues may include:

- Giving or lending money to a client

- Misrepresenting your professional training, skills, or capacity

- Physical contact with a client

- Romantic or sexual involvement with a client
- Managing dual or multiple relationships with clients

A **dual or multiple relationship** exists when a CHW has another type of relationship with a client. For example, your client could be a former co-worker, the son or daughter of a dear friend, a neighbor, or a member of your faith community.

CHWs encounter potential boundary dilemmas frequently, including offers of gifts from clients, requests for financial assistance or babysitting, or invitations for romantic relationships. Whether it is an invitation to a wedding or seeing clients regularly at the local grocery store, it is sometimes difficult to know what to do.

- *Can you think of other situations that present professional boundary dilemmas?*

What Do YOU Think?

Not every boundary crossing is unethical. Because CHWs often work in the same community where they live, it is difficult to avoid dual relationships with clients. In fact, those relationships may be part of what makes the CHW a trusted member of the community. CHWs must stay aware of their influential position with respect to clients, protect the confidentiality of the information they share, and avoid exploiting the trust of clients. Understand that some dual relationships can impair professional judgment or increase the risk of harm to clients. The guiding principle here should be: What is in the best interest of the client? If it could be harmful for a client to work with a CHW with whom the client has a dual relationship (such as a former romantic partner), then the CHW should refer that client to a colleague.

SETTING PROFESSIONAL BOUNDARIES. (*Source:* Foundations for Community Health Workers/ http://youtu.be/WXn-tvVILbY/last accessed 21 September 2023.)

Please watch the following video [▶] interview about the challenge of setting professional boundaries.

Please watch the following videos [▶] that show a CHW working to set a professional boundary with a client. In the Counter Role Play, the CHW struggles to establish a clear boundary. In the Role Play Demo, the CHW does a better job of establishing a clear boundary.

- *What type of professional boundary was this CHW trying to establish?*
- *How well did the CHW establish a clear professional boundary in the Counter and Demo videos?*
- *What would you do differently to establish a boundary with this client?*

SETTING BOUNDARIES WITH CLIENTS: ROLE PLAY, COUNTER

(*Source:* Foundations for Community Health Workers/ http://youtu.be/kziHCHrwtzo/ last accessed 21 September 2023.)

Taking time to review the CHW Code of Ethics can help to clarify the boundary issue you are facing. There are also questions that you can ask yourself as you reflect on the boundary dilemma:

- Why am I considering this crossing of boundaries?
- Who benefits from the boundary crossing?
- Is the boundary crossing necessary or are there other actions you could take?
- How will the boundary crossing affect the professional relationship?
- Is there a cultural context to consider?
- Is this boundary crossing something that I would share with my supervisor or a document in writing? Why? Why not?

SETTING BOUNDARIES WITH CLIENTS: ROLE PLAY, DEMO

(*Source:* Foundations for Community Health Workers/ http://youtu.be/pX9x_w8ME9s/ last accessed 21 September 2023.)

- What might be the impact of crossing this boundary on me, my client, my other clients, and my organization?
- What are the most likely and worst-case scenarios for crossing this boundary?

If you have doubts or concerns about the risk of crossing a professional boundary, consult with your supervisor or another senior colleague. Don't make the decision on your own.

SELF-DISCLOSURE

Self-disclosure is when a CHW—or other health or social service provider—reveals personal or private information about themselves to a client. Examples of this include telling a client HIV status, discussing your own mental health challenges, or talking about a diagnosis of cancer or another disease. It can also include revealing life experiences like homelessness, incarceration, or trauma.

Self-disclosure is a controversial issue and organizations and professionals have different opinions about it (Dalton, 2020). Some would say it is never a good idea to self-disclose. Others would argue that a limited amount of self-disclosure helps the client/provider relationship. Some say it also can help reduce the stigma and isolation that a client may be experiencing.

There are different types of self-disclosure. Personal information is sometimes disclosed to others in an accidental or unavoidable manner. Some disclosure of information is unavoidable, such as revealing to clients that you are pregnant or disabled and using a wheelchair. A CHW may also disclose personal information in an accidental way, such as through unplanned contact with a client outside of the office (e.g., when a CHW sees a client at church or in another member organization). However, most self-disclosure is deliberate: the provider decides to share personal information with the clients and communities they are working with.

Potential Risks of Self-Disclosure

The key reason why health and human service providers do not disclose personal information to clients is due to the potential risks and harms that could result. Risks may include:

- Self-disclosure may shift the focus from the client to the provider. It may interrupt or take time away from the client's story or concerns.
- A provider's self-disclosure may imply or unintentionally send a message that the client should think, feel, or make choices that are the same or similar (i.e., take the same path to recovery from substance use).
- It may leave the CHW/provider vulnerable to further inquiries about their personal life.
- It may change the nature of the relationship between the client and the provider. For example, some clients may want to develop a friendship with the CHW, and self-disclosure may lead them to believe that this is possible.

Keep in mind that while the CHW Code of Ethics and organizational policies protect the client's confidentiality, there is no obligation for your clients to maintain confidentiality about what you choose to disclose to them. They are free to share with anyone whatever you have said to them.

- *Can you think of other potential risks of self-disclosure?*

What Do
YOU?
Think

Potential Benefits of Self-Disclosure

There is a strong tradition within the CHW profession in practicing limited self-disclosure. Limited self-disclosure can be beneficial when clients face stigma, shame or isolation, and related challenges in accessing services and support. For example, clients may be struggling with issues such as addiction, incarceration, schizophrenia or depression, cancer, HIV disease, sexual orientation, or surviving trauma experiences. Sometimes it can be helpful to the client for a service provider to briefly disclose that they have faced similar experiences and issues in their own life. For example, a CHW might say, "*I was in prison too,*" or "*I have HIV disease.*" Without going on to provide any further details, this type of self-disclosure can help clients feel more comfortable talking about their own lives and sharing their thoughts, concerns, and feelings. If the client continues to ask questions about the CHW/provider's experience, the CHW can always explain and shift the focus back to the client's experience: *"This is a place to focus on your experience and concerns, not mine. Can you tell me more about what you have been going through?"*

- *Can you think of other potential benefits to self-disclosure?*

Important Considerations for Self-Disclosure

We encourage you to consider the following questions as you determine if, when, and how you may share personal information with clients.

1. **Benefit:** How might your client benefit from your self-disclosure? How might you benefit? Whose needs are being met?

2. **Alternatives:** Are there alternative ways that you can support the client other than disclosing personal information about yourself? Have you tried using person-centered skills like motivational interviewing?

3. **Burden on your client:** Will your self-disclosure shift the focus of your work away from the client's experience and priorities? Will the nature of your self-disclosure place a burden on your client?

4. **Nature of information that is being disclosed:** Is the information related to the topic that the client is discussing?

5. **Context:** What is happening at the moment when you are considering self-disclosure? What has been the primary focus of the meetings? Is your self-disclosure consistent with the client's priority and goals?

6. **Condition of the client:** What is the client's emotional state? Are they highly distressed or vulnerable? Are they addressing issues in a state of anxiety or in a comfortable, safe state?

7. **Timing:** At what point in the relationship are you thinking of disclosing personal information? Is it at the beginning, the middle, or at the end of your work with the client? Is the timing of your self-disclosure appropriate? Is it about you or about them? Why are you considering self-disclosure at this time?

If you choose to self-disclose, keep in mind that you are opening yourself up to further questions from clients who may want to know more about your life. You may need to explain the organization's policy on self-disclosure and why you can't and won't share more information. Be prepared to explain that your work and primary goal is to support clients in making their own decisions, and you don't want to impose your beliefs, values, and situation on others.

Suggested Guidelines for Self-Disclosure

In general, we suggest that you err on the side of not disclosing personal information with those that you work with. In this way, you avoid the potential harms highlighted above.

If you are unsure about why you are disclosing and how it benefits the client, please don't disclose.

While it may be tempting, don't use self-disclosure simply as a short cut to establish rapport and gain trust. There are other evidence-based methods that help deepen the connection with a client. Use person-centered approaches including cultural humility and motivational interviewing skills (covered in Chapters 7 and 9).

If you do decide to disclose personal information to a client (once you have weighed the options), here are some guidelines:

- **Keep it brief:** Don't go on and on providing additional information about your identity or experience. The best self-disclosure is done with just a few words (*"I was unhoused too"*).

- **Keep it limited:** Don't get into the details of your treatment for any health condition. Don't give specific dates, times, reasons for incarceration, or other events. The focus of your work is not your own challenges, experiences, beliefs, or values. Keep the focus on the client.

- **Refocus the discussion as quickly as possible** to address the concerns and priorities of the client (*"What are your priorities right now?"*).

Please watch the following videos, including role plays and an interview, on the topic of self-disclosure.

- *What personal information did the CHW disclose to the client, and why?*

- *What did the CHW do well—and not-so-well—in terms of self-disclosure?*

- *What would you have done differently if you were the CHW working with this client?*

- *What are your guidelines for providing self-disclosure to the clients or communities you work with?*

5.5 Multidisciplinary Teamwork

CHWs often work as part of a team with colleagues who have received formal education in different disciplines, such as nurses, social workers, psychologists, alcohol and drug recovery coaches, peer specialists, physician assistants, nurse practitioners, and physicians. Sometimes, CHWs comprise a large part of the team, while in other settings, you may be the only CHW on the team.

An added benefit of being a member of a multidisciplinary team is that you will discover how people with different professional specializations view and approach a particular topic or problem. You will have an opportunity to understand the different lenses your colleagues are looking through and offer your own perspective. As a valued member of the team, this is an opportunity for you to demonstrate your own professional expertise, which may be rooted in your unique understanding of the communities being served.

SELF-DISCLOSURE: ROLE PLAY, COUNTER
(*Source:* Foundations for Community Health Workers/http://youtu.be/7CpFvjXO-rs/last accessed 21 September 2023.)

SELF-DISCLOSURE: ROLE PLAY, DEMO
(*Source:* Foundations for Community Health Workers/http://youtu.be/12s4zgUUJFs/last accessed 21 September 2023.)

SELF-DISCLOSURE, FACULTY INTERVIEW
(*Source:* Foundations for Community Health Workers/http://youtu.be/ihcr6GvBAAg/last accessed 21 September 2023.)

> **Paul Mendes:** I may not have a fancy college degree and a bunch of letters behind my name, but I have a Ph.D. when it comes to understanding life on the streets and addiction.

CHWs are hired to work as part of a multidisciplinary team in health care settings, such as in primary health care clinics that focus on serving low-income patients. CHWs are valuable team members who contribute to achieving goals of improving patient outcomes, improving the patient experience of care, and reducing health care costs. A 2023 report on the effectiveness of CHWs provides clear evidence that "Community health workers (CHWs) are critical to improving individual and community health through their ability to build trust and relationships and deepen communication between patients and providers" (The Association of State and Territorial Health Officials, 2023). This report offers a summary of several research studies demonstrating CHW effectiveness in rural and urban settings addressing a wide array of health issues.

Understanding the value of your contributions and learning how to work effectively as part of a team is critical for achieving long-term success as a CHW.

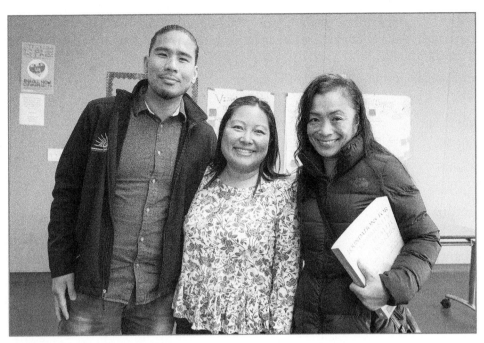

CHWs always work as part of a team.

THE USE OF CLINICAL TEAMS IN HEALTH CARE SETTINGS

Clinical teams are increasingly used to provide primary health care, especially in busy clinics that serve a high volume of patients living with chronic health conditions. The use of health care teams is defined as: "A team-based model of care strives to meet patient needs and preferences by actively engaging patients as full participants in their care, while encouraging and supporting all health care professionals to function to the full extent of their education, certification, and licensure" (American College of Physicians, 2023).

Providing primary care services through a team-based model is a way to address common health care challenges such as:

- A large ratio of patients to licensed clinicians
- The lack of sufficient time allotted for physicians and other licensed providers to spend with patients
- Physicians serving historically marginalized communities are less likely to reflect the populations they serve and may experience more obstacles to gaining the patient's trust.
- Many patients have a difficult time understanding health information (health literacy). Research shows that nearly 36% of adults have low health literacy and just 12% of patients have a proficient level of health literacy. Disproportionate rates of low health literacy are found among patients who are older, have limited education, lower income, chronic conditions, and those who are non-native English speakers (Hickey & Masterson Creber, 2018).
- The increasing complexity of modern medicine and insufficient collaboration and communication among providers.
- Increasing rates of chronic conditions such as diabetes and hypertension.
- The number of Americans aged 65 and older makes up an increasing share of the population. With this has come a steep increase in the number of people with Alzheimer's disease, osteoporosis, and other ailments often associated with aging.
- The needs of patients living with chronic diseases for more intensive care to manage symptoms, change behaviors, and take any prescribed medications properly
- Addressing patient's challenges associated with managing many different medications for co-occurring medical conditions.
- Rising health care costs

There are many ways to organize primary health care teams. Some teams are quite small, and others are quite large, depending upon the needs of the health care practice and the patients they serve. In general, primary health care teams include:

- The patient (the most important member of the team)
- The patient's family and close social circle
- One or more physicians
- One or more nurses
- A medical assistant

Some teams also include:

- Community health workers
- Nurse practitioners
- Physician assistants
- Licensed mental health providers such as social workers or psychologists
- Front-desk staff
- Peer specialists
- Peer recovery coaches
- Pharmacists
- Nutritionists
- Other providers

THE BENEFITS OF TEAM-BASED CARE

There are many benefits to a team-based approach to the delivery of primary health care. Teams can improve the coordination of health care services for patients, their families, and providers and often provide more timely access to health care (it is easier for patients to get an appointment with one of the team members). Team-based practice promotes greater collaboration and consultation among health care providers and has been shown to result in improved health outcomes for patients and their families. Team-based care is effective in achieving what is known as the quadruple aim—improving quality of care, patient experience, staff well-being, and cost savings (Santoro, 2021).

KEY CHARACTERISTICS OF EFFECTIVE TEAM-BASED CARE

As the use of health care teams has increased, a new literature has emerged that is striving to research, identify and promote the key characteristics of successful teams. The Community Workforce Institute gathered data nationally from over 200 supervisors and identified characteristics of successful teamwork (Community Workforce Institute, unpublished results) including:

A shared vision and mission: A shared vision is essential for teams to work together effectively. All team members should share the same understanding of their collective purpose and common goals. This includes a shared understanding of the organization's core values and beliefs.

Role clarity: Clear roles and responsibilities prevent confusion and conflict among team members. The CHWs and everyone else on the team need to have a clear understanding of their own roles and responsibilities, as well as those of their colleagues. This includes clarity and adherence to the organization's established guidelines, policies, and protocols. This helps to ensure that the team is working toward a common goal and knows precisely what is expected of them.

Open and respectful communication: High-functioning teams regularly engage in open communication to share ideas and discuss challenges and progress. All members should be encouraged to share their thoughts openly and respectfully. Approaching each other with honesty, curiosity, respect, and empathy is what builds trust and cohesiveness among the team.

A culture of unity: Unity cannot be demanded; it is built over time only when people feel truly safe with each other. The workplace climate needs to be one where everyone feels supported. Effective organizational leaders, just like effective CHWs, establish a supportive environment where people can identify challenges or problems, celebrate successes, and work together to overcome obstacles and improve both the work environment and the quality of services they provide.

Growth opportunities: To ensure quality health care services, every member of the multidisciplinary team needs to keep up to date with the latest information, evidence-based practices, and technologies in their respective fields. This includes investing in professional development opportunities. Sometimes supervisors are reluctant to have CHWs attend training because of staffing shortages or concerns about clients not having their needs met. Other times, it is the CHWs themselves who feel guilty about being away from work when so many people need their assistance.

Measurable processes and outcomes: Data are gathered and analyzed on an ongoing basis to identify patient or client needs, risks, and outcomes. Patient outcomes are analyzed over time and this drives the continuous improvement of team systems and services.

Data gathering provides an opportunity to objectively evaluate the success of an activity or intervention at the individual or group level. This evidence can help to determine if a program or services are having the desired effect. For example, data may indicate low flu vaccination rates in a specific community. By gathering and analyzing this data, health care teams can develop or revise culturally responsive approaches to boost vaccination rates. The effectiveness of the new or revised intervention is then evaluated once again based on gathering new data on vaccination rates in the prioritized community.

If You Are Working as Part of a Clinical Team

Take a moment to reflect on your experience working as part of a clinical team.

- Does the team clearly identify common values?
- Are the roles and responsibilities of all team members clearly identified?
- How does the team work to develop and maintain trust?
- How often, and how well, does the team communicate with one another (including the patient)?
- Does the team welcome communication that identifies potential challenges and problems?
- What data does the team use to measure processes (policies and protocols) and health outcomes? Are these data used to improve team systems and the delivery of patient-centered health care?

THE ROLE OF THE CHW WITHIN HEALTH CARE TEAMS

The role of the CHW as a member of a primary health care team will vary depending upon the size and composition of the team. It will also depend upon the training and skills of the CHW. In general, however, CHWs serve on the front lines and typically provide the following types of services:

- **Outreach** to recruit new patients and maintain contact with existing patients
- **Communication** with patients (via phone, text, email, and regular mail) and reminders about appointments, medications, behavior change, etc.
- **Patient education** (such as providing and reinforcing information about how to manage chronic conditions)
- **Person-centered case management services**, including the development and monitoring of Action Plans
- **Chronic conditions management** including supporting patients with the self-management of chronic health conditions through action planning and person-centered coaching/counseling
- **Medication management** (this may include showing someone how to properly use an inhaler or help come up with creative solutions to remember taking medications)

- **Home visits** (when patients are too ill to come to the clinic or are out of communication with the clinic)
- **Other:** *What other services may CHWs provide?*

CHWs often spend more time with patients than other members of the health care team. This is particularly true if the CHW conducts patient education, counseling, and case management services. This, in turn, frees up physicians and other licensed providers to see more patients, and to focus on issues of diagnosis and treatment. Because the CHW may spend more time with patients, visit them at home or in other community settings, and engage in more frequent email, text, and/or phone and telehealth communications, the CHW often has a better understanding of the patient's current health risks and concerns, and can play a vital role in sharing this valuable information with the rest of the team.

THE CHALLENGES OF TEAMWORK

While an increasing number of organizations have figured out how to successfully integrate CHWs into their teams, in some settings, there is still confusion and misunderstanding about the roles, competencies, and tasks of CHWs. The problem may be more pronounced in settings where most team members spend all their time at the clinic and the CHWs spend a considerable amount of time out in the community. This sometimes leads people to make negative assumptions about how CHWs use their time.

> **Anonymous:** Sometimes it's like people at the office think that I am at home all day watching Netflix while they are stuck inside working! They have no idea how much I am actually out there helping their patients manage chronic conditions and make sure that they show up for medical appointments.

Teamwork in any workplace setting can be challenging. However, CHWs are likely to face unique challenges due to their professional roles. These challenges may include:

- Being treated, at times, with less respect than other members of the team, particularly those who are licensed providers
- A perception that CHWs are more closely allied with clients than with the agency, program, or other providers
- A lack of understanding and respect for the services that CHWs provide outside of the agency office or clinic (such as outreach, accompaniment, and home visits).

> **Yemisrach Kibret:** A lot of times, others on the team don't really know what we do. They think we are just something warm and fuzzy and don't know what to make of us. You can count how many blood draws a phlebotomist makes or how many vaccinations a nurse gives. What they sometime don't see is how we help make sure people get enough to eat and don't get evicted. Without food and shelter, there is no good health. Not to mention, we are a big part of why the patient chooses to show up at the appointment in the first place.

- **Hierarchies:** Workplaces in general are hierarchical and the health care field is no different. Often medical doctors sit at or near the top of the hierarchy and CHWs toward or at the bottom. Hierarchies often operate in a way that makes those at the bottom feel like less-valued members of the team.
- A lack of information and understanding about the CHW SOP and qualifications. As a result, CHWs may have to spend extra time explaining their role and job duties to their colleagues.

- Less job security arising from the way that services and provider positions are financed and paid for. For example, many organizations still rely upon limited-time grant funds to pay for CHW positions.
- **Workload equity:** Many programs are structured so that each CHW has an equal number of people they serve. However, some CHWs may work with client populations that require additional assistance and time. Bilingual and multi-lingual CHW may be asked to provide additional services (sometimes without additional compensation) such as translation and interpretation or to cover the front desk. It is important for organizations to be aware that when a CHW is pulled away for tasks that are outside of their scope of work, it leaves less time to serve patients.

- *Can you think of other types of challenges that CHWs may face?*
- *Have you faced other challenges as a member of a health care team?*

SUCCESS STRATEGIES FOR EFFECTIVE TEAMWORK

As a CHW, you will always be working with some type of team. Learning how to be a valued team member is critical for the long-term success of your career. Strive to become the type of professional that others can rely on and are excited to work with day to day. Consider the following suggestions for successful teamwork:

- Know your job description, SOP, and what is expected of you in the workplace day-to-day
- If you don't understand some aspect of your job or organization, speak up and ask for clarification and guidance
- Bring a positive attitude and your "best self" to work every day
- Participate actively in team meetings. If you tend to be quiet in meetings, try and take the opportunity to have your voice heard and gradually work toward saying more as your comfort level increases
- Provide culturally responsive services and share your expertise and community knowledge with other team members who will benefit from what you know about the communities they serve.
- Keep up to date with your documentation
- Learn how to switch codes and adapt to the codes of the professional workplace including, for example, codes for dress, language, mode of communication, time management, etc. What is considered professional may also vary from one organization to the next (see Chapter 14 on Professional Skills).
- Maintain close communication with your direct supervisor
- Reach out and ask for the support and guidance that you want and need
- Take responsibility for the mistakes that you make and view them as learning opportunities
- Learn how to receive and provide critical feedback professionally
- Be a systems thinker and avoid blaming others for problems. Work to understand the context of the problem. Recognize that problems never exist in isolation; they are surrounded by other problems that need to be understood in order to find effective solutions
- Don't avoid big or persistent problems in the workplace; find a professional and respectful way to raise them with your colleagues in the appropriate forum (a meeting with your supervisor, a team meeting, huddle or case conference, etc.)
- **Broadcast stories of ingenuity:** CHWs have so many unheard stories of where they played a major role in helping vastly improve the well-being of patients. While medical professionals may be credited with positive health outcomes, behind the scenes, a CHW may have worked tirelessly to make it possible for their client to show up at medical appointments and adhere to the prescribed treatment regimen. As such stories are conveyed, it will assist in raising your stature and the stature of the CHW profession.

- *What else might be helpful guidance for working effectively with a multidisciplinary health care team?*

Chapter Review

To review your understanding of the concepts and skills addressed in Chapter 5, please review the questions provided below and consider how you would answer them.

SELF-AWARENESS

- Why is self-awareness an essential quality for CHWs and other helping professionals?
- What populations are you less familiar with and least prepared to work with?
- What health topics and other issues do you feel least prepared to address with clients and community members?
- What steps can you take to enhance your self-knowledge and self-awareness?

ETHICAL GUIDELINES

- What is the purpose of a code of ethics?
- What are three ethical guidelines from the CHW Code of Ethics?
- How—and when—will you explain the principle of confidentiality to clients?
- What are the limits to confidentiality policies?
- What types of client information must you report to your supervisor or other third-party agencies?

SCOPE OF PRACTICE

- What is Scope of Practice and why is it important for CHWs to understand?
- What may happen when CHWs exceed their Scope of Practice?
- Identify at least three tasks or services that are clearly within the CHW SOP.
- Identify at least three tasks or services that are outside of the CHW SOP.
- What factors may determine whether this task is within the CHW's SOP?
- What will you do if you are uncertain about whether a specific task is within your SOP?

PROFESSIONAL BOUNDARIES

- What are professional boundaries and why are they important for CHWs to maintain?
- What are some of the potential risks and harms of crossing professional boundaries?
- How will you communicate your professional boundaries to a client who doesn't understand them?
- What can you do if you face a situation in which you are uncertain about your professional boundaries?

SUCCESSFUL TEAMWORK

- What are some of the key characteristics of successful teams?
- What are some of the common challenges that you may face when working as a member of a multidisciplinary team?
- Identify at least three key strategies for successful teamwork.

References

American College of Physicians (ACP). (2023). Team Based Model of Care Toolkit. https://www.acponline.org/ practice-resources/patient-and-interprofessional-education/team-based-care-toolkit#:~:text=Academy%20of%20Medicine-,What%20Is%20Team%2DBased%20 Care%3F,education%2C%20certification%2C%20and%20licensure (accessed 7 May 2023).

Association of State and Territorial Health Officials (ASTHO) & National Association of Community Health Workers (NACHW). (2023). Community Health Workers—Evidence of Their Effectiveness. https://www. astho.org/globalassets/pdf/community-health-workers-summary-evidence.pdf (accessed 7 May 2023).

Centers for Disease Control and Prevention. (2022). Health Insurance Portability and Accountability Act of 1996 (HIPAA). https://www.cdc.gov/phlp/publications/topic/hipaa.html#:~:text=The%20Health%20 Insurance%20Portability%20and,the%20patient's%20consent%20or%20knowledge (accessed 4 May 2023).

Dalton, K. (2020). Self-Disclosure: The Risks and the Benefits. https://medium.com/@daltonk002/ self-disclosure-the-risks-benefits-94649a1ada44 (accessed 14 December 2022).

Goleman, D., Kaplan, R.S., David, S., & Eurich, T. (2018). *Self-awareness (HBR emotional intelligence series)*. Harvard Business Press (accessed 12 December 2022).

Hickey, K. T. & Masterson Creber, R. (2018). Low health literacy: implications for managing cardiac patients in practice. *The Journal for Nurse Practitioners*. https://pubmed.ncbi.nlm.nih.gov/30028773/ (accessed 7 May 2023).

Santoro, H. (2021). Patients, clinicians benefit from team-based care model, study finds. *Stanford Medicine*. https://med.stanford.edu/news/all-news/2021/12/team-based-care-physician-burnout.html (accessed 6 May 2023).

Additional Resources

A Day in the Life of a Community Health Worker. https://youtu.be/MXpgGABXfx0 (accessed 11 January 2023).

Alvarez-Hernandez, L. R., Bermúdez, J. M., Orpinas, P., Matthew, R., Calva, A., & Darbisi, C. (2021). "No queremos quedar mal": A qualitative analysis of a boundary setting training among Latina community health workers. *Journal of Latinx Psychology*, 9(4), 315.

American Association of Community Health Workers Code of Ethics. CHW_Code_of_Ethics.pdf (in.gov).

Ashley, G. C. & Reiter-Palmon, R. (2012). Self-awareness and the evolution of leaders: The need for a better measure of self-awareness. *Journal of Behavioral and Applied Management*, 14(1), 2–17.

Association of State and Territorial Health Officials (ASTHO) and National Association of Community Health Workers (NACHW). (2023). Community Health Workers: Summary of Evidence. https://www.astho.org/ globalassets/pdf/community-health-workers-summary-evidence.pdf.

Boston University School of Social Work—Center for Innovation in Social Work. (2023). A Training Curriculum for Community Health Workers|Core Competencies, Establishing and Supporting Professional Boundaries. https://ciswh.org/chw-curriculum/establishing-and-supporting-professional-boundaries/.

Community Health Worker Code of Ethics Toolkit. https://chwcentral.org/resources/community-health-worker-code-of-ethics-toolkit/.

Community Health Works. (2018). Building a community health worker program: The key to better care. *Better Outcomes & Lower Costs*. https://www.aha.org/system/files/2018-10/chw-program-manual-2018-toolkit-final.pdf.

Duval, S. & Wicklund, R. A. (1972). *A theory of objective self awareness*. Academic Press ()

Kilpatrick, S., Cheers, B., Gilles, M., & Taylor, J. (2009). Boundary crossers, communities, and health: exploring the role of rural health professionals. *Health & Place*, 15(1), 284–290.

Laurenzi, C. A., Skeen, S., Rabie, S., Coetzee, B. J., Notholi, V., Bishop, J., Chademana, E., & Tomlinson, M. (2021). Balancing roles and blurring boundaries: Community health workers' experiences of navigating the crossroads between personal and professional life in rural South Africa. *Health & Social Care in the Community*, 29(5), 1249–1259.

Logan, R. I. (2022). *Boundaries of care: Community health workers in the United States*. Rowman & Littlefield.

Musoke, D., Ssemugabo, C., Ndejjo, R., Molyneux, S., & Ekirapa-Kiracho, E. (2020). Ethical practice in my work: community health workers' perspectives using photovoice in Wakiso district, Uganda. *BMC Medical Ethics*, 21(1), 1–10.

Social Work License Map. (2023). Engaging in Self-Awareness: How Not to Judge When Helping Others. Retrieved from https://socialworklicensemap.com/blog/self-awareness-how-to-avoid-judgment-when-helping-others/.

Utah Broad-Based Community Health Worker Coalition (CHWC). (2023). CHW Scope of Practice. https://nachw.org/chw_resources/chw-scope-of-practice/ (accessed 12 January 2023).

Zeng, F., Ye, Q., Li, J., & Yang, Z. (2021). Does self-disclosure matter? A dynamic two-stage perspective for the personalization-privacy paradox. *Journal of Business Research*, 124, 667–675.

Behavior Change and Person-centered Practice

Tim Berthold

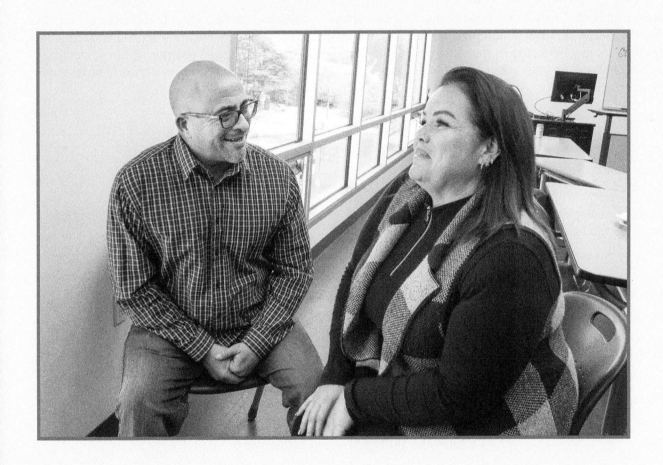

Foundations for Community Health Workers, Third Edition. Edited by Tim Berthold and Darouny Somsanith.
© 2024 John Wiley & Sons, Inc. Published 2024 by John Wiley & Sons, Inc.
Companion website: http://www.wiley.com/go/communityhealthworkers3E

Introduction

This chapter introduces two topics that are essential to your success as a community health worker:

- Understanding Behavior Change and
- Person-centered Practice

As a CHW, you are likely to work closely with clients who want to change a health-related behavior in order to promote their wellness and improve their quality of life. To be successful in this work, you must understand the factors that get in the way of and facilitate behavior change.

Professionals and service providers in the fields of health care, social services, and education are gradually shifting away from traditional approaches that emphasized the knowledge, skills, and authority of the provider. Increasingly, these traditional approaches are being replaced by person-centered models—including patient-centered health care, person-centered counseling, and student-centered learning—that honor and emphasize the knowledge; skills; values; identities; and priorities of clients, patients, and students. Person-centered approaches are more effective in supporting clients to achieve behavior change and positive health outcomes. They also promote the independence, self-confidence, and resilience of clients. We will continue to address person-centered practice concepts and skills throughout the book.

WHAT YOU WILL LEARN

By studying the information in this chapter, you will be able to:

Behavior Change

- Identify behaviors that clients typically seek to change
- Apply an ecological model to analyze individual, family, community, and societal factors that influence behavior and behavior change
- Discuss and analyze four common mistakes that CHWs make when supporting clients to change behaviors

Person-centered Practice

- Discuss essential concepts of person-centered practice
- Compare and contrast traditional or provider-centered practice with emerging person-centered practice models
- Explain the value of a strength-based approach to working with clients
- Discuss implicit theory and how you will develop your own theory of behavior change

C3 Roles and Skills Addressed in Chapter 6

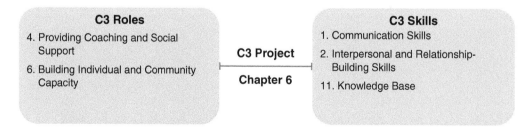

C3 Roles		**C3 Skills**
4. Providing Coaching and Social Support	**C3 Project**	1. Communication Skills
6. Building Individual and Community Capacity	**Chapter 6**	2. Interpersonal and Relationship-Building Skills
		11. Knowledge Base

WORDS TO KNOW

Implicit Theory   Unconditional Positive Regard

Strength-based Approach

6.1 Understanding Behavior Change

One of the most common roles for CHWs is supporting clients to modify behaviors that influence their health. While supporting people to change behaviors may sound relatively straightforward, the process of changing behavior and the art of supporting others in doing so are complex and challenging. For these reasons, we will review some basic information and guiding principles about the behavior change process. We will build on this information in Chapters 9, 16, and 17 and provide more skills—such as motivational interviewing—for supporting clients to successfully change health-related behaviors.

WHICH BEHAVIORS DO PEOPLE TYPICALLY ATTEMPT TO CHANGE?

These behaviors may include:

- Patterns of eating and drinking
- Physical activity or exercise
- Smoking, alcohol, and drug use
- Stress management
- Building greater social support and connection to family, friends, or community
- Adherence or compliance with treatment guidelines (such as remembering to take medications at the proper times and in the proper doses)
- Sexual behaviors (such as regular and effective contraceptive use and safer sex practices)
- Anger management
- Parenting practices (such as effective communication and discipline)
- Screening for cancer and other health conditions
- Adjusting behaviors to prevent COVID-19 infections such as wearing masks, physical distancing, and vaccination.

- *Can you think of other behaviors to add to this list?*

What Do
YOU?
Think

Most of us have attempted to change a behavior: to stop smoking, to regularly engage in physical activity, to eat healthier foods, to turn in homework assignments on time, or to change the way we talk with loved ones when we are angry. We know from our own experience how challenging and frustrating it can be to make and sustain behavior change. If it were easy to change behavior, our society wouldn't experience such high rates of heart disease, diabetes, COVID-19, or sexually transmitted infections.

Your Experience with Behavior Change

Before considering how to support *others* in changing *their* behaviors, please reflect on *your own experiences*. If possible, take time to discuss your responses with a friend or colleague.

- Which behaviors have you tried to change?
- What motivated you to change your behavior?
- Was it easy to make changes?
- What factors supported you in making change?
- What got in the way of successful behavior change?
- Were you able to maintain change over time?
- Did you ever relapse or return to the old behavior you had hoped to change? If so, what influenced this? How did you feel when you relapsed?

FACTORS THAT INFLUENCE BEHAVIOR: DEVELOPING AN ECOLOGICAL APPROACH

Imagine that you are working with a client who has expressed the desire to:

- Change their diet in order to manage diabetes or prevent heart disease
- Use condoms regularly to reduce the risks of sexually transmitted infections
- Leave an abusive relationship

Despite good intentions, people sometimes fail to meet their own expectations and may relapse to the very behaviors or situations they were attempting to change. *Why is changing behavior so difficult? What gets in the way?*

Table 6.1 identifies some of the factors that may get in the way of successful behavior change. These factors correspond to the ecological model presented in Chapter 3 and are categorized at the level of the individual, family and friends, neighborhood or community, and the broader society.

The table illustrates how a wide range of factors may influence people's health and complicate their efforts to change behaviors. These factors always depend on a person's identity (including life experiences, age, ethnicity, nationality, immigration status, primary language, sexual orientation, gender identity, disability status, and so on) and social context. Social context refers to the reality in which people live and includes their families, friends, workplaces, homes, and economic, cultural, and political dynamics and policies affecting their neighborhood, city, state, or nation.

The list of factors provided in Table 6.1 is not meant to be exhaustive; it doesn't include every possibility. When CHW students at City College of San Francisco brainstorm a list of factors that influence behavior, the list typically fills up six to eight large pieces of flip chart paper and includes dozens of distinct items. Additional factors that influence people's ability to successfully change behaviors include the following:

Table 6.1 Factors That Get in the Way of Behavior Change: An Ecological Model

CLIENT EXAMPLE	INDIVIDUAL FACTORS	FACTORS RELATED TO FAMILY AND FRIENDS	NEIGHBORHOOD AND COMMUNITY FACTORS	SOCIETAL FACTORS: MEDIA, ECONOMICS, AND POLITICS
R. wants to eat healthier foods in order to manage their type 2 diabetes.	R. works at a low-wage job and lacks funds to purchase healthier foods Lack of knowledge about healthier foods R. craves the less healthy foods they grew up with Usually drinks soda Lack of cooking experience Lack of self-esteem Loneliness and history of eating less healthy foods to manage depression *Other possibilities?*	R. eats several meals a month with family R's family traditions don't feature healthier foods R's children are used to processed and fast foods and don't like to eat vegetables Pressure from family and friends to eat "regular" foods that are less healthy *Other possibilities?*	Lives in a neighborhood that lacks grocery stores and access to affordable healthier foods Neighborhoods where the client lives and works are full of fast-food restaurants and convenience stores *Other possibilities?*	Advertising and promotion of foods high in sugar, fats, and carbohydrates (fast foods and processed foods) Judgement about people who don't "promote their own health." Lack of government policies and programs providing access to affordable and healthy foods to low-income communities Government policies do not adequately promote and protect a living wage for all workers *Other possibilities?*

Individual Factors

- Emotions, such as embarrassment, shame, guilt, fear, love, or loneliness
- Desire for love, intimacy, and a sense of belonging
- Dependency—economic or emotional—on others
- Lack of confidence in the ability to succeed
- Thoughts, including self-defeating thoughts (such as *"I always mess up," "I won't be able to," "I don't care what happens …"*)
- Self-esteem (how we think and feel about ourselves)
- Pleasure (the desire for pleasure, including pleasure from food, sex, alcohol, and drug use)
- Spiritual, religious, or metaphysical/philosophical faith, meaning, or purpose
- Knowledge relevant to behavior change (such as information about healthier foods)
- History—what has happened before—including history of successful behavior change and history of trauma such as domestic violence and sexual assault
- Long-established patterns of behavior, including risk behaviors such as drinking or using drugs when under stress

Family and Friends

- Level of family support and conflict
- Isolation
- Cultural identity, values, and traditions
- Peer pressure—from friends and family
- Sense of belonging
- Healthy romantic and sexual relationships
- Exposure to violence or abuse in relationships with family or others

Neighborhood and Community Factors

- Social identity and sense of belonging to a defined community
- Availability of community-based resources such as health and social services agencies, good schools, faith-based institutions including churches and mosques, recreational and cultural programs including parks and after-school programs for youths, affordable and healthy food, public transportation, and affordable housing
- Working conditions, including exposure to hazardous chemicals, low pay and lack of benefits, conflict with management, and other sources of stress
- Exposure to potentially harmful resources or dynamics such drug sales, police violence, and other forms of violence
- Support from helping professionals or harmful interactions with helping professionals
- Cultural or religious support or rejection
- Community norms and expectations
- Stigma and prejudice against one's identity or behaviors

Societal Factors

- Prejudice and discrimination based on ethnicity, nationality, immigration status, language, gender, gender-identity, sexual orientation, weight or size, level of education, disability, age, history of incarceration, and so forth
- Government policies, including those determining access to essential services such as safe housing, healthy nutrition, effective schools, school-based meals, after-school programs, health insurance, employment, drug treatment programs, residency or citizenship, health education programs, and civil rights

- Criminal justice approach to drug use, rather than a harm-reduction approach (people are sentenced to criminal justice facilities for using drugs rather than provided with treatment and services to reduce harm)
- Economic policies and forces influencing wages, working conditions, employment benefits, and access to resources
- Corporate promotion of products such as processed or fast foods and soda, alcohol and tobacco, or guns
- Media promotion of harmful attitudes, behaviors, and products
- Political events such as armed conflict, war, pandemics, and economic crisis
- Natural events—often influenced by human actions—such as drought, famine, fire, and hurricanes

- *What other factors influence our ability to successful change our behavior?*

What Do YOU Think?

As discussed in Chapter 3, public health research has demonstrated that social and ecological factors have a much more significant influence on human health than genetics, knowledge, or individual behaviors. An ecological approach to understanding and facilitating behavior change examines both the factors that individuals may be able to control and the broader social, economic, cultural, and political factors that influence their choices, behavior, and health. We encourage CHWs to view individual clients within the broad social context in which they live.

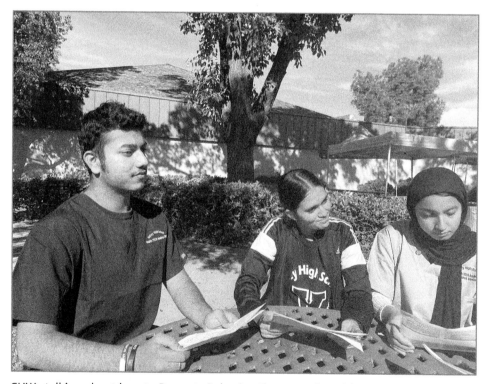

CHWs talking about how to Promote Behavior Change and Healthy Eating in their Community.

COMMON MISTAKES IN ATTEMPTING TO FACILITATE BEHAVIOR CHANGE

We want to highlight several common mistakes that health and helping professionals often make when addressing the challenge of behavior change. We encourage you to understand what these mistakes are and why we suggest that they may undermine your work with clients. The four common mistakes are:

1. Relying on information alone
2. Giving advice

3. Blaming the client
4. Failing to address issues of accountability

Common Mistake #1: Relying on Information Alone

Helping professionals often assume that if they provide people with clear and accurate information about a health condition, and what they can do to prevent the condition or improve their health, then clients will apply that information and change their behavior.

For example, a CHW may provide a client living with high blood pressure with information about their condition, their risks for stroke and heart attack, and guidelines for the management of their condition including medication management and guidelines for healthy eating and physical activity levels. Sometimes, helping professionals spend most of a visit providing information to the client.

While the information provided may be accurate, it is unlikely to result in immediate, significant, and lasting behavior change. It is likely that the client has heard the information before, especially if they have been living with the health condition or the health risks for some time. For most people, the problem isn't that they lack knowledge about health risks or guidelines for promoting their health (most of us know something about healthier eating and the benefits of physical activity, for example). Rather, other factors—such as stress, lack of time and money, self-esteem, familiar health habits, and family obligations—complicate our ability to adopt healthier behaviors.

- *Have you ever encountered a health care or other helping professional who focused exclusively on providing you with health information?*

- *How does this type of approach work for you?*

- *Do you think that this type of approach will be effective with most clients? Why or why not?*

We don't recommend this approach because:
- It is unlikely to result in effective and lasting behavior change.
- It assumes that people don't have complete or accurate knowledge about the health issue.
- The CHW provides information, dominates the session, and does not make space for the client to share their own knowledge, questions, concerns, and ideas.
- The client may feel disrespected or "talked-down-to."
- It minimizes the difficulty of making changes in behaviors and doesn't provide meaningful support to assist in that process.
- The client may feel frustrated by the encounter and less likely to return to this or other similar providers in the future.

Please note: We want to underscore that this critique is not about the value of providing health information. Indeed, a vital role of CHWs is to educate clients about health conditions under the guidance of other health professionals and within their scope of practice. The problem arises when CHWs don't first assess what the client already knows and when they assume that accurate health information alone is sufficient to support their clients in making healthy and lasting behavior changes.

Mistake #2: Giving Advice

Many helping professionals provide advice to clients about what they should and shouldn't do, and sometimes what they should think and feel.

For example, a CHW working with a client living with a chronic condition such as high blood pressure may offer advice about what they "should" do to manage their health. Advice may include how and where to store medications, what types of physical activity are best to engage in, how to eat healthier foods, how to stop smoking cigarettes, and how to prevent and reduce stress.

- *Have you ever encountered a health care or other helping professional who liked to give you advice?*

- *How does this type of approach work for you?*

- *Do you think that this type of approach will be effective with most clients? Why or why not?*

<u>We don't recommend this approach because:</u>

- It is unlikely to result in effective and lasting behavior changes.

- It assumes that clients lack knowledge about how to promote their health or manage a health condition

- It assumes that clients require an "expert" to guide their behavior.

- Advice and guidance are often offered without first assessing the client's relevant knowledge, skills, and experience promoting their own health

- It may undermine the client's autonomy and sense of competency. It fosters dependence on others.

- Most people don't like to be told what to do. This approach may cause them to lose trust in and respect for health care and other helping professionals and could result in avoiding services in the future.

Sometimes, we fall into a pattern of giving advice without even noticing it, generally out of a desire to be supportive. While providing advice may be an appropriate thing to do in your family or with your friends, it isn't something that we recommend you do with clients. Be aware of the words you use and cautious about the times when you find yourself using phrases such as:

- *You should ... .*

- *You need to ... .*

- *I'd like you to ... .*

Please note: There are many occasions when we encourage CHWs to share suggestions with clients. Rather than telling a client what to do, however, we encourage you to present your ideas as options for the client to consider. Instead of saying "You should," try saying something like:

- *Have you thought about?*

- *Have you considered?*

- *What do you think about ... .?*

- *I have a suggestion for how to increase your physical activity. Only you can decide if it is something that could be useful to you. Is it okay with you if I go ahead and share this idea?*

Please watch the following videos ▶️ that show a CHW working with a client. In the Counter Role Play, the CHW provides the client with advice in a way that we don't recommend. In the Demo Role Play, the CHW shares information with the client in a different way.

- *What classic mistake does the CHW make in the Counter Role Play?*

  - *How may this impact or affect the client?*

- *What does the CHW do differently in the Demo Role Play?*

- *What would you do differently if you were working with this client, and why?*

Mistake #3: Blaming the Client

Helping professionals sometimes focus primarily on what clients do that may increase their health risks. This focus is sometimes accompanied by a tendency to blame clients for their illnesses or disabilities. This approach is deeply influenced by social, political, and media messages that tend to blame people for unfortunate circumstances, including poverty and poor health outcomes.

GIVING ADVICE: ROLE PLAY, COUNTER
(*Source:* Foundations for Community Health Workers/ https://youtu.be/ Our62-cD0gk/last accessed 21 September 2023.)

GIVING ADVICE: ROLE PLAY, DEMO
(*Source:* Foundations for Community Health Workers/ https://youtu.be/ J8Jn_okskAM/last accessed 21 September 2023.)

For example, when people engage in risky behaviors, others blame them. When people try but don't succeed in changing behaviors, they may be blamed again. Sometimes when people are diagnosed with diabetes, COVID-19, HIV disease, or other health conditions, they are judged yet again.

Blaming the client is manifested both in the tone that a provider uses to communicate with a client and the content of what they say. Providers may question or judge clients for missing appointments or medications, for not leaving abusive relationships, for failing to engage in enough exercise, for failing to cut down on processed and fast foods, or for strictly following a healthier diet. They may blame clients for not trying hard enough, for not caring enough, or for lacking motivation or concern for their future or their families.

What Do YOU? Think

- *Have you ever encountered a health care or other helping professional who seemed to judge or blame you or a family member in some way?*

- *How does this type of approach work for you? Does it motivate you to change behaviors?*

- *Do you think that this type of approach will be effective with most clients? Why or why not?*

We don't recommend this approach because:

- It is unlikely to result in effective and lasting behavior changes.
- It isn't the proper role of CHWs to pass judgment on clients.
- It is likely to provoke feelings of embarrassment, shame, or anger in the client, especially if they have often been judged by others in the past.
- It fails to recognize how difficult it can be to change behaviors such as diet, exercise, alcohol and drug use, and sexual behaviors.
- It is likely to prevent the formation of a trusting, supportive, and lasting relationship with the CHW.
- It fails to recognize social, political, economic, and cultural relationships and dynamics that influence our choices and access to resources.
- It may discourage a client from returning to the same agency for services or from accessing services elsewhere.
- It may be harmful to your client. Blaming people for poor health or for the inability to change behaviors is generally counterproductive; it contributes to a lack of confidence and may diminish their hope in the possibility of change. One of the key roles of CHWs is to carry hope for positive change for the clients and communities you work with, especially during difficult times when they are discouraged.

Ramona Benson: I don't put the blame on the client when she doesn't do something. She's probably blaming herself already. I look at the whole picture. I look at the system, too. Did the health care system treat her right? Give her an appointment on time? Cancel that appointment? Get her a prescription that she needed for her baby? Charge her too much? Mix up her health insurance?

Mistake #4: Failing to Address Issues of Accountability

Many people engage in behaviors that may be harmful to their health or the health of others. When a client reveals that they are engaging in harmful behavior, how will you respond?

Helping professionals sometimes fail to take this opportunity to engage clients in talking further about these potential harms. This common mistake is the flip side of "blaming the client." In order to avoid making judgments about clients, the CHW may stay silent about potential harm, may focus the discussion on what clients are doing well to promote their health, or may otherwise avoid the conversation.

Some of the reasons for making this common mistake may include:

- A mistaken notion that the role of the CHW is to accept and support everything their client *does* (rather than always accepting and supporting *the client*, but not necessarily the behavior or choices)

- Being uncomfortable with confrontation or conflict
- Fear of insulting, angering, shaming, or otherwise harming the relationship with the client

- *Have you ever encountered a health care or other helping professional who failed to talk with you about things that you were doing that could be harmful to yourself or others?*

- *How does this type of approach work for you?*

- *Do you think that this type of approach will be effective with most clients? Why or why not?*

We don't recommend this approach because:

- It is unlikely to result in effective and lasting behavior changes.
- It deprives the client of an opportunity to reflect in a deep way about behaviors that may be harmful to themselves or others.
- It does not respect your client's ability to address challenging issues.
- It sends and reinforces a message that the client should not discuss these issues.
- It may result in increased shame and guilt regarding the behaviors.
- It increases the likelihood that clients will continue to engage in the behavior and will indeed cause harm to themselves or others (imagine, e.g., that your client has untreated gonorrhea and is continuing to have unprotected sex with others).
- It violates your code of ethics to do no harm to the client or others.
- It may discourage a client from returning to the same agency for services or even from accessing services elsewhere.

6.2 Person-centered Practice

In Section 6.1, we presented four common mistakes to avoid when working with clients who want to change a behavior to enhance their health. In this section, we will introduce the overarching concept of person-centered practice *that we recommend* to guide your work with clients and communities.

Person-centered practice is not a unified theory. It draws upon a wide variety of models, approaches, theories, concepts, and skills. These include the work of Carl Rogers, the field of humanistic psychology, models of person-centered counseling promoted by leading public health organizations such as the Centers for Disease Control and Prevention and the World Health Organization, harm reduction, cultural humility, motivational interviewing, self-determination theory, and the wellness and recovery model. Person-centered approaches have been applied to the fields of medicine and education, and standards for patient-centered health care (or patient-centered care) and student-centered learning are now common.

The concept of person-centered practice was developed in reaction to traditional models of providing services in health care, counseling, social services, and related fields.

Carl Rogers is often cited as one of the founders of person-centered practice. As a young psychologist in the 1930s, Carl Rogers began to question his training and assumptions that he should direct counseling sessions with patients and offer special insight or guidance about their lives and the challenges they face. He developed what he called a "nondirective" approach that supported clients in examining their own lives, identifying their own challenges and strategies for growth and change.

Person-centered practice can be contrasted to more traditional models for service delivery that are provider-centered.

Provider-centered models of practice typically establish a professional relationship in which providers such as physicians, social workers and counselors are viewed as an authority with expertise in the health and social issues that clients are facing. The traditional role of providers is to assess and identify (or in the case of physicians and other licensed health care providers, to diagnose) illness, health conditions, or challenges and to dispense advice regarding what the client *should do* to improve their health and wellness. In traditional provider-centered models, the role of clients is to follow the advice of providers. Clients are not supposed to question or challenge the wisdom, expertise, or advice of providers.

Person-centered models turn this traditional power dynamic around, placing the client in the role of expert and the provider in the role of facilitator. Person-centered models acknowledge that clients are the only true experts regarding their own lives, cultural identities, and beliefs. The role of providers is to honor and respect the client's knowledge, experience, skills, and priorities and to support them in making informed decisions about how best to create change and enhance their health and wellness. A goal for person-centered practice models is to support and enhance the client's resilience and self-reliance or independence.

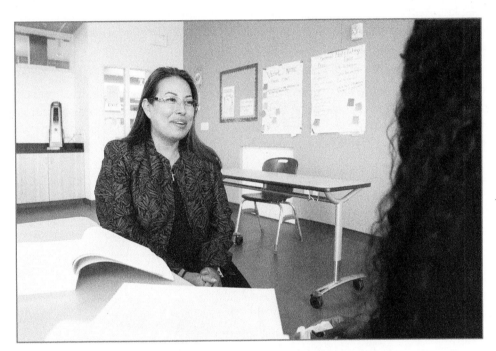

A CHW listening to a Client.

Person-centered concepts and skills can guide all of the services that CHWs provide including health outreach and home visiting, case management, health education, counseling, and chronic conditions management. It can be used to facilitate trainings, group-based work, and community organizing efforts. The concepts are relevant when working with individuals, families, groups, or at the community level.

Carl Rogers promoted the concept of unconditional positive regard as an essential component of person-centered work. **Unconditional positive regard** means demonstrating support and acceptance of people no matter who they are, what they say, or what they do. It requires not passing judgment about the people we work with and the choices they make.

While person-centered practice standards and the concept of unconditional positive regard encourage us to accept and support every client or community member we work with, it does not imply that we should be passive if we witness a client making decisions that could be harmful to themselves or others. While every client has the right to make decisions about their own life and health, CHWs and other providers also have an obligation to speak up—in a respectful way—if they have concerns about the choices that clients are considering. For example, if you learn that clients are suicidal or that members of their household are experiencing abuse, you have an ethical obligation to address these concerns and to report them to a supervisor or to a crisis response team member or another agency (see Chapter 5). If clients suddenly stop taking medications or participating in treatment, if they continue to engage in unprotected sex after testing positive for a sexually transmitted infection, or if they are sharing syringes and works when injecting drugs or engaging in other behaviors that place their health or the health of others at risk, we must directly and respectfully communicate with them about these topics.

Explaining Person-Centered Practice to Clients

Clients have a right to understand the values and principles that guide your work. Most clients will appreciate your person-centered approach, especially those who have prior experience with providers who imposed their own beliefs, knowledge, expectations, and judgments. Sharing a few words about your approach can encourage clients to claim control of your work together, setting their own priorities and goals, and talking about the issues most important to them.

For example, a CHW might say something like:

CHW: "It isn't my role to tell you what I think you should do to promote your health. I want to work in a way that respects your experience, knowledge, and accomplishments. My role is to support you in identifying your key priorities and goals, and to decide what actions you want to take to reach your goals. So, to get started, let me ask: What brings you to our clinic? What priority concerns are you hoping to address?"

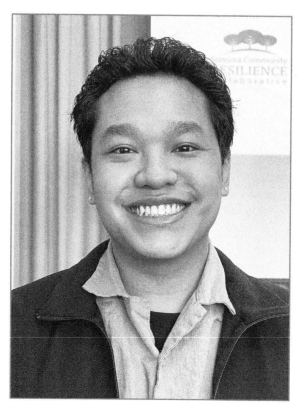

A CHW trained in person-centered practice.

VIDEOS ON PERSON-CENTERED PRACTICE

The *Foundations for CHWs* team developed a series of short video interviews and role-plays designed to highlight person-centered concepts and skills. Please take a few minutes to watch the following videos and consider the questions that we pose about the highlighted concepts.

BIG EYES, BIG EARS, AND A SMALL MOUTH

HIV prevention groups in Zimbabwe (International Training and Education Center on HIV, unpublished curriculum) developed the following image (Figure 6.1) to represent person-centered practice.

This diagram illustrates a CHW working with a client. The Big Ears represent a CHW who is listening carefully and deeply to the client. The Big Eyes indicate that the CHW is carefully observing the client and the surrounding world (the client's social context). The small mouth indicates that the CHW is careful not to talk too much during the session. Rather than dominating the discussion, the CHW uses person-centered techniques such as asking open-ended questions to provide clients with an opportunity to reflect upon and talk about their life and their health.

Please watch the following video interview about the concept of a CHW with Big Eyes, Big Ears, and a small mouth.

- *What do you think about the image of a CHW with Big Eyes, Big Ears, and a small mouth?*

- *How could you apply this concept to your work with clients?*

WHEN PROVIDERS DOMINATE CONVERSATIONS WITH CLIENTS

Please watch the following video that shows a CHW working with a client and making the common mistake of talking too much.

- *In this video, what information is the CHW trying to share with the client?*

- *Why might this CHW—or other helping professionals—make the mistake of talking too much when working with a client?*

- *How may talking too much impact or affect your work with a client?*

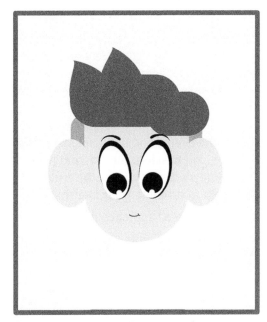

Figure 6.1 Big Ears, Big Eyes

BIG EARS, BIG EYES.

(*Source:* Foundations for Community Health Workers/http://youtu.be/ffFXsvPAKkAhttp://youtu.be/jE9uNHRhLA4/last accessed 21 September 2023.)

TALKING TOO MUCH: ROLE PLAY, COUNTER.

(*Source:* Foundations for Community Health Workers/http://youtu.be/VhDFNaFow6c/last accessed 21 September 2023c.)

THE STRENGTH-BASED APPROACH

Person-centered practice is also strength-based. While traditional models for providing direct services often focus primarily or exclusively on the client's risk behaviors and lack of resources, a person-centered approach seeks greater balance. A **strength-based approach** emphasizes the internal and external resources that a client already has. External resources are often easier to identify. They are the resources that lie outside of the client and may include family and friends, stable housing, a trusted primary health care provider, spiritual faith or religious tradition, or a secure job at a living wage. Internal resources reside within the client, and may include knowledge, skills, talents, experiences, values, cultural identity, wisdom, courage, compassion, humor, and past accomplishments. A person-centered practitioner always looks for and acknowledges a client's internal and external resources and supports clients to draw upon these resources to promote their health.

A strength-based approach has several potential benefits:

- Talking with clients about their strengths and accomplishments helps to build a positive rapport and professional relationship

- It identifies key internal and external resources that will support the client in addressing current challenges and promoting their health

- It builds the self-esteem, confidence, and resilience of clients

- It promotes the independence and autonomy of clients

Please watch the following video interview about strength-based practice.

- *Why is a strength-based approach important for working with clients?*

- *As a CHW, what else can you do or say to support clients to identify and build upon their resources and strengths?*

STRENGTH-BASED PRACTICE: FACULTY INTERVIEW.

(*Source:* Foundations for Community Health Workers/http://youtu.be/ Cq4PX89tlZE/last accessed 21 September 2023.)

ARE YOU DOING PERSON-CENTERED WORK?

We encourage you to regularly evaluate the quality of your work. To assess whether or not you are doing person-centered work, reflect on the following questions:

- Are you dominating meetings or discussions with clients? Are you talking more than the clients are? Are you stepping in to offer advice instead of first asking clients for their own ideas for what they want to do?

- Are you providing clients with the space and the opportunity to voice their true feelings and opinions?

- Are clients making health decisions that reflect their own ideas, values, and reality?

- Are you assessing and acknowledging client strengths such as their knowledge, skills, values, and achievements?

- Are you bringing your own agenda into your work with clients?

- Are you having difficulty listening to clients or focusing on what they are sharing with you? If so, what is getting in the way of your ability to truly listen to clients?

For more information about how to assess or evaluate the quality of your work with clients, please see Chapter 9.

CHW Profile

Cristina Arellano, she/her

Case Manager/Housing Navigator

Lifelong Medical Care/Supportive Housing Program

Whole Person Care/Wraparound Services

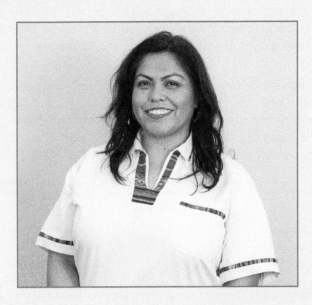

My parents immigrated from Mexico. I advocated for the family from a young age. I was the interpreter for the family, signing us up for community programs for low-income families. I've always enjoyed getting to know people and their stories. I believe in people, and I learn something from each client I support. I tell clients, if you get evicted, if you relapse, I'll still be here. I'll be supportive.

Lifelong Medical Care provides comprehensive primary care and behavioral health services. I work with vulnerable clients in Alameda County who are in crisis and unhoused, or who were previously unhoused. As a Housing Navigator, I get referrals from the County and my job is to connect them with housing. I help them complete documentation that has to be submitted to various housing authorities and landlords. The clients have to qualify for housing subsidies or vouchers to get on waitlists. Then it can take six months to two years before an apartment opens up. The real work begins once the client is housed because staying in housing can be even more difficult than getting housing.

As a Case Manager, I support people who were previously unhoused to stay in housing. A lot of them are elders and most of them spent years living on the street, in encampments, cars, or RVs. Many of them have substance use histories and posttraumatic stress. I help them get connected with primary health care, with managing their chronic health conditions, connecting them to resources in the community like meals and groceries, cell phones, in-home support so that they can live independently. I help clients develop Care Plans and set goals for 30–60 days, 90 days, 6 months, and so on.

I met Mr. Torres about eight months ago. He was 63 years old and living in hotel. He wanted to leave because there is a lot of drug use in the hotels, and he is in recovery. He had been homeless for six years and was finally matched with an apartment. So I worked with Mr. Torres to make it possible for him to move into the apartment. He didn't open up much at first. I helped him with independent living skills like how to clean and pay bills. I got him connected to Meals on Wheels and they deliver two meals a day Monday through

(continues)

CHW Profile

(continued)

Friday. I helped him get an EBT (Food Stamps) card. Now that he has a place he feels more at peace. He is able to set new goals. He is opening up more. He suffers from depression and anxiety and gets very nervous about medical visits. I accompany him and that helps. He is beginning to talk more about his life and his needs and even to advocate for himself.

My work and training as a CHW have been profound and eye-opening. It helped me to make clearer sense of my own experiences and to name things like systemic racism and social injustice. In general, I ask more questions now about what is going on in the world and why, and I am more involved in my local community.

My own tip for new CHWs is boundaries, boundaries, boundaries! I don't think it is talked about enough. It's something I emphasize with new CHWs or case managers on our team. I talk with them about maintaining professional boundaries, being careful about what you disclose to clients. It is for your own safety as well as the safety and well-being of the client. And it's not just about maintaining boundaries with clients, but also with the organization you work for. When you clock out, really clock out. Leave work behind. Live your life.

IMPLICIT THEORY

When most people think of theory, they think of formal theories that have been researched and published in books and articles. **Implicit theory** refers to the concepts that each of us develops based on our own life and work experience. Over time, CHWs develop implicit theories about behavior change and how best to work with clients based on their work experience.

The Implicit Theories Project investigated beliefs about behavior change among CHWs doing HIV prevention work in the San Francisco Bay Area. Researchers from the University of California, San Francisco (UCSF) reported that CHWs develop their own theories about risk behaviors and the factors that influence behavior change based on their work with clients and communities (Freedman et al., 2006). The theories developed by CHWs often shared common ideas, including an emphasis on the influence of social context (or ecological factors) and the importance for clients of having a sense of community. Researchers also highlighted the importance of implicit theories for the development of effective community-based programs and services.

We strongly encourage you to develop your own implicit theories as you build your career in the community health field. We encourage you to reflect deeply about the question of why people behave the way they do and what supports people to change behaviors. Consider the following resources for developing your own theories:

- Examine your own biases and reflect on how your own identity, experience, and culture may influence your ideas about behavior and behavior change (you may wish to refer to Chapter 7 on Cultural Humility).
- Research and read about theories of behavior change.
- Attend local workshops and classes that address issues related to behavior change.
- Notice the factors and approaches that seem to get in the way of clients' ability to change behavior. Identify the factors that seem to play a part in supporting them to successfully change behaviors.
- Ask your colleagues what they have found works in supporting the behavior change of clients.
- Share your implicit theories with colleagues, engaging in dialogue and refining your beliefs over time.

- *Most importantly, don't forget to ask about and to listen carefully to what your clients believe helps them to make meaningful life changes that promote their health and wellness. We predict that the clients you work with will be your most important teachers.*

You will learn more about person-centered practice and how to apply it in your work with clients in Parts 2 and 4 of the *Foundations* book.

Please watch the following video interview about the process of developing your own approach to person-centered practice.

- *What influences your work as a CHW and your approach to supporting clients to promote their health and wellness?*

YOUR APPROACH TO PERSON-CENTERED COUNSELING.

(*Source:* Foundations for Community Health Workers/http://youtu.be/yHIf0qqkxJI/last accessed 21 September 2023.)

Chapter Review

To review your understanding of the concepts addressed in Chapter 6, please consider your answers to the questions presented below.

PROMOTING BEHAVIOR CHANGE

Imagine that you have been assigned to train and mentor a new CHW. They have never provided direct services to clients before. How would you explain the four classic mistakes that can get in the way of supporting clients to change behaviors?

Imagine you are working with a client who is living with chronic health conditions. The client wants to increase their level of physical activity or exercise but is finding it difficult to change their behavior. Apply the ecological model to identify the types of factors that may influence the client's behavior at each of the following levels:

- The Individual
- Family and Friends
- Neighborhood and Community
- Society or Nation

PERSON-CENTERED PRACTICE

It is important for CHWs to communicate with confidence about the key concepts and skills that guide their work. This will permit you to participate actively in discussions within your own agency and to advocate for the type of programs and values you believe are most valuable for the communities you serve. It will also advance your career and open up new professional opportunities.

Take a few minutes to test your knowledge by answering the following questions:

- How do you define or explain the concept of person-centered practice?
- How does person-centered practice differ from more traditional provider-centered models?
- How can you apply a strength-based approach to your work with clients and community members? How will a strength-based approach benefit the people you work with?
- How will you demonstrate a person-centered approach when working with clients and community members? What will you do? What will you avoid doing?
- How will you assess whether or not you are providing person-centered services?

Reference

Freedman, B., Binson, D., Ekstrand, M., Galvez, S., Woods, W. J., & Grinstead, O. (2006). Uncovering implicit theories of HIV prevention providers: It takes a community. *AIDS Education and Prevention 18*(3), 216–226. https://doi:10.1521/aeap.2006.18.3.216.

Additional Resources

Rogers, C. R. (1951). *Client-Centered therapy: Its current practice, implications and theory.* Boston. Houghton Mifflin.

Rogers, C. R. (1961). *On becoming a person: A therapist's View of Psychotherapy.* Boston: Houghton Mifflin.

Practicing Cultural Humility

Alberta Rincón and Pau I. Crego

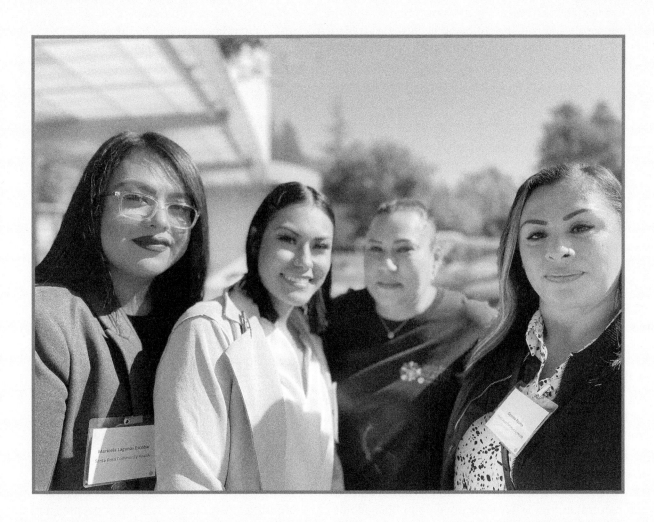

Foundations for Community Health Workers, Third Edition. Edited by Tim Berthold and Darouny Somsanith.
© 2024 John Wiley & Sons, Inc. Published 2024 by John Wiley & Sons, Inc.
Companion website: http://www.wiley.com/go/communityhealthworkers3E

Client Scenario: Luisa M.

Luisa M. is a new client at the agency where you work as a CHW. You are the first staff member to meet with her.

Luisa is a recently arrived immigrant from Honduras who currently works as a domestic helper during the day and washes dishes at a restaurant at night. She has three children, all living with her mother in Honduras. She has limited English language proficiency, wants to take ESL classes, and thinks she might be pregnant.

As you conduct an initial meeting and assessment with Luisa, you learn that she has undocumented immigrant status and is fearful of being deported. Luisa is also worried about being unable to support her family back home. As a result she has trouble sleeping at night and suffers from severe stomach aches.

Finally, you learn that one of the reasons she left Honduras was to escape from a domestic violence situation and now has severe anxiety, which she refers to as *nervios* (nervousness).

If you were a CHW working with Luisa M., how would you answer the following questions?

- How will you honor and respect Luisa's cultural identities, values and beliefs?
- How will you work with Luisa in a way that does not impose your own cultural assumptions or prejudices?
- How will work with Luisa in a way that promotes her autonomy or independence?

Introduction

Community Health Workers and Promotores de Salud are committed to becoming culturally humble providers to people of all backgrounds and identities. One chapter will not make you an expert in cultural humility. However, studying cultural humility concepts and skills will enhance your understanding and ability to respond to the challenges and opportunities of cultural diversity. This chapter invites you to become a lifelong learner and practitioner of cultural humility.

All CHWs provide services to clients and communities who have cultural backgrounds and identities that are different from their own. Even if you work in your own community, some of the clients you encounter will come from a different generational, economic, ethnic, religious, or linguistic background, or will have a different gender identity, gender expression, and/or sexual orientation.

The rich cultural diversity that surrounds us can pose challenges for CHWs and other helping professionals. How can we learn to work effectively with all clients and communities? What if we don't know much about a particular cultural group? What if we grew up in households or communities that taught us to view people from different communities with bias or prejudice?

Cultural humility is an approach to providing services that emphasizes an awareness of our cultural perspectives and an acknowledgment of the risks of imposing our own beliefs on other people. It provides a framework for demonstrating respect for the cultural identities of every person you work with, and for interacting in ways that promotes their health and supports their autonomy. We believe that cultural humility is a foundational concept to guide the work of CHWs.

Cultural Humility is often framed within an umbrella term called Diversity, Equity, Inclusion, Belonging and Justice (DEIBJ). Many organizations are addressing DEIBJ as part of their vision and mission, to ensure that programs and services are accessible and effective for all people. These organizations acknowledge injustices, unequal treatment, and inequities in access, delivery of care and services and health outcomes. They work to ensure that all clients and communities are included, valued and celebrated.

To be effective in your work, CHWs must not only be culturally humble, but also an advocate for the larger perspective of DEIBJ.

WHAT YOU WILL LEARN

By studying this chapter, you will be able to:

- Define the concept of cultural humility

- Discuss how cultural humility fits within the DEIBJ framework

- Explain the concept of unconscious bias

- Describe the changing population in the United States and how this affects the work of CHWs

- Discuss how historical and institutional discrimination affects the health of vulnerable communities and influences their work with public health providers

- Analyze the importance of becoming lifelong learners and practitioners of cultural humility

- Discuss and analyze concepts of traditional health beliefs and practices and how they may influence the delivery of services to clients

- Identify, analyze, and apply models for practicing cultural humility and conducting person-centered interviews regarding health issues

- Develop a plan to enhance your knowledge and skills as a culturally humble CHW

C3 Roles & Skills Addressed in Chapter 7

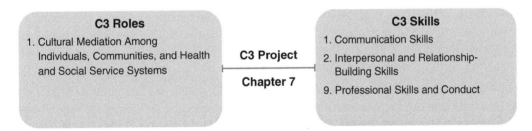

WORDS TO KNOW

Gender Identity	Sexual Orientation
Heterogeneity	Structural Discrimination
Intersectionality	Structural Racism

7.1 Defining and Understanding Culture

In essence, culture includes the beliefs, behaviors, attitudes, and practices that are learned, shared, and passed on by members of a particular group. Medical anthropologist C. G. Helman defines culture as: "a set of guidelines, (both explicit and implicit) that individuals inherit as members of a particular society, and that tell them how to view the world, how to experience it emotionally, and how to behave in it in relation to other people, to supernatural forces and gods, and the natural environment." (Helman, 2007)

According to Judith Carmen Nine Curt (1984):

- Culture cannot be shed.

- Every cultural detail is incredibly old.

- Culture functions in "out-of-awareness."

- In order to understand others, we must first understand our own culture.

- Culture is better understood by observing and studying the cultures of others.

- Cultures are neither better nor worse, simply different.

- Every human being is bound by their culture.

- In order to be free from the hidden constraints of culture, we must study it.

- This study is new in our society and our educational world.
- Behind the differences among people, there are basic similarities, such as love, family, loyalty, friendship, joy, and the belief in transcendence.

Culture is not static—it doesn't stand still. It is dynamic, constantly changing and evolving with us. Culture is also multifaceted. It incorporates and includes ethnic identity, immigration status and experience, sexual orientation, gender identity, religion or spirituality, social class, family background, language, physical ability, traditions, and much more.

Because culture is multifaceted and dynamic, there is a lot of diversity within any culturally defined community (**heterogeneity**). It is important to keep in mind that there may be as many differences within the community as there are similarities.

- *What are some of the differences between people within the communities you belong to?*
- *As a CHW, why is it important to understand that differences exist within communities who share a common culture?*

It is not unusual for people to have more than one ethnic identity. For example, someone who has an Ethiopian parent and a Vietnamese parent may identify with both Ethiopian and Vietnamese ethnic communities. But is this person's cultural identity based solely on ethnic roots and traditions? Probably not. This same individual may have other cultural affiliations that have stronger ties other than ethnic identity (for example, gender identity, socioeconomic status, immigration status). For instance, an elderly, gay, Latino man potentially shares experiences with multiple cultural groups depending on his identities, his current and past experiences, and the historical and cultural moments he has lived through.

This is also known as intersectionality. As humans, we are multifaceted and have many identities and cannot be categorized into only one group. **Intersectionality**—a theory coined by Dr. Kimberlé Crenshaw—acknowledges the interconnected nature of social categorizations such as race, class and gender; and recognizes that the unique combination of our social categorizations affect how we are viewed, understood, and treated (Crenshaw, 1989). Going back to the previous example, an elderly gay Latino man may have similar experiences to elderly Latino men who are heterosexual and to young gay Latino men, but he is viewed and treated different from those other groups because of the unique intersection of his identities and social categories (elderly, Latino, male, and gay).

It is important to note that culture not only refers to the cultural guidelines that are typically passed on from parents to children; it also refers to the practices and traditions of the communities that we become a part of based on our identities. For example, lesbian, gay, bisexual, transgender, queer, intersex, asexual and other (LGBTQIA+) communities (and many subgroups within the LGBTQIA+ community) have a rich history and specific cultural guidelines that influence how these communities engage with the world around them. However, because most LGBTQIA+ people don't have parents or children who also openly identify as LGBTQIA+, this history and culture is transferred from LGBTQIA+ elders to younger generations through storytelling, art, and chosen family bonds (as opposed to the families we are born into and grow up with). As you work with diverse communities, it is crucial to recognize that culture and family can take many different forms, and as CHWs it is critical to do your best to unlearn the assumptions that you may bring based on your own cultures and family experiences.

- *Have you ever had someone ask you, "Where are you from?" or "What are you?"*
- *Have you ever had someone mistakenly assume one of your cultural identities?*
  - *How did this make you feel?*
  - *How did you react?*
- *How do you define your cultural identities?*
- *Does this change depending upon the circumstances?*

7.2 Defining Cultural Humility

Melanie Tervalon defines cultural humility: *"More than a concept, Cultural Humility is a communal reflection to analyze the root causes of suffering and create a broader, more inclusive view of the world ... Cultural Humility is now used in public health, social work, education, and non-profit management. It is a daily practice for people to deal with hierarchical relationships, changing organizational policy and building relationships built on trust"* (Tervalon & Murray-Garcia, 1998).

Cultural humility:

* Is essential for working effectively with diverse clients and communities.
* Acknowledges histories of discrimination and current dynamics of power and privilege.
* Asks health care and social services providers to examine their own biases in order not to impose assumptions—about behaviors, beliefs or values—onto the clients with whom they work.
* Guides us in flipping traditional power dynamics between providers and clients.
* Emphasizes the limits of our ability to know or truly understand the culture of others.
* Advances values of equity and an understanding that no cultural identity or tradition has more or less value than another.
* Is designed to challenge and prevent the type of cultural arrogance that has led individuals, communities, organizations and nations to impose their own beliefs and standards upon others.

A good place to start when studying the concept of cultural humility, is with the meaning of the word "humility." Humility signifies not raising one's own significance or value too high, or above the value of others. It implies recognizing the limits of one's own wisdom and skills, and acknowledging and appreciating the wisdom, value and skills of others. When your work is guided by cultural humility, you will recognize that the client is the expert of their own life (including their cultural identities, values and beliefs). Leading with cultural humility enhances client autonomy and opportunities for empowerment.

Cultural Humility and Person-Centered Practice

Cultural humility is a foundational concept and skill for guiding the work of CHWs. We will refer to cultural humility throughout this textbook, drawing connections with other key concepts and skills. For example, cultural humility informs all of the work that CHWs do directly with clients and communities. It is also a key component of the person-centered approach (addressed in Chapters 8 through 10) which is designed to support a client's autonomy and self-determination.

Cultural humility goes beyond previously taught concepts—such as cultural competence or cross-cultural work—that emphasize the importance of learning about other cultures in order to provide services. What is the difference between cultural competence and cultural humility?

According to Melanie Tervalon and Jane Murray-Garcia, *"Cultural humility incorporates a lifelong commitment to self-evaluation and critique, to redressing the power imbalances in the physician-patient dynamic, and to developing mutually beneficial and non-paternalistic partnerships with communities on behalf of individuals and defined populations"* (Tervalon & Murray-Garcia, 1998, p. 123).

THE LIMITS OF OUR KNOWLEDGE ABOUT OTHER CULTURES: A WORD OF CAUTION

Some resources designed to promote an appreciation of cultural diversity and skills for working across cultural identities may do more harm than good. They teach seemingly definitive information about specific cultural groups. The assumption is that once people have learned about Mexican Americans and related health issues such as diet, death and dying, or sexuality, they will then know how to provide more sensitive or culturally competent services to members of that community.

There are several key problems with this approach:

- It stereotypes culture by assuming that there is such a thing as *the* Mexican American culture or *the* Mexican American diet. In reality, there is tremendous diversity within Mexican American or Chicano cultures, just like there is diversity within Vietnamese cultures, Italian American cultures, or any cultural group or community.

- It fails to recognize, honor, and appreciate the tremendous richness and complexity of what we call culture (and the tremendous diversity *within* cultures).

- It promotes the idea that cultural communities and identities can be deeply and accurately understood by participating in trainings or another course of study.

- It may foster stereotypes.

- It focuses on knowing specific information about the cultures, beliefs, and customs of others rather than the process and interaction between providers and the clients and communities they serve.

- It ignores power imbalances between people of different identities or cultural backgrounds (such as a helping professional and a client).

- It fails to focus our attention on our own cultural traditions, values, and beliefs, and how these may cause us, unintentionally, to make assumptions about the beliefs, values, feelings, and behaviors of others.

While learning about different cultures can certainly strengthen your understanding of the communities you work with, assuming that we understand or know something definitive about other cultures can be harmful. When we assume that we understand where others are coming from, we may fail to ask for, or to listen to, the information that they provide, and we may offer guidance that is based on faulty assumptions or misinformation.

To illustrate, let's consider the following scenario. Your agency sends you to a training that focuses on the Cultural Health Beliefs and Practices of the Hmong Community. The training is two days in length and exposes you to knowledgeable speakers, including leaders from the Hmong community, social workers, CHWs, and anthropologists. Detailed information is presented about Hmong history, culture, and customs and the challenges Hmong immigrants face in the United States. You leave with a sense of understanding key aspects of Hmong culture, their history in the United States, and some of the most pressing health issues the community currently faces. However, there is a risk that the next time you encounter a Hmong client, you may assume to know a lot about them. As a result, you may not ask appropriate questions and fail to learn important information about the client and their health. The client may not receive an accurate assessment, relevant health education, case management services, or referrals from you.

While there is considerable value in learning as much as possible about the cultures of the communities that you will work with, we encourage you to balance your desire for learning with a cultural humility framework. Cultural humility reminds you of the limits of our own knowledge or understanding about the lives of others and guides you in highlighting the expertise of the clients and communities with whom you work.

7.3 Practicing Cultural Humility

Many clients and communities face bias and discrimination in the process of accessing health and social services and, as a result, receive fewer services and services of poorer quality. As we addressed in Chapter 4, this is a significant reason for persistent health inequities. In order to be successful in promoting health equity and social justice, you must develop your capacity to reach and provide quality services to people from many different backgrounds, cultures and identities.

As a CHW, it's important to acknowledge what you don't know about cultural diversity. This is the first step toward improving your ability to work with people effectively, regardless of their identity and life experience. To better understand cultures and identities different from your own, you must undertake a personal journey. Learning how to work effectively across cultures is not just an intellectual endeavor: In order to develop cultural humility, you must open your heart as well as your mind.

This process requires a willingness to acknowledge your pain and past hurts and those of others, as well as acknowledge your own biases and judgments about people who are different from you. This may be uncomfortable and provoke strong emotions. In these moments, it can be helpful to stay humble and remember that we have all made mistakes and are capable of personal growth and change. Learning about cultural humility can be a challenging, lifelong, and transformative journey.

Practicing cultural humility requires:

- Studying histories of oppression and discrimination.
- Examining our own assumptions and prejudices about people who come from different communities than our own.
- Engaging respectfully with all clients and recognizing that they are our guides in determining their own cultural identities, values, knowledge, behaviors, and decisions.
- Engaging in self-reflection and self-critique, including reflection about our own assumptions and biases in our interactions with clients.
- Understanding that our own culture is no better than any other. All cultures deserve our respect.
- Learning to be comfortable with not knowing about the experience, culture, identities, values or beliefs of others.
- Recognizing that only the client is the expert about their own culture, identities, values, and beliefs.
- Placing our assumptions aside when working with others and asking clients and communities to share their own experiences, knowledge, resources, needs, and priorities with us so that we may best support their health and well-being.

By practicing cultural humility with clients, we build a welcoming and respectful working partnership. In this partnership, we recognize that we need to learn about a client's experience, culture, identities, values, beliefs, and behaviors, and we remember that the way to do that is to ask and to listen deeply to what they tell us.

Estela Munoz de Cardenas: With my clients, I want to know about their cultures and their stories. As CHWs, we need to be listeners more than talkers. We all come from different backgrounds so if you don't understand something they tell you, that's okay. Speak up and ask with respect and compassion about anything you don't understand.

CHW Profile

Kim Lien Tran (she/her)

Program Coordinator/Community Health Worker

Boat People SOS (BPSOS)

Vietnamese Community

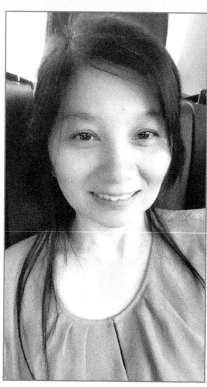

Most of my youth I was doing church related things and helping people through the youth group. When I grew up, I was working at Providence Hospital doing medical billing and coding. A doctor called me and said they had a Vietnamese interpreter job, did I want to come? So, I did, and it was a really short job, but I had fallen in love with the community and the people. And then my old supervisor called and told me there was CHW training, it was just like, okay, I didn't even have to think twice. It was like a second chance for me to come back and help my community.

I am a CHW at Boat People SOS (BPSOS) in Bayou La Batre, Alabama. We serve mainly the Vietnamese community. It's a rural area, so there's not a lot of resources down this way. Most of our resources are in Mobile, 45 minutes away. Transportation is a big issue. We live in a food desert, there's one grocery store and a Dollar store. So, there is food insecurity and employment insecurity. A majority of people here are fishermen or work in the seafood industry, so work comes and goes, it's up and down all the time. And most don't have health insurance.

What I do is healthcare accessibility. I go with them and interpret for them at the doctor's office. I help them understand the healthcare system. We have two small clinics here, but the closest hospital is 45 minutes away. I help them with immigration, applying for citizenship, registering to vote. Many are not comfortable with social services, so I help them get food stamps, translate their mail, show them how to pay bills and show them the different resources that we know.

One of the successful things we did was starting a health resource fair. It was after the British Petroleum oil spill and the Gulf Region funded us and two local clinics. They wanted to hold a town meeting and I told

(continues)

CHW Profile
(continued)

them I think down here they're kind of tired with town meetings, and I don't know if they'll want to just hear people talk. So, I said how about we do a health fair.

The first year we had 35 vendors, organizations came down and brought their resources, and did health screenings. Over 300 people showed up! Some got help, like a glucose test or a blood pressure test, and then a referral to a doctor to follow up. And we showcased our community, the organizations learned about us, so they know and are aware of our needs.

Being a CHW has made me become more open. I'm very timid, very quiet. But now I can talk about anything, all day if I need to. Now, if you just say, hey, come talk about something, I can do it. The community is so comfortable with me now, they just come to say hi, or just to chat or if they have something going on, or their kids are graduating. It's a rewarding job, but it's not even a job because it's like I have the biggest extended family.

I think first, when you start working, it could get overwhelming for some time. People will call you when they have every little issue and you're on call 24/7. And I just want to help people and serve my community. That takes a toll because it's a lot. We just have to take a step back and make sure we make some time for ourselves, for self-care. You want to help everybody but sometimes you forget that you need time for you.

7.4 The Culturally Diverse Context for Community Health Work

Ismael Reed said that, as a society, the United States is unique in the world because "the world is here." In America, "the cultures of the world crisscross" on a daily basis (Takaki, 1993, p. 16).

- *Where do you fit in to this multicultural mix?*

- *Were you born in the United States?*

- *What about your parents and grandparents?*

- *What about your neighbors, the people you encounter at the grocery store, the bank, in your children's schools?*

- *What are the languages, cultures, and other identities of the students in your classes and the people in your community?*

- *What identities do you have in common with your family of origin, and which identities are different?*

- *What are the cultural identities of your local politicians or those in charge of large businesses and government institutions?*

The population of the United States is rapidly changing and growing. This includes the number of languages spoken, the number of people who identify as bi-racial and multi-racial, the types of available food, the range of cultural, religious and community-based organizations, and the increasing number of people who feel safer to openly identify with a variety of sexual orientations and gender identities in today's society.

The U.S. is continuing to become more diverse in all racial and ethnic categories. As of June 2022, the fastest growing populations in the United States are Native Hawaiians, Pacific Islanders and Hispanic populations (U.S. Census Bureau, 2022a). Not only is the United States becoming more diverse in all racial and ethnic groups but also becoming older (Ibid).

The majority of children born in the United States today are people of color (US Census Bureau, 2022a). Communities of color are the majority of the population in 49 of 366 metropolitan regions in the United States, and in four states: California, Hawaii, New Mexico and Texas. Data and analysis from the US Census Bureau predicts that by the early 2040s, whites will no longer be a majority and will constitute less than 50% of America's population. (US Census Bureau, 2022a). Contrary to popular belief, the increase of communities of color in the US is not the result of more immigration but is due to more births within the communities of color that are already here. This is especially true for Latine/a/o and Asian populations.

Each of the categories of the Census Bureau includes a wide array of ancestral countries of origin, cultural backgrounds, tribal affiliations, customs, religions, and life experiences. The U.S. has a rich linguistic diversity as well: it is estimated that between 350 and 430 languages are spoken (US Census Bureau, 2018). This adds to the rich diversity of cultures the differences emerging from life experiences and opportunities, such as poverty, political experience, and educational opportunity, and individual differences, such as gender identity, disability, family history, or sexual orientation.

While the U.S. Census is an important source of information about the demographic makeup of the country and how populations are changing, it has some limitations as a result of historical and current bias. One of those limitations is that the U.S. Census does not capture sexual orientation and gender identity beyond the binary, which in practice means that LGBTQIA+ identities are not counted. Due to this unfortunate gap in the U.S. Census data, we rely on other studies to determine population estimates for LGBTQIA+ communities. In 2021, the Gallup Daily tracking survey found that 7.1% of people in the U.S. identified as LGBTQIA+, or something other than cisgender and heterosexual (Jones, 2022). LGBTQIA+ communities are a growing population, as LGBTQIA+ identification has doubled since Gallup started to ask this question (3.5% in 2012). This demographic change occurs because younger generations tend to identify as LGBTQIA+ more so than older generations. For example, a Gallup survey found that roughly 21% of Generation Z adults (born between 1997 and 2003) identify as LGBTQIA+, compared to 10.5% of Millennials (born between 1981 and 1996) and 4.2% of Generation X (born 1965–1980) (Jones, 2022).

Transgender and nonbinary communities are increasing in the U.S. (for key concepts related to transgender and nonbinary identities, read Chapter 4). This is also because younger adults are more likely to identify with a gender other than the one they were assigned at birth: in the U.S., 5.1% of adults under 30 years old identify as transgender and/or nonbinary, compared to 1.6% of adults of all ages (Brown, 2022). It is important to note that—although more people openly identify as LGBTQIA+ than ever before, likely as a result of access to information and positive role models—the rights of LGBTQIA+ communities continue to be heavily contested in this country. In recent years, an increase in anti-transgender sentiment has led to multiple states passing laws that target transgender and nonbinary adults and children in schools, sports, public accommodations, and more. This is an example of how discrimination can be ingrained into the systems of our society.

The diversity of our nation's population, including sexual orientation and gender identity, is a tremendous strength that contributes to our nation's economy. Richard Florida has noted, "the evidence is mounting that geographical openness and cultural diversity and tolerance are not by-products but key drivers of economic progress" (Florida, 2011).

IMMIGRANT COMMUNITIES

- Almost 48 million immigrants or people born in other nations are in the United States as of September 2022, according to the Census Bureau's monthly Current Population Survey (Camarota & Zeigler, 2022; US Census Bureau, 2022b), a record high in American history.

- Of the 48 million immigrants in the country 61% (29.4 million) were employed (Camarota & Zeigler, 2022; US Census Bureau, 2022b).

- The United States has more immigrants than any other nation in the world.

- The majority of immigrants come from four nations, in this order: China, India, Mexico and the Philippines (Budiman, 2020).

- The states with the highest number of immigrants are California, Texas, and Florida and New York (Ibid).

Most immigrant communities have faced prejudice and discrimination as they struggled to establish themselves in the United States. Unfortunately, there is still a strong backlash against immigrants today. Some people argue that immigrants are a drain on the U.S. economy, taking away resources. However, research has consistently demonstrated the immigrants make significant contributions to the U.S economy (Rouse, Barrow, Rinz, & Soltas, 2021; Sherman, Trisi, Stone, Gonzales, & Parrott, 2019). The Institute on Taxation and Economic Policy states: *"In fact, like all others living and working in the United States, undocumented immigrants are taxpayers too and collectively contribute an estimated $11.74 billion to state and local coffers each year via a combination of sales and excise, personal income, and property taxes"* (Institute on Taxation and Economic Policy, 2017).

7.5 Histories of Discrimination

As CHWs, it's important to know the histories and current experiences of discrimination that diverse communities in the U.S. experience. Your ability to work effectively with diverse communities will also depend on your willingness to examine how larger societal policies and practices influence health status. CHWs must be ready to understand the impact of discrimination based on ethnicity, nationality, immigration status, sex, gender identity, sexual orientation, and other identities on the lives and health status of the clients and communities with whom you work.

Racial discrimination is a historical fact. African American/Black people, Latine/a/o communities, Native Americans, Pacific Islanders, and some Asian groups are disproportionately represented in the lower socioeconomic ranks of our society. Racial discrimination across generations has also meant that a greater majority of children of color attend lower-quality schools; more adults of color work in lower-paying jobs; and disproportionate percentages of Black and Latino men end up in our prison systems. Ultimately, racial discrimination results in higher rates of illness, lower life expectancy and excess deaths (see Chapter 4) for communities of color. The government and institutional policies that created these inequities in the past—and that sustain them in the present—are referred to as structural racism. Structural racism means that inequities are built into the key systems of a society, such as the educational, legal, employment, housing, and health care systems.

Other groups in the United States have also experienced individual and structural discrimination. For example, women still experience high levels of domestic violence. In the workforce, they receive less pay and fewer opportunities for promotion and experience higher rates of sexual harassment.

Another example of this type of discrimination is structural transphobia. Many transgender and nonbinary people choose to update their legal name and/or gender marker to ensure their official documents better reflect their identities. However, in many states in the U.S., changing one's legal information is a burdensome and expensive process. This has serious consequences for the livelihood and health of this community because, for many people, having identification documents that do not reflect the correct name and gender identity leads to being "outed" in school, employment settings, health care spaces, and more. Being 'outed' is a safety issue, as it can make a person vulnerable to harassment and violence in a world that is still all-too-often unsafe for transgender and nonbinary people.

- *Can you think of other examples of structural racism or structural discrimination?*

- *How might structural discrimination affect a client?*

- *Have you ever experienced structural discrimination?*

EXAMPLES OF DISCRIMINATION IN PUBLIC HEALTH

The fields of medicine and public health harbor notorious instances of racism and other forms of discrimination that have led some people to have a deep mistrust of the public health and health care systems.

Throughout medical history, LGBTQIA+ communities have been classified as having mental health disorders on the basis of their identities. The American Psychiatric Association considered being gay/lesbian a mental health condition until 1973, and since 1980, classified being transgender or nonbinary as a mental health disorder. In recent years, transgender and nonbinary people are no longer categorized as having a mental health disorder based on their gender identities; however, those in need of gender transition-related care are still deemed to have the mental health condition of "gender dysphoria" (American Psychiatric Association, 2023). This legacy results in LGBTQIA+ people being afraid to access medical and mental health services, in LGBTQIA+ patients being turned away by healthcare providers, and most alarmingly, in some mental health providers subjecting LGBTQIA+ adults and minors to harmful conversion "therapies" that attempt to change the person's sexual orientation or gender identity.

One of the most horrific examples of discrimination in public health was a clinical study of the effects of untreated syphilis conducted on Black men in Mason County, Georgia. In 1932, the Public Health Service, a branch of the U.S. government, carried out an infamous study known as the "Tuskegee Study of Untreated Syphilis in the Negro Male" (Brawley, 1998). For more than 40 years, Black men who had the disease were given a placebo (a treatment that the patient does not know is ineffective) for what they were told by the U.S. government was "bad blood." They were each given $50 to participate in the study, offered a decent burial when they died, and were under the impression that the treatment for "bad blood" was helpful. Even though in 1942 it was well known that penicillin could cure syphilis, it was never offered to the men in the study. As a result, many of the men died, and others became disabled.

The Tuskegee study officially ended in 1972 after it was exposed and publicized by the media. However, the memory of this unethical study, a blatant form of anti-Black racism, remains strong in many African American communities. On May 16, 1997, President Bill Clinton issued a formal apology on behalf of the nation to the family members of the men who took part in this study.

A more recent example is the systemic response to the 2020 Covid-19 pandemic that touched every country in the world. The impacts of the pandemic on different groups exposed the continuation of health inequities in a glaring and alarming manner. As of late fall 2022, almost 1.1 million people died from Covid-19 in the United States. People of color had higher rates of COVID-19 infection, hospitalization, and death. Data collected by the United States demonstrates that the COVID-19 death rate for Black communities is more than double that of other racial groups (Vasquez Reyes, 2020). These glaring impacts prompted UN Commissioner Michelle Bachelet to warn that "Covid-19 exposed other inequalities that are often ignored in the United States." Bachelet went on to note that the inequities are not only in health but also in education and employment (Bachelet, 2020).

Public health experts also acknowledge that "vaccine hesitancy"—or reluctance to trust the efficacy of vaccines—also played a role in COVID-19 infections and deaths. More specifically, the legacy of past racist public health practices such as the Tuskegee study fueled a hesitancy among people of color to obtain the recommended vaccines due to a deep distrust of the medical establishment.

This and other inequities are fueled by systemic issues, including the lack of access to health care, culturally uninformed and discriminatory health care policies, and unequal economic and social conditions that primarily impact people of color in the U.S.

Discriminatory policies and practices such as the ones described above destroy public trust and create barriers between the communities who have experienced discrimination and our public health system. While you don't have the power to undo history, as a CHW you can work to ensure that gaps in your own knowledge, attitudes, and professional competencies do not cause further harm to your clients.

- *What are your thoughts and feelings about the government-sanctioned Tuskegee study and the systemic discrimination of LGBTQIA+ communities?*

- *Are you aware of current structural or institutional injustices that harm people of color or other communities?*

- *How might these injustices influence your work as a CHW?*

- *How can you build trusting relationships with communities that have experienced such injustices?*

7.6 Building Capacity as Culturally Effective CHWS

With time, study, training and self-reflection, you will enhance your understanding of cultural humility and your ability to demonstrate it in your working relationships.

TRANSFERENCE OF POWER

An important component of cultural humility is a heightened awareness of the transference of power when clients work with caregivers. Traditionally, during a health care appointment, the health care provider asks most of the questions and leads the appointment with what they think is most important to assess and talk about.

Reflect on your last appointment with your health care service provider:

- *Who asked most of the questions?*
- *Were you able to fully express yourself, ask questions and assert your priorities?*

Changing our approach can make it possible for an appointment – or any type of direct service - to be person-centered and to support clients to take the lead in identifying the concerns that are most important to them. This is what is known as a transference of power. While some questions need to be asked to begin an initial client intake or interviewing session, we want to create an atmosphere that invites and supports the client to tell their story and assert their needs. This transference of power allows the client to be the expert and the CHW or other caregiver to be the student. This produces a powerful change in the caregiver-client dynamic.

How can CHWs facilitate this transference of power? Person-centered counseling skills such as Motivational Interviewing are the best approaches for changing the power dynamic. This is a skill based on the concept of cultural humility. Chapters 8 through 11 provide detailed information about the person-centered approach.

Unconscious Bias

Unconscious bias, also called Implicit Bias, are terms used to acknowledge our personal prejudices and stereotypes about people who come from communities other than their own. Forming these prejudices, biases and stereotypes happens "unconsciously"—we are not even aware we are doing it. Everyone has unconscious bias, informed by our past experiences and how our family, friends and community leaders talked about other people, often reinforcing stereotypes. Human nature lends itself to "categorizing people" but this often leads to discrimination, unfair and unequal treatment and perpetuates historical racism, homophobia, sexism and other forms of oppression.

As a culturally humble CHW, it's important to "check" yourself and to intentionally work with each person as they present themselves to you. Disregard previous assumptions and beliefs about the community that the person belongs to. Remember, their experiences are unique to them. They will teach you about themselves. You will learn from each person you work with. Acknowledge when you have learned something new, and when you make a mistake. This is the ongoing, transformative work of being culturally humble.

Please reflect on your own experiences:

- *Can you think of a time when someone stereotyped you? How did you feel?*
- *Can you think of a time when you stereotyped someone and later learned it was untrue?*
- *Name one action you can take to reduce unconscious bias*

Building capacity as a culturally effective CHW takes commitment and guidance provided by professional resources for interacting with clients. Some resources to help you demonstrate cultural humility in a person-centered intake session include tools to elicit health beliefs and the LEARN model which is often used by providers in health care settings. These are examples of how to apply cultural humility in a person-oriented intake session. Keep in mind that these tools and many of the questions may be adapted as best defined by CHWs in the work setting.

CULTURAL SELF-AWARENESS

Take a few minutes to answer the following questions:

1. What types of clients/communities do you think might have the greatest difficulties in accessing health or social services? Why?

2. What types of clients and communities do you lack experience with and knowledge about?

3. What types of clients or communities may you be less comfortable working with? Why?

4. How can you keep your personal attitudes and feelings from influencing the way you work with diverse clients?

5. What can you do to acknowledge your own stereotypes and prejudices? Why is this an important step to becoming an effective CHW?

6. Is it okay to be uncomfortable at times with clients of a particular cultural identity, or does this make you an unskilled CHW?

7. Is it okay to talk with your colleagues when you find that you are challenged in working with a client?

8. How can you learn to accept constructive feedback about your work with diverse clients?

Reflect on your answers. Becoming aware of your own perceptions of others, your attitudes and behaviors, will aid you to work and live in a more culturally sensitive manner. All of us have ideas and beliefs about people based on our upbringing and the prejudices that were passed on to us.

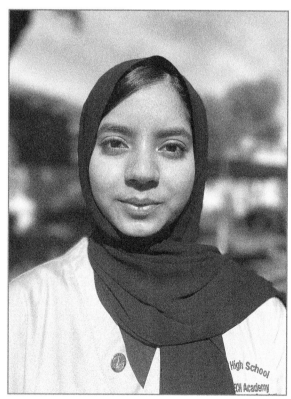

A young CHW starting her career.

Self-reflection is a powerful process for understanding our own cultural backgrounds and identities, as well as our own "hot-button issues"—the strong feelings, attitudes, and values that may arise during our work with others and that can have a negative influence on our ability to effectively support a client.

Taking the additional step of acknowledging when the communities you belong to are the beneficiaries of unearned privilege in our society (for example, White people, men, heterosexuals and the physically able) may be more challenging, because we are socialized to assume that our experiences are shared by others around us—that everyone has access to the same level of benefits as we do. Consider where you have privilege in our society, and where you may lack it. These dynamics of power and privilege are not abstract or theoretical: they may well influence your working relationships with clients, communities and colleagues.

Cultivating a high degree of self-awareness is the first step in becoming a culturally effective CHW.

Please view the following video interview with Abby Rincon, the author of this chapter. Ms. Rincon talks about the challenge and the value of developing your skills for practicing cultural humility.

CULTURAL HUMILITY:

(*Source:* Foundations for Community Health Workers/http://youtu.be/yV3DxgK5pn4/last accessed 21 September 2023.)

WHAT IF YOU MAKE A MISTAKE?

Cultural humility is an approach that acknowledges the limits of our understanding and our tendency to make mistakes when working with clients. Consider the following scenario:

A CHW is working with a client in a health education session. The client has diabetes that is not yet under control. The client is from a cultural group that is different from that of the CHW. Throughout the session, the CHW is compassionate; however the client reacts negatively to the manner in which the CHW explains certain health information, particularly the information about healthy nutrition and eating. While the client doesn't say anything, the information the CHW presents is directly in conflict with the client's dietary traditions and family practices. The client feels that the CHW is trying to change her diet and doesn't understand or respect her traditions. Visibly offended and upset, the client leaves the session early.

Afterward, the CHW spends time thinking about what happened with the client and talks with his supervisor. Through an examination of the session, the CHW and the supervisor determine it is likely that the client was offended. The CHW realizes that he did not take time to ask the client about her own dietary beliefs and practices before presenting her with guidelines for a healthy diet and is committed to doing so when working with future clients.

The CHW demonstrated cultural humility by acknowledging his mistake and desiring to learn and improve his skills. In this case, the CHW is "flexible and humble enough to then re-assess anew the cultural dimensions of the experiences of each client" (Tervalon & Murray-Garcia, 1998).

What Do YOU? Think :

- *Have you ever been offended by assumptions that a health care or social services provider made about you or a family member?*

- *What could you do to demonstrate cultural humility in working with the client described above?*

Please view the following short video that shows a CHW working with a client who wants to change her diet and to control her diabetes. *In this video, the CHW does not do a good job of demonstrating cultural Humility.*

- *What happened between the client and the CHW in this role play?*
- *What mistakes did the CHW make in terms of demonstrating cultural humility?*
- *How could the CHW's mistakes affect the client?*
- *What would you do differently to support this client?*
- *How would you demonstrate cultural humility?*

NUTRITION AND CULTURE, ROLE PLAY, COUNTER:

(*Source:* Foundations for Community Health Workers/http://youtu.be/2Ck3V4johPM/last accessed 21 September 2023.)

In summary, CHWs have the opportunity to enhance their cultural humility skills each time they interact with a community member or client. This is a life-long transformational learning process. Utilizing empathy, compassion and courage will create trusting and important relationships for those you serve.

7.7 Cultural Health Beliefs

Every cultural group has its own beliefs, values, attitudes and practices related to health issues, such as pregnancy and birth, death and dying, gender roles, familial responsibility, disease causation, religion and spirituality, traditional healing, and alternative healing practices. Your cultural community(ies) is no exception to this rule.

What Do YOU Think?

- *What are the health beliefs in your family or culture?*

- *Where did your family go to receive health care?*

- *What were the home remedies for illnesses?*

- *How were they used?*

- *What do you still practice today?*

- *Were there health topics or issues that were considered "taboo" or were forbidden to discuss?*

Earlier we discussed why CHWs must exercise caution and not generalize or stereotype people from any cultural group. Yet CHWs must still acknowledge and appreciate that individuals are indeed members of one or more cultural groups and may hold values rooted in those cultures. As CHWs, our goal should be to bring an open mind and to listen deeply to "where the client is coming from."

TRADITIONAL HEALTH PRACTICES

Many people turn to traditional health practices when they or a family member becomes ill. Traditional health practices are often different from the biomedical or Western medicine approaches used by most healthcare providers in the United States. Interestingly, many of today's biomedical treatments for disease are derived from traditional healing practices throughout the world, though this is not widely understood or acknowledged. Traditional health practices are often discounted or viewed as dangerous by Western medical providers. However, the recognition of traditional health practices is growing in the United States in two ways:

1. **Alternative medicine**: Traditional health practices are used instead of Western medicine (in the United States, the medical profession classifies any health practice that is different from its own biomedical model as "alternative"). Examples of alternative medicine are the use of acupuncture to treat asthma and the use of a special diet and herbs to treat cancer instead of being treated with radiation or chemotherapy.

2. **Complementary medicine**: In this approach, Western or biomedical practices are integrated and provided along with one or more other health traditions (such as Ayurvedic, chiropractic, acupuncture, or Chinese medicine). Some medical schools and hospitals in the United States are beginning to recognize and support complementary medicine.

What Do YOU Think?

- *What traditional health practices are you familiar with?*

- *Do you know of clinics or hospitals in your area that practice complementary medicine?*

- *What has your experience been with biomedical and alternative medical traditions?*

A Culturally—Focused Approach to Medication Assisted Treatment for Opioid Use

The Friendship House Association of American Indians (FH) has been providing culturally-focused residential substance abuse treatment since 1963, serving over 6,000 American Indians/Alaska Natives (AI/AN). The mission of FH is to promote healing and wellness in the American Indian community by providing high quality substance abuse prevention, treatment and recovery services while integrating cultural and spiritual traditions.

Friendship House believes that recovery begins with culture and fostering healthy connections as the foundation for healing. Native traditional practices, spiritual space, and cultural interventions are integrated with evidence-based practices such as the Twelve Steps of AA/NA, the Red Road, and peer-peer support model. Love, tolerance, reciprocity, humility, and respect for all life inform and lay a foundation for their major programs.

Friendship House provides:

- **The Healing Center** is an eighty-bed adult residential substance abuse treatment program for men and women for up to one year.
- **The Women's Lodge** is a nine-bed residential treatment program for AI/AN women and their children (under age 5), supporting the parental connection between mother and child, establishing a healthy family-bond and promoting positive child development.
- **AI/AN community events and gatherings** are hosted throughout the year to provide sober and safe gatherings for our local AI/AN relatives, to recognize and celebrate Native cultures and traditions.
- **The Friendship House Youth Program** provides culturally relevant afterschool and summer programs geared toward AI/AN children, youth, and young adults up to age 24.

During the past four years, FH has integrated Medication Assisted Treatment (MAT) as a component of evidence-based practice to treat opioid addictions. Opioid misuse is a leading cause of overdose for AI/ANs and has significantly increased during the past three years due to the COVID-19 pandemic. FH garnered grant funding with California Consortium for Urban Indian Health and other funding to advance opioid treatment methods sensitive to AI/AN that integrate traditional healing principles and practices.

Michelle James, FH MAT Project Coordinator/HIV Project Director, and the FH clinical team, have developed and implemented a successful MAT treatment and support services program. The program includes screening;

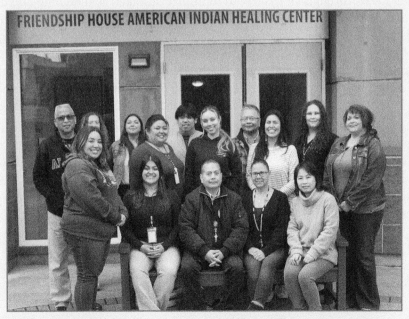

Staff at The Friendship House American Indian Healing Center.

(continues)

A Culturally—Focused Approach to Medication Assisted Treatment for Opioid Use

(continued)

assessment; care coordination; establishing key medical partners; leading a culturally-based community readiness assessment; and providing critical harm reduction trainings on the use of Naloxone. Naloxone is a life-saving opioid reversal medication that has saved countless lives. Ms. James is a local champion and the key change agent for reducing harm and developing person-centered care in coordination with local medical partners. She is a Community Health Worker who believes in healing and is a compassionate recovery advocate dismantling shame and stigma.

To learn more about the work of Friendship House, go to https://www.friendshiphousesf.org/

The following scenarios illustrate how traditional healing practices or cultural health beliefs may affect the care provided by health institutions.

1. A young Cambodian mother brings her eight-year-old daughter to a health center with a fever and bad cough. Upon the physical examination, the clinician discovers multiple red marks across the child's chest and back. The clinician could mistake this as a sign of parental child abuse. However, it is not. The mother practices "coining," a traditional, common practice in Southeast Asia. Coining entails rubbing heated oil on the skin and vigorously rubbing a coin over the area in a linear fashion until a red mark is seen. This is used to allow a path by which a "bad wind" can be released from the body. People use this method to treat a variety of minor ailments, including fever, chills, headache, colds, and cough.

2. At a hospital, the nursing staff alerts a doctor about a patient who is agitated. The nurses want the doctor to order medication to calm the patient down, since he does not want to stay in bed. He is an elderly Japanese man who became upset and "uncooperative" because his bed was situated in the direction used to lay out the deceased in traditional Japan.

3. A patient is seen at a health clinic for persistent, abdominal pain. The clinician suspects a stomach ulcer, prescribes medication, and sends the patient to speak with the CHW about following a new dietary regimen, eating several small meals throughout the day to minimize stomach acid buildup and pain. As the CHW explains the diet prescribed by the doctor, the patient remains quiet and appears uninterested. Finally, at the end of the session, the CHW asks if he has any questions. The man doesn't have any questions, but states that he is Muslim, this is Ramadan, and he cannot follow the prescribed diet. Ramadan is the ninth month of the Islamic lunar calendar, and every day during this month, Muslims around the world spend the daylight hours in a complete fast. Muslims abstain from food, drink, and other physical needs during the daylight hours as a time to purify the soul, refocus attention on God, and practice self-sacrifice.

Having the awareness and sensitivity to work effectively with people of all cultural identities is a critical skill for the twenty-first century. CHWs often play a vital role in aiding clients to access alternative or complementary medicine and to advocate for these choices with Western or biomedical providers. As cultural brokers who build "bridges" between poor and underserved communities and health care providers, CHWs can play an important role in assisting to foster a mutually respectful and cooperative partnership or understanding between biomedical providers and providers of other traditions.

THE LEARN MODEL

Another useful model for working with diverse clients is the LEARN model of Cross Cultural Encounter Guidelines for Health Practitioners (Ladha, Zubairi, Hunter, Audcent, & Johnstone, 2018):

LEARN:

L: Listen with sympathy and understanding to the client's perception of the problem

E: Explain your perceptions of the problem

A: Acknowledge and discuss the differences and similarities between the perceptions of the client and the CHW

R: Recommend resources

N: Negotiate agreement

The LEARN model acknowledges the cultural health beliefs of clients and allows for CHWs to share what they know about a specific health condition. Neither perception is negated or devalued, and both are acknowledged and incorporated into the session. Both are taken into consideration as clients choose a course of action to promote their health.

As CHWs engage with their clients in this manner they are aiding their clients to preserve their own cultural health belief systems. Remember, however, that what may be true about some or most individuals from a particular cultural group, region, or country may not be true of all people who come from the same background. According to the Provider's Guide to Quality and Culture (Management Systems for Health, 2023), as you work with diverse clients, keep the following in mind:

- People from rural areas may have been living a more traditional lifestyle than people who have been living in urban areas.
- Economic status and education vary greatly among people within a cultural group or people who come from the same country.
- People from the same country may have migrated to the United States for very different reasons, including seeking economic opportunity, escaping religious or ethnic persecution, fleeing civil strife, or joining relatives in America.
- Generational differences may exist among people of different ages within the same cultural group and may include different belief systems.

Client Scenario: Luisa M. (continued)

Review the scenario about Luisa M. presented at the beginning of the chapter. Note that even if you share some aspects of Luisa's cultural identity and experience, you are unlikely to share every aspect. Remember that cultural humility guides us in working with *all* clients including those who share some of our own cultural identity.

The CHW who met with Luisa started the interview primarily concerned with her pregnancy and wanted to connect her to prenatal care. However, as the CHW listens to Luisa with cultural humility, they realize there are other issues to learn more about.

For example, the CHW considers how they can learn more about Luisa's *nervios*. This is a new term for the CHW. Might her *nervios* be a sign of post-traumatic stress and, if so, what her views and beliefs about trauma and recovery? Would Luisa be open to meeting with a trained counselor or social worker? What if the counselor was Latina and bilingual? The CHW says, "*Luisa, I'm not familiar with the term nervios. Would you tell me more about what you're experiencing and feeling?*"

By practicing cultural humility and striving to learn about a client's reality as part of your core competencies, a client will feel more comfortable sharing her multiple cultural identities. Only she is qualified to tell you what is most important to her. Listening in a nonjudgmental and compassionate manner, as well as validating her, will be critical to establishing trust, learning what is really going on for her, and creating a positive encounter so that she will return for a follow-up visit.

For Luisa M., how well the CHW listens and demonstrates cultural humility may determine how much of her story she tells, whether she returns to the clinic, and if she is connected to licensed colleague who can provide prenatal care and address her nervios and severe stomach ache.

7.8 Professional Roles of Culturally Effective CHWs

In Chapter 1, you read about the core roles of CHWs. Here, we look at some of those roles again and provide an example or idea for how to apply cultural humility. As you read, think of examples of your own.

1. **Cultural Mediation between Communities and Health and Social Services Systems**

   - Help clients to better understand the nature of the services, treatments and systems they access. Clients may also need support in expressing key concerns or posing questions.

   - Support other providers to demonstrate cultural humility as they work with diverse clients. Encourage them to refrain from making assumptions about the lives and health-related behaviors of new clients, and to consult directly with clients to better understand their priorities, values and goals.

   - If possible, encourage your colleagues or agency to participate in a training about cultural humility, and to examine how they can put key concepts and skills into practice.

     - *What else might you do, in your role as cultural mediator?*

2. **Providing Culturally Appropriate Health Education and Information**

   - Participate in local community and cultural events and opportunities to increase your knowledge and cultural humility skills.

   - Support clients to understand their health and medical care by providing easy-to-understand health information and health education materials in the appropriate language and literacy level. Don't assume everyone can read.

   - Create a checklist to guide you in providing health education. For example, did you remember to ask the client how she understands her illness? Did you acknowledge his cultural traditions respectfully? Did you avoid professional jargon and technical words that the client may not understand?

     - *What else might you do while providing health education and information?*

5. **Advocating for Individuals and Communities**

   - Consider how well the program and agency you work for demonstrates cultural humility. Are agency policies and practices inclusive and supportive of diverse cultural backgrounds and identities? Does the agency have a good reputation of respecting the cultures and identities of the clients or customers they serve? If necessary, advocate within the agency you work for and ask for additional professional development regarding cultural humility. Support your colleagues and your agency to improve the quality of services to diverse clients and communities.

   - Advocate for your agency to expand its capacity to provide services in multiple languages and to use qualified health care interpreters.

   - Advocate for agency forms and policies to be changed to be inclusive of lesbian, gay, bisexual, transgender, and intersex identities.

     - *What else might you do to advocate for your clients' and communities' cultural needs?*

6. **Building Individual and Community Capacity**

   - Invite community members to provide input into the design of the services you provide. Facilitate a focus group to determine, for example, if the community is comfortable with the idea of support groups, or would social groups or events be a better way to build mutual support? Adapt programs and services to what will work for *this* community.

   - Work with community members to learn new concepts and skills—such as community organizing and advocacy skills—that will enhance their capacity to take action to promote their own health.

     - *What else might come up as you work to build individual and community capacity? How might you address those cultural differences effectively?*

> **Nilda Palacios:** I work with a diverse ethnic and gender population. I am open to people from different cultures and learning about their unique experiences. I do my best to be transparent and inclusive in my communication and engagement with consumers and community members. Working with cultural humility allows people to be open to expressing themselves without a fear of judgment.

7. **Providing Direct Services**

   - As you provide services to clients, carefully consider if the questions you ask or the suggestions you provide are culturally biased. For example, when talking about diet and nutrition, are you referring to dietary guidelines that are inclusive of diverse cultural traditions? Are your questions inclusive of the client's experience, culture and behaviors?

   - Become familiar with referral resources in the community that are culturally and linguistically appropriate. Assist your clients in navigating the system in the best way possible for them. Know which languages are spoken at various agencies for your clients who have limited English proficiency.

     - *What else might you do, in your role providing services and referrals?*

Please view these short videos that show a CHW working with a client with depression. In the counter video, the CHW does **not** do a great job of demonstrating cultural humility. In the demonstration, the CHW does a much better job.

- *What mistakes did the CHW make in the counter role play?*
- *How may the lack of cultural humility impact this client, or the relationship between the client and the CHW?*
- *What did the CHW do differently in the demonstration video?*
- *What else would you do to demonstrate cultural humility and support this client?*

DEPRESSION, RELIGION AND CULTURAL HUMILITY: COUNTER ROLE PLAY

(*Source*: Foundations for Community Health Workers/http://youtu.be/y6d-GdXi8go/last accessed 21 September 2023.)

DEPRESSION, RELIGION AND CULTURAL HUMILITY: DEMONSTRATION ROLE PLAY:

(*Source*: Foundations for Community Health Workers/http://youtu.be/Bgr6TXWknQQ/last accessed 21 September 2023.)

CULTURAL DIVERSITY: IT'S PERSONAL, IT'S PROFESSIONAL, AND IT'S RIGHT

Cultural diversity isn't something to tolerate, but rather to embrace and celebrate. Diversity brings richness to our society and keeps our work as CHWs fascinating, dynamic, and rewarding.

As you continue to advance in your career, remember to keep an open mind and an open heart. Respect and honor the differences of the clients and communities you have the opportunity to work with. Demonstrate compassion and a nonjudgmental perspective along the way.

We encourage you to expand your understanding of what cultural diversity means. Ask hard questions of yourself, examining your own cultural upbringing and values, including any bias that you may have towards others. Learn to acknowledge and accept your own limitations and mistakes. At times you may not be comfortable as you examine your own life and attitudes and expand your horizons to study the history and perspectives of others. But the very moments when you are most uncomfortable may be your greatest opportunities for personal and professional growth.

Chapter Review

As in any other area of professional development, building our capacity to practice cultural humility requires planning. Spend some time answering the preliminary questions. Then identify specific steps or actions you will take to strengthen your knowledge and skills over the next three to six months.

1. What three strengths do I bring to this work on cultural humility? In what ways could I build on these strengths?

2. What three gaps (or challenges) do I want to work on?

3. Did any data, discussions, definitions, principles, or questions in this chapter provoke a strong emotional reaction for me? What are those feelings? What can I do to respond to my feelings in a way that honors my own experiences and perspectives and at the same time assists me to understand and honor the experiences or perspectives that are provoking those feelings?

4. Over the next six months to a year, what activities could I undertake to strengthen my capacity to work across differences of race, class, culture, and language?

    a. Read the following books or articles: _____

    _____

    _____

    b. View the following films or videos (in fictional movies, look especially for movies made *by* members of a culture, *about* their own culture): _____

    _____

    _____

    c. Meet with and discuss these issues with: _____

    _____

    _____

    d. Attend a lecture or presentation on: _____

    _____

    _____

    e. Participate in the following training or workshops: _____

    _____

    _____

    f. Participate in the following cross-cultural community events: _____

    _____

    _____

    g. Join or organize a small discussion or study group focused on: _____

    _____

    _____

    h. Volunteer with the following organization that promotes or organizes cross-cultural work in my community: _____

    _____

    _____

i. Join or support the work of the following organization that advocates or organizes for the cultural diversity or equity concerns of a group that is marginalized or discriminated against in my community: _____

_____

_____

j. Other activities: _____

5. What resources would I draw on to assist me in these activities? Who can I go to in my organization or agency to seek support and guidance in carrying out my learning plan? Which friends, family members and colleagues do I feel most comfortable talking with about these issues, and why?

6. I will sit down again on the following date to evaluate my progress and development and to update my learning plan: _____

References

American Psychiatric Association. (2023). What is Gender Dysphoria? https://www.psychiatry.org/patients-families/gender-dysphoria/what-is-gender-dysphoria#:~:text=Gender%20dysphoria%3A%20A%20concept%20designated,and%2For%20secondary%20sex%20characteristics. (accessed 5 May 2023).

Bachelet, M. (2020). Our Health Depends on each Other. That's why we need to fight this threat together. *Time Magazine*. April 15.

Brawley, O. W. (1998). The study of untreated syphilis in the negro male. International Journal of Radiation Oncology Biology *Physics*. doi: 10.1016/s0360-3016(97)00835-3.

Brown, A. (2022). About 5% of Young Adults in the U.S. say their Gender is Different from their Sex Assigned at Birth. *Pew Research Center*. June 7.

Budiman, A. (2020). Key Findings about U.S. Immigrants. *Pew Research Center*. August 20.

Camarota, S. A. & Zeigler, K. (2022). Foreign-born Population hits 48 Million in September 2022. *Center for Immigration Studies*. October 27.

Crenshaw, K. (1989). Demarginalizing the intersection of race and sex: A black feminist critique of antidiscrimination doctrine, feminist theory and antiracist politics. *University of Chicago Legal Forum*, 1989 (8): 139–167.

Curt, C. J. N. 1984. *Non-Verbal communication in Puerto Rico* (2nd ed.). Cambridge, MA: Evaluation, Dissemination, and Assessment Center.

Florida, R. (2011). How Diversity Leads to Economic Growth. *Bloomberg*. December 12.

Helman, C. (2007). *Culture, health and illness*. London, UK: CRC Press.

Institute on Taxation and Economic Policy (ITEP) (2017). Undocumented Immigrants' State and Local Tax Contributions Report.

Jones, J. M. (2022). LGBT Identification in U.S. Ticks up to 7.1%. *Gallup News*. February 17.

Ladha, T., Zubairi, M., Hunter, A., Audcent, T., & Johnstone, J. (2018). Cross-cultural Communication: Tools for Working with Families and Children. Paediatrics & Child Health, 23(1), 66–69. >https://doi:10.1093/pch/pxx126.

Management Systems for Health. (2023). A Provider's Guide to Quality and Culture. https://uceddclctraining.org/resources/a-providers-guide-to-quality-and-culture (accessed 5 May 2023).

Rouse, C., Barrow, L., Rinz, K., & Soltas, E. (2021). The Economic Benefits of Extending Permanent Legal Status to Unauthorized Immigrants. *The White House*. September 17.

Sherman, A., Trisi, D., Stone, C., Gonzales, S., & Parrott, S. (2019). Immigrants Contribute Greatly to U.S. Economy, Despite Administration's "Public Charge" Rule Rationale. *Center on Budget and Policy Priorities*. August 15.

Takaki, R. (1993). *A different mirror*. New York, NY: Little, Brown.

Tervalon, M. & Murray-Garcia, J. (1998). Cultural humility versus cultural competence: a critical distinction in defining physician training outcomes in multicultural education. *Journal of Health Care for the Poor and Underserved*, 9(2), 117–125.

U.S. Census Bureau. (2018). American Community Survey. www.census.gov/programs-surveys/acs/data.html (accessed 18 March 2023).

U.S. Census Bureau. (2022a). 2020 Census Results. www.census.gov/programs-surveys/decennial-census/decade/2020/2020-census-results.html (accessed 18 March 2023).

U.S. Census Bureau. (2022b). Current Population Survey September 2022. www.census.gov/programs-surveys/cps.html (accessed 18 March 2023).

Vasquez, Reyes M. (2020). The Disproportional Impact of COVID-19 on African Americans. *Health and Human Rights*, 22(2), 299–307.

Additional Resources

Chavez, Vivian. (2013). Cultural Humility: People, Principles & Practices. A Video. www.youtube.com/watch?v=SaSHLbS1V4w.

Miss Evers' Boys. (1997). A Movie. www.imdb.com/title/tt0119679/.

Conducting Initial Client Assessments

8

Tim Berthold and Lorena Carmona

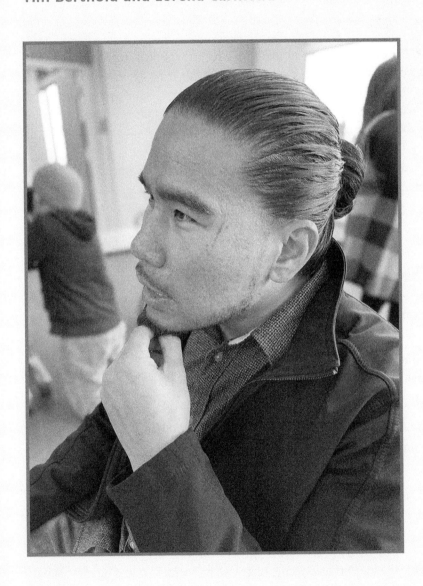

Foundations for Community Health Workers, Third Edition. Edited by Tim Berthold and Darouny Somsanith.
© 2024 John Wiley & Sons, Inc. Published 2024 by John Wiley & Sons, Inc.
Companion website: http://www.wiley.com/go/communityhealthworkers3E

Client Scenario: Maria Nguyen

Maria Nguyen is 29 years old. She worked as a housekeeper for a downtown hotel but was laid-off (lost her job) during the COVID-19 pandemic due to a downturn in the economy.

When Maria lost her job, she also lost her employer-provided health insurance. Maria has type-two diabetes but can't afford to purchase medications. She is also struggling to afford rent and food.

Maria is anxious about her health and worried that if she doesn't find work quickly, she may lose her apartment.

Maria went to the emergency department of the county hospital. A nurse checked her blood glucose levels, provided Maria with a prescription for her diabetes medication, and arranged for her to meet with a social worker. The social worker enrolled Maria in Medicaid and referred her to the Eastside Neighborhood Health Center (Eastside) to get connected with a primary health care provider.

Maria has worked steadily since she was 15, starting out in her family's restaurant in another state. She never thought it would take so long to find a new job. Maria is feeling ashamed that she is still unemployed and struggling financially.

As Maria sits in the waiting room of the Eastside Neighborhood Health Center, she is feeling anxious.

If you were the CHW who meets with Maria Nguyen to conduct an initial assessment, how would you answer the following questions?

- *How may Maria Nguyen be feeling as she sits in the waiting room? What types of worries or concerns may she have?*
- *How will you greet Maria?*
- *What are your key goals for conducting an initial assessment with Maria? What do you hope to a accomplish?*
- *How will you explain your role as a CHW and the purpose of an initial assessment?*
- *How will you explain your agency's confidentiality policy?*
- *What topics will you assess when you talk with Maria? How will you gather this information?*
- *How will you conduct an initial assessment that is person-centered?*
- *How will you document the initial assessment?*
- *How will you end the initial assessment?*

Introduction

Think about a time when you were a new client or a patient at a clinic, hospital, or social services agency. What was your initial intake or assessment like? How did you feel during the assessment, and how did you feel about the clinic or agency afterward? What did the person who was interviewing you say or do to make the assessment more (or less) comfortable and effective?

This chapter addresses how to conduct an initial interview or assessment (sometimes also referred to as an intake) with a new client who may be interested in participating in a particular program, service, or research study. These assessments are often the first contact that a client has with an agency, and a CHW's first opportunity to develop a positive connection or rapport with that individual or family.

For the purposes of this chapter, we will focus on conducting initial assessments to determine eligibility and participation in a particular health-focused program or service such as primary health care, case management services, or a residential treatment program.

WHAT YOU WILL LEARN

By studying the information in this chapter, you will be able to:

- Describe the purpose of initial client assessments
- Explain confidentiality policies
- Discuss and demonstrate how to build rapport with a new client
- Conduct a person-centered assessment, including the use of open and closed-ended questions
- Assess key health and wellness topics, including the social determinants of health
- Explain the value of the strength-based approach, and demonstrate how to conduct a strength-based assessment
- Explain the importance of documentation and specific strategies for taking notes during an assessment
- Close or end an initial assessment

C3 Roles and Skills Addressed in Chapter 8

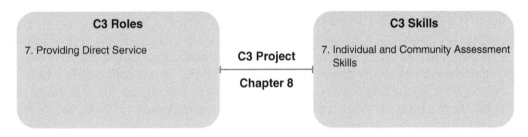

WORDS TO KNOW

Closed-Ended Question

Open-Ended Question

8.1 An Overview of Initial Client Assessments

In general, CHWs conduct initial assessments with new clients in order to:

- Assess and determine whether the client is eligible for and interested in participating in the services provided by a particular agency or program
- Identify the client's resources, risks, and priority concerns

The questions that you will ask, the length of the assessment, and the forms used to document information about clients will vary depending on where you work and the type of program the client is interested in. Initial assessments may be simple or complex and may consist of ten to fifty or more questions. Some assessments are conducted in one session lasting 15–45 minutes or longer, and others take place during more than one meeting.

During an initial assessment, you will gather a range of information from the client. Typically, you will gather basic demographic data such as the client's date of birth, gender, gender identity, ethnicity, primary languages, address, health insurance status, employment status, income, and family status.

If you are working in a healthcare setting or for a program focused on health conditions, you may also ask questions about the client's health status, including questions about their knowledge, attitudes, and behaviors in relation to a specific health condition or concern such as diabetes, hepatitis C, or a type of cancer. *Note that in healthcare settings, licensed providers will conduct separate assessments regarding a patient's health history and to diagnose current health conditions and discuss available treatments.*

Assessments also include questions about the client's social support system; their access to food, housing and other essential resources; prior experience with similar programs and agencies; the client's current concerns and goals; and the client's expectations regarding the program or service your organization offers.

The type of questions you ask during initial assessments will vary depending on the program you are working for. The questions asked by CHWs working with a domestic violence agency will be different from those working for a perinatal health, drug counseling, diabetes management, or mental health program. Some questions may be highly personal in nature. For example, some assessments include questions about a client's sexual behaviors and use of drugs and alcohol.

You will use a form or forms, provided by your employer, to document the information you learn from the client. You may complete these forms online as part of an electronic health record or electronic data system.

Initial assessments can be stressful for clients. They may be worried that they—or their family members—won't qualify for services. They may have faced rude or discriminatory treatment from health or social services providers in the past and feel anxious about how they will be viewed and treated by you and the agency you work for. Clients may have engaged in activities that are classified as illegal, such as drug use or prostitution, and be worried that you or your colleagues will judge or discriminate against them as a result. Undocumented immigrants may be worried about their security and the possibility that they will be reported to immigration authorities.

- *Can you think of other concerns or sources of anxiety for new clients?*

A REMINDER ABOUT SCOPE OF PRACTICE

Your scope of practice (see Chapter 5) may limit the type of questions you ask and the type of information you gather during an assessment. For example, when CHWs conduct a client assessment at a hospital or health center, medical providers will assess and document medical conditions. In this context, the role of the CHW is to work in partnership with licensed healthcare providers who will be responsible for diagnosing medical conditions and prescribing treatment. When working as part of a team, be sure to clarify your role and scope of practice with your supervisor and your teammates.

THE STRUCTURE OF A CLIENT ASSESSMENT

A client assessment, like a good story, has a distinct beginning, middle, and end.

The *beginning* of the client assessment is likely to include:

- Welcoming the client and assisting the person to feel as comfortable as possible
- Introducing yourself, your agency and program, and the purpose of the assessment
- Explaining the assessment process and the types of information that you hope to gather
- Explaining confidentiality and its limits
- Obtaining informed consent to conduct the assessment and initiate services
- Building rapport

The *middle phase* of the assessment generally includes:

- Gathering information from the client required in order to determine eligibility for the health program, service, or research study
- Assessing a broad range of topics that influence a client's health and wellness including social determinants of health such as housing, food security and personal safety
- Answering the client's questions and concerns
- Assessing the client's risk factors, their priority concerns, and the internal and external resources they bring to the task of improving their health
- Building rapport or a positive connection with the client

The *ending phase* of the assessment generally includes:

- Determining enrollment or participation in the program or service in question
- Providing referrals, as appropriate
- Identifying the next steps for the client (such as scheduling a follow-up appointment)
- Asking if the client still has any outstanding questions or concerns

- Continuing to build rapport
- Ending the assessment in a way that affirms and respects the client

JUGGLING ALL THE ELEMENTS OF THE ASSESSMENT

It can be challenging to juggle all the essential elements of an initial client assessment; you have a lot to accomplish in a relatively short period of time. As you conduct an assessment and document the key information that the client shares with you, you also want to apply person-centered concepts and skills. You want to listen carefully and respectfully to the client's priority concerns. While you may feel pressure from your employer to complete the assessment and all the required paperwork, if you pressure the client to answer your questions and respond to your priorities, you may undermine rapport and trust. Be patient with the client and yourself. If necessary, you can always schedule another time to complete your intake questions and forms.

8.2 The Beginning of The Assessment

In most cases, the assessment will serve as your first interaction with a prospective client. It may also be the client's first interaction with anyone from the agency you work for. Making a positive first impression is vital. It is the first step toward establishing an ongoing working relationship, and it increases the chances that the client will return to the agency to participate in the services you provide.

What Do YOU Think?

- *What makes you feel comfortable and welcomed when you go to a new agency for services?*

- *Have you ever had a negative experience during an initial assessment or meeting at a new agency or program?*

  - *What happened during the assessment?*

  - *How did you feel about the agency/program after the assessment?*

Please view the following video ▶ interview about the importance of providing a new client with a warm welcome.

- *What else do you want to do or say to welcome a new client to the program or agency you work for?*

WELCOMING A CLIENT:
(*Source:* Foundations for Community Health Workers/http://youtu.be/iQrImzhjAIs/ last accessed 21 September 2023.)

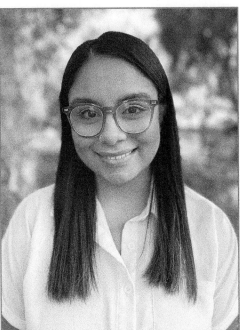

CHWs welcome clients like an honored guest to their home.

BUILDING A POSITIVE CONNECTION OR RAPPORT

Your success as a CHW will be influenced by your ability to create and maintain a positive, trusting relationship with clients. While trust takes time to establish, it will largely be based on the quality of services that you and your organization provide, and how clients feel treated by you and others who deliver services. Your own style or approach to your work as a CHW also contributes to building a positive professional relationship. This personal style may include, for example, your tone of voice, your smile and sense of humor, and how you listen to clients and acknowledge their accomplishments and their challenges. Clients can tell when service providers are not comfortable or being themselves. Learn to work in a way that embraces your authentic self; be true to your own experience, values, and personality.

Many clients have also had negative experiences with helping professionals in the past, and these experiences may influence their interactions with you. Some clients will observe you closely to see if you are going to be yet another person who in some way disappoints or disrespects them. While you can't do anything to change the past, you can treat all clients with respect and dignity and work to build a professional alliance that supports their health. We cannot emphasize enough the vital importance of building a warm and respectful relationship with your clients: it is the foundation for all the work that you will do together.

- *How do you demonstrate respect for the clients you work with?*

THE INTERVIEW SPACE

Not all client assessments take place in a quiet, comfortable, and private meeting room. Sometimes initial assessments take place in the middle of waiting rooms, in homes, in shelters or jail—or even outside, on the street or in a park. No matter where the assessment takes place, find ways to make the best of a less than private situation to assist the client feel safer and more comfortable.

If you are working in a setting that is not ideal for conducting an assessment, acknowledge this and ask the client to assist in determining the best location for your conversation. For example, if you meet a client in a public space, such as a park, you might say:

> **CHW:** *"How about sitting down together on that bench over there in the corner: it seems a little less noisy and more private. Would that work for you? Do you have another suggestion for where we can talk?"*

If you have access to an office for conducting assessments, think about what you can do with the materials and budget at hand to make it as inviting as possible. Does the office have a comfortable chair for clients? Can you decorate the space? Is there a place for a client's children to sit and play while you conduct an assessment? Can you purchase or seek donations of children's books or toys? Can you offer clients a glass of water, a cup of tea, or a snack?

This attention to detail can be meaningful in conveying your commitment and concern for clients and your work. Seating arrangements are also important to consider. For example, asking a client to sit on the other side of your imposing desk may create a feeling of formality and distance that could get in the way of building rapport or connection. Sitting next to a client during an assessment may create a more relaxed atmosphere and allow the information you write down to be shared. Think about the options available to you and talk with colleagues about how they set up their meeting space.

- *What kind of office makes you feel most comfortable?*

- *How would you decorate an office—with very little money!—where you conduct client assessments?*

Conducting a Telehealth Assessment

Increasingly, service providers meet with clients remotely via a telehealth platform that permits videoconferencing. The challenge is not to let the technology get in the way of your work with the client, including your efforts to build a warm and positive connection or rapport. The same concepts that work in-person can usually be applied when using technology. Convey your warmth and interest in connecting with the client with your voice and—if you are using videoconferencing—your body language. Smile. Listen patiently and don't interrupt the client. Ask open-ended questions that invite the client to share their concerns, questions and their knowledge and accomplishments. Validate the client's concerns and achievements. Summarize key information shared during the meeting and check with the client for their understanding: *"Maria, I want to make sure that I did a good job explaining our primary healthcare services. Can you repeat what you understand about the services that we provide?"*

INTRODUCING YOURSELF

Remember to introduce yourself to clients: tell them your name, job title, what you will cover during your meeting, and how you would like to be addressed. For example:

> **CHW:** *"Hello, it's a pleasure to meet you. My name is Lucy Chang, and I'm a Community Health Worker here at the Eastside Neighborhood Health Center. I use she/her pronouns, and I'll be talking with you today about the services we provide. Please call me Lucy."*

Sometimes people try to use a so-called "professional" tone of voice that may seem impersonal, cold, or robotic to a client. We encourage you to be yourself, and to welcome a new client like you would a valued guest to your home. Smile. Reach out to shake hands if appropriate. Use a warm and friendly tone of voice.

Greet the client, and if you know it, call them by name—it may be written down in your agency's appointment schedule. It is important to call people by their proper name and the best way to be sure that you do this is to ask. We also strongly recommend asking each client which pronouns they use to avoid offending or misgendering them (see Chapter 7). If the client is using a different name from the one you have written on the appointment form, clarify which name they would like to use in the documents you prepare and what name they would like to be called by. If you are ever unclear as to how to address new clients, ask them how they would like to be addressed.

> **CHW:** *"What name would you like me to call you as work together? And what pronouns—such as she, he or they—do you use?"*
>
> **Maria Nguyen:** *"Please call me Maria. I go by she/her."*

By asking the clients what name they would like to be called, and what pronouns they use, you are demonstrating respect and cultural humility. This sets a positive tone for a person-centered assessment. Asking about pronouns is vital in conveying respect to transgender and non-binary clients, and to helping them feel welcomed at the agency or program where you work.

DETERMINE THE LANGUAGE OF SERVICE

You may be conducting an assessment in English, American Sign Language, Farsi, Spanish, Cantonese, or another language. Be sure to ask clients what their primary language is. You may need to provide them with a trained healthcare interpreter, if available, or find someone who speaks their language to conduct the assessment. Don't proceed with an assessment if you are not truly fluent in the language of service to prevent making mistakes that could be harmful to the client's health or welfare. See Chapter 1 for more information about how to work with an interpreter.

ASK CLIENTS WHAT THEY WANT TO ACHIEVE

A good way to begin an initial assessment is to ask some version of: *"What brings you to _____ (name of your agency) today?"* This gives clients an opportunity to share what they hope to get out of the meeting. It also conveys your interest in the client's priority concerns.

> **Maria Nguyen:** *"Well, I need to see a doctor. I have diabetes and I haven't been able to afford my medications, so I haven't been taking them. And—I'm not sure if you can help me with this—but I lost my job and I need help finding employment."*

EXPLAIN THE ASSESSMENT

Let the client know what to expect from the initial assessment by clearly explaining:

- The purpose of the assessment
- How long the assessment may take
- The type of information you will ask them for
- How this information will be used

You will speak more at the beginning of the assessment and should take time to explain the assessment process. You will also explain confidentiality and obtain informed consent.

Client Scenario: Maria Nguyen (continued)

CHW: Maria, I understand that you were referred to our clinic by the county hospital. I'm going to explain the services that we provide at the Eastside Neighborhood Health Center, review some of our policies, and gather some information from you that will help us to better support you. This first meeting will take about 50 minutes. Do you have that much time today?

Maria Nguyen: Yes, that's okay. Thank you.

CHW: I have a number of questions to ask about your health and about housing, employment, access to food and other services. Here's a copy of the form that we use to gather information from a new patient. [The CHW gives Maria a copy of the Eastside Health Center Assessment Form]

Maria: [Looks at the Assessment form] Okay.

CHW: I'll be writing down the information that you share with me on the client intake form. At the end of the assessment, you can decide if you want to become a patient at our health center and, if you do, I can schedule a first appointment with one of our nurse practitioners or doctors. If you do decide to participate in the program, the information I document will be placed in your new health record to be shared with our healthcare provider. Do you have any questions about the assessment before we begin?

Lorena Carmona: When I'm conducting an initial assessment, I start by explaining the purpose. I tell the client that I'm gathering information so that I can better understand their life circumstances and their resources, needs and priorities. That way, I can support them to develop a plan to meet their most important concerns like getting access to health care or housing or food.

I always like to ask the client how much time they have to meet with me. I explain that an assessment could take anywhere from 45 minutes to an hour and half. I tell them that we can always get started and finish up the assessment at another meeting or over the phone. I let them know that they can take their time, they can think over certain questions and answer them later.

EXPLAIN THE CONFIDENTIALITY POLICY

Confidentiality was introduced in Chapter 5 as an important ethical obligation for CHWs. Part of this obligation is learning how to clearly explain confidentiality and its limits to clients. You must do this at the beginning of your first session or assessment with new clients, before they have an opportunity to tell you something that you may have to report to others. Check with your supervisor to be sure that you understand the confidentiality policy and protocols at your agency.

The Health Insurance Portability and Accountability Act (HIPAA)

If you work in a healthcare setting, every new client or patient will be asked to read and sign a Health Insurance Portability and Accountability Act (HIPAA) form. HIPAA is a federal law that requires the protection and confidential handling of health information. To read more about HIPAA, please see the resource provided at the end of this chapter.

Telling a client that an appointment or services are confidential is not sufficient. Clearly explain what confidentiality means.

While in general you are able to promise that the client's information will be kept private, there are important exceptions to this rule. For example, if you learn that any of your clients have harmed or are intending to do harm to themselves or others, or have been harmed by others, you have a duty to report this information. The harms that we refer to include suicide, child abuse, elder abuse, sexual abuse, physical assault, or threats. Please note that reportable exceptions to confidentiality vary from state to state. Check carefully with your employer to be certain that you explain each type of "harm" that must be reported, and to whom.

Earlier, we suggested that when you welcome a new client, you ask: *"What brings you to the clinic today?"* However, if clients begin to talk about a subject that you may need to report to legal authorities, we suggest that you interrupt them and take time to clearly explain the limits of confidentiality. If you don't explain this up front, and a client discloses a situation that you have a legal and ethical obligation to report, it is likely that they client may feel set up or betrayed. This is likely to destroy all hope of establishing trust.

> CHW: *"Maria, I want to hear more about what brings you to the health center and the type of services and support you are looking for. But before we start to talk about that in greater detail, I need to explain our policy on confidentiality."*
>
> *"Everything that you tell me will be kept private and confidential. If you decide to join our health center as a patient, the information will go into your patient file here. Only your service providers here at Eastside will have access to the information in your file. They can't share this information with other service providers unless they talk with you first, and you sign a form giving them permission to share this information with others."*

Take your time. Don't rush this. Maintain eye contact and a friendly tone of voice. Pay attention to your client's body language and signs that the person may not understand you.

> CHW: *"However, there are a couple of exceptions to the confidentiality policy that I need to discuss with every new client. If a client tells me that they are harming themselves or others or are being hurt by someone else, then by law I have to tell my supervisor, and they may have to report the information to a crisis team or an agency such as Child Protective Services or the police. By hurting themselves or others we mean things like suicide or sexual or physical abuse. As a health worker, if I learn that someone is in danger, I can't keep silent. The only ethical consideration that is even stronger than my commitment to protecting your privacy is our commitment to protecting you and others from harm.*
>
> *Do you understand these guidelines? Do you have any questions about the privacy of what we talk about today?"*

To be certain that clients fully understand the privacy or confidentiality policy, ask them to explain it to you. This is the best way to be certain that you have been clear.

> CHW: *"Maria, I want to make sure that I have explained our policy clearly. Can you tell me what you understand about our confidentiality policy?"*

For more information about confidentiality and ethics, please refer to Chapter 5 and, most importantly, remember to share any questions or concerns you may have with your supervisor.

Preserving Confidentiality by Phone or Telehealth Platforms

You may conduct client assessments remotely by phone call or a telehealth platform (meeting with a client via a videoconferencing program). Regardless of how you meet with a client, you must safeguard their confidentiality and comply with HIPAA requirements.

When meeting with clients by phone, CHWs should be in an isolated environment where no one can overhear the conversation. Encourage clients to find a place where they can also talk with you privately. Always use a work phone for these calls and under no circumstances should you share personal contact information with the client, such as your personal phone number or email address. If you use a personal cell phone to call clients, make sure that you block your number from being revealed.

If you meet with clients via a telehealth platform, you can schedule appointments through your agency's electronic health record system or set up a friendly reminder via text messages. The telehealth system you use will typically send a link to the client so that they can join the appointment with a single click without the need to access an app or portal or to login for the call. Telehealth appointments can be conducted on laptops, desktops, tablets or phones. When the person clicks the link to join the session, they are taken to a virtual waiting room where they can confirm that their system and network settings are ready to go.

OBTAIN INFORMED CONSENT

Before you conduct an initial assessment or provide services to a new client, you need to obtain their informed consent. Informed consent means that the client understands what the assessment or service will consist of and gives permission to participate in the assessment, research interview or program in question. Generally, the client is asked to give informed consent in writing.

In order to be certain that clients understand what the interview will consist of, explain it to them in simple language and ask them to repeat back what they understand.

> **CHW:** *"Maria, we want to make sure that clients understand the goals, services and guidelines for the Eastside Neighborhood Health Center before they decide whether or not to participate. I'll review our services and guidelines for patients. Please stop me along the way if you don't understand something that I say and I'll try to explain it in a different way. Please also let me know if you have any questions or concerns about the program."*

Clearly describe the services that will be provided, any eligibility guidelines or criteria if they exist, any payments or fees that the client will have to pay, and any guidelines for participation. For example, some health education or support groups ask clients to participate in a certain number of sessions, and residential programs may have policies regarding participation in services and when clients can leave the premises.

If a client doesn't fully understand the services that the agency will provide, slow down and review the information again. Check to see if they have any questions or concerns: *"I don't want to rush you. Before we begin the assessment, do you have any questions for me?"*

Note: Review your agency's policies about informed consent. Depending on the program you work for, there may be an age of consent for minors and guidelines for working with people with certain disabilities or health conditions. In some instances, a parent or legal guardian must be consulted. People who are noticeably drunk or high on drugs cannot provide consent for services.

BE AWARE OF BODY LANGUAGE AND TONE OF VOICE

We communicate not only with words, but also through body language and tone of voice. Our facial expressions, how close we sit to others, how we hold our body and our arms, and the degree of eye contact we maintain often convey important messages about what we are thinking or feeling. The tone of our voice also tends to change with emotion and may invite connection or create distance. A voice can be warm, or cold, scolding or inviting. Try to build an awareness of the tone of voice and body language that you and your clients use.

Be cautious, however, about assuming that you understand what is meant by a particular physical expression such as avoiding eye contact, crossing arms over the chest, frowning, or rolling the eyes. Body language is influenced by cultural as well as individual differences. With experience, you will become more skilled in noticing the body language of others, and as appropriate, talking with your clients about them. For example: *"I'm wondering if there is anything else you'd like to say or ask about residential treatment programs?"* Remember that many people are unaware of their body language. Don't push clients to talk further about this, or anything else, if they don't want to.

COMMUNICATING WITH BODY LANGUAGE: ROLE PLAY, COUNTER

(*Source:* Foundations for Community Health Workers/http://youtu.be/DbsgG-LObPE/last accessed 21 September 2023.)

What Do **YOU**? Think

- *How might your tone of voice and body language work to build a connection with clients?*

- *How might it get in the way of building a connection?*

Please view the following videos that show a CHW talking with a client. In the first counter role play video, the CHW does not do a good job of communicating with body language. In the second video, the CHW does a much better job.

- *What mistakes did the CHW make in the first counter video in terms of communicating with body language? How may the CHWs behavior have impacted the client?*

- *What did the CHW do differently in the Demo video?*

- *What would you do differently if you were the CHW working with this client? How do you use body language to communicate with the clients you work with?*

COMMUNICATING WITH BODY LANGUAGE: ROLE PLAY, DEMO

(*Source:* Foundations for Community Health Workers/http://youtu.be/WDV2OPRzfYo/last accessed 21 September 2023.)

CHW Profile

Sengthong S. Sithounnolat (She/her)

Job Title: Health Ambassador

Agency: Urban YMCA

Underserved communities in the Hunters Point Neighborhood, San Francisco

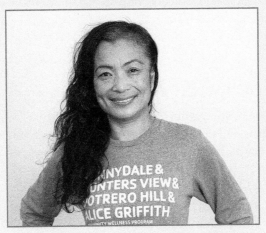

(continues)

CHW Profile

(continued)

What motivated me to become a CHW is being a refugee from Laos and surviving the civil war. When I was in the refugee camp in the Philippines, there was a lot of support from CHWs and social workers. When my family arrived in San Francisco we had help from interpreters. There was a Lao interpreter who went with my family to doctor's appointments. When I got older, I was my parent's interpreter and CHW. Ever since my childhood, I knew I wanted to help others like they helped my family. I have a passion to give back.

I work as an Ambassador for the San Francisco Urban YMCA in the Hunters Point neighborhood. I work with individuals and groups. I do intakes, provide referrals and case management services. People tell me what their needs are, and I try to help them. I assist clients to schedule medical appointments, to talk about their concerns, to apply for benefits, whatever they need. A lot of our clients are seniors, and I help them with using the computer and understanding their benefits.

I co-facilitate a number of groups including a woman's group, a group for seniors, a walking group, a group for children, and a group on trauma called the Resident Warriors. For the women's group, we always do arts and crafts together as we talk about whatever questions or concerns they may have. I lead discussions about health topics such as stress or trauma or healthy eating. I also co-facilitate a Walking Group with a nurse. We start out walking short distances and little by little we walk the Herion Park trails (down the hill) to the ocean. With the seniors, we help them to bring their questions and concerns to the Hunter's Point Community Council. I also work with Resident Warriors. We focus on trauma and provide education so that people can talk about their experience, recognize how it affects them and what do when they or their family needs help. We let our stories be heard, we support each other.

A client came to the office for help. I met with her and did an intake and ended up working as her case manager. Her husband was sick with cancer. They owed $18,000 in back rent and were at risk of losing their housing. She was really upset and needed a shoulder to cry on. I learned that she didn't always get along with others, but we got along just fine. I was patient with her. I helped her to apply for COVID-19 rental assistance and she was approved and was able to clear her debt. This gave her peace of mind. She was so grateful. I felt proud to be able to help her.

Being a CHW has influenced me to be more patient. Before I would interrupt people or be too fast to respond back. Now I listen to the details when helping a client and I know how to have a moment of silence in case there is something else they want to tell me. Being a CHW and having an influence in peoples' lives also makes me more humble. I'm more appreciative of the things that I have, a roof over my head, and my family.

When things get rough or you're not having a good day, just remember what brings us to this work. For me, it's a passion to help others. Somedays it's just about talking with people and showing that we care, you know? So many people are lonely and isolated, and just talking with someone can make a big difference to them.

8.3 The Middle of The Initial Assessment

The middle of the assessment is when you gather information about the client's health and social circumstances as well as their key concerns and priorities. This information sets the stage for any services that will be provided to the client by you or your colleagues.

LISTEN TO AND FOCUS ON THE CLIENT

Gathering the right information is an important part of providing quality services to clients. However, you don't have to be rigid in the way you gather information. Your focus should be on the client or family in front of you rather than on the form waiting to be filled out. Ask the questions on the form and document what you learn as the conversation flows. Maintain eye contact periodically while taking notes and be sure to explain why you are taking notes. For example, *"I want to make sure I accurately record the information you share with me."*

> **TG:** The forms are not the most important part of the interview. I want to make sure my families are doing okay. I check in with them first, and we talk. Most of the time, I get all the information I need by just talking with them. No one wants to be grilled with question after question.

Before you begin an initial assessment, carefully review the forms and data systems that your organization uses for language and categories that could make someone uncomfortable, such as assumptions about gender, gender identity, or who makes a family. If are concerned that the forms you have been asked to use may be biased, talk with your supervisor. When you are working with your clients, practice cultural humility. Frame your questions in ways that respect all kinds of individuals, and all kinds of families. Asking a client to tell you about their family, for example, is preferable to asking: *"Are you married or single?"*

> **Lorena Carmona:** Completing an initial assessment isn't just for my organization. It's always about the person in front of me. Don't be pushy about completing an assessment. It's more important to go at the client's pace and make a good connection. Completing an assessment is just another type of service, and it needs to be person-centered like everything else you do.
>
> Sometimes I have to put the forms aside and just get to know the client. Really listen to them. Maybe we need to take a walk. I slow the process down to the client's pace. Sometimes people take a long time to open up about their life and an assessment may not be completed in a day, or a week. Sometimes it can take several months to gather all the information, but this is okay if you are also building a connection with the client and helping them with some immediate concerns. Always put the person in front of you first, not your organization or the assessment forms you need to complete.

USE LANGUAGE THAT IS ACCESSIBLE TO THE CLIENT

If you use words or phrases that a client doesn't understand, you will undermine the accuracy and effectiveness of the initial assessment. Similarly, if you present detailed information that a client already understands, you may also undermine rapport. A good way to start is to ask clients what they already know about a topic. For example: *"Can you tell me what you already know about when and how to use your asthma inhaler?"* or *"Can you tell me what you remember about the HIV antibody test?"* If you use medical terms, such as mammogram, sputum, or antibody test, be sure to explain them using everyday language. Try to avoid using acronyms (initials or words made from initials, like SSDI or WIC), at least until you have first spelled them out and explained them (Social Security Disability Insurance; Women, Infants, and Children). As you talk with clients, periodically check in to see whether they understand, by asking them to explain the information to you.

DEMONSTRATE YOUR CONCERN FOR THE CLIENT

Create an atmosphere of mutual respect and trust by showing genuine interest, concern, and empathy. Ask questions that provide clients with an opportunity to talk with about their lives, key resources, and priority concerns. If the client sounds upset, check in with them:

> *Would you like to take a break before we move on?*

or

> *I'm really sorry to hear that you had such a bad experience at the emergency department. Is this something that you'd feel comfortable talking about? If it is okay with you, I'd like to better understand what happened. Maybe we can help to prevent similar problems in the future.*

GATHERING DEMOGRAPHIC INFORMATION

The demographic information that you document (information such as date of birth, nationality, ethnicity, sex, gender identity, family status, address, income, health insurance status, and so on) can be highly sensitive for some clients.

For these reasons, we suggest that you don't start an interview by asking for demographic information. Even though these questions tend to be placed at the beginning of the forms you use, you may want to leave them until later in the interview, after you have established a connection with the client. You could also ask clients to fill out the information themselves and then review it together (although keep in mind that not all your clients will be able to read or write). As always, be respectful of the client's right not to answer any of the questions that you ask.

> **Francis Julian Montgomery:** I know I'm asking for a lot of personal information during an intake or assessment, so I try to make it more of a dialogue instead of an interrogation. I don't just read questions off an intake list. I want to create a natural conversation, and I make sure to listen because clients will often tell me things in response to one question that fills in answers to other questions as well.

TIME MANAGEMENT

Part of your job is to juggle providing person-centered services with the need to complete the assessment, all within the time frame that you and the client have allotted for your meeting. With practice, you will learn to listen to your client and to be aware of the time that remains in your session. If you scheduled 50 minutes, are you on track to finish the interview on time? Would it be possible to finish on time without unduly interrupting the client's agenda or damaging your rapport? If so, call this to the client's attention and make this decision together: *"Maria, I'm sorry to interrupt, but we have about 15 minutes left, and I think we can complete the intake form in that time. Should we move on to the next set of questions?"*

Sometimes, priority issues may emerge for the client during the course of the interview, and these are the most important issues for you to address in the moment. If this occurs, acknowledge this to the client. *"Maria, we have about 15 minutes left, and I'd like to keep talking with you about your family. Is it okay if we schedule another meeting time to complete the interview form?"*

RESPECT YOUR CLIENT'S RIGHT TO PRIVACY

While it's your job to ask questions, clients have a right to decide what information they will and won't share with you. This is especially true with questions about immigration, welfare, substance use, sexual orientation, gender identity, traumatic experiences, and any issue that may have legal consequences that may range from loss of housing to deportation. If you ask a sensitive question and you sense that the client is uncomfortable, move on—don't try to push or force an answer.

   CHW: *"Maria, these questions can be difficult to talk about. Would you like to move on to the next question?"*

ASSESSING CLIENT RESOURCES: A STRENGTH-BASED APPROACH

You will be asked to assess clients' health risks and current needs including, for example, their needs for housing, legal assistance, mental health counseling, and health education.

At appropriate points in the assessment, ask questions and create opportunities to focus on the client's strengths. There are many ways to do this. For example, ask clients about their past accomplishments, key relationships, their knowledge and skills, what they most care about and who or what keeps them going. Listen closely to the information they share with you. Remember to inquire about and to document a client's external and internal resources, even if this is not part of your agency's assessment form.

Affirm the resources and strengths that you observe in your client (you will read more about this in Chapter 9). For example, you might say something like: *"You mentioned that you quit smoking. That seems like a really big accomplishment to me. What did you learn that you might be able to apply to your current health goals?"* or *"You've survived a lot. It takes a lot of strength to keep going after losing so much."* A few kind words can mean a lot to a client who is struggling and acknowledging a client's strengths often makes it more possible for that person to do so as well. These words must be authentic, though, and true to the strengths you observe in a client.

These strengths are often the most important resources that a client has for making changes in their life to promote their health. Every client you will work with has both external and internal resources, though, at times, it may be difficult for the client or the CHW to notice these resources.

One of the key roles for CHWs is to hold onto hope for clients, even in times when they can't hold it for themselves. Recognizing a client's strengths—and assisting them to apply those strengths to enhance their health—should underlie all your interactions with clients.

Noticing and Acknowledging a Client's Strengths

During a class at City College of San Francisco, a CHW student raised her hand to say: *"All this stuff about strengths sounds good in theory, but I'm working with homeless heroin addicts. I'm working with one man who has been out on the streets for almost 10 years. He doesn't have any of these resources."* In response, the other students offered support ("sometimes it is really hard to see the positive things") and suggestions for how to move forward with the client. For example, classmates asked:

- "He must have been doing something right just to survive the streets for so long. What's kept this man alive on the streets for 10 years?"
- "What do you like about this client?"
- "If he isn't in touch with any of his family, does he have any friends out on the streets?"
- "What else—other than heroin—is important to this client? What else does he really care about?"

As a consequence of this classroom discussion, the student began to shift her view of the client and to understand that he did, indeed, have both internal and external resources. For example, the client had developed strong survival skills from living on the streets for so long. He had a tremendous capacity to be kind to others: no matter how bad he was doing, he always asked the CHW how *they* were doing. He also had a best friend and they watched out for each other on the street, sharing places to sleep, drugs, and food.

ASKING EFFECTIVE QUESTIONS

The effectiveness of an initial assessment depends not only on the type of questions you ask, but also on the ease of communication between you and the client. You want to create a smooth conversation. Using a combination of open-ended and closed-ended questions can assist you to accomplish this goal.

Closed-Ended Questions

Closed-ended questions can be answered with a few words, such as *yes* or *no*. They are used when you want to focus the conversation and gather specific information.

> *"Do you have your diabetes medication?"*

> *"Did you have a chance to communicate with the counselor at the job assistance center?*

Open-Ended Questions

An **open-ended question** invites the client to respond with more than a *yes* or *no* answer. It encourages people to talk about their health and their lives.

> *What motivated you to come to the health center today?"*

"What concerns or questions do you have about the diabetes management group?"

"How did you feel when ....?"

"Who are the people that you reach out to when you need support?"

"What are some the challenges that you are facing in terms of eating a healthier diet?

Questions at the Beginning of the Appointment

Asking a broad open-ended question, such as *"How have things been since we last talked?"* or *"What would you like to talk about today?"* opens up discussion and leaves plenty of room for dialogue.

Questions for Gathering Additional Information

There are times when clients will share information that is vague or unclear, such as: *"Things could be better,"* or *"I wasn't feeling well."* To get a more accurate assessment of the issue or problem, you will need to follow-up by asking an open-ended question.

"What do you mean when you say that things could be better?"

"When you say that you weren't feeling well, what was going on for you?"

If the information clients share is vague or unclear, there may be other reasons for this. If you press for more information and they are still resistant, check in and make sure you're not making them uncomfortable. For example: *"Would you prefer to move on with the rest of the assessment and we can come back to the subject later?"*

Questions for a More Accurate Assessment

During initial assessments, you will gather information about a wide range of issues that influence the client's health and wellness. The *who, what, when, where, how,* and *why* series of questions can serve as a guide to aid you in asking questions for a more accurate assessment.

WHO: *"Who do you reach out to if you are facing a challenge?"*

WHAT: *"What happened next?" "What is it that you are most worried about? What else could you do to find out about work opportunities?" "What have you done in the past that was helpful when you felt depressed?"*

WHEN: *"When did you first notice that ....?" "When were you first diagnosed with type 2 diabetes?" "When you notice signs that you may have low blood sugar, what do you do?"*

WHERE: *"Where are you staying now?" "Where is your family based; do they live locally?"*

HOW: *"How are you feeling right now, as we talk about this?" "How did you manage your diabetes in the past?" "How does your depression affect other aspects of your life—such as working and relationships?"*

WHY: *"Why do you think it was difficult for you to ... ?" "Why are you feeling hesitant about going to the diabetes management group?"*

Don't Interrogate!

Avoid the interrogation style of interviewing or asking a series of blunt questions at a relatively fast pace. Asking too many questions too quickly like that can make clients feel uneasy and defensive.

Don't Ask More Than One Question at a Time

Asking several questions at once can be confusing. *"When did your daughter first show signs of asthma? Was it before or after the episode on the playground at school? Did your family physician ever notice symptoms or speak to you about asthma?"* Ask one question at a time!

Pace Yourself

Building a positive relationship with the client is more important than finishing your intake or assessment form. You don't need to ask every question during one meeting. Slow things down to make sure that clients have a chance to reflect before answering a more complicated question. Listen patiently. You might say something like: *"Take your time answering these questions."* Or, as appropriate: *"Let's put the form aside for a few minutes. Would you like to talk further about ___ (whatever the issue is that seems to be a priority for the client)?"*

ASSESSING KEY HEALTH AND WELLNESS ISSUES

Most assessments seek to gather information about a variety of topics or issues that impact a client's health and wellness. The assessment forms that you use typically separate these issues into distinct categories such as:

- **Healthcare and health conditions:** This includes access to health insurance and healthcare services and any previously diagnosed health condition, including mental health conditions and disabilities. It also includes any medications or other treatments that the client is taking or has had in the past. Ask the client if they have any immediate or urgent health concerns.

- **Substance use:** Assess the client's current and past history of alcohol and drug use. For example, does the client use alcohol or other substances or have a history of substance use? Has the client participated in substance use treatment services in the past? Is the client currently concerned about substance use or interested in accessing substance use treatment services including harm reduction services?

- **Social support:** A person's level of social support often plays a key role in their health status. Social support includes the client's most important relationships, especially the people who they can count on for support when they need it. It may include family, friends or organizations they are connected to.

- **Housing status:** Access to stable, affordable and safe housing is an essential prerequisite for good health. During an assessment, you want to determine where the client is currently living. Is there housing stable and safe? Are they unhoused? Who do they live with? Are there any modifications that need to be made to the home to accommodate the client and any disabilities they may have (Medicaid and Medicare may cover these costs)?

- **Access to food and clothing:** Does the client experience food insecurity or times of the month when they cannot afford food? Do they have access to healthier foods such as fresh fruits and vegetables? Do they qualify and are they interested in accessing available benefits and resources such as SNAP (previously called Food Stamps), Special Supplemental Nutrition Program for Women, Infants and Children (WIC), food pantries and organizations that serve free hot meals? Does the client or their family need clothing? Does the client need professional clothing for job interviews or employment?

- **Employment and income:** Assessments typically include questions about a client's employment status. For example, are they currently employed and, if so, what is their monthly or annual income? If they are not working, do they have other forms of income such as social security, veterans or disability payments or other benefits? Is the client able to cover the costs of essentials including housing, food, transportation, and clothing?

- **Mobility/Transportation:** Does the client experience any difficulty with mobility and use or need access to any mobility support such as a cane, walker, scooter or other support? How does the client typically travel? Do they use a bus or subway system, a car or bicycle? Do they have difficulty getting to key locations such as work, school, grocery stores or health services?

- **Legal issues:** Is the client facing any legal difficulties such as custody, immigration or criminal justice charges? Is the client on parole or probation?

- **Personal safety:** Exposure to violence, abuse and other forms of trauma have a significant impact on our health (for more information about this topic, please see Chapter 18). The assessments you conduct may address these topics. For example, is the client safe in their home or housing situation and in their intimate relationships? Has the client experienced violence or other trauma that is impacting their health in the present?

- **Other topics:** A good assessment always leaves room for other issues or topics that may be influencing a client's health and wellness. *"Are there other topics that we did not ask you about that you would like to talk about? Is there anything else that you would like to share that will help us to provide quality services to you?"*

Case Study: The Vital Signs Life Assessment

Roots Community Health Center provides medical and behavioral health care and related services at multiple sites throughout the San Francisco Bay Area of California (Roots Community Health Center, 2023). At Roots, CHWs and other providers use a Vital Signs Life Assessment to gather and document information about the social determinants of health.

The Vital Signs Life Assessment (see Figure 8.1) includes 10 different domains or areas of health to be discussed with clients. These ten domains are: Housing, Financial Security, Employment/Education, Mobility/Communication, Healthcare, Social Support, Legal Status, Mental Health, Substance Use, and Food Access.

CHWs start a conversation with clients about each domain or topic area, identifying key resources that the client already has access to and resources that they currently lack and want to access—such as stable housing.

Each domain is rated with a Risk Score that ranges from "In Crisis" to "Struggling" to "At-Risk" to "Secure." Risk scoring is determined by the information that clients share about their current circumstances. For example, a "secure" rating for the housing domain indicates that a client is living in affordable and secure housing. An "at-risk" rating could indicate that a client is about to lose their housing or employment. A rating of "struggling" could indicate that a client is having difficulty paying their rent and or bills. A rating of "in crisis" could indicate that a client does not have regular access to food or is unhoused and living on the streets.

For each domain, CHWs ask clients to identify their goals, actions to be taken (such as securing a place in a local shelter or applying to get on a list for transitional or permanent housing opportunities), and a deadline or target date to complete the actions. These conversations create an opportunity to get to know the client's priority concerns and goals, and the actions they want to take to reach these goals. It is also an opportunity to build rapport or a positive connection with each client.

At Roots, the client's electronic health record has been updated to include space to document their Vital Signs.

For CHWs or other providers who provide on-going services to clients, such as case management services, the Vital Signs Life Assessment forms can be revisited overtime to assess progress in reaching goals and identifying emerging challenges and priorities.

Lorena Carmona: I like to share the Vital Signs Life Assessment form with clients and let them know the domains or topics that we are going to be talking about. They can review a blank form and I explain that I'll be asking them about each of these topics including their housing situation and their access to food and transportation. This helps clients know what the assessment will be about and gives them a chance to think about what topics they want to start talking about, and what their priorities are. I also tell clients that they get to decide what we talk about, and they have a right not to talk about any of these topics if they don't want to. It helps to put them more at ease. It lets them know that we'll meet them where they're at.

I really like using the Vital Signs Life Assessment form because it keeps me organized and gives me a structure for what types of information to ask clients about. Vital Signs also provides a way of ranking the client's needs in certain areas. It shows where their priorities are or if they are in crisis, and this is a road map to guide my work with clients. It helps me to have key information all in one place so that I can track it over time, and I don't have to start from scratch with any type of assessment. You don't want to waste the client's time by asking the same questions over again.

RATING	HOUSING
SECURE	• *I live with my family* • *I live in my own home or apartment* • *The conditions in my home are safe and livable* • *I own a home or have a long-term lease* • *Less than a third of my income is spent on housing*
AT RISK	• *I won't be able to stay in my current place long term* • *My home is over-crowded* • *I spend between a third and half of my income on housing* • *I moved more than one time in the last year*
STRUGGLING	• *I spend more than half my income on housing* • *I am behind on my rent or mortgage* • *I live temporarily with friends or family* • *I moved more than 3 times in the past year*
IN CRISIS	• *I am being evicted* • *I am living in a car, a shelter, a park or on the street*

RATING	FINANICAL SECURITY
SECURE	• *My income is enough to meet basic needs including housing, food, transportation, clothing, childcare and healthcare* • *I spend money on "extras" once in a while* • *I have enough money saved to cover 3 months of expenses*
AT RISK	• *My income is barely enough to cover my basic needs* • *I can't spend money on any extras* • *I don't have much money saved* • *I rely on public benefits for at least one basic need like food, housing or childcare*
STRUGGLING	• *My income isn't enough to meet my basic needs* • *I rely on public support for most basic needs like food and housing* • *I owe money for essentials like rent or utilities*
IN CRISIS	• *I don't have a regular source of income* • *I am dependent on others for basic needs like food and housing*

RATING	EMPLOYMENT
SECURE	• *I have a secure full-time job* • *I have worked regularly for over 2 years* • *I can take time off from work if I need to* • *I have skills or experience in 2 or more industries or occupations*
AT RISK	• *I work less than 20 hours a week* • *My job is temporary* • *I have not worked regularly in the past 2 years* • *I have skills in only one occupation or industry*
STRUGGLING	• *I work off and on* • *I have been unemployed for more than 6 months* • *I don't have many work skills* • *I have a hard time keeping a job*
IN CRISIS	• *I haven't worked for over a year* • *I stopped looking for work*

Figure 8.1 Vital Signs Life Assessment and Rating Form

RATING	MOBILITY
SECURE	• *I don't have any problems getting around* • *I have access to my own car* • *Public transportation gets me where I need to go*
AT RISK	• *It is sometimes hard to get places* • *Public transportation isn't reliable where I live*
STRUGGLING	• *I have a lot of difficulty getting to the places I need to go* • *I am often late or don't show up because of transportation problems*
IN CRISIS	• *I don't really go places because I don't have a way to get around* • *I can't afford to pay for the bus or the train*

RATING	HEALTHCARE
SECURE	• *I have health insurance* • *I can see a doctor when I need to* • *My out of pocket payments for healthcare visits and medications are affordable* • *I am pursuing one or more personal health goals*
AT RISK	• *I have basic health insurance but have to pay a lot for out-of-pocket expenses* • *I rely on public support for healthcare* • *I am not able to see a doctor as often as I need to*
STRUGGLING	• *My health insurance doesn't cover some of the care that I need* • *Transportation or finances makes accessing health care difficult* • *I sometimes skip getting the medical care that I need*
IN CRISIS	• *I have serious and chronic health problems but don't have a way to access health care*

RATING	COMMUNICATION
SECURE	• *I can communicate my needs and questions to others without difficulty* • *I can understand most things that I read or hear without assistance or language interpretation*
AT RISK	• *Understanding and communicating information is easier with some help or language interpretation*
STRUGGLING	• *I usually need some help to understand or communicate*
IN CRISIS	• *I am not able to communicate what I need without assistance*

RATING	LEGAL STATUS
SECURE	• *I have no legal issues*
AT RISK	• *I have been denied an application for public benefits (SSI, TANF)* • *I have delinquent child support or alimony payments* • *I have been denied an application for housing* • *I have debt that I am unable to pay back*
STRUGGLING	• *I am being pursued for debts I can't pay back* • *I am on parole or probation* • *I have a suspended driver's license* • *My employer owes me wages*
IN CRISIS	• *I am on bail waiting for a hearing or a trial* • *I have a deportation order* • *I have an imminent or current need for a restraining order* • *I am being evicted*

Figure 8.1 (Continued)

RATING	PERSONAL SAFETY
SECURE	• There are no threats to my physical or emotional safety • I feel safe and secure
AT RISK	• I have experienced physical or emotional abuse in the past (but not now)
STRUGGLING	• I am vulnerable to emotional or physical abuse • I am regularly exposed to violence in my neighborhood
IN CRISIS	• I am experiencing physical or emotional abuse now • I am witnessing abuse happen in my home

RATING	INTERPERSONAL SUPPORT
SECURE	• I have at least 3 people in my life who can help me out • I have people who will listen to me if I'm having a problem • I am able to support my friends and family when they need help
AT RISK	• I have one person in my life who helps me out if I'm having a problem
STRUGGLING	• I have friends and family members but cannot rely on them to be there if I need help or support
IN CRISIS	• I don't have anyone who I can ask for help

RATING	COMMUNITY INVOLVEMENT
SECURE	• I do something with family, friends or social or religious/spiritual groups at least once a week
AT RISK	• I do something with friends, family or social groups at least once a month but not every week
STRUGGLING	• I do something with friends, family or social or religious/spiritual groups less than once a month
IN CRISIS	• I rarely participate in social or community activities

RATING	FAMILY WELLBEING
SECURE	• My children are well supervised when I am not with them • I can afford the cost of childcare • I have enough time to support my child's academic and developmental needs • My children are rarely absent from school
AT RISK	• I wish my children had better supervision when I am not with them • I worry about the costs of childcare • My children miss school more often than I would like • I wish I could do more to support my child's educational or developmental needs
STRUGGLING	• I can't afford childcare • I have too little time to meet my child's educational or developmental needs • My children are not meeting academic or developmental standards • My children are often absent from school
IN CRISIS	• My children are unsupervised sometimes • My child has been arrested or had problems with the law • My child has been suspended or expelled from school

Figure 8.1 (Continued)

RATING	PHYSICAL ABILITIES
SECURE	• I don't have any physical problems that limit my abilities or daily activities
AT RISK	• I have a physical condition that limits what I can do • I am partially disabled
STRUGGLING	• I am unable to engage in daily activities without assistance • I have a physical condition that limits or interferes with daily activities several days a month • I am significantly disabled
IN CRISIS	• I can't perform regular activities most days due to a physical health condition • I am fully disabled

RATING	MENTAL HEALTH
SECURE	• I have no mental, emotional or psychological limitations
AT RISK	• I have emotional or psychological conditions that limit my regular activity more than one day a week
STRUGGLING	• I have emotional or psychological conditions that limit my activities several days every month
IN CRISIS	• I don't feel safe right now • I feel that I can be a danger to myself or others at times

RATING	SUBSTANCE USE
SECURE	• I have no concerns about alcohol or drug use
AT RISK	• I used to have a problem with alcohol or drug use
STRUGGLING	• I have problems with use of alcohol or drugs like heroin, meth or cocaine • I use hard drugs from time to time
IN CRISIS	• I am afraid of what might happen if can't get the drugs that I use

RATING	INDEPENENCE OR AUTONOMY
SECURE	• I understand my choices and make decisions about the paths I choose in life • I am usually able to influence important things in my life
AT RISK	• I can make decisions for myself but I don't always make good choices • Sometimes I don't feel confident that I can manage the problems in my life
STRUGGLING	• I am choosing between options that aren't good for me • I have more problems in life than I can manage
IN CRISIS	• I don't know what I'm going to do about the problems in my life • I don't have control over where my life is going

RATING	FOOD SECURITY
SECURE	• I can afford the foods of my choice for myself and my dependents • I have a kitchen in my home • I prepare or eat healthy foods most of the time
AT RISK	• I can't afford the foods I want • Getting or preparing healthy foods is difficult for me
STRUGGLING	• Some months there are days when I skip meals or go hungry • I am dependent on public food subsidies and other free food resources
IN CRISIS	• I skip meals or go hungry at least once a week

Figure 8.1 (Continued)

Client Scenario: Maria Nguyen (continued)

CHW: Maria, part of the assessment process is to check in with clients about how they're doing financially. You said that you lost your job at the _____ Hotel and haven't been able to find work since then?

Maria Nguyen: Yes. [Maria nods and looks down]

CHW: I'm so sorry to hear that, Maria. So many people have lost their jobs recently. How long ago did you lose your job?

Maria: It's been eight months.

CHW: How have you been managing financially?

Maria: It's hard. My unemployment is running out. I'm worried about rent and I don't really have enough money to cover food. Honestly, I've mostly been eating Ramen noodles.

CHW: Do you know about the rental assistance that is available to people who lost employment?

Maria: No, what is that?

The CHW talks with Maria about a program that provides rental assistance for people who lost employment due to the COVID-19 pandemic. After reviewing the criteria for the program, Maria decides to apply for assistance and asks the CHW to help her with the application forms.

CHW: Maria, before we fill out your application for rental assistance, I also wanted to ask if how your job search is going.

Maria: It's hard. The hotel is starting to hire back some people, but not as many as before, and I had fewer years at the job, so there isn't an opening for me. I tried to apply at some of the other hotels too, but they aren't taking on new staff.

CHW: What type of job are you hoping for?

Maria: Well, I don't mind working in the hotels, but I want to get a job that pays better than housekeeping.

CHW: We partner with a non-profit that helps people find work. They help with resumes, job searches, preparing people for interviews—they do a lot really. The services are free. Would you be interested in learning more about it?

Maria: Yes, I need help figuring this out.

The CHW provides Maria with detailed information about The JobHub including the address, website, and hours of operation. The CHW gives Maria a card for a colleague who works at The JobHub. Maria indicates that she will stop by The JobHub by the end of the week. Maria and the CHW will talk about her visit to JobHub during their next meeting.

ASK FOR CLARIFICATION

Sometimes CHWs feel shy about interrupting a client or admitting they didn't understand what a client said. However, it's much worse to pretend to understand when you don't, to miss the opportunity to document important information, or to record misinformation. If you don't fully understand what a client is saying, and are unable to record the information accurately, ask! You might say something like: *"I'm not sure that I fully understood what you told me about the situation with your sister. Could you tell me again?"* or *"I want to make sure I fully understand what you are saying about your housing situation. Did you say that your landlord has sent you an eviction notice? When did this happen?"*

SUMMARIZE WHAT YOU HAVE HEARD

Depending on the nature of the assessment, you may want to review some of what you learned in order to be certain that you are accurately documenting what the client shared with you. For example, you might say something like: *"I just want to make sure that I've documented everything correctly. You said that you attended a diabetes education group before and would be interested in joining our diabetes management group. You want assistance signing up for SNAP (Food Stamps) benefits. You are interested in a referral to an agency that can assist you with finding employment. Did I get that right? Is there anything that you'd like to add or correct?"*

DOES THE CLIENT HAVE QUESTIONS OR CONCERNS?

Check in regularly to see if your clients have questions or concerns, particularly if you sense that they may be confused or upset. Taking the time to address their questions as you go helps to build trust. Talking with clients about their questions or concerns is likely to provide you with important information about their health and social circumstances so that you can assist them to access relevant programs and services.

Client Scenario: Maria Nguyen *(continued)*

CHW: Maria, with every client, we want to learn about their social support network, or the people they are close to and can get support from when they need it. These could be family or friends, or people you know from a group or organization that you belong to. Can you tell me a little bit about the people or groups that you're closest to right now? For example, is there anyone that you've been able to talk with about the stress you are experiencing since you lost your job?

Maria Nguyen: I was worried about losing my apartment, so I thought I should find a roommate. I asked some of my old co-workers and my friend Tina moved in. She's still working for the hotel; she helps with reservations. She stays in the bedroom now and I sleep in the living room. She helps with the rent and ... it's just better now.

CHW: It sounds like you found a good solution to help you save money on your rent. And it sounds like it's working out with Tina.

Maria: Yes, she's more than a roommate now, she's a friend.

CHW: Other than Tina, is there anyone else who is supportive to you such as family members?

Maria: I'm divorced. [Maria pauses]. I moved here with my husband, but we divorced about ... three years ago. It was [Maria sighs]. . . It was really difficult, and I don't really talk to him or his family now. My family is in _____ [another state], so I haven't seen them for too long.

CHW: Are you close to your family? Have you talked with them about what you're going through?

Maria: They were worried about me moving so far away and then I got divorced. They didn't understand why I had to divorce. I couldn't tell them everything. Then I lost my job, and I just didn't want to tell them all of that. My father had a stroke, so he needs a lot of help and ... I just don't want to add to their worries.

CHW: You don't want to worry your family.

Maria: Yes, they have enough to handle now. They have to run the restaurant without my dad.

CHW: It sounds like you've been kind of on your own since your divorce.

Maria: Yes. I used to rely on my husband and his family. But after the divorce, I was really alone.

CHW: You lost part of your support system when you divorced. [Maria nods] You say that you and Tina have become friends. Can you talk to her about what you've been through and about your family?

(continues)

Client Scenario: Maria Nguyen *(continued)*

Maria: Yes, we talk with each other. She's had her difficult times too.

CHW: I'm really glad to hear that you can talk about things with Tina. I want to let you know that I'm also here to support you. And we have a wonderful team of counselors here at Eastside. They can offer support for people who are going through difficult times in their life. Would you be interested in talking with a counselor?

Maria: I don't know.

CHW: Okay, well, if you are interested you can always talk with me about it, and you can also talk with the Nurse Practitioner when you have your appointment.

Maria: Okay. I am feeling better since Tina moved back in. I've gotten to know her sister Tran too.

CHW: I'm glad that you reached out to Tina and created these friendships, Maria.

8.4 The End of the Assessment

Don't rush the end of an initial assessment: this is the time to review questions, concerns, or decisions that the client has made. You don't want to undermine a good assessment by rushing the client out the door or leaving the person confused about what steps to take next.

TIME MANAGEMENT

Toward the end of your appointment, check the time to see if it's possible to complete the initial assessment. You may need to allow time to schedule a follow-up appointment. If you need more time, you may be able to continue the assessment for an extra ten or 15 minutes.

If you routinely find that you need extra time to complete initial client assessments, in spite of effective time management, you may wish to talk with your agency to see if it is possible to schedule longer appointments.

REVIEW DECISIONS MADE AND NEXT STEPS

The assessment may or may not have clarified the client's eligibility and interest in participating in a particular program or service. If decisions have been made, be sure to review them together. If the client has decided to participate in follow-up meetings or services, be sure to provide a written copy of this plan, including when and where to access services, who their contact person or service provider will be, and how best to contact that person.

> **CHW:** *"Okay, Maria, thank you so much for your time today. We have completed your initial assessment. I'm glad you decided to become a patient here at Eastside. You have a first appointment with Nancy Ly, one of our Nurse Practitioners, on September 3 at 9:30 AM. Nancy will talk with you in more detail about your diabetes and your medications. Should I give you an appointment card or could I text you to remind you about this appointment?"*
>
> **Maria Nguyen:** *"A text would be great."*
>
> **CHW:** *"You and I are scheduled for a follow-up meeting the next week, September 9 at 1:30 PM. I'll text you this appointment too. We can follow-up on your appointment with Nancy and talk about other needs that you have, such as finding a job. I will also start the paperwork for you to be enrolled in the SNAP Program. That will be a big help in being able to purchase food. Do you have any questions about our next steps or any other questions for me?"*

PROVIDE REFERRALS

In some cases, you will offer referrals to clients who have expressed an interest in additional services, such as transitional housing, legal or employment assistance. Review what the referral is for and provide them with clear information about where to go and who to contact.

> **CHW:** *"Maria, you said you might be interested in The JobHub, the organization I mentioned that helps people find employment. They help people with creating or revising a resume, job interview skills, finding employment opportunities and applying to available jobs. They're located right on Market near 6th Street and are open six days a week from 11:00 AM to 7:00 PM. Do you know the location?"*

> **Maria Nguyen:** *"Yes, I know the area."*

> **CHW:** *"I wrote down the name of one of their counselors here on the back of this card. Her name is Stella C_____ and I've heard great things about her from other clients. Do you have any questions about the referral?"*

For more information regarding how to make an effective referral, please see Chapter 10.

ASK CLIENTS IF THEY HAVE ANY REMAINING QUESTIONS OR CONCERNS

Check in one last time to see if clients have any outstanding questions or concerns that they would like to talk about. Even if the answer is no, asking the question communicates your concern for their welfare.

> **CHW:** *"Maria, is there anything else that you would like to ask or to share with me?"*

THANK THE CLIENT

Regardless of how the initial assessment went, and whether or not the client ultimately decided to enroll in a particular program or service, the person invested significant time and effort talking with you. Thank them and leave them with an encouraging word. For example:

> **CHW:** *"Maria, thank you for meeting with me today. It's been a pleasure getting to know you. I appreciate all you shared with me. I hope everything goes well for you at The JobHub and they are able to help you find employment soon. I'll look forward to hearing about this at our next meeting."*

PROVIDE YOUR CONTACT INFORMATION

If it is appropriate for clients to contact you in the future, give them your business card and contact information.

> *CHW: "Maria, here's my card. Don't hesitate to call or text me if you think I can be helpful. I won't always be able to get back to you right away, but I promise I'll always call or text you back."*

8.5 Documenting Client Assessments

The primary purpose of documentation is to provide information that will be used to guide the delivery of care and services for clients. The information you provide is also required by the organizations that fund (and accredit) the organization or program you work for. The information you document may also be used to evaluate services and programs with the purpose of improving the quality of services that clients receive. If you can't provide timely, clear, and accurate documentation of the services you provide, including initial client assessments, this could be harmful to the client and to your career.

BECOME FAMILIAR WITH THE FORMS AND DATA SYSTEMS YOU USE

The forms and electronic data systems that you use to document client information will vary depending on the nature of the assessments you conduct and the program and agency you work for. A good starting point is to carefully review all the forms and systems that your agency or program uses, not just the ones you are responsible for completing. Review each question on every form. You should understand all the terms used, why each question is being asked, how to document a variety of common responses, how the information you document will be used, and how it may impact the health of the client.

Talk with a colleague or supervisor to clarify anything that you don't fully understand and couldn't explain to a client. Ask an experienced colleague to show you how they use the forms and document client information. The more familiar you are with the forms, the better you will be able to focus on talking with and listening to clients during an assessment without constantly referring to the paperwork.

Lorena Carmona: Filling out forms and applications for benefits or resources can be tricky. You really have to focus on the details and make sure you fill everything out correctly. In the county where I work, they'll reject certain applications—like housing applications—if the forms aren't completed the way they want them. So, I spend time getting to know what the county wants because I don't want a client's applications for resources like housing to be rejected. A lot of this comes down to making sure that clients are what we call "document ready." They need to have an identification card, such as a driver's license, a social security card and proof of income (such as a paycheck, disability, veterans or social security payments). Without these three documents, a lot of applications will be considered incomplete and be rejected. So, I work with clients to make sure they have these documents and, if they don't, I help them to get them.

EXPLAIN THE FORMS TO CLIENTS

Let clients know that you will be documenting the information they share with you on forms or in data systems provided by your agency. Consider providing clients with a printout or copy of the key forms that you will complete together during the initial assessment (please also remind those who use one how to access information in their electronic health record). Depending on the nature of the assessment and the literacy level of clients, you may ask them to fill out part of the form on their own and review it with them later.

Take time to clearly explain why you are using forms to document the interview, and how the information will be used in the future. Be prepared for clients to stop you during an appointment to ask something like: *"Why do you need to know that?"* For example, clients may be concerned about why you need to know their Social Security number, or what may happen if they tell you that they are experiencing domestic violence at home. Learn to view these moments as opportunities for deeper engagement with a client. Affirm their right not to answer a particular question. It may or may not be essential for determining their eligibility and participation in services, and you may be able to return to these issues in the future once trust has been established. Most

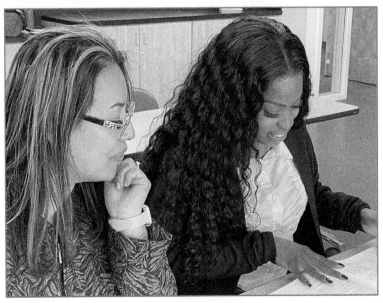

A CHW reviews required forms with a client.

importantly, be prepared to respond to questions honestly and accurately. If you aren't sure, say so, and if possible, find someone who can answer their question.

Please watch the following video ▶ that shows a CHW talking with a client about how and why she will be taking notes during their meeting.

● *What did the CHW do well in explaining note taking to the client?*

● *What else might you want to do and say to a client to help them understand the notes you take during a session?*

TAKING NOTES: ROLE PLAY, DEMO.

(*Source:* Foundations for Community Health Workers/http://youtu.be/yZ6FiTr3O4o/last accessed 21 September 2023.)

HOW AND WHEN TO FILL OUT THE FORMS

We strongly encourage you to take detailed notes and, if possible, to fill out the relevant assessment forms as you talk with clients. This is the best way to ensure that the information you record is accurate. If you wait to fill out forms until after your meeting with a client, you may not remember all they shared with you, and you may misrepresent important information. You may end up unintentionally harming clients.

Especially if you meet with many clients in a workday, schedule these meetings with time allotted to write or enter your notes at the end of each session (as well as some time to stand, walk, stretch and ground yourself before the next appointment). If you find that you are rushing to complete notes or finishing your note-taking responsibilities at the end of the day or after work, talk with your supervisor to negotiate time during each workday for you to complete this essential task.

> **TG:** I made mistakes in the past by delaying writing up client notes, thinking that I would remember it all. Now I always document client information while we talk. I explain what I'm doing and why I'm doing it. It has never been a problem with a client.

Most forms ask for specific information: name, address, phone number, medical history, and so on. Some forms, especially those used during home visits, will ask for more descriptive information, such as about conditions in the home. This is where your observation skills will be essential. Some agencies use a specific note-taking system or approach such as DAP, SOAP or APSO Notes. These are discussed in greater detail in Chapter 10 on Case Management.

Chapter Review

Imagine that you are a CHW at the Eastside Neighborhood Health Center and are scheduled to meet with Maria Nguyen, the client described at the beginning of this chapter—to conduct an initial client assessment. Based on what you have learned, *and in your own words:*

● How will you welcome Maria Nguyen to the Eastside Neighborhood Health Center?

● How will you explain the purpose of your meeting and the initial assessment?

● How will you explain your agency's confidentiality policy?

● What will you do and say to keep the assessment person-centered?

● What key issues or topics will you assess as you meet with Maria?

● What types of open-ended questions might you ask Maria?

● How will you document the information that Maria tells you, and how will you explain this process to her?

- What will you say when Maria tells you that she is embarrassed and ashamed to be unemployed?
- What types of referrals might you provide to Maria?
- What will you say to end your meeting with Maria?

Reference

Roots Community Health Center (2023). https://rootsclinic.org/ (accessed 9 May 2023).

Additional Resources

The Centers for Disease Control and Prevention. (2022). Health Insurance Portability and Accountability Act of 1996 (HIPAA). https://www.cdc.gov/phlp/publications/topic/hipaa.html (accessed 19 November 2022).

U.S. Department of Health & Human Services. Health information privacy. Retrieved from http://www.hhs.gov/ocr/privacy/ (accessed 19 November 2022).

Person-Centered Counseling and Motivational Interviewing

Tim Berthold and Darouny Somsanith

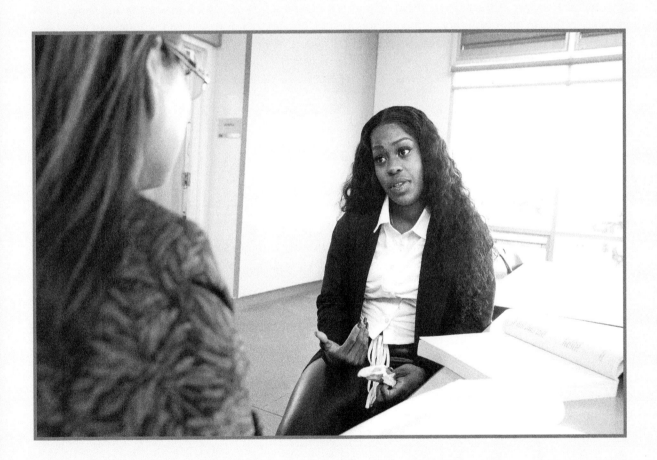

Foundations for Community Health Workers, Third Edition. Edited by Tim Berthold and Darouny Somsanith.
© 2024 John Wiley & Sons, Inc. Published 2024 by John Wiley & Sons, Inc.
Companion website: http://www.wiley.com/go/communityhealthworkers3E

Client Scenario: Mr. Boun Somchanh

Mr. Boun Somchanh was referred to meet with you by Dr. Chen, your colleague at the Northside Community Health Center. Your role as a Community Health Worker (CHW) at Northside is to provide person-centered counseling and case management services to people living with chronic health conditions.

You are meeting Mr. Somchanh for the first time. He is a 60-year-old Laotian refugee who came to the United States in the mid-1980s via Thailand. He's been a patient at the clinic for over 20 years. The receptionist and one of the nurses at Northside are Laotion and speak his language, but the clinic does not yet have any CHWs who speak Laotion.

Mr. Somchanh was diagnosed with high blood pressure a year ago. Dr. Chen prescribed medication and advised Mr. Somchanh to change his diet to manage his high blood pressure. Since his diagnosis of hypertension, Mr. Somchanh dreads coming to the health center for his annual check-up. After seeing Dr. Chen, Mr. Somchanh was told to meet with you to review his plan for managing his blood pressure.

When Mr. Somchanh arrives at the health center, he politely asks for you. You greet him warmly and show him to a private office. In his health record, there is a note that Mr. Somchanh speaks Lao at home, so you ask if he would like a medical interpreter. Mr. Somchanh tells you that he doesn't need an interpreter and would prefer to speak English with you.

If you were a CHW working with Mr. Samchanh:

- *How would you support Mr. Somchanh to talk about his health?*
- *What concepts would guide your work?*
- *What counseling or coaching skills would you use?*
- *What questions will you ask Mr. Somchanh?*
- *What personal experiences, values, or beliefs might influence your work with Mr. Somchanh?*
- *How will you assess the quality of the services that you provide to Mr. Somchanh?*

Introduction

This chapter provides a brief introduction to key concepts and skills for providing person-centered counseling. CHWs apply person-centered counseling skills every time they communicate with clients and community members. This chapter builds upon information from Chapters 3, 5, 6, 7, and 8 including person-centered practice concepts, an understanding of behavior change, the use of ecological models, cultural humility, and conducting an initial assessment with a new client. We encourage you to review these concepts before reading this chapter.

WHAT YOU WILL LEARN

By studying the information in this chapter, you will be able to

- Define person-centered counseling
- Discuss person-centered counseling concepts, skills, and resources including harm reduction and action planning
- Explain key concepts and techniques for Motivational Interviewing
- Identify common challenges to providing person-centered counseling
- Evaluate your own performance in providing person-centered counseling
- Create a professional development plan to enhance your counseling knowledge and skills

C3 Roles and Skills Addressed in Chapter 9

C3 Roles		C3 Skills
4. Providing Coaching and Social Support	**C3 Project**	1. Communication Skills
6. Building Individual and Community Capacity		2. Interpersonal and Relationship-Building Skills
8. Implementing Individual and Community Assessments	**Chapter 9**	4. Capacity Building Skills
		7. Individual and Community Assessment Skills

WORDS TO KNOW

Ambivalence

Harm reduction

Motivational interviewing

Person-centered counseling

Relapse and relapse prevention

Risk-reduction counseling

Stages of change model

9.1 An Overview of Person-Centered Counseling

Person-centered counseling is a form of person-centered practice (sometimes called client-centered practice) (see Chapter 6). It incorporates a wide variety of theories, models, concepts, and skills including the work of Carl Rogers, concepts and models of harm reduction, cultural humility, motivational interviewing, self-determination theory, and wellness and recovery models.

The essence of person-centered counseling is to honor and enhance the client's autonomy or independence. It emphasizes the experience, ideas, beliefs, goals, and feelings of the client. The role of a person-centered counselor is to be a facilitator who supports clients to make desired changes that promote their health. For these changes to be meaningful, effective, and long-lasting, they should come from the client, not from providers or outside "experts."

> **Precious Beddell:** With person-centered counseling, the client is in the driver's seat. Providers are like the signs along the road that offer compassionate support to help the driver reach their destination. If the driver veers off course, they can consult a CHW or other provider who will always ask if they require support or resources to get back on track to continue their journey.

WHO PROVIDES PERSON-CENTERED COUNSELING?

Person-centered counseling is provided throughout the world by people with a wide range of training including licensed health and mental health providers such as nurses, physicians, counselors, and social workers. Unlicensed providers also use person-centered counseling to support clients with behavior change and other goals. These unlicensed and front-line providers include CHWs, health educators, HIV prevention workers, mental health peer specialists, drug and alcohol counselors, and sexual assault and domestic violence counselors.

CHWs provide person-centered counseling in a variety of settings including community-based organizations, hospitals, clinics, substance use treatment programs, and local health departments.

CHWs apply person-centered counseling to address all health issues including nutrition and physical activity; infectious diseases such as hepatitis, COVID-19, and HIV disease; mental health challenges; tobacco, alcohol, and drug use; reproductive health; and the management of chronic health conditions such as diabetes, cancer, or hypertension. Typically, person-centered counseling is used to support clients to make and sustain behavior changes designed to promote or enhance their health and wellness.

RESEARCH ON THE EFFECTIVENESS OF PERSON-CENTERED COUNSELING

Research studies have demonstrated the effectiveness of person-centered counseling. For example, Motivational Interviewing (MI) is effective in supporting patients to enhance their motivation for behavior change for a broad range of health conditions and behaviors including substance use, treatment adherence, and physical activity levels (Bischof, Bischof, & Rumpf, 2021). Motivational interviewing provided both in-person and telephonically was shown to increase the uptake of breast and cancer screenings (Chan & So, 2021). MI improved motivation among stroke patients for participating in rehabilitation (Chen et al., 2020) and resulted in improved lung function and reduced hospitalization for patients with Chronic Obstructive Pulmonary Disorder (Wang, Liu, Sun, Yin, & Tang, 2022). The federal Substance Abuse and Mental Health Services Administration (SAMHSA) endorses the use of MI for treating people with substance use conditions (SAMHSA, 2019).

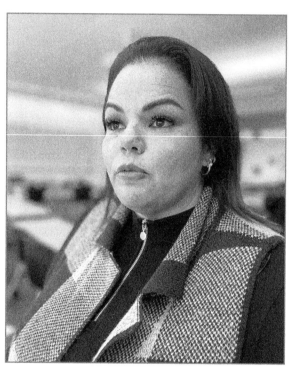

CHWs are highly skilled at providing person-centered counseling.

SCOPE OF PRACTICE CONCERNS

It is important to distinguish person-centered counseling from therapy. Person-centered counseling (or coaching) is provided by public health and health care professionals of all levels. It is typically applied to support clients in changing behaviors related to a specific health issue. The emphasis is on *what the client can do now* to enhance their health in the near future (such as within 3–12 months). It does not focus on past issues.

In contrast, therapy is provided only by licensed health and mental health professionals (such as licensed counselors, social workers, psychologists, and psychiatrists) with extensive training and the required skills to address the client's history and more challenging issues such as trauma and crisis. Licensed health and mental health professionals are qualified to diagnose mental health conditions, address complex and urgent challenges, and offer and provide recommendations for treatment.

CHWs who provide person-centered counseling or coaching should receive on-going supervision and regularly consult with colleagues to monitor the scope of practice concerns. When clients face issues that are beyond the CHW's training level, skill, and scope of practice, they should be referred to a colleague with more advanced training and skills such as a physician or licensed mental health professional.

ON-GOING PROFESSIONAL DEVELOPMENT

Professional development is a commitment to keep enhancing your knowledge and skills with the goal of improving the quality of the services you provide to clients. We strongly encourage you to seek out opportunities to enhance your person-centered counseling skills over the course of your career. There are many ways to do this. You may ask to shadow or sit in and observe a more experienced colleague as they provide person-centered counseling services. Supervision meetings and case conferences are opportunities to pose questions, discuss challenges, and learn from your colleagues. Free and low-cost training opportunities may exist in the city or county where you live such as with suicide prevention/crisis intervention, domestic violence, and rape crisis centers. Not only will you receive training in vital areas, and in some cases certification, but you will also have an opportunity to volunteer, practice your skills, and receive supervision. Community-based organizations, community colleges, and universities also provide affordable in-person and online workshops and classes that will enhance your counseling knowledge and skills.

- *What training have you already received in person-centered skills such as Motivational Interviewing?*

- *What opportunities for additional training exist in the area where you live?*

CHARACTERISTICS OF SUCCESSFUL PERSON-CENTERED COUNSELORS

Your work will be guided by concepts and skills of person-centered counseling. It will also be influenced by personal qualities that support your ability to build connections with the communities you serve. The following list of qualities and characteristics of successful counselors is adapted from a curriculum designed to train CHWs working to respond to the HIV epidemic in Zimbabwe (International Training and Education Center on HIV, unpublished curriculum).

- Belief in the wisdom of their clients
- The desire to learn something new from each client and counseling session
- The ability to set aside personal issues, concerns, and beliefs when working with clients
- Cultural humility
- The ability to honor the life experience, feelings, opinions, and values of the client
- Acceptance of their own limitations and mistakes
- A deep commitment not to discriminate against clients on the basis of their identity, beliefs, behavior, or any other reason
- Acceptance of a client's ambivalence to change
- Understanding that resistance to change is natural and common
- The expression of empathy in a visible and authentic manner

- *What qualities or characteristics would you add to this list?*

- *Which of these qualities do you possess?*

Client Scenario: Boun Somchanh (*continued*)

CHW: Hello Mr. Somchanh, it's good to see you again. I see from your health record that you're here to work on managing your hypertension. Is that correct?

Mr. Somchanh: Yes, but I don't understand why my blood pressure is still up. That doctor keeps saying I need to go on a diet. I have a diet, but they say it's no good! Every time I come, she always finds something wrong with me. I don't know what to do and why she sends me to you.

CHW: Well, I'm glad you came to see me. Let me tell you what I do here at the Northside Health Center. I'm a Community Health Worker and I help people create a plan to improve their health. Doctors don't always have a lot of time to meet with patients, so they ask our team of CHWs to work with them.

Mr. Somchanh: So, are you like a nurse?

CHW: No, we don't have the same training. I have a different role. I work closely with the nurses and doctors here and provide health education and connect people to services or resources they need in our clinic and in the community. I help patients to develop individual plans that will help make them healthier. But I want to be clear that you are in charge of your plan and any decisions you want to make about your health. Can we talk a bit more about your health and then see if we can come up with a plan for getting you healthier? Does this sound like something you want to try?

Mr. Somchanh: Okay, I'll try.

CHW: Will you tell me what you know about hypertension or high blood pressure?

Mr. Somchanh: My doctor said it can give me a heart attack and make me go blind, and that it's related to the food I eat. My wife and I have been talking about it and she tries to cook fish for me and put less salt in our food. She yells at me if she thinks I'm eating something bad when we go to the temple. Usually, she comes to the doctor's appointment with me, but today she couldn't get off work.

CHW: I'm so glad that your wife is supporting you Mr. Somchanh. You're right that the foods that we eat can increase our risk for hypertension and make it harder to control. There are many factors that influence hypertension including diet, physical activity, stress, and taking medications correctly as the doctor prescribes.

Mr. Somchanh: (crosses his arms over his chest) … Oh really.

CHW: Yes. Hypertension is one of the most common illnesses in the United States. Many people have it, and many people struggle to control it too. That's what we're here to help you with. It's important to get your blood pressure down because of those risks that you mentioned, like heart attack or stroke or even losing your vision.

Mr. Somchanh: So, it can be serious then?

CHW: Yes. That may be why your wife is so worried about you and trying to help you keep to a healthier diet. [Mr. Somchanh uncrosses his arms] So I can support you, can I ask you to tell me more about your life? I'll be asking some questions about your home life and your diet, your work, and things like that. For example, are you working now?

Mr. Somchanh: I do cleaning for the University for over 20 years. The job is hard, but I like it and my co-workers are very friendly. I'm always moving all over the campus. I have to stand and walk a lot, but it pays good, and I get good benefits.

CHW: Well congratulations on working at the University for over 20 years! It sounds like you probably get lots of physical activity on your job and even if it's demanding it's probably also good for your health and your hypertension. Getting regular physical activity is something that some people with hypertension struggle with.

Mr. Somchanh: That's no problem for me. You have to be strong to do my job.

(continues)

Client Scenario: Boun Somchanh *(continued)*

CHW: Can you tell me about your living situation and family life?

Mr. Somchanh: I live with my wife and my two kids. My oldest daughter doesn't live with us no more. She is with her fiancé and is about to get married [smiling proudly].

CHW: Oh, congratulations on your daughter's engagement. Your family must be so excited. [Mr. Somchanh smiles] Let's talk a bit more about your diet. Who prepares the food in your house, and what kinds of food do you like to eat?

Mr. Somchanh: My wife works at this company that makes plastics for hospitals. She usually cooks and sometimes I help out too if I'm not too tired. I work from 2 to 10 AM, so when I come home I just eat the leftovers and then do some work around the house and go to bed. We like to eat Lao food.

CHW: I've heard of Lao food. It is similar to Thai, right?

Mr. Somchanh: Yes, yes! Do you know about Thai or Lao food?

CHW: Yes, some of my co-workers are Lao and they sometimes bring in food to share with us. And of course, Thai food is very popular around here.

Mr. Somchanh: Oh ... good! Where are you from?

CHW: I was born here. My family is originally from Mexico. Thai and Lao food is spicy like Mexican food, right?

Mr. Somchanh: I know, it's good! We're like cousins, very similar. I have a lot of Mexican co-workers too.

CHW: (Smiling). What types of food do you usually eat and how is it prepared?

Mr. Somchanh: We make sticky rice or jasmine rice, soup with vegetables, stir fry, or grill beef or chicken. Also, once a week we make larp (mincemeat with spices and herbs).

CHW: That sounds delicious. And so good to be eating home-cooked meals instead of fast foods, right?

Mr. Somchanh: No, we don't eat much fast food. If there was Lao fast food, maybe I would eat it! [laughing]

CHW: Your wife is mindful of your hypertension and cooking healthier foods with less salt.

Mr. Somchanh: Yes, she's in charge of cooking for the family, and she met with Dr. Chen. So, she is using less salt and more vegetables. We are also eating less sweets. But, for some reason, my pressure is still high, and I don't know what else to do. I don't really like to take the medicine.

CHW: You said you don't like to take the medicine. What are your concerns about the high blood pressure medication?

Mr. Somchanh: I don't want to be dependent on it and I want to see if I can bring my pressures down with diet. Also, I heard from my friends that it's bad for my liver and I pee a lot when I take it. When I start to feel better, I cut back on the pills.

CHW: It's important to share this with Dr. Chen—your concerns about side effects and that you sometimes don't take the full dosage of your medications. Have you talked with her about this?

Mr. Somchanh: It's not like I cut back every day. And sometimes I just forget, so it's not like I don't take it on purpose. I'm working a lot of overtime because I want to help my daughter have a good wedding, so sometimes I forget to take it.

The CHW continues to talk with Mr. Somchanh and to learn more about his life, his knowledge, and what he has been doing to manage his hypertension. The CHW also reinforces how important it is to take medications as prescribed and to share any questions or concerns directly with the doctor. She schedules an appointment for Mr. Somchanh and his wife to meet with Dr. Chen to talk about his hypertension medications.

9.2 Developing an Action Plan

Person-centered counseling typically involves supporting clients to develop an individualized action plan or behavior change plan. The plan documents the client's goals and outlines a set of specific and realistic actions or behaviors to reach these goals (the format of the action plan is also used when providing case management and is discussed in greater detail in Chapter 10).

The first step to developing a plan is to support the client in identifying their current challenges, risks, and needs (see Chapters 8 and 10). Next, the client will prioritize these concerns to identity a goal or goals that they can work toward in the next three to six months or so. You will also support the client in identifying their internal and external resources, also known as strengths (see Chapter 12), and to discuss how they can build upon resources as they implement their action plan.

Sometimes, you will conduct person-centered counseling with a client who has been referred to your program to address a specific health risk or issue such as smoking, depression, or pregnancy. At other times, the issues that the client is most concerned about will emerge during the assessment.

Organizations use a variety of forms and structures for developing and documenting an action plan (this may be called by different names such as a risk-reduction plan, treatment plan, health plan, etc.). Ideally, the form will have a place to clearly document the following information:

- Client demographic information (including name, address, date of birth, sex/gender identity, primary language, and so on)
- Health conditions and risk factors (such as diagnosis with depression, being unhoused, experiencing food insecurity, etc.)
- Strengths or internal and external resources including social support from family and friends and individual knowledge, skills, and accomplishments
- Goals, such as to prevent pregnancy or manage a chronic condition such as depression or high blood pressure
- Actions or steps to reach the goal, such as consistent use of contraception, taking medications as prescribed and directed, eating a healthier diet, or reducing asthma triggers—such as dust, tobacco smoke, or animal dander—in the home.
- Notes or comments about the counseling session
- Follow-up appointments and referrals to resources such as a food pantry, substance use treatment, or employment assistance program

The action plan may be completed at the beginning of a session, but typically, the client's needs, strengths, and goals are identified over the course of one or more sessions.

> **TG:** You might think you are going to sit down and do this all at once in some logical order—assess risks and resources, come up with goals and a plan. But that isn't how it usually goes, at least for me. Especially when I first meet with clients, I want to follow their lead about what is most important to talk about. I know that if the client decides that they want to keep working with me—we will develop this plan together, and I will write it down. Like everything, it's a process, and the plan keeps developing. That's a good thing, because new goals or priorities come up, or the client realizes that some of their action steps are just too unrealistic.

Client Scenario: Boun Somchanh *(continued)*

The CHW greets Mr. Somchanh at Northside Community Health Center and reminds him that the agenda for today's meeting is to develop his personalized Health Action Plan.

CHW: Today we can begin to develop your plan for managing your hypertension and promoting your health. Let's start by talking about the things that are most affecting your blood pressure. Then you can choose one of these topics to be the first focus of your health plan. This will be your main priority for improving your health.

Mr. Somchanh: Okay.

CHW: These circles [places a Bubble Chart in front of Mr. Somchanh] represent different things that have an impact on your hypertension and your health overall. We can fill them together. From what you have told me already, I imagine that one of the bubbles could be eating healthier foods at home, is that right?

Mr. Somchanh: Yes, but that is the hardest one!

CHW: [smiles and writes "Healthy Food" in one of the bubbles] What else effects your health and hypertension?

Mr. Somchanh: My medications. We met with the doctor, and she explained more to me, I am taking the pills every morning now. My wife leaves them out for me, and I take them when I get back from work.

CHW: That's great Mr. Somchanh [fills in another bubble with "Take Medications"]. And if you start to experience side effects or have concerns about your medications, what will you do then?

Mr. Somchanh: I'll talk with the Dr. And if I don't, my wife will tell the doctor [he laughs].

CHW: [laughing] Wonderful, you're doing a great job with your medications and communication with Dr. Chen. Okay, what else effects your hypertension?

Mr. Somchanh: We said before that exercise is good for the heart, and I do get a lot of exercise because of my job at the University.

CHW: Yes, you do more physical activity than most of us Mr. Somchanh [writes down "Physical Activity" in the Bubble Chart]. Remember we talked about how stress or worries can impact our health and blood pressure? [Mr. Somchanh nods] What are the biggest stresses in your life now?

Mr. Somchanh: Oh, family! I'm working overtime to pay for my daughter's wedding and my wife is busy planning. But we are worried about our son.

CHW: What is worrying you about your son? Oh, and what is his name?

Mr. Somchanh: His name is Seng. He's not going to school. He stays in his room all the time sleeping. We are worried he may not graduate high school. Then what will happen? He used to be so good at school!

CHW: Who does Seng still talk to or confide in? Has he spoken to anyone about what he's experiencing?

Mr. Somchanh: He's not talking, only yelling. My wife and my daughter tell me I yell too much. But he yells too, so where's the respect?

CHW: You're finding it hard to communicate with your son.

Mr. Somchanh: Yes, so tell me, what has he got to be depressed about? No war, no refugee camps—only opportunities. We do everything for him!

CHW: Well, depression also happens to people who have good families and good opportunities. It isn't something that people choose or that they can control.

(continues)

Client Scenario: Boun Somchanh *(continued)*

Mr. Somchanh: Ha! [crosses his arms again]

CHW: Here at Northside, we think of depression just like hypertension. It's another illness. It's also a very common illness, and, like hypertension, it can be serious. You must be worried about Seng.

Mr. Somchanh: We are very worried. We don't sleep so good. Sometimes my wife and I are fighting about what to do because we don't know what to do.

CHW: You and your wife are very worried about Seng, and you don't know what to do.

Mr. Somchanh: Yes [uncrosses his arms].

CHW: Is there anyone you can reach out to who could help Seng? Is there anyone in the extended family or the community that he might talk with?

Mr. Somchanh: I don't know. He was such a happy boy before. Always good at school. A good son. He always went to the International House for study groups and basketball.

CHW: We work a lot with International House. They have a great team of counselors there. Do you think Seng would feel more comfortable meeting with a counselor here at Northside or at International House?

Mr. Somchanh: I think International House. He goes there since he was little. He already knows people there.

CHW: Okay. Is there anyone at International House whom he particularly trusts? Someone who might meet with him there or at your home, or talk with him by phone?

Mr. Somchanh and the CHW talk about possible resources at International House, a trusted local nonprofit agency that provides a wide range of services to the local Lao community. International House refers the community to Northside for primary health care services, and Northside refers patients to International House for employment readiness and English classes, counseling and case management services, and after-school youth services. The CHW adds two new circles to Mr. Somchanh's Bubble Chart and writes in "Stress" and "Worries about his son, Seng."

CHW: Looking at the Bubble Chart you created, what is your biggest priority right now? What is the factor that is most affecting your health?

Mr. Somchanh: My son. He's our priority. Seng needs help and that has to be number one.

Mr. Somchanh asks the CHW to call International House to request an urgent referral for his son Seng. Mr. Somchanh will ask his wife and daughter to speak with Seng to encourage him to speak with a counselor from International House.

The Northside Community Health Center, Health Action Plan

Client's Name: Mr. Boun Somchanh

Client Case Number: _____

Demographic information (such as date of birth, address, gender identity, ethnicity, primary language): Male. Married. 37a Birchwood Drive, Central City, _____. 07/01/1960. Laotion. Lao, Thai and English.

(continues)

The Northside Community Health Center, Health Action Plan (continued)

Health Goals

- To manage hypertension and prevent further progression of the disease
- To find support for his son Seng, who is no longer attending high school

Health Risks

- Not taking medications regularly. Sometimes skips or splits doses. Concerned about side effects.
- Diet. Mr. Somchanh is trying to change his diet. His wife prepares food at home and is willing to adapt to a heart-healthy diet.
- Stress. Mr. Somchanh experiences stress in his physically demanding job at the University of _____, and at home. His daughter is getting married and his son, Seng, has stopped going to high school (may be depressed).

Internal Resources

- Engages in regular physical activity through his job
- Willing to talk about his hypertension and to develop an action plan
- Resilience. Survived flight from Laos, years in a refugee camp, resettling in the United States, learning English, supporting his family.
- Speaks three languages.
- Other: _____

External Resources

- Strong family and community bonds
- Mr. Somchanh's wife supports her husband by attending medical appointments, putting out his medication and cooking healthy meals
- Has a good job with good benefits. Is proud of his employment.
- Other: _____

Action Plan

- Priority is to get help for his 17-year-old son, Seng, who has stopped going to school.
- Mr. Somchanh has agreed to take his hypertension medications daily, as prescribed
- Mr. Somchanh has agreed to talk about other actions after we address his urgent concern for his son
- Other: _____

Comments_____

Follow-up meeting scheduled

___x___ Yes _____ No   When? 10/9/_____ 6:00 PM

Referrals Provided: Referral made to International House, Counseling Services, requesting outreach to Seng Somchanh to assess his mental health status. Requested an appointment with the Northside Nutritionist for Mr. Somchanh and his wife.

The client and the CHW (or other health provider) may revise an action plan many times over the course of their work together. Goals and actions may be updated according to the progress and shifting priorities of the client.

Working with Refugee and Immigrant Communities

The United States is one of the most diverse countries in the world with immigrants and refugees looking to resettle for better economic opportunities or to find refuge due to conflict or human rights violations in their home country. The United Nations estimates that in 2022 alone more than 100 million people were forcibly displaced worldwide (United Nations News, 2022). Immigration will be the primary driver for population grown in the United States by 2030 (U.S. Census Bureau, 2022).

The Census Bureau estimates that the immigrant population will continue to increase in the next several decades, with an estimated 69 million immigrants living in the United States by 2060, comprising 17% of the population (Ibid). As newcomers resettle, they will be looking for health services and social support through public agencies, health clinics, and local community–based organizations—organizations that often employ CHWs. As you work with immigrants and refugees, consider the following:

- Learn about the changing demographics and needs of the communities you serve.
- Practice your cultural humility skills and keep an open mind.
- Keep in mind that how immigrant communities access health care and their home country may be quite different from how health care services are accessed in the United States. You will have to play the role of a cultural broker and a cultural bridge between immigrant clients and local service providers.
- Stay informed about local, state, and federal criteria for public program benefits such as WIC, EBT, Medi-Caid, and Medicare, as well as workforce and English language programs.
- Continue to network and learn about resources provided by and for refugee communities. Almost all county government has a program for refugee resettlement and many faith-based program exists to help new immigrants.
- Continue to practice and enhance your person-centered skills.

CHWs Support Refugee Communities: The Newcomers Health Program

Across the globe, refugees and asylees flee their home countries due to war, or persecution based on race, religion, gender, political opinion, or membership in a particular group, and seek legal protection in the United States. They are individuals and families who have experienced arduous journeys, physical and emotional trauma, family separation, and neglected health care. Many are fearful of obtaining services, including healthcare, and supportive social services because of fear of negative immigration consequences and a history of mistrust of the government.

The Community Health Workers with the San Francisco Department of Public Health's Newcomers Health Program have been providing healthcare access and linkages for refugee populations in San Francisco since 1980 (Newcomers Health Program, 2023). The San Francisco Department of Public Health's Newcomers Health Program partners with the Family Health Center based at Zuckerberg San Francisco General Hospital and supports access and linkage to comprehensive health assessments and ongoing primary care for newly arrived refugee populations in San Francisco.

Multi-lingual and trauma-informed CHWs play a key role in warmly welcoming those who have fled home to find refuge in the United States. The bilingual and bicultural skills of the CHWs enable supportive communication channels to better assess individual needs and provide direct support and linkages, including how

(continues)

CHWs Support Refugee Communities: The Newcomers Health Program
(continued)

to enroll in health insurance, support for job training, studying English, ongoing education options in San Francisco and the United States, as well as legal services and mental health support.

Luis, a CHW with the Newcomers Health Program first met Marco (the client's name has been changed to preserve confidentiality) when he was granted asylum status and referred by his lawyer for healthcare. Luis first talked to Marco by phone to welcome and help him understand the support services available to him. Luis used Motivational Interviewing skills to help Marco identify his needs. Luis helped Marco through the application process for Medi-Cal (California's Medicaid health insurance program), CalFresh (SNAP or Food Stamps), and CalWorks (public assistance benefits). They made phone calls together, navigated complex phone-tree systems, and built a trusting relationship. Once Marco's Medi-Cal coverage was established, Luis helped him make a healthcare appointment and provided interpreting during the appointment where Marco felt comfortable sharing the trauma he experienced and how it still caused him anxiety and stress. Marco shared that he was forced to flee his home country because of family violence and abused based on his sexual orientation. During his journey to the United States, Marco was kidnapped and abused again. He felt guilty for the money that some family members paid to release him from hostage. When he finally arrived in the United States, Marco found a pro-bono lawyer to help his case, who then connected him to the Newcomers Health Program. Marco was referred to therapy with an agency specialized in trauma support. Luis providing ongoing support for Marco with appointments and interpreting for psychological screening and therapy sessions.

Luis had to keep his CHW role and interpreting role separate, which was emotionally heavy and challenging. Luis' supervisor provides space to debrief and share feelings and support Luis and other CHWs to acknowledge challenges, keep successful outcomes in mind, help and encourage others, and manage expectations.

Through this collective effort of support, Marco regained physical and emotional health, started a job, and achieved a stable living situation. He is applying for his Green Card and hopes to eventually become a US Citizen.

For more information about the Newcomers Health Program, please go to https://zuckerbergsanfrancisco-general.org/refugee-services/

9.3 Knowledge and Skills for Person-Centered Counseling

There is a wide range of skills and resources that can be used to conduct person-centered counseling. The skills you use will depend upon the topics you address, the agency or program you work for, your own level of knowledge and experience, and your scope of practice.

CULTURAL HUMILITY

Chapter 7 introduced Cultural humility. It is a foundational concept for providing person-centered counseling and other services. Cultural humility guides us in working with others in a way that honors their cultural identities, traditions, values, beliefs, wisdom, and priorities. It involves working with clients without imposing our own judgments, privileges, assumptions, or cultural values. To accomplish this, we need to develop an awareness of our own identities, values, and beliefs and moments when we may be at risk of imposing them on others.

HARM-REDUCTION AND RISK-REDUCTION COUNSELING

Harm-reduction and risk-reduction counseling offer practical strategies for person-centered work and are commonly used by CHWs.

Harm reduction is a philosophy about life and health, as well as an approach to behavior change that was developed by people who inject drugs. This community objected to the "abstinence-only" philosophy that usually guides programs and services for people who use alcohol and drugs. The goal of abstinence-based programs is to encourage people to stop using drugs as quickly as possible. Because abstinence-based programs focus exclusively on supporting people to stop using drugs or alcohol completely, they offer little or nothing to clients who may not (or may not yet) want to quit using. The National Harm Reduction Coalition defines **harm reduction** as: "a set of practical strategies and ideas aimed at reducing negative consequences associated with drug use. Harm reduction is also a movement for social justice built on a belief in, and respect for, the rights of people who use drugs." (NHRC, 2022).

The harm-reduction philosophy and approach can be applied to many health-related issues, not just to issues of substance use (Hawk et al., 2017). For example, harm reduction can be applied to support clients to reduce their risks for diabetes, the flu or COVID-19, sexually transmitted diseases, depression, or cancer. Essentially any action that reduces potential harm to ourselves or to others is viewed as beneficial. Not everyone will quit smoking, stop drinking sugary soda, or eating "fast" food completely. However, if they change their behavior and reduce their use in some way, they can also reduce health risks. For example, if someone who drinks four to five sodas a day reduces this to two sodas a day, they can reduce risks for heart disease, diabetes, and other chronic conditions. People who inject drugs can reduce potential harm by reducing their use of drugs or using in other ways such as no longer sharing syringes and works (depending on the drug, this may include cottons and cookers, for example) with others. All of these actions can significantly reduce their exposure to pathogens that cause infections and diseases such as HIV and Hepatitis C. Harm reduction strategies depend upon local and state policies and may include the use of medication assisted treatment (MAT) for people using opioids. MAT combines behavioral health services with the use of medications that help to relieve drug cravings and block drug effects. Some cities and states have considered opening supervised injection sites (SIS) or places where people can inject drugs under the supervision of health providers to help prevent and respond to potential risks and harms such as overdose and to link users with available resource referrals.

Harm reduction is a realistic and person-centered approach to preventing risks and promoting health. It recognizes how difficult it can be to change potentially harmful behaviors, especially behaviors that are longstanding and pleasurable. It also acknowledges that not everyone who engages in behaviors that are associated with health risks will want to—or be able to—stop these behaviors. Harm reduction recognizes and respects peoples' autonomy or independence and their right to make decisions for themselves regarding their behaviors and health.

Harm reduction remains a controversial practice in the United States in relation to drug use. Some cities and states have embraced harm reduction policies and programs, and others have not. Drug policies in the United States are predominately based on a criminal justice approach. In countries such as Canada, Portugal, and the United Kingdom; however, governments have developed policies guided by harm reduction. In some cases, these governments have decriminalized drug use, addressing it as a health issue rather than a criminal justice issue. Local government programs sometimes provide injection drug users with clean syringes along with counseling, employment assistance, and other social services. These policies and programs have been shown to dramatically reduce the harms associated with injection drug use, including rates of HIV infection, overdose and death, unemployment, and loss of family and home.

- *What is your opinion about the philosophy and practice of harm reduction?*

- *How can harm reduction strategies and programs benefit the communities that you work with and belong to?*

- *How does harm reduction apply in your life: what actions do you take that assist you in reducing health risks?*

Risk-reduction counseling is a person-centered form of behavior change counseling that is widely used to address issues such as HIV and other sexually transmitted infections (STIs). Clients identify behaviors that place their health at risk, such as unprotected sex. CHWs assist clients to identify options for reducing these risks by changing behaviors, such as having less sex or different types of sex, taking pre-exposure prophylaxis or PrEP (taking antiretroviral medications to prevent infection with HIV), using condoms or other safer sex strategies. This is the predominant person-centered approach to HIV prevention throughout the world.

Harm-reduction and risk-reduction counseling are frequently used along with the Stages of Change theory and motivational interviewing (introduced next).

STAGES OF CHANGE THEORY

The Stages of Change theory is a framework for understanding behavior change (Prochaska, Norcross, & DiClemente, 1999). The model is still widely used and describes behavior change as a process that typically involves many steps rather than a single event. It highlights the fact that behavior change may be marked by both progress and setbacks, including relapse or returning to prior patterns of behavior. The model has been used to understand behavior change related to different health concerns including substance use, HIV/AIDS, nutrition, diabetes, mental health challenges, and other chronic conditions.

The Stages of Change theory (Table 9.1) is often used with motivational interviewing and other person-centered counseling skills and techniques. It can guide clients and CHWs in identifying where the client is in terms of their own process of behavior change.

Table 9.1 The Stages of Change

STAGE OF CHANGE	DEFINITION	BEHAVIORAL DESCRIPTION	ROLE OF THE CHW
Precontemplation	The individual is not thinking about the health risks of their current behaviors (such as the risks of unprotected sex).	The individual is not planning to change their behavior within the next six months.	To encourage clients to begin thinking about health risks and possible behavior change.
Contemplation	The individual is thinking about change in the near future (such as trying PrEP or condoms).	The individual is planning to change within the next six months.	To support clients to talk about how they want to change their behavior.
Preparation	The individual is ready and making a plan to change (for example, has purchased condoms and lube and has planned for how to use them).	The individual is actively preparing to make changes within the next month.	To support clients to develop an individualized and realistic plan for behavior change.
Action	The individual has started making changes (for example, talking with partners and using condoms and lube for vaginal and anal sex).	The individual has made the change for more than one day and less than six months.	To encourage and support clients to take action and change behaviors in accordance with their plan.
Maintenance	The individual has committed to the change long term (practicing safer sex regularly, including the use of condoms and lube for sex).	The individual has maintained this change for more than six months.	To support clients in maintaining new behaviors, and to prevent relapse to the previous risk behaviors.
Relapse	Individual has "relapsed" to previous patterns and risk behaviors (has stopped taking PrEP or is having sex without using condoms).	Individual found it hard to maintain new behaviors or faced challenges that made it difficult to be consistent with the new behavior. May have relapsed due to relationships, trauma, loss, doubt, or other factors.	To support clients to consider relapse as a common part of the behavior change process. To support clients to identify the factors that influenced their relapse, and what they want to do now. Clients may revise their behavior change plan.
Return to precontemplation or action	Behavior change is a complicated process, and people frequently have to keep trying before they are able to maintain new behaviors.	As described above.	As described above, CHWs support clients to continue to think about and take actions to reduce health risks.

TG: The stages of change are useful because the whole belief of harm-reduction and person-centered counseling is that you have to meet the client where they are. Stages of change help me to understand where the client is so that we can build from there.

What Do
YOU?
Think

- *What do you think about the Stages of Change model?*

- *Are you trying to change a behavior? If so, where are you on the Stages of Change?*

- *Where is Mr. Somchanh in terms of the Stages of Change?*

RELAPSE PREVENTION

Relapse is a common and natural part of the behavior change process. **Relapse** means returning to the behavior that the client has been trying to change. For example, a client may relapse and start to drink alcohol again, stop exercising, skip their medications, or return to eating a less healthy diet.

Relapse prevention is working with clients to help them anticipate and prevent relapse, as well as to plan for how they may recover from a relapse. We recommend talking with clients about relapse as a common part of the behavior change process. This helps to "normalize" relapse and may support clients to feel more comfortable talking with you or others if they do relapse. For example, a CHW might ask: *"What factors could make you more vulnerable to returning to _____ (the behavior they are trying to change)? In the past, what types of factors have prompted you to return to _____?"*

RELAPSE PREVENTION, ROLE PLAY DEMO

(*Source:* Foundations for Community Health Workers/http://youtu.be/g7UiLRJ-QkE)

As a CHW, you can also help clients anticipate the possibility of relapse and to come up with a plan for what to do next. For example, you could ask the client: *"How do you want to respond if you do relapse? Who could you reach out and talk with if you do relapse?"* This provides the client with an opportunity to come up with a plan that may help them to recover from a relapse more quickly and to either resume or revise their behavior change plan.

Please watch the following video [▶] that shows a CHW talking with a client about on Relapse Prevention:

- *In this video role play, how did the CHW support the client with relapse prevention?*

- *What else would do—or do differently—if you were working with this client?*

Please also watch the following video interview [▶] about Relapse Prevention:

THE CONCEPT OF FALLIBILITY

Fallibility is the recognition that we are all imperfect human beings prone to making mistakes. Accepting our own fallibility means recognizing the limitations of our own knowledge, awareness, and skills, and acknowledging that we will make mistakes in our work with clients. CHWs and other service providers will inevitably say the wrong thing, assume something that isn't true, offer a suggestion that isn't appreciated, or provide information or a referral that isn't up-to-date.

RELAPSE PREVENTION.

(*Source:* http://youtu.be/EaXhsT6B8y8.)

Embracing the concept of fallibility can help us to let go of internal expectations to "know it all." This is particularly valuable in the moments when clients or community members point out our mistakes. When we are able to demonstrate accountability for our errors of understanding or practice with grace and kindness, it often helps to restore a positive working alliance with clients.

Integrating the concept of fallibility into our work requires learning how to say, *"I don't know about _____,"* and *"I'm not certain about that, let me check with my colleagues,"* and *"I was wrong about _____; I'm sorry."*

These may seem like minor or inconsequential statements, but they help to present ourselves as fallible and accessible human beings who are doing our best and sometimes falling short of the mark.

CHWs who have embraced the concept of fallibility report working with less anxiety about making mistakes, and greater confidence that they can recover when they do make mistakes.

- *What do you think about the concept of fallibility? Can it be helpful in guiding your work?*

- *How do you want to respond when you make mistakes in your work with clients?*

9.4 Motivational Interviewing

Motivational interviewing (MI) is a form of person-centered counseling widely used throughout the world to support clients to change behaviors and enhance their health. First used to counsel clients about alcohol use, today MI is applied to a wide variety of health-related behaviors and issues including the management of chronic health conditions, prevention of infectious disease, sexual behaviors, healthy eating, physical activity, and other topics. All types and levels of health and social services providers use MI, including CHWs, health educators, social workers, therapists, nurses, and physicians.

We recommend MI as one of the most important resources for CHWs to use in their daily work with individual clients, families, groups, and communities.

Please note that we can only provide a brief introduction to motivational interviewing in the Foundations textbook. The literature on MI is large, complex, and always developing. With further study and on-going practice, you will increase your understanding and skills for practicing MI. For further study, please see the additional resources provided at the end of this chapter.

Motivational Interviewing is defined as "a collaborative, goal-oriented type of communication with particular attention to the language of change. It is designed to strengthen a person's motivation for and commitment to a specific goal by eliciting and exploring the person's own reasons for change within an atmosphere of acceptance and compassion." (Miller & Rollnick, 2013).

KEY CONCEPTS FOR MOTIVATIONAL INTERVIEWING

Like all forms of person-centered counseling, MI aims to support the autonomy or independence of people to make informed decisions about their health, and their lives more broadly. Motivational interviewing is specifically used to support people in the process of changing behaviors to promote their health and improve the condition of their lives. Before introducing MI techniques, we will review several key concepts.

Responding to Ambivalence

Motivational interviewing acknowledges that changing behavior can be difficult. Behavior change implies giving up something that we have become used to and that may provide pleasure, comfort, or a sense of meaning or identity. It is natural that people feel **ambivalent** or uncertain or have doubts or mixed thoughts and emotions about behavior change. Let's consider smoking cigarettes as an example. On the one hand, people may want to quit smoking to promote their health and wellness, and, on the other hand, they may be uncertain about giving up the perceived benefits of smoking which could include stress reduction or social connections to other smokers. Motivational interviewing not only accepts ambivalence to change as natural, but it encourages clients to explore their ambivalence as a key part of the behavior change process. The techniques described later in this chapter—including the use of OARS and Rolling with Resistance—support the client in addressing and, if possible, resolving their ambivalence and challenges related to behavior change.

> **TG:** I worked for a long time in the gay community, and I think we made some mistakes early on in the AIDS epidemic. We kind of pushed safer sex and condom use, and we didn't stop to acknowledge what a big change this was. I mean, sexual freedom and sexual pleasure are really important to most of the community. Motivational interviewing is a great resource for me to use when I counsel gay men, because it is a way to focus on what makes it so hard to change, how they feel about it, and what they really want in their lives.

What Do YOU Think?

- *What behaviors have you tried to change over the course of your life?*

- *What did you have to give up to make these changes?*

- *Did you ever feel ambivalent or have doubts about changing these behaviors?*

The Spirit of Motivational Interviewing

Practitioners of MI caution against focusing too much on its techniques alone. For MI techniques to be effective, they must be guided by the *spirit* of motivational interviewing. The spirit of motivational interviewing emphasizes the quality of the relationship between counselor and client, the importance of addressing ambivalence, and supporting the client's autonomy. The four key components of MI spirit or way of being with people are (Motivational Interviewing Network of Trainers, 2022):

- **Partnership:** Motivational interviewing is a collaborative process. The MI practitioner is an expert in helping people change; people are the experts of their own lives.

- **Evocation:** People have within themselves the resources and skills needed for change. MI draws out the person's priorities, values, and wisdom to explore reasons for change and support success.

- **Acceptance:** The MI practitioner takes a nonjudgmental stance, seeks to understand the person's perspectives and experiences, expresses empathy, highlights strengths, and respects a person's right to make informed choices about changing or not changing.

- **Compassion:** The MI practitioner actively promotes and prioritizes clients' welfare and well-being in a selfless manner.

> **TG:** Motivational interviewing is a lot different from the kind of counseling I got when I was going through recovery [from drug use]. In those days, they used a much more aggressive strategy to kind of break you down—to make you see and admit that you needed to change. However, motivational interviewing doesn't force anything on the client, and I like that. I still ask clients what is keeping them from making the changes that they want to make. But they can choose to talk about it with me or not. Motivational interviewing gives me the tools to do this in a much better way.

What Do YOU Think?

- *How does the spirit of MI fit with other concepts for person-centered practice, including cultural humility?*

Enhancing Motivation

Motivational interviewing highlights the way that a client's motivation for change is shaped and influenced by the quality of the relationship and interactions between a client and a service provider or counselor. MI was developed with an understanding that the approach that counselors take—the skills they use, and the choices they make—can enhance or undermine a client's motivation for change. In other words, what you say and do when working with clients can make a *significant difference* in whether they make progress in understanding and changing health-related behaviors. Some of these factors are represented in Figure 9.1 below.

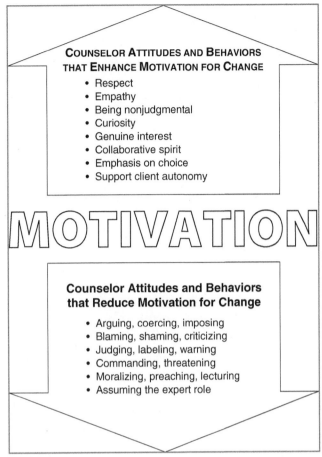

Figure 9.1 Factors that Enhance and Reduce Motivation for Change.
Source: Centers for Disease Control and Prevention (2009).

What Do
YOU?
Think :

- *What else might CHWs do to diminish or enhance a client's motivation for change?*

- *Has your motivation for change ever been influenced by a counselor or other type of helping professional? In what ways?*

The Four Processes

Motivational interviewing highlights four key processes (Motivational Interviewing Network of Trainers, 2010):

- **Engaging**: Together the client and the helping professional begin to establish a productive working relationship based on respect for the client's identity, expertise, and autonomy. The relationship is nonjudgmental and strength-based.

- **Focusing**: Working together, the client and provider identify a common purpose and goal for their work. The client identifies the type of change they want to work toward.

- **Evoking**: The client reflects upon their reasons and motivations for changing behaviors. Providers use OARS (see below) and other techniques designed to encourage clients to reflect and talk about the factors that prompt them to seek changes in their lives. Clients' ambivalence or uncertainty about change is anticipated, accepted, and explored without judgment and, as a result, may be resolved by the client.

- **Planning**: This is when the client actively explores how they wish to change their behavior by developing a realistic and specific plan of the actions they will take. Plans must be based on the client's own ideas, insights, and expertise.

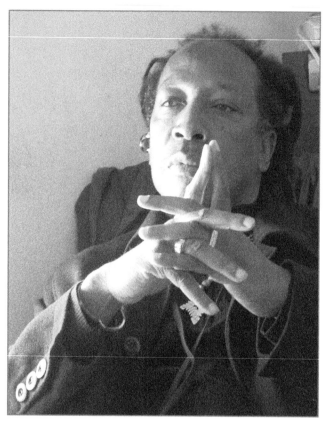

A CHW listens closely to a client's story.

MOTIVATIONAL INTERVIEWING TECHNIQUES

Motivational interviewing features a variety of person-centered counseling techniques and resources. We highlight three techniques in this chapter.

The Use of OARS

OARS are skills that CHWs can use to guide conversations with clients. OARS stands for:

Open-ended questions

Affirmations

Reflections or Reflective Listening

Summarizing

Open-Ended Questions

Open and closed-ended questions were discussed in Chapter 8. Closed-ended questions generally prompt yes, no, or one-word answers from clients. They may be used to gather or verify information, but when they are used too often in the context of behavior change counseling, they tend to shut down dialogue rather than open it up.

In the Client Scenario, the CHW asks Mr. Somchanh several closed-ended questions: *"I see from your health record that you're here to work on better managing your hypertension. Is this correct?"* and *"Have you talked with Dr. Chen about this* [medications side effects]*?"*

Open-ended questions encourage a client to reflect and talk in a detailed way about their life experiences, feelings, and beliefs.

In the Client Scenario, the CHW asks Mr. Somchanh several open-ended questions:

- *"What have you learned about hypertension or high blood pressure?"*
- *"Where are you working now and what type of work do you do?"*

- *"What types of food do you usually eat?"*
- *"You said you don't like to take the high blood pressure medicine. What are your concerns about the medication?"*
- *"If you start to experience side effects or have concerns about your medication, what will you do then?"*
- *"What are the biggest stresses in your life now?"*
- *"What is worrying you about your son?"*

Open-ended questions encourage clients to talk about health risks, their readiness to change behaviors, and any ambivalence or resistance they may have about these changes. Providing space for dialogue without judgment also builds trust. Open-ended questions provide clients with opportunities to talk about sensitive health topics while honoring their independence and supporting their decisions about which information they are willing to share with a provider. As always, the client must drive the behavior change process, and the solutions by which behavior change can happen must come from them.

Examples of other open-ended questions include:

- *What motivates you to think about changing _____ (a specific behavior)?*
- *What are you feeling right now? What's it like for you to talk about these issues?*
- *What would you like to do about that?*
- *What else can you tell me about that?*
  - *Such as? How so? What happened then? What did you do then?*
- *What happened the last time that you _____?*
- *What would it be like for you to try _____? How might you begin?*
- *What gets in the way of making these changes?*
- *You say that in the past you were successful with _____. How did you accomplish this? What skills and resources did you bring to this situation?*
- *What have you learned from prior challenges and experiences that are similar to what you are facing now? What is different now?*

  - *Why are open-ended questions particularly helpful for clients?*

  - *What are some of your favorite open-ended questions to ask clients?*

What Do YOU? Think

> **TG:** My favorite questions are simple ones like: "What's going on?" or "What are your thoughts about this?" or "What was that like?"

Affirmations

Many people rarely receive an acknowledgment of their strengths, internal resources, and accomplishments. Sometimes, when clients work with service providers, the focus is on what isn't working in their lives (rising blood pressure, a cancer diagnosis, a domestic violence situation), the "mistakes" they may have made, the risks they are facing, and their outstanding needs. Motivational interviewing places an emphasis on recognizing and affirming people's positive qualities, intentions, and accomplishments. These strengths are often the most important resources to support a client to enhance their health.

Affirming statements provide clients with direct and immediate positive feedback for their efforts and accomplishments and encourage them to continue reflecting about, planning for, and taking steps to change behavior.

Be cautious about providing affirmations too frequently or for more routine accomplishments, because they may begin to lose their value for the client. Provide affirmations in an authentic manner about important client accomplishments and strengths in the moments you determine that they might be most valuable, such as when clients are expressing self-doubt.

In the Client Scenario, the CHW shares the following affirming statements with Mr. Somchanh:

"You and your wife clearly have a strong partnership—it is wonderful that she is so supportive in promoting your health."

"Wonderful, you're doing a great job with your medications and communicating with Dr. Chen."

Other examples of affirming statements include:

- *I respect how open you are to considering these changes _____ (behavior that the client is thinking about changing).*
- *It sounds like it took a lot of _____ (courage, strength, willpower) to _____ (talk with him, go to the meeting, and so forth).*
- *You have a lot of insight into the factors that influence your health.*
- *Things didn't turn out like you expected, but you did your best in a difficult situation.*
- *You've survived some really difficult things in the past, and I trust that you can figure this out too.*
- *You have been very generous in supporting _____ (your friend or family member)*

  - *Can you think of other examples of affirming statements?*

  - *Are affirmative statements important to you and for your own attempts to change behaviors?*

What Do YOU Think?

Please watch the following video ▶ of a CHW working with a client and providing an affirmation:

- *How well did this CHW provide an Affirmation to the client?*
- *How may this Affirmation have benefited the client?*
- *What value have Affirmations had in your own life?*
- *When do you provide an Affirmation to others?*

PROVIDING AN AFFIRMATION: ROLE PLAY, DEMO.

(*Source:* http://youtu.be/FrggzUE7Z_I.)

Reflections/Reflective Listening

This is the art and the skill of reflecting back to clients what they have shared with you about their experiences, beliefs, feelings, behavior, and intentions. By reflecting back on what clients say, you can:

- Clarify what clients have said, preventing miscommunication and inaccurate assumptions
- Let clients know that they are being heard and understood
- Provide clients with an opportunity to hear and reflect upon their own insights and statements
- Build and deepen a conversation

Sharing reflections isn't always easy to do—it requires commitment, concentration, patience, and cultural humility. There are different types of reflections that a CHW may share with a client, including those that attempt to echo back precisely or similarly what the client has said, and reflections that may add an interpretation or emphasis for the client to consider.

Different types of reflections include:

a. *Repeating:* Repeating back as precisely as possible words or phrases that the client has said. For example, in the Client Scenario, Mr. Somchanh says: *"We are so worried. We don't sleep so good. Sometimes my wife and I are fighting about what to do, because we don't know what to do."*

   The CHW says: *"You and your wife are very worried about Seng, and you don't know what to do."*

   However, we caution you against repeating what a client tells you too often. If the CHW repeats exactly what the client says too many times, it can be irritating and may begin to undermine the connection or rapport you are building with the client.

b. *Rephrasing*: Using different words to try to express the same meaning that the client has expressed. For example, in the Client Scenario, the CHW rephrases information several times. The CHW says: *Your wife is mindful of your hypertension and cooking healthier foods with less salt,"* and, *"You're finding it hard to communicate with your son."*

c. *Paraphrasing*: This is a step beyond rephrasing in which the person-centered counselor attempts to interpret and summarize what the speaker means. The purpose is to assist the client to better understand their own experience, feelings, and meaning.

   For example, the CHW working with Mr. Somchanh might say something like: *"You're worried about your son and finding it difficult to talk with him. You and Seng often end up yelling at each other which isn't helping his situation."*

d. *Reflection of emotion or meaning*: This is an attempt to assess and reflect a possible emotion or meaning connected to what a client is saying. It represents an educated guess about what the client *might* be feeling or thinking and could be correct or incorrect. Either way, it provides clients with an opportunity to further refine what they are thinking and feeling. This is a more complex type of reflection and should be used sparingly at first.

   For example, in the Client Scenario, the CHW might share the following reflections with Mr. Somchanh:

   ● *"You're frustrated with the doctor because she doesn't seem to acknowledge the positive things you and your wife are doing to eat healthier food,"*

   ● *"You don't understand why your son is depressed,"*

   ● *"You don't understand why Seng is depressed because his life has been easier than yours was"*

You don't have to get the emotion or meaning "right." Right or wrong, you present clients with an opportunity to clarify for themselves what they are feeling. You may intentionally amplify an emotion to assist clients to clarify what they are feeling.

> TG: Sometimes when I use the OARS and I reflect on something that a client said, it helps them to really hear their own words, the feeling and meaning of what they said. Even when I get it wrong it can help because if the client says, "No, that's not what I said!"—then I have an opportunity to show that I want to listen, I want to understand.

e. *Reframing*: Reframing is to take information given by the client and reflect it back with a different emphasis or interpretation. The goal is to suggest a different way of viewing or thinking about an experience or an issue—one that may be more affirming or supportive to their behavior change efforts. Reframing can be particularly useful in terms of changing patterns of negative thinking that undermine a client's efforts. As always, the client is free to accept, to reject, or to change any suggestion you offer for how to reframe an experience (see Table 9.2).

Table 9.2 Examples of the Use of Reframing in Behavior Change Counseling

CLIENT SAYS:	CHW REFLECTS AND REFRAMES AS:
I just don't know what to do anymore …	You feel like you don't know what to do. But I see that you *are* doing something—you came here to talk with me and to ask for support.
I know I should start exercising, but I just can't fit it in. After work, taking care of my kids, and making dinner, I'm just too exhausted. I just don't have the motivation.	You feel like you don't have any motivation. But you clearly have a lot of motivation to work and raise a family. What motivates you to do these things so well?

- *What benefit do you see to sharing reflective statements with clients?*

- *In what situations might you share reflective statements?*

Summarizing

Summarizing is a way to reflect back on the main concerns, priorities, feelings, or decisions that a client shares with you. It is another way to demonstrate that you are listening deeply and that you have understood the most important information a client shared with you. It can be used to transition from one main idea or stage of change to another, to reflect the client's natural ambivalence about and resistance to change, and to clarify key decisions that the client has made.

For example, in the Client Scenario, the CHW might say to Mr. Somchanh:

- *"I understand that you want to lower your blood pressure but, at the same time, you haven't been taking your medication consistently."*

- *"You have concerns about taking the medication that the doctor prescribed but you haven't shared these concerns with the doctor yet."*

- *"You have been reducing the amount of salt in your diet but aren't sure what else you can do to improve your diet to manage your blood pressure."*

- *"You're very concerned about your son Seng, but don't know how to help him right now."*

- *"You're open to a referral to International House to see if they can reach out and help your son."*

Other examples of summaries may include:

- *"You're not ready to stop using _____ (an injectable drug), but you do think that you can stop sharing syringes with friends. Is that right?"*

- *"You want to change your diet, but you are worried about giving up your favorite foods."*

- *"Let me see if I have heard you correctly: you really want to bring your blood pressure down, and you'd like to be able to manage it without using medications. But you aren't sure what changes you can realistically make right now to control your blood pressure."*

Use of a Readiness or Motivation Scale

A resource that is sometimes used to support motivational interviewing and other forms of person-centered counseling is a simple scale from 0 to 10 (Figure 9.2). The scale can be used to assess how important it is for clients to change their behavior, how ready they are to make a change, and how confident they are that they will succeed in making changes.

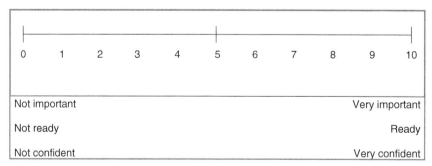

Figure 9.2 A Simple Scale

The following guidelines come from Thomas Bodenheimer, a physician, researcher, and advocate of new primary health care models that feature a central role for CHWs. He promoted the use of the 0–10 scale in working with clients or patients with diabetes and other chronic conditions (Bodenheimer & Laing, 2007).

The 0–10 scale may be used to assess how important a particular issue is to the client. If the level of importance to the client is relatively high (a 7 or higher), the CHW can move on to explore risk-reduction steps and the client's confidence in putting them into action. But if the level of importance is low, the CHW may take time to talk about the issue further, providing the client with information about the risks that the issue may pose to the client's health.

When clients develop behavior change or action plans, the scale may be used to assess how confident they are in putting the plan into action. If the client's confidence level is relatively low, such as a four, the CHW might ask the client why they rate their confidence at a four rather than a one. This can aid in identifying what the client *is* confident about changing. The CHW might also ask the client what would make it possible for the person to move up the scale in confidence from a lower score, such as a four, to a higher score, such as an eight or nine. This may assist the client to reflect further about behavior change, what is getting in the way, and what the client may need to keep moving forward.

If there is a high enough level of importance and confidence to make the behavior change, the CHW should suggest discussing an action plan. The action plan should be tailored to the importance and confidence level of the client.

For example, the CHW working with Mr. Somchanh could ask him to rate his motivation, on a scale from 0 to 10, for managing his hypertension. The CHW could also ask how ready Mr. Somchanh is, on a scale from 0 to 10, to start taking his hypertension medications each day as prescribed. If Mr. Somchanh answers with a six or below, the CHW should revisit the topic. For example, the CHW might say, *"Mr. Somchanh, what could we change about your plan that would make you feel more prepared to take your hypertension medications as prescribed?"*

Please watch the following videos that show a CHW using a Motivation Scale as they work with a client:

- *How did the CHW use a Motivation Scale in her work with this client?*

- *How might the use of a motivation scale be beneficial to this client?*

- *How and when do you like to use a motivation scale in your work with clients?*

SAFER SEX AND USING A MOTIVATION SCALE: ROLE PLAY, DEMO.

(*Source:* Foundations for Community Health Workers/http:// youtu.be/ h9MP3W4vFFE)

Rolling with Resistance

Rolling with Resistance is a technique for supporting clients who are experiencing ambivalence or doubts as part of the behavior change process.

When people face challenges in changing behaviors, providers sometimes respond in ways that are ineffective or harmful. Providers may judge, lecture, or attempt to persuade clients what they should do or feel. Providers may say something like:

"Lots of people eat healthier foods every day, it isn't so hard."

"If you keep eating fast food and processed foods your diabetes is going to worsen and you could face a health crisis."

"I've had lots of clients manage their diabetes through a healthier diet. If they can do it, you can do it."

While the provider is attempting to help the client, they aren't responding directly to the doubts or ambivalence that the client is experiencing in the moment. Attempts from providers to lecture, encourage, or persuade clients may backfire. Clients may feel discounted, ashamed, or angry. They may discontinue services and resume older patterns of behavior that pose risks for their behavior.

Motivational interviewing is a collaborative partnership between clients and providers that rejects attempts to persuade, coerce, or impose change. In contrast, MI encourages us to 'Roll with Resistance" in the moments when clients experience ambivalence. In these moments, use your OARS to provide clients with a nonjudgmental space and an opportunity to reflect on their own thoughts, feelings, experiences, and desires for change.

It can be difficult to respond to a client's ambivalence by rolling with resistance. The MI literature acknowledges this and encourages providers to *"resist the righting reflex"* or the impulse to resist ambivalence with attempts to persuade clients or control the dialogue. Watch for signs—such as impatience, judgment, or frustration—that you may be resisting the client's natural ambivalence and use your OARS to let the client guide the way. If necessary, take a brief break to collect yourself and re-commit to honoring the client's autonomy or independence.

Try acknowledging that change is difficult: *"It's common for all of us to face moments when we feel discouraged or uncertain about changing behaviors. Behavior change is hard."*

Ask Open-ended questions and share Reflective statements that invite clients to share more of their story.

> *"You want to eat healthier to manage your diabetes and protect your health, but you also miss the types of food that you used to eat."*
>
> *"You really miss going to a fast food drive through. What do you miss most about this?"*
>
> *"You doubt that you're strong enough to maintain a healthier diet. I know you did have some success with eating healthier in the past. What do you think helped you to accomplish this before?"*
>
> *"What are some of the benefits and the drawbacks of your new plan for healthy eating?"*

The technique of rolling with resistance honors the client's right to self-determination and offers a safer place to explore difficult emotions, relationships, and choices. With time to reflect on their behavior change experience and their health and life goals, people can move past ambivalence and determine what choices and actions they wish to take next.

> **TG:** Sometimes, when a client is resistant to change—and haven't we all been resistant to change?—a counselor kind of digs in there, or the client and counselor can become kind of stuck. The counselor might think their job is to help to convince a client to change anyway, but for some clients—most of my clients—that will only make them even more resistant. So, rolling with resistance is just acknowledging that the client is having a hard time making these changes, or is having second thoughts, and just kind of normalizing that. I feel like talking about it in this way kind of takes some of the power or the energy away and makes it easier to talk about whatever the client is facing.

Please watch the following videos that show a CHW working with a client who is experiencing ambivalence about how to move forward and promote his own health.

- *In the Counter Role Play, how did the CHW respond to the client's ambivalence? How did the CHW's response impact the client?*

- *In the Demo Role Play, what did the CHW do differently to roll with resistance? What was the impact of the CHW's approach on the client?*

- *How would you demonstrate rolling with resistance in working with this client?*

ROLLING WITH RESISTANCE, COUNTER ROLE PLAY

(*Source:* Foundations for Community Health Workers/http://youtu.be/x_hyIMRMy7A)

ROLLING WITH RESISTANCE, ROLE PLAY DEMO

(*Source:* Foundations for Community Health Workers/http://youtu.be/rgqrusY2MJI)

Now please watch the following interview about Rolling with Resistance:

- *What are your thoughts about the technique of rolling with resistance? Is this a technique that you plan to use when working with clients?*

We encourage you to seek out opportunities for additional training and education on Motivational Interviewing.

ROLLING WITH RESISTANCE, FACULTY INTERVIEW

(*Source:* Foundations for Community Health Workers/http://youtu.be/9vNeWuNUflo)

CHW Profile

Michelle James, She/Her

Medication-Assisted Treatment (MAT) Project Coordinator

Friendship House Association of American Indians, San Francisco CA

Indigenous-led Social Services Agency

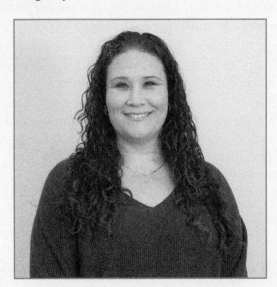

What motivated me to be a CHW is my own background. I grew up poor, I witnessed and experienced domestic violence, I was homeless, and had to utilize the system to get help. The most important challenge I had to overcome was my substance use addiction. There were so many amazing people along the way that played a huge part in helping me get back on my feet. I want to be that support for the next person out there today who needs guidance and support.

For the past five years, I have been working with the Friendship House Association of American Indians, a Native American substance abuse rehabilitation center in the heart of the Mission District in San Francisco. Friendship House integrates Native American cultural and spiritual healing principles, practices, and interventions as its fundamental approach to recovery and wellness. We have an 80-bed facility in San Francisco with 40 beds for men and 40 beds for women, and another 9 bed facility for women with children in Oakland. The length of stay is anywhere from 90 days to a year.

(continues)

CHW Profile

(continued)

I've had a number of positions at Friendship House including Case Manager, Health Educator, Medication Assisted Treatment (MAT) Program Coordinator, and Intake Staff Supervisor. Currently, I am the MAT Project Coordinator. I develop program policies and train our staff. I facilitate an eight-week support group based on the Medicine Wheel: we address the mental, emotional, physical, and spiritual aspects of health and recovery. I teach the group about drug use, the effects of opioids, and how medication assisted treatment works.

I facilitate trainings for staff and community members on how to use Narcan (a treatment for opioid over-dose). In the past six months, our team provided Narcan to two people experiencing overdose, saving their lives.

As the Intake Staff Supervisor, I supervise the team that welcomes and assesses all new incoming clients. I perform HIV and Hepatitis C testing for new clients and link them to care and services.

As a case manager, I worked with a client who was in active withdrawal in the early phase of her recovery. I walked with her every day to the clinic where she could dose (take suboxone to help with opioid withdrawal and treatment) and helped her enroll for health insurance. She was just 20 years old, from a small reservation, and had been in a domestic violence situation. A lot of people doubted she was going to make it. All four of her children were taken away by Child Protective Services. She stayed in treatment for a full year. She was accepted into low-income housing away from the city and she got all her kids back. She's still clean today, she's been clean for five years. I still remember the first day I met her.

Being a CHW has played a huge role in my own sobriety. It keeps me humble. I am able to use my lived experiences and my education to inform communities on a wide range of topics including mental health, HIV/Hepatitis C prevention, trafficking, medication assisted treatment, Narcan, and so much more. My work gives me a sense of purpose and meaning.

My biggest tip for new CHWs is to really get to know motivational interviewing and the importance of cultural humility. You can apply it to any situation that you face. For me, it has been the most powerful tool I have for working with clients, helping them to reflect and talk about their lives, understanding where they are coming from, and meeting each person where they are.

9.5 Additional Resources for Person-Centered Counseling

There are a number of other person-centered resources and techniques that CHWs use to support clients to change behaviors and promote wellness. At City College of San Francisco, we encourage CHWs to customize a virtual "CHW Toolkit" with the most important concepts and skills they will use when working with clients. You might want to consider adding the following resources to your own CHW Toolkit.

USING A BUBBLE CHART

Bubble charts are used to assist clients in identifying options for reducing risks and promoting their health. These charts show a number of blank circles or bubbles that represent possible issues that a client may want to prioritize or actions the client may want to take (see Figure 9.3 below). The bubbles may be left completely blank for the client to identify or may be presented with some options already filled in. The tasks are to identify a wide range of actions that the client can take, and for the client to decide which of these options are best to begin with (Bodenheimer & Laing, 2007).

Not everyone uses a Bubble Chart as part of an initial assessment with a new client or to develop an action or case management plan, but it can be a helpful visual resource for documenting key concerns and identifying priorities for action.

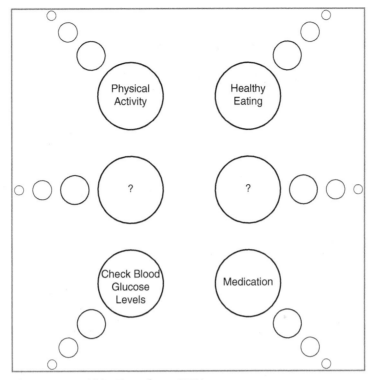

Figure 9.3 Bubble Chart from CHW.
Source: Adapted from Bodenheimer and Laing (2007).

In the Client Scenario about Boun Somchanh, the CHW uses a Bubble Chart to support Mr. Somchanh in developing an action plan to manage his hypertension. The CHW asks Mr. Somchanh to identify key factors that affect his hypertension and his health and writes these items down in the Bubble Chart (Figure 9.3).

After Mr. Somchanh identifies several key factors that influence his health status, the CHW asks, "What is your biggest priority right now? Which of these factors [pointing to the Bubble Chart] is most affecting your health?"

In this way, the CHW uses a Bubble Chart to identify client concerns and to select an item to serve as the first priority for their action plan. Mr. Somchanh decides that his first priority is to get help for his son Seng who may be experiencing depression.

The Use of Silence

A moment of silence can provide an opportunity for clients to reflect on a question or decision, to identify their thoughts and feelings, and to find the words to express them. Some providers become unsettled by silence and rush to fill it with their own words. In these moments, learn to pause, breathe, observe, and if necessary, count to 10 (or 20!) before you say something. Give the client space and time to think and feel. If the silence continues, you might comment on the process (see below) and seek clarification about how the client would like to proceed. For example, you might say something like: *"Do you want more time to think about the question I asked, or would you like to move on to another topic?"*

Please watch the following videos on the Use of Silence that show a CHW working with a client:

THE USE OF SILENCE, COUNTER ROLE PLAY

(*Source:* Foundations for Community Health Workers/http://youtu.be/ e98joohaQwU)

- *How well did the CHW use silence in working with this client?*

- *How would you have used silence in working with this client?*

Please watch the following video interview about the Use of Silence:

- *What are your thoughts about the use of silence? When and how may you use silence in working with clients?*

THE USE OF SILENCE, ROLE PLAY DEMO

(*Source:* Foundations for Community Health Workers/http://youtu.be/N5NyZ7OLcMA)

Commenting on the Process

Commenting on the process draws the client's attention to what is happening at the moment and often highlights the dynamics between the client and the service provider. It can help to identify or resolve difficulties that the client may be experiencing in their work with you, and to shift the conversation or working dynamic in a more productive direction.

If you sense a client's change of mood when a particular topic is raised or a discrepancy between the client's verbal and nonverbal communication, you may wish to comment on the process. For example: *"I notice that each time we talk about your husband, your voice drops to a whisper,"* or *"You say that everything is fine at home, but when you talk about it your eyes fill with tears."*

THE USE OF SILENCE, FACULTY INTERVIEW

(*Source:* Foundations for Community Health Workers/http://youtu.be/DZNOeVxZfIs)

Commenting on the process is also a way to acknowledge what a client has been through, while at the same time highlighting their strengths: *"I am really impressed that you have been able to cope on your own for so long. How have you managed to do it?"*

Finally, commenting can also highlight aspects of your interaction with the client:

CHW: *"How are you feeling about the work that we're doing together?"*

"Would you like to talk about a different topic?"

"I notice that you keep shifting the focus of our conversation to ask me questions about my own life."

"I'm wondering if you are feeling frustrated or upset with me because of something I've said or done. I'm open to hearing feedback from you if you want to share it, and to improving the way that we work together"

Widening the System

When people are facing challenges, they often forget that others may be able to assist them. "Widening the system" refers to reminding clients about their external resources, including friends, family, and others who may be able to provide meaningful support. For example:

- *"Have you shared your concern with anyone else?"*
- *"Who do you usually turn to for support or to talk about issues like this?"*
- *"What would it be like to talk with a family member or friend about what you are going through?"*
- *"What additional support would be helpful to you right now?"*

Role-Playing and the Empty Chair Technique

Instead of continuing to talk about a situation or challenge, consider asking the client to role-play or act it out in some way. This technique can assist clients to think through and prepare for challenging situations. For example, you might help a client to role-play how they will talk with a family member about a personal matter or health issue, or how they will advocate for themselves with another health or social services provider: *"What will you say when ...."*

The Empty Chair technique is a form of role-playing. An empty chair represents another person in the client's life. You can ask a client to imagine that this other person (a parent, partner, child, service provider, or other significant person in their life) is sitting in the chair and ask them what they would like to say to them: *"If your boyfriend/spouse/partner was sitting in this chair, what would you like to say?"* This technique can assist clients to rehearse difficult conversations and practice effective communication skills in a safer environment.

Clients may also try sitting in the chair to role-play the responses of the other person. For example, the CHW might say: *"I wonder if you would consider sitting in the chair for a moment and playing the role of your partner. I'm curious what you think she might say about the situation. Is this something you would like to try?"* Taking on the role of another person in their life can sometimes help clients to better understand their circumstances, or their own relationship with that person.

Role-playing is not for everyone, and these techniques should be offered as a suggestion to the client. Try practicing with colleagues before you introduce the technique to clients.

When done correctly, role-playing can assist a client to "get in touch" with certain experiences, thoughts, and emotions that may otherwise be hard for them to identify or talk about.

Client Scenario: Boun Somchanh (continued)

Mr. Somchanh and the CHW are discussing his relationship with his son Seng.

CHW: You've been having difficulty talking with Seng lately, and sometimes you end up yelling at each other, is that right?

Mr. Somchanh: Yes, we never had problems before. I don't know how to talk with him now. He's getting worse and worse. I worry about his future.

CHW: So, you're very worried about Seng. Have you tried to tell him this?

Mr. Somchanh: [thinking] Maybe I get so worried I start to yell too much.

CHW: What happens when you yell at Seng?

Mr. Somchanh: He stops talking to me, or he yells back.

CHW: So, what you've been saying hasn't been effective in opening up communication with Seng.

Mr. Somchanh: No, like I said, I don't know what to do!

CHW: You want to help your son but aren't sure what to say. I think a lot of parents often feel this way. What if we practiced a bit together? You could pretend that Seng is sitting over there [points to another chair] and practice what you want to say to him.

Mr. Somchanh: Like pretend?

CHW: Yes, pretend to talk with him here. There is nothing to lose in this situation so maybe you can find a way to better way communicate with him.

Mr. Somchanh: You mean like *right now?*

CHW: [laughs] Yes, but only if you want to. If Seng was here, what would say to him?

Mr. Somchanh thinks and begins to talk as if he is speaking with his son Seng.

What Do YOU Think?

- *Which of the techniques described above have you used before?*

- *How do you feel about role-playing or the empty chair technique?*

- *What other counseling, communication, or active listening skills might you use when conducting behavior change counseling?*

9.6 Common Challenges

CHWs work with clients who face difficult life challenges and health conditions. You will work with clients returning home from prison, struggling with substance use or depression, who are unhoused or have lost a beloved family member. Supporting people who are facing challenges, or a crisis can be difficult work. It can also be deeply inspiring and rewarding.

MAKING MISTAKES

People who are training to become a CHW often say, *"I just don't want to make a mistake!"* They don't want to do or say something that may be hurtful, disrespectful, or harmful to a client's health. However, despite your knowledge, skills, ethics, and best intentions, *you will make mistakes: everyone does.*

Anticipate that you will make mistakes and consider how to respond when you do. Listen and observe clients carefully for signs that you may have said or done something that they find hurtful or disrespectful. Hopefully, the client will tell you by saying something like: *"That is not what I meant: don't put words in my mouth!"* In this moment, don't become defensive. Place your own issues and reactions aside and focus on the client's experience. Learn the art of offering an authentic apology. Apologizing can restore your connection with the client and can even deepen it. A sincere apology can create a foundation for deeper work (for more information on the Art of Apology, please see Chapter 13).

NOT UNDERSTANDING THE CLIENT

Helping professionals sometimes feel embarrassed to admit that they haven't understood something that a client says. If you don't stop to clarify what they said, you risk misunderstanding something important and continuing to work with a false assumption. When you don't understand something that the client has told you, *ask them about it*. If a client talks about a particular topic or issue that you are unfamiliar with, ask for an explanation: *"I'm not familiar with _____. Could you tell me more about it?"* Asking questions demonstrates your interest in the client and your desire to learn more about their life.

SCOPE OF PRACTICE

Keep your scope of practice in mind as you work with clients. Identify any situations in which you may be at risk of working beyond your scope of practice due, for example, to factors such as the health risks that the client is facing or their level of distress. This may include issues such as mental health challenges, trauma, suicidal thoughts, or any issue that you have not been properly trained to address or services that you are not approved to provide. Consult immediately with a supervisor. Together you may determine that it would be best for the client to be referred to work with a colleague who has more training and skills, such as a licensed mental health professional. More information about scope of practice is provided in Chapter 5.

ANGER, AGGRESSION, AND CONFLICT

There are many reasons why people may feel frustrated or angry. The clients you work with may sometimes express anger or other emotions in ways that seem disrespectful or even threatening. Feeling anger is natural and learning to express it can be a powerful and positive resource for self-knowledge and behavior change. Yelling at or threatening a counselor, however, is not. When this happens, the challenge for the CHW is to de-escalate the conflict and to support the client to express themselves in a different way. If you are unable to de-escalate a situation, end the session as quickly as possible. Your work should never be done at the expense of your own safety. To read more about handling anger and conflict, please read Chapter 13.

CRISIS

You may work with clients who are in crisis. They may stop using the medications they need, become homeless or incarcerated, or face domestic violence. These are the moments to remember your scope of practice and to consult with a supervisor or make an immediate referral. Over the course of your career, seek out opportunities for additional training on working with clients in crisis.

Wellness and Recovery Action Plans (WRAP) are a great resource for supporting clients to anticipate and plan for how to respond to crisis. WRAP asks clients to reflect upon past challenges and crisis, to identify early warning signs that they may be heading toward and a crisis, and to detail specific steps that they can take in these circumstances. For more information about WRAP, please refer to Chapter 10.

Mandatory Reporting

As discussed in Chapter 5, there are limits to client confidentiality. You have a legal and ethical duty to report certain kinds of behaviors and events. If you learn that a client is harming or threatening harm to themselves or others, you must immediately report this to your supervisor and to appropriate law enforcement authorities. These events and behaviors include physical or sexual abuse of a minor, assault or threats of assault on others, and plans or attempts to kill oneself. Again, if you face these circumstances, *immediately contact your supervisor* for assistance in reporting these risks to a third party such as a local crisis response team, the police, or child protection agencies. Your supervisor will also guide you in determining your next steps with the client, such as making an appropriate referral. Assessing a client's risks for suicide are addressed in Chapter 18.

- *Have you experienced these types of challenges with clients?*

- *Can you think of other types of challenges that you may face as a counselor?*

9.7 Teamwork and Supervision

All CHWs work in team settings (see Chapter 5), and many work as a member of a multidisciplinary team. Teamwork implies both benefits and challenges for all members of the team, including clients and CHWs.

Do your best to develop and maintain positive relationships with all members of your team, and to consult them regularly as you face questions or challenges in your work. Your teammates can help to determine how best to support a client, can serve as the basis for a referral, and can help you to enhance your skills over time.

Working with supervisors is addressed throughout this textbook, including in Chapters 5, 14, and 16. If you provide person-centered counseling, your employer should arrange for you to receive on-going supervision provided by an experienced counselor or mental health provider (see Chapter 12). Supervision is an opportunity to support you to provide quality person-centered counseling by addressing issues such as:

- Ethics including confidentiality and scope of practice
- Safety and mandatory reporting
- Stress and burnout prevention and management
- Referrals
- Practicing cultural humility
- Challenges with documentation
- Personal issues that arise during or after counseling
- Understanding and resolving counseling challenges
- Counseling goals and developing risk-reduction or behavior-change plans
- Counseling skills and techniques such as the use of motivational interviewing

You have an ethical duty to accurately describe your work to your supervisor. Don't waste valuable time by avoiding difficult issues. If you are confused, uncertain, or struggling in your work with a particular client or bothered by personal issues, memories, or emotions, talk about these topics. The purpose of supervision is to protect the welfare of clients (and support a positive work environment). It also supports your continued professional development and your well-being so that you can continue to provide person-centered services.

9.8 Self-Awareness

Providing direct services to others will naturally touch upon your own life experiences, identity, values, feelings, and beliefs. You have an obligation to ensure that your own issues do not get in the way of your work with clients. If your own cultural assumptions and beliefs, values, or emotional needs start to guide your work, you risk doing harm to your clients. If you become aware that this is happening, seek consultation.

Signs that your own issues may be getting in the way of your work may include:

- Finding it difficult to listen to the client
- A strong need to talk about your own ideas or experiences
- Asking questions that are more related to your own needs and interests than those of the client
- Inability to demonstrate interest, curiosity, and inter-personal warmth to the clients you work with
- Becoming overwhelmed or distracted by difficult memories and emotions
- Having strong judgments about the client, their behaviors, or decisions
- A desire to tell the client what to do
- Providing less counseling, or poorer-quality counseling, to certain clients (discriminatory treatment)
- Difficulty listening to particular types of issues (such as sexual issues or trauma experiences)
- Listening to a client's trauma story awakens or activates part of your own trauma experience, making it difficult to focus on your professional role
- Difficulty providing affirmations to a client
- Becoming defensive with a client
- Treating a client with anger, disrespect, or contempt

- *How else might a CHW's own issues get in the way of their ability to provide effective person-centered counseling?*

Many service providers are challenged to keep their own issues from interfering with their work with clients. Good supervision, as discussed above, should focus not only on the challenges that clients face but also on your own issues that arise during counseling. If, for example, you are working with a client who is the victim of domestic violence, and you grew up in a home characterized by domestic violence, talk about this with your supervisor, another colleague, a counselor, or a friend. Don't talk about it with clients. For further discussion of these issues and guidelines for self-disclosure (if or when to share personal information with a client), please see Chapters 5 and 18.

- *What issues may be particularly difficult for you to discuss with a client?*

9.9 Self-Assessment

In addition to the supervision you receive, and the evaluation of your counseling work by others (including clients and colleagues), we recommend that you regularly evaluate your own work to assess whether or not you are providing person-centered services. Every month or so, after you end a meeting with a client, or at the end of the day, use the following Self-Assessment resource (see Table 9.3) to evaluate your work. You may want to do this with a trusted colleague and talk together about your work with clients more broadly.

- *When and how might you use this self-assessment?*

- *What else would you add to this checklist?*

Table 9.3 Self-Assessment for Person-centered Counseling

COUNSELING SKILL	YES	NO	COMMENTS AND SKILLS TO IMPROVE:
1. Did the client identify their own health goals and risks?			
2. Did I assess client strengths (internal and external resources)?			
3. Did the client develop their own action or behavior change plan?			
4. Did I apply a harm-reduction approach?			
5. Did the client speak as much or more than I did?			
6. Did I ask open-ended questions?			
7. Did I provide the client with affirmations?			
8. Did I practice reflective listening?			
9. Did I summarize appropriately?			
10. Did I roll with resistance?			
11. Did I share appropriate referrals?			
12. Did I document this counseling session for the client and the program?			
13. Did my own agenda, values, or beliefs get in the way of person-centered practice?			
14. Did I identify personal issues that I should address in supervision?			
15. Were any ethical or scope of practice concerns identified that require follow-up?			
16. Other?			

9.10 Creating a Professional Development Plan

Throughout your career, you will continue to enhance your skills. Figure 9.4 shows a sample Professional Development Plan to establish goals for building your person-centered counseling skills. There are many ways to engage in professional development activities, such as:

- Research and read about behavior change and person-centered counseling and related issues including books, articles, and online resources
- Attend classes, workshops, conferences, and trainings

Professional Development Plan

Name:_____

Identify one or more health topics that you would like to learn more about:	
Identity one or more communities that you would like to learn more about:	
What I will do to enhance my counselling skills:	When I will do it:

Figure 9.4 Professional Development Plan

- Participate in case conferences (see Chapter 10 for more information)
- Shadow another counselor
- Ask to sit in and observe an experienced counselor at work. The client must give permission for you to observe before you join the session.
- Self-reflection
  - Make time to think about your own work. Keep a journal. Talk with family and friends about your professional accomplishments and the challenges you face. Use the self-assessment provided in Table 9.3.
- Debrief with colleagues
- Talk with a trusted colleague about your work, particularly the challenges you face and the personal issues that may get in the way of person-centered practice.
- Participate in supervision

- Participate in ongoing supervision with an experienced behavior change counselor or therapist.
- Learn from clients
- *This may be the most valuable way to continue to enhance your skills.* Listen to the feedback that clients provide about your approach, style, and skills. Pay particular attention to any critical feedback that you receive. Try not to be defensive, but to reflect on what you may want to change about the way you work.

  - *Have you participated in any of these professional development activities before?*

  - *Can you think of other strategies and opportunities for professional development?*

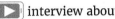

Please watch the following video 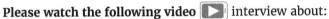 **interview about:**

- *What types of concepts and resources guide your approach to providing person-centered counseling?*

- *What questions and concerns do you have about person-centered counseling?*

- *What is your strategy for continuing to enhance your skills for doing person-centered work?*

DEVELOPING YOUR CLIENT-CENTERED PRACTICE

(*Source:* Foundations for Community Health Workers/http://youtu.be/A71MPjMuYh8)

Chapter Review

Gerald is 38 years old. He has been smoking cigarettes since he was sixteen. He smokes approximately half a pack of cigarettes a day. Gerald's wife and children have been trying to persuade him to stop smoking for many years. Recently, his good friend and neighbor died of lung cancer, and Gerald is newly motivated to stop. He has tried to stop smoking on his own, but never lasted longer than a month or two. He says: *"Smoking has been a part of my life for so long, I don't know what I'd do without it. It helps me to relax. It's what I do."*

You are a CHW working with Gerald. He shares the following information with you:

- *"I just don't want to let my family down, particularly my wife. I know she's scared I could get sick."*

- *"You think I'm bad now. I tell you, when I was younger, I used to smoke a pack a day or more."*

- *"You know, I wasn't gonna say anything, but I used to drink too much. It almost ruined my marriage. My wife, she asked me to move out at one point. She told me she wouldn't take me back if I kept it up. And I did it. I quit, and I haven't had alcohol in nine years."*

- *"Is it gonna make any difference now—quitting? I've probably done enough damage already. Sometimes I lie awake at night, and I worry that cancer is already there."*

- *"I don't know if I can quit. I used to think I'd give it up by the time I was thirty or forty, but I just never did. It embarrasses me, but I don't know if I've got what it takes to do this. When I stopped before, all I thought about was smoking."*

Please practice answering the following questions about how you would work to support Gerald:

1. Where is Gerald on the Stages of Change in relation to stopping smoking?

2. What is an example of a harm-reduction strategy or approach that Gerald might take?

3. Use your OARS. Based on the information provided above, provide at least two examples of each of the following that you would ask or share with Gerald:
   - Open-ended questions
   - Affirming statements
   - Reflective statements
   - Summaries

4. Explain two different ways that you could use a 0–10 scale when working with Gerald.

5. Gerald says to you: *"I know my wife wants me to quit, but I don't think I can. I've smoked for too many years, and what good is quitting now gonna do me now anyway?"* How would you respond in a way that demonstrates rolling with resistance?

6. What will you do if you become aware that your own issues are interfering with your ability to provide person-centered counseling?

7. Identify at least three things that you will do to continue to enhance your person-centered counseling skills, and when you will do them.

References

Bischof, G., Bischof, A., Rumpf, H. J. (2021). Motivational interviewing: An evidence-based approach for use in medical practice. Deutsches Ärzteblatt *International*, 118(7): 109–115. https://doi: 10.3238/arztebl. m2021.0014.

Bodenheimer, T., Laing, B. Y. (2007). The teamlet model of primary care. *Annals of Family Medicine*, 5(5),457–461. https:// doi: 10.1370/afm.731.

Centers for Disease Control and Prevention. (2009). YES WE CAN Children's Asthma Program. https://www.cdc.gov/asthma/interventions/yes_we_can_toolkit.htm.

Chan, D. N. S. & So, W. K. W. (2021). Effectiveness of motivational interviewing in enhancing cancer screening update amongst average-risk individuals; A systematic review. *International Journal of Nursing Studies*, 113. https://doi.org/10.1016/j.injurstu.2020.103786.

Chen, H-M., Lee, H-L., Yang, F-C., Chiu, Y-W, Chao S-Y. (2020). Effectiveness of motivational interviewing in regard to activities of daily living and motivation for rehabilitation among stroke patients. *International Journal of Environmental Research and Public Health* 17(8), 2755. https://doi.org/10.3390/ijerph17082755.

Hawk, M., Coulter, R. W. S., Egan, J. E., Fisk, S., Friedman, M. R., Tula, M., Kinsky, S. (2017). Harm reduction principles for healthcare settings. *Harm Reduction Journal* 14, 70. https://doi.org/10.1186/s12954-017-0196-4.

Miller, W. R. & Rollnick, S. (2013). *Motivational interviewing: Helping people change*, 3rd ed. New York: Guilford Press.

Motivational Interviewing Network of Trainers. (2010). Four Fundamental Processes in MI. https://www.motivationalinterviewing.org/sites/default/files/Four%20Fundamental%20Processes%20in%20MI-REV%20w%20definition.pdf (accessed 15 November 2022).

Motivational Interviewing Network of Trainers. (2022). Understanding Motivational Interviewing. https://motivationalinterviewing.org/understanding-motivational-interviewing (accessed 15 November 2022).

National Harm Reduction Coalition. (2022). Principles of Harm Reduction. https://harmreduction.org/about-us/principles-of-harm-reduction/ (accessed 15 November 2022).

Newcomers Health Program. (2023). San Francisco Department of Public Health. https://zuckerbergsanfranciscogeneral.org/refugee-services/ (accessed 13 May 2023).

Prochaska, J., Norcross, J., & DiClemente, C. (1999). *Changing for good: A revolutionary six-stage program for overcoming bad habits and moving your life positively forward.* New York: Avon Books.

Substance Abuse & Mental Health Services Administration. (2019). Using motivational interviewing in substance use disorder treatment. *Treatment Improvement Protocol (TIP)*, 35. https://store.samhsa.gov/sites/default/files/SAMHSA_Digital_Download/PEP20-02-02-014.pdf (accessed 15 November 2022).

United Nations News. (2022). More than 100 Million now Forcibly Displaced: UNHCR Report. United Nations. https://news.un.org/en/story/2022/06/1120542 (accessed 19 December 2022).

United States Census Bureau. (2022). Demographic Turning Points for the United States: Populations Projections for 2020 to 2060. https://www.census.gov/content/dam/Census/library/publications/2020/demo/p25-1144.pdf (accessed 30 December 2022).

Wang, C., Liu, K., Sun, X., Yin, Y., & Tang, T. (2022). Effectiveness of motivational interviewing among patients with COPD: A systematic review with meta-analysis and trial sequential analysis of randomized controlled trials. *Patient Education and Counseling.* https://doi.org/10.1016/j.pec.2022.07.019.

Additional Resources

Hartney, E. (2021). What is Motivational Interviewing. verywellmind. https://www.verywellmind.com/what-is-motivational-interviewing-22378.

Health Leads. (2018). Patient-Centered Care: Elements, Benefits, Examples. https://healthleadsusa.org/resources/patient-centered-care-elements-benefits-and-examples/.

Miller, W. R. & Rollnick, S. (1991). *Motivational interviewing: preparing people to change addictive behavior.* New York, NY: Guilford Press.

Motivational Interviewing Network of Trainers. https://motivationalinterviewing.org/about_mint (accessed 15 November 2022).

Portillo, E. M., Vasquez, D., & Brown, L. D. (2020). Promoting hispanic immigrant health via community health workers and motivational interviewing. *International Quarterly of Community Health Education*, 41(1), 3–6. https://doi:10.1177/0272684X19896731.

Rollnick, S., & Miller, W. R. (1995). *What is motivational interviewing? Behavioral and Cognitive Psychotherapy*, 23, 325–334.

Santana, M. J., Manalili, K., Jolley, R. J., Zelinsky, S., Quan, H., & Lu, M. (2018). How to practice person-centred care: A conceptual framework. *Health Expectations*, 21(2), 429–440. https://doi: 10.1111/hex.12640.

University of North Caroline Center for AIDS Research. Motivational Interviewing Components: Spirit of Motivational Interviewing. https://uncmotivationalinterviewing.wordpress.com/2016/12/31/motivational-interviewing-components-spirit-of-motivational-interviewing/ (accessed 15 November 2022).

Urban Alliance. (2022). An Introduction to Motivational Interviewing. https://www.urbanalliance.com/Customer-Content/www/CMS/files/covid_temp/MotivationalInterviewing_Rev7_11_19.pdf (accessed 15 November 2022).

World Health Organization. People-centered health care: a policy framework. (2013). https://www.who.int/publications/i/item/9789290613176 (accessed 15 November 2022).

World Health Organization. (n.d.). HIV/AIDS Training. http://www.who.int/hiv/topics/vct/toolkit/components/training/en/index4.html (accessed 15 November 2022).

Case Management

Tim Berthold and Cristina Arellano

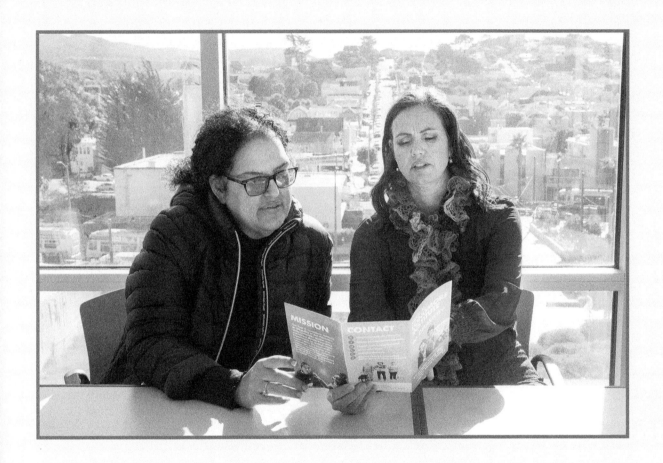

Foundations for Community Health Workers, Third Edition. Edited by Tim Berthold and Darouny Somsanith.
© 2024 John Wiley & Sons, Inc. Published 2024 by John Wiley & Sons, Inc.
Companion website: http://www.wiley.com/go/communityhealthworkers3E

Client Scenario: Marcos Bernales

Marcos Bernales is thirty-eight and unhoused. Three years ago, Marcos lost his job and had to move out of his apartment. Marcos sold most of his belongings and lived in his car until it was towed away for having too many unpaid parking tickets. Since then, he has been sleeping in an encampment under a freeway overpass or in the doorway of a local restaurant.

Marcos used to live with his younger brother but moved out four years ago after his niece was born. Marcos says that he hasn't been in touch with his brother since he lost his job and his apartment: "*I don't want to bother them with my troubles.*"

A city outreach worker refers Marcos to WrapAround Health to meet with a case manager. WrapAround Health is a neighborhood health center that provides primary health care, behavioral health care, and social support services.

Marcos meets with a case manager for an initial intake. Marcos wears a pair of large, dark sunglasses, even inside the health center. When Marcos takes his glasses off to look at a flyer about housing options, the case manager notices a large scar over his left eye. When asked about the scar over his eye, Marcos says, "*It's nothing to worry about.*"

Marcos doesn't share much during the first meeting. He wants help finding work and a safe place to live. When the case manager asks him if he is willing to go to a shelter and if he is interested in a transitional housing program, Marcos says: "*Either one. Anything. I never thought I'd be living on the streets this long.*" The case manager asks, "*Can I ask where you were living before you were living on the streets, Marcos?*"

Marcos shakes his head and changes the subject, "*Can I get into a shelter tonight?*"

The case manager calls a colleague who works at SafeSpace and is able to reserve a shelter bed for Marcos in three days. "*Unfortunately, they don't have a bed for you tonight. You can always check in with them again tomorrow, but you have a guaranteed space starting on Thursday.*" Marcos knows where SafeSpace is, "*I've stayed there before.*" The case manager provides Marcos with a transportation voucher and the name of the colleague at SafeSpace and encourages him to check in with her.

Marcos is also placed on a waiting list for transitional housing. The case manager explains that it can sometimes take many months before a transitional housing opportunity opens up and, when it does, he will have to be interviewed and approved before he can move in. Marcos and the case manager schedule a follow-up meeting 10 days later.

If you were the Community Health Worker assigned to work with Marcos Bernales, how would you answer the following questions:

- What types of services can you provide as a case manager?
- How might Marcos Bernales benefit from case management services?
- What health risks and challenges is Marcos facing?
- What strengths and resources does Marcos possess?
- What additional information are you hoping to learn from Marcos?
- What types of referrals might you share with Marcos, and how will you share them (what will you say)?
- How will you document your work?

Introduction

This chapter provides an introduction to basic knowledge and skills for providing case management services. As a case manager, you will support clients in creating a realistic plan to promote their own health and well-being and to take action to implement their plan. You will link clients to resources, programs, and services to enhance their health and safety. You may also help them with navigating systems (such as health care and health insurance), advocacy and self-empowerment, and short- and long-term goal planning.

WHAT YOU WILL LEARN

By studying the information in this chapter, you will be able to:

- Define case management
- Explain your scope of practice as a case manager
- Demonstrate a strength-based approach to working with clients
- Support clients to develop a detailed case management plan designed to promote their health and well-being
- Identify and provide meaningful referrals to community resources
- Discuss when and how to advocate with or for a client
- Clearly document the case management services you provide
- Identify opportunities for team-based practice and consultation with your supervisor

C3 Roles and Skills Addressed in Chapter 10

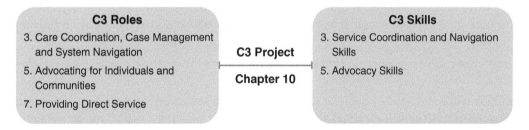

WORDS TO KNOW

Action Plans	SMART Goals
Case Management	Warm Handoff
Caseload	Wellness and Recovery Action Plan
Electronic Health Record	

10.1 Defining Case Management

Because we live in a society characterized by inequitable access to basic resources, rights, and opportunities, many people face significant barriers to health and wellness. Clients who participate in case management develop and implement a plan (we will refer to this as an Action Plan) to improve their health. A key goal for case management is to support the autonomy or independence of clients and to enhance their skills and confidence for managing health and social challenges independently.

Case management services are provided in a wide variety of settings including health care, social services, academic, and legal/criminal justice settings. Case management services are provided by a broad range of helping professionals such as nurses, physicians, social workers, licensed counselors, and CHWs. There are case management associations and trainings at the state, national and international levels. Some of these associations serve specific professions or types of organizations (such as schools or maternal and child health programs) and others are more inclusive. Many of these organizations provide trainings, certifications, and standards of practice to members. To learn more, please go to the section on Additional Resources at the end of this chapter.

As we conducted research for this chapter, we found dozens of definitions of case management. The following definition comes from the Case Management Society of America:

> *Case Management is a collaborative process of assessment, planning, facilitation, care coordination, evaluation and advocacy for options and services to meet an individual's and family's comprehensive health needs through communication and available resources to promote patient safety, quality of care, and cost effective outcomes. (CMSA, 2022)*

Please note that several different terms are used to describe these services including case management, care management, care coordination, and systems navigation. As a working CHW, the agency that employs you will orient you to the language, policies, and protocols that they use to provide these services. For the purposes of this chapter, we will use the term case management.

What Is the "Case" to Be "Managed"?

Some people object to the term *case management* because it may be interpreted to suggest that clients are "cases" who need to be "managed." That view of people would clearly undermine the person-centered practice of CHWs, who work to support the autonomy and self-determination of clients. We view the "case" that requires management as the social context that creates health inequities and limits access to essential resources. Case management supports clients to overcome existing barriers and gain improved access to essential resources.

CHW case managers work for a wide variety of public and private sector agencies and with programs that address a wide range of health issues such as primary health care, housing, mental health, domestic violence, maternal and child health, infectious diseases such as tuberculosis or HIV/AIDS, and chronic conditions such as diabetes or asthma.

Case management services are provided in varied locations such as an agency office, a client's home, in the hospital, in jails or prison, in a homeless shelter, soup kitchen, residential drug recovery program, on the streets, or through phone or internet connections.

Case management services are generally provided on an ongoing basis. It takes time for clients to develop and implement an action plan and to gain access to new resources and services. For example, it typically takes many months to gain access to stable housing. Case managers may work with clients from two to three months to a year or more. Some people experience ongoing needs for support and some agencies provide case management services without a time limit.

TG: At my agency, we are supposed to work with clients for about six months, but some of my clients need more time, and sometimes I don't see them for a while and then I start working with them again. One of my clients, we've been working together for 18 months. He just got out of jail and then went into the hospital, and he called me from there. I'm just glad that he keeps calling and reaching out to me, and even if he doesn't always succeed, I know that he wants a better life.

Your **caseload**—or the number of clients you work with at one time—can range widely from 20 to fifty or more, depending on the nature of the program you work for, the level of complexity and severity of a client's circumstances, relevant policies, and how frequently you have contact with clients.

Cristina Arellano: As a supportive housing case manager, my caseload is usually 26 but has gone up to as high as 32. The clients are referred to our program through the county. They are considered our community's most vulnerable population due to age, chronic conditions, and years spent unhoused. Because of the complexity of the clients' circumstances, I am considered their long-term case manager. The goal is for them to become stable enough not to need me week-to-week. The reality is that many of them will always need a case manager, especially as they age and their health declines. I talk with some clients three to four times a week. Others, I may only see once or twice a month, depending on their needs.

One of the challenges with the concept of case management is that it seems to imply that the services and resources that clients need actually exist in all local communities. *The reality, however, is that many communities lack essential resources* such as transitional or affordable housing options, food assistance programs, mental health services, legal services, and educational or employment opportunities.

* *What types of services and resources are lacking or most difficult to access in the places where you live and work?*

What Do YOU? Think

RESEARCH ON THE ROLE OF CHWS IN CONDUCTING CASE MANAGEMENT

Research studies from the United States and other nations indicate that case management services provided by CHWs have a positive impact on health and social outcomes for the patients and families they serve.

The Centers for Disease Control and Prevention released a report in 2015 on the role of CHWs in addressing chronic health conditions. The effectiveness of CHW case management was measured in high-risk or priority populations, which often do not receive or benefit from services they need. This report highlights the unique role of CHWs as "culturally competent mediators, . . . between providers of health services and the members of diverse communities" (National Center for Chronic Disease Prevention and Health Promotion, 2015). The CDC findings support the integration of CHWs in the role of case managers in health care teams, including in the prevention and control of various chronic health conditions such as hypertension, cardiovascular disease, breast, cervical, colorectal and prostate cancers, diabetes, and asthma.

Research has also highlighted the effectiveness of case management services provided by CHWs in improving health outcomes related to the management of pediatric asthma (Coutinho, Subzwari, McQuaid, & Koinis-Mitchell, 2020), sickle cell disease (Smith et al., 2019), malaria (Paintain et al., 2014), and mental health conditions (Weaver & Lapidos, 2018).

CHW Profile

Nilda Palacios. She/Her

Community Health Worker, Behavioral Health

Lifelong Medical Care, William Jenkins Health Center, Urgent Care

Health and social services to people of all ages, pediatrics to geriatrics

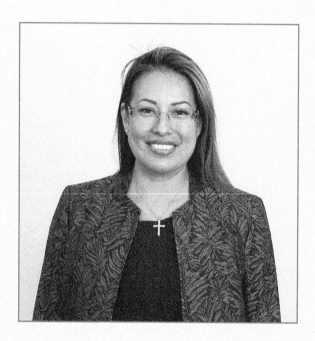

As a formerly incarcerated individual, I was able to connect with the Transitions Clinic. They provide health care to people coming home from prison. As a patient, I met a team of CHWs and observed the work they do. I witnessed the sincere compassion, respect, and dignity they show people, their caring and way of being non-judgmental. I asked them how I could do what they do. The next school semester, I registered for CHW classes at the local community college.

As a CHW with Lifelong Medical Care in Richmond, California, I serve families in the urgent care department, folks experiencing mental health issues, individuals and families who do not qualify for Medi-Cal and want to enroll in Covered California and Family Pack (health insurance programs in California) and Contra Costa CARES (a county program that covers immigrant adults). I help out at the food drives on Wednesdays from 10 AM until all the food /groceries are gone. I get to meet the families who come and to tell them about some of our other services such as our wellness and fitness groups, our women's health services, our group for pregnant mothers, and help with getting health insurance. We don't deny anyone services, whether they are working or not or have insurance or not.

I worked with a patient who was 65 years of age and unhoused, who came to our urgent care department with shortness of breath. He was diagnosed with asthma and prescribed an inhaler. When I met the patient, I noticed he did not have a source of communication like an Obama phone (free cell phone plans for people living near the poverty line). I asked the patient if we could call Medi-Cal to get his health insurance up to date so that he could get his medication. Then we worked on getting him a phone, housing, and food. Working with this patient, he was able to get his medication through Medi-Cal, and he received an Obama phone and eventually got housing with Senior Living. He was able to register for the Marin Food Bank to deliver food to his new home.

(continues)

CHW Profile

(continued)

Working as a CHW has helped me to be spiritually grounded and to connect with people like myself who have mental health needs. I remember how much I struggled when I first got out of prison. With time, I was able to trust CHWs as they guided me through connecting with health care and searching for housing. I have been home now for four years, and there are many things I have overcome. I used to have anxiety and a phobia about crowds and people, but now I help people to manage their anxiety and panic attacks. I still face a few challenges but working as a CHW has helped me to work through these challenges and improve my own health.

A few tips that come to mind for new CHWs. Maintain distinctive and clear boundaries and meet clients with empathy and patience. Sometimes, clients rely upon us for answers, and they will keep calling us to help them with everything. Clients sometimes give up on themselves too soon, and they need extra encouragement and support. It is important that they find their own strength and abilities to meet their goals. You can help them to find their own way. When I started out, I was hard on myself and it was difficult to admit my mistakes. Now I now there is always room for improvement; I am still learning. As CHWs, allow yourself to keep learning and improving. Making mistakes is just part of improving.

10.2 Basic Case Management Concepts

The approach to case management provided in this chapter draws on concepts of health equity, cultural humility, and person-centered practice discussed in other Chapters of the *Foundations* textbook.

The Case Management Society of America promotes the following philosophy of case management:

> *The underlying premise of case management is based in the fact that when an individual reaches the optimum level of wellness and functional capability, everyone benefits: the individuals being served, their support systems, the health care delivery systems and the various reimbursement sources. Case management serves as a means for achieving client wellness and autonomy through advocacy, communication, education, identification of service resources and service facilitation. The case manager helps identify appropriate providers and facilities throughout the continuum of services, while ensuring that available resources are being used in a timely and cost-effective manner in order to obtain optimum value for both the client and the reimbursement source. Case management services are best offered in a climate that allows direct communication between the case manager, the client, and appropriate service personnel, in order to optimize the outcome for all concerned. (Case Management Society of America, 2022)*

The Global Social Service Workforce Alliance is an international network of licensed and unlicensed social services providers dedicated to "alleviate poverty, challenge and reduce discrimination, promote social justice and human rights, and prevent and respond to violence and family separation" (GSSWA, 2022). The Alliance website includes resources for case managers and other social service workers and programs. This includes a list of Guiding Principles for Case Management. While these Guiding Principles overlap considerably with the list of key elements provided above, we wish to highlight several of the principles here (GSSWA, 2018):

- **Resilience:** Case management services should work to increase the resilience of the client, "an ability to better withstand shocks and adversities that arise without negative or debilitating consequences."
- **Cultural humility:** Case managers "should know about and respect the local cultures and tradition that apply in the area in which they are working. Respect for diversity, culture and tradition also means looking for local solutions and using community resources where possible when setting goals and case planning."
- **Client consent:** Case management "requires a clear explanation of the case management process, roles and responsibilities, and an opportunity for the client ... to provide verbal or written consent."
- **Supervision:** "Supportive supervision involves regular meetings between the supervisor and social service worker performing case management to agree on work plans, carry out individual case review, support decision making, provide support to cope with stress, and identity on-the-job training and professional development opportunities."

SCOPE OF PRACTICE AND WORKING AS PART OF A TEAM

As a case manager, you will work as part of a team. *The most important member of any team is always the client.* Teams may also include the client's family and always include additional health or social services providers such as social workers, counselors, teachers, occupational or physical therapists, health care interpreters, chaplains or other faith-based leaders, nurses, or physicians. If you are working as part of a larger team, take time to clarify and understand the roles and scope of practice of each team member (review Chapter 5 for more on scope of practice and working with teams).

Ideally, your team will meet regularly to discuss your work, the client's progress, and how best to collaborate in order to promote the client's health and wellness. The agency and program you work for should provide you with clear written policies and protocols to guide your work as a member of a team. These generally include participating in team meetings to discuss the welfare of specific clients (sometimes called "case conferences"), described at the end of this chapter.

Sometimes you will question whether a certain aspect of case management is your responsibility or if it should be provided by another member of the team. Remember to consult with your colleagues to clarify these concerns.

COMMON STAGES OF CASE MANAGEMENT

Case management generally consists of several distinct stages including:

- The initial assessment of a client's strengths, needs, and priorities.
  - As a CHW, you may conduct part of this assessment. Your colleagues will assess other aspects of the client's health and life circumstances. Physicians or nurse practitioners, for example, will assess the client's health status, diagnose health conditions, and prescribe treatments.
- Development of a case management or action plan.
- Implementation of the action plan.
- Monitoring progress and revise key elements of the plan based on the client's experience, progress, and shifting priorities or needs.
- The end or completion of case management (sometimes referred to as discharge or termination).
- Evaluation of case management services and outcomes
  - Evaluation seeks to determine how effective case management services are in promoting the health and well-being of clients, to identify challenges or problems and opportunities to strengthen the quality of services.

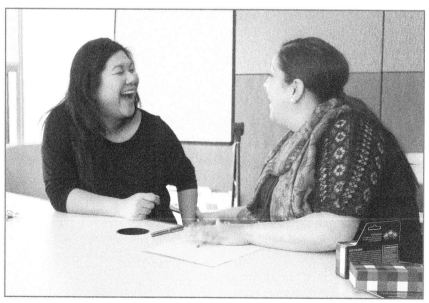

A client connects with a CHW.

10.3 Developing the Case Management Plan

The focus of case management is to develop a person-centered plan documenting the strengths, needs, goals, and actions that will be taken to promote the client's health and well-being. Depending on where you are working, this document may be called an action plan, care plan, treatment plan, care coordination plan, service plan, case management plan, self-care plan, or other terms. For the purposes of this chapter, we will refer to it as an action plan.

Action plans are varied and use different electronic data systems, forms, categories, and language. Some action plans are designed to be broad and comprehensive in nature, while others may focus on particular health or social issues such as mental health concerns, substance abuse, housing, or pregnancy and parenting. Some plans are elaborate and may require many pages of documentation, including an extensive assessment. Others are more focused and require fewer details. The type of plan you develop with clients will depend on the agency and the program you work for, the funding source for that program, the primary topic or health issue the program is concerned with (such as housing, perinatal health, or substance use), and the population you serve. Despite these differences, most case management plans include the following:

- An assessment of the client's strengths and existing resources, current health conditions and challenges, their priority concerns, and goals. For more information about conducting an initial assessment with a new client, please see Chapter 8.
- The development of a detailed action plan outlining practical steps designed to reach identified goals.
- Documentation of who is responsible for putting each step into action (client, care manager, or other professional).
- Release of information forms signed by clients and the agencies they work with to permit agencies and providers to share specific information about the client. Note that with the emergence of electronic health records, client information is more commonly shared between agencies and programs (always with the client's permission).
- Documentation of referrals provided and accessed, and outcomes.
- Progress notes.
- Documentation of the end of case management services (also known as discharge or termination).

An action plan is a working document to keep everyone focused on the client's desired goals and steps to achieve them. After the plan is developed, it is usually signed by the client or family, the case manager, and sometimes by another member of a team who you may be working with, such as a nurse or social worker. As a working document, the plan can and is likely to be revised and updated over time, based on the experience, and needs of the client.

You can find hundreds of examples of case management plans online (search for case management plans).

THE FIRST MEETING BETWEEN CLIENT AND CASE MANAGER

Before starting to conduct an assessment or to develop a case management plan, apply the skills you learned in Chapter 8 to:

- Welcome the client warmly
- Build rapport and the beginning of a trusting relationship with the client
- Explain the nature and the extent of the services that you can provide as a case manager
- Describe any program restrictions and/or costs
- Clearly explain the limits of client confidentiality and other essential program policies
  - This may include asking clients to review or sign Release of Information forms to permit sharing information with other providers and agencies
- Obtain informed consent (and HIPAA if working in a health care setting) to proceed with the assessment process
- Answer the client's questions and concerns

Take time to clearly explain your role as a case manager, the types of questions you will ask as part of the assessment, and the purpose of asking such questions, as in the example that follows.

> **Cristina Arellano:** When I meet clients in my office, I offer them something to drink from the lunchroom. I ask if they have eaten that day. Whenever I meet with a client for an initial intake, I have a bag of canned nonperishable food items in my office—things that don't require a lot of cooking. Clients rarely turn down this bag of food. I can tell that a lot of people really appreciate it, and it starts a conversation about where and how they get their food, if they have access to cooking facilities, and if they are comfortable preparing meals. It is also a way of showing I care about their well-being. It lets them know that I can be a supportive resource. Providing food bags or referrals to a local food pantry or program that serves hot meals is a tangible benefit for clients.

Client Scenario: Marcos Bernales *(continued)*

CHW: Marcos, I'd like to spend some time today reviewing and developing your action plan. This will involve talking about some of the important resources that you already have, some of your priority concerns and goals, and resources and services that you hope to access. How does this sound?

Marcos Bernales: That's okay.

CHW: I want to make sure that I'm accurately documenting what you already shared with me during our first meeting. I wrote down that you want to find safe and stable housing and a new job, and to complete your GED. Is this right?

Marcos: Yes, I really want to get off the streets. A safer place to stay is my number one priority.

CHW: Okay, we'll prioritize housing. You're staying at the SafeSpace shelter now, correct?

Marcos: Yeah, I've been staying there, but I don't want to stay there too long.

CHW: You also applied for transitional housing, so you're on the wait list. The problem is that there are too few available places for all the people who need housing. It may take several months, maybe longer, for a housing option to open up for you. And, as I hope I explained before, you would still need to interview with the housing manager or landlord before they offer you a place.

Marcos: I understand. I've been waiting awhile so. . . I'll just try to keep waiting.

CHW: I appreciate your patience Marcos, and we'll keep checking in about the status of your application each time we meet. I can also help you with other goals or concerns. Here's a copy of the form that we use to create your plan [The CHW hands Marcos a copy of the plan]. If you have any questions about any of this just let me know, okay?

[Marcos nods]

CHW: The most important thing I want to say is that this is your plan. I'll make suggestions from time to time, about resources or actions that I think may be helpful, but please know that these are just suggestions for you to consider and to accept or reject as you wish.

Marcos: Thanks, that sounds good. I have a pretty good idea of what I need.

CHW: So your first priority goal is to access stable housing, and the actions that you are implementing include staying at SafeSpace and submitting an application to the city for transitional housing. You've already completed both of these actions. What would you like to focus on next? We could talk about getting your GED and a new job, or any other goal or priority that you have.

Marcos: Well, let me think. [Marcos pauses] Let's talk about _____

CONDUCTING AN ASSESSMENT

The purpose of an assessment is to establish a clear common understanding of the client's primary concerns, strengths, priorities, and goals. This information is then used to guide the development of an action plan designed to meet the client's goals and promote their health.

The assessment typically consists of gathering four types of information from clients:

1. Basic demographic information
2. The client's strengths (or internal and external resources)
3. The client's current risks and needs (including the need for additional resources)
4. The client's concerns and goals

In Chapter 8, we discussed how asking for demographic information—the client's date of birth, address, family status, employment status, gender, ethnicity, and so forth—can create an uncomfortable distance between you and a client at the very moment when you are trying to establish a positive professional connection. For this reason, we suggest that you don't begin the assessment by gathering all the required demographic data. Instead, start with questions that are more likely to put clients at ease and may be most important to them, such as: *"How can we support you?" "What are your current concerns and priorities?"*

When Forms Don't Recognize People's Identities

Review the forms at your agency. Are they inclusive of the identities of all people? Do they provide options other than single, married, and divorced to document relationship status? Do the forms recognize gender identities other than female and male? Do they recognize multiracial identities or instead force people to identify with just one ethnic category? If the questions we ask and the forms we use to document information aren't inclusive of the diverse identities of the clients we serve, we risk offending them and undermining our ability to work together successfully.

ASSESSING THE CLIENT'S STRENGTHS AND AVAILABLE RESOURCES

Person-centered practice emphasizes the importance of assessing, valuing, and building on a client's strengths. Starting from a person's strengths means recognizing and valuing what they have, rather than what they don't have; what they can do, rather than what they can't do; and what they've accomplished, rather than their perceived mistakes or failures. Focusing on strengths guides you and clients in identifying *all* of the resources available to assist in enhancing their health and independence.

Assessment typically doesn't happen all at once during one interview. Rather, you will learn more about the client's strengths as you establish your working relationship.

TG: I don't always start with a big assessment. I'll ask a few questions but come back to the rest later as I get to know the client. Generally, I want to listen first to what is on their mind. They almost always have an idea of something they want, or want to change, or some resource that they need. If I can start by learning about that and working to help them out—like helping them find a good doc (doctor) or some clean clothes or something to eat—then they're more likely to open up and answer the questions I want to ask.

We encourage you to use a combination of open-ended and closed-ended questions to conduct your assessment of both strengths and needs, as explained in Chapters 8 and 9. The program you work for and the policies, protocols, and forms that you use will provide a certain degree of guidance about how to conduct your assessment and how to identify the client's strengths. Strengths include the client's own knowledge, skills, accomplishments, and beliefs (internal resources) as well as their connection to external resources such as family and friends, housing, employment, health care, and social, cultural, and spiritual or religious groups and organizations. More information about internal and external resources is provided in Chapter 12.

Over time, you will gain a deeper understanding of the client's strengths. One of the pleasures of case management is that you will often have the opportunity to witness clients developing new strengths along the way.

ASSESSING CLIENT RISKS AND NEEDS FOR ADDITIONAL RESOURCES

Case managers also ask questions to guide people in identifying current life challenges, risks, and the need for additional resources. The client's needs and interest in accessing resources such as housing, interpretation services, drug or alcohol treatment, employment, legal assistance, and health care are also addressed.

Open-ended questions (see Chapter 9) are particularly helpful because they provide the client with an opportunity to identify needs that you may not ask about. Open-ended questions might include: *"What are you most concerned about right now?" "What are you hoping to achieve through our work together?" "What is the biggest challenge that you face right now?" "What do you most want to change about your life?" "What resources do you most need in your life?" "What are the biggest risks to your health right now?"*

Finally, the client is asked to prioritize the risks and needs identified during the assessment. The case manager asks which of these issues or problems the client is most concerned about and what resources they most want to access. For example, Marcos might say that a steady job and a safe place to live are his highest priorities. He might also talk about his headaches, the assault he survived, his difficulty sleeping, or his lack of contact with his family. The client's priorities are then used to create their action plan.

(*Source:* Foundations for Community Health Workers/ http://youtu.be/ isOQoAF4kAA/ last accessed 21 September 2023.)

Please watch the following video ▶ interview on *Establishing Client Priorities*.

IDENTIFYING CASE MANAGEMENT GOALS

> **Martha Shearer:** Each individual comes with so many different issues. I had a 72-year-old patient who was gone [incarcerated] for 30 years. His parents died while he was gone. He needed food stamps, medication, possibly housing, help with reintegration into society, and clothes. At first, I thought, "this is more than I should take on," but then I realized, "but who else will do it?" It takes a lot for a person to be reintegrated—they may need help advocating with family, with parole, and with housing, and that is the perfect job for a CHW!

Based on the assessment, you will support the client to identify one or more specific goals for their action plan. While it is often meaningful for clients to talk about their ultimate life goals (working as a counselor, reuniting with and living near children or grandchildren, owning their own home, and finding a sense of peace), the purpose of case management is typically to address more immediate concerns. The goals should come from the client, not the case manager, and should be specific and realistic. For example, while a client may not be able to purchase their own home in the next 6–12 months, the client may be able to find stable housing or a place in a transitional housing program. If goals are too unrealistic, this may set the client up for disappointment or a sense of failure. A key task of the case manager is to guide and support clients to develop goals that they can realistically work toward within a specified time frame such as three or six months. Other goals may include, for example, securing a part-time or full-time job, entering a drug treatment program, getting school clothes for their children, reducing blood pressure, or working to reestablish contact with family members.

Smart Action Plans

Health and social services providers often use the SMART system for developing health or case management goals. For action plans to be most effective in supporting clients to reach their goals, they should be:

i. **Specific:** the goal or objective clearly states what the client wants to achieve in a way that anyone who reads it can understand.
   a. An example of a goal that is not specific enough: To improve my health.
   b. An example of a specific goal: To keep my blood pressure within a healthy range or less than 120/80.

(continues)

Smart Action Plans
(continued)

2. **Measurable**: Action plans should be measurable in order for the client and their provider to be able to assess their progress. A plan to "walk as much as possible," or to "go to the gym," or "to eat healthier" is harder to assess. Encourage the client to set more measurable actions such as "Walk 3 times a week for at least 60 minutes."

3. **Attainable**: Action plans should be possible for clients to implement or achieve. Actions such as jogging 10 miles a week may not be attainable, especially for clients who don't have experience running. A more attainable goal might be to start with walking around the block, or to the corner, or whatever the client is able to do now. As the client is successful in implementing smaller actions or steps, they can gradually increase their goals, building for continued success.

4. **Relevant**: Does the plan address goals and actions that are meaningful to the client? Does the plan fit with the client's values, cultural identity, and current resources?

5. **Timely (or Time-bound)**: The goals and actions should clearly specify when they will be completed. Vague statements such as "Walk as much as possible when I can" are less likely to be completed. Start with some specific times, such as: "Walk to the dog park and back on Saturday morning. Walk for at least 20 minutes."

SMART Goal Worksheet

Today's Date: _____ Target Date: _____ Start Date:_____

Date Achieved: _____

Goal:_____

Verify that your goal is SMART

Specific: *What exactly will you accomplish?*

_____
_____

Measurable: How will you know when you have reached this goal?

_____
_____
_____

Achievable: *Is achieving this goal realistic with effort and commitment? Do you have the resources to achieve this goal? If not, how will you get them?*

_____
_____
_____

Relevant: *Why is this goal significant to your life?*

_____
_____
_____

(continues)

SMART Goal Worksheet
(continued)

Timely: *When will you achieve this goal? How frequently will you take these actions?*

_____
_____
_____

This goal is important because:

_____
_____

The benefits of achieving this goal will be:

_____
_____
_____

Take Action!

Potential Obstacles	Potential Solutions
_____	_____
_____	_____
_____	_____
_____	_____
_____	_____

Who are the people you will ask to help you?

_____
_____
_____

Specific Action Steps: *What steps need to be taken to get you to your goal?*

What Steps?	Expected Completion Date
_____	_____
_____	_____
_____	_____
_____	_____

ENSURING THAT PLANS REFLECT THE PRIORITIES OF CLIENTS

When you provide case management services and work with a client to develop and implement an action plan, you will establish priority issues or goals to work on. The issues that you as a case manager view as priorities may be different from those of the client. *Always work in a way that honors and respects the client's wishes; it is their plan, after all, not yours.*

As you work together, you will offer information, referrals, and options for the client to consider for how to meet their goals. A soft touch is required here; clients will notice and often resist if you try to push your own agenda. Keep in mind that clients are much more likely to have success if their action plans reflect their own ideas, respect their boundaries, and honor their limitations. One way to share a resource or an option with a client is as a suggestion for them to consider: *"Marcos, there is a local organization called The JobStop that helps people with getting their GED and finding employment. They have helped a lot of the clients I work with. Their services are free. Would you be interested in learning more about this resource?"* Pose this as an idea that may or may not be of interest to the client.

CHWs are often employed by programs that focus on specific health issues and outcomes. For example, you may work for a primary care clinic with the goal of supporting patients to manage chronic health conditions such as diabetes and hypertension. Your employer may want you to prioritize actions such as medication management and healthy eating to reduce the client's blood pressure and improve their blood glucose levels. However, some of the clients you work with may have other more immediate priorities that pose risks to their health or the health of their families. They may be unhoused, experiencing food insecurity or domestic violence. They may be taking care of family members with even greater health needs. Follow the client's lead and support them to develop an action plan that addresses their first priority concerns. If we don't address a client's true priorities, they may choose to stop working with us. When we support clients to meet their immediate concerns, we build a closer professional relationship. Addressing one priority issue at a time and accomplishing some sort of meaningful change—such as providing them with free groceries or assisting them to apply for transitional housing—will make it that much easier to establish trust and to move forward to address the next priority issue. Keep harm reduction in mind: anything that the client accomplishes that reduces risks for themselves and their family is a good thing. Make sure to acknowledge and celebrate the progress that your clients make.

TG: My clients wouldn't need case management if everything was working out for them. But they are dealing with big problems like HIV disease and on top of that maybe they're homeless, or they lost their job, or they relapsed and started using drugs again, or their boyfriend beats them up and sometimes all of this combined together. And sometimes what I'm paid to do—like get them to follow through with their antiretroviral therapy—may not be a big concern to them. They almost always have other priorities—like being safe, or getting something to eat, or finding a place to stay. If I don't listen to what they want, then why should they listen to me? And if I'm not listening in the first place, then why am I working as a CHW?

DEVELOPING AN ACTION PLAN

The next step is to support the client to identify the actions that they will take to reach their stated goal(s).

Clients may choose to take the following types of actions: changing patterns of diet or exercise; practicing a new stress management technique; reducing their use of alcohol or other drugs; attending support groups; applying for transitional housing or a new job; enrolling in a community college class; or calling or writing letters to their mothers, grandchildren, nephews, or sisters.

Each goal and action should be linked to a specific time frame. The time it takes to complete specific actions will depend upon how difficult the steps in the action plan are and the client's existing knowledge, skills, and motivation. We recommend including action steps with a variety of time frames such as actions that are scheduled to be completed in the next few days, weeks, and months. If the timeline is too long, it increases the likelihood that the actions won't be accomplished. Start with steps that are less intimidating and seem most possible to put into action quickly.

Client Scenario: Marcos Bernales *(continued)*

Actions that Marcos may take include:

- Go to SafeSpace on Thursday September _____ to get a shelter bed.
- Make an appointment to meet with a counselor at The JobStop by next Tuesday (09/___/___).

(continues)

Client Scenario: Marcos Bernales *(continued)*

- Develop a list of his key accomplishments and strengths and most important health and life goals (by the end of September)
- Schedule an appointment ASAP with a WrapAroundHealth physician to assess the injury to Marcos' eye and his persistent headaches
- Consider meeting with a WrapAroundHealth counselor to talk about the assault he survived, his intrusive memories, and difficulties sleeping
- Attend GED classes regularly at The JobStop on Mondays and Wednesdays at noon
- Consider reconnecting with his brother
- Schedule a follow-up meeting with his WrapAroundHealth case manager

Actions that the case manager may take include:

- Before the next appointment, review and identify local resources, including culturally competent mental health counselors, agencies, and services that focus on working with transgender and gender-variant clients.
- Call the eye clinic by _____ to advocate for an earlier appointment for Marcos (current appointment is in three months)
- Continue to monitor – at the beginning of each month – the wait list for transitional housing and keep Marcos informed
- At the next appointment, talk with Marcos about preparing a release of information to talk with other service providers about how best to coordinate efforts.

Wellness and Recovery Action Plans (Wrap)

Wellness and Recovery Action Plans or WRAP are used extensively by peer specialists and CHWs working with clients living with mental health conditions and disabilities. WRAP Plans include several features that may be helpful for any client seeking to create behavior changes or other types of changes in their life.

WRAP Plans ask clients to identify and anticipate events and circumstances that could lead to worsening health conditions or crisis, as well as actions that could prevent or help to manage these circumstances. Clients are asked to reflect on past experiences that were challenging and resulted in a relapse or crisis. By better understanding risk factors they faced in the past, and actions and resources that helped to promote their wellness, clients can more effectively plan for the future.

WRAP Plans include (National Health Service Foundation Trust, 2022):

- A focus on identifying events or circumstances (referred to as "triggers") that may prompt thoughts, feelings, or behaviors that could be harmful to the client's health and well-being.
- Actions that can be taken to avoid or limit exposure to triggering circumstances or events
- Coping strategies that may prevent triggering events from getting worse
- Early Warning Signs "what are the subtle signs of change that indicate you may need to take action to avoid a worsening of your condition of situation?"
- Response Plan for Early Warning Signs
- Signs of a potential Crisis or "when things start breaking down or getting worse—what happens when the situation has become uncomfortable, serious, or even dangerous, but you are still able to take action on your own behalf?"

(continues)

Wellness and Recovery Action Plans (Wrap)
(continued)

- Reducing signs of potential crisis or "what will help you to reduce your signs and symptoms when they have progressed to this point?"
- Crisis Plan. These plans are created in partnership with providers and include guidance about what actions and services can best help the client if they are in crisis.

You can incorporate elements of WRAP Plans into general case management or action plans for clients living with mental health and other chronic health conditions, drug or alcohol use challenges, and other similar issues that may be accompanied by cycles of progress or setbacks, relapse, or crisis.

To learn more about WRAP please see refer to Additional Resources included at the end of this chapter.

COORDINATE WITH OTHER CASE MANAGEMENT TEAM MEMBERS

If you are working as part of a professional team, the client's action plan should be developed collaboratively. The plan will clearly detail which team member and service provider is responsible for which steps. All team members should attend regular meetings to monitor progress and any need to revise the case management plan.

PLANS CAN AND DO CHANGE

Sometimes, clients will feel that part (or all) of their action plan is not working for them. Clients have the right to change their action plans and to withdraw at any time from services or programs that they feel are not working for them. Sometimes new needs emerge that are more important to address than the issues identified in the original action plan. For example, a client may become unhoused or actively suicidal, be arrested, have a death in the family, or relapse and start using drugs again. These circumstances are likely to cause the immediate focus of case management to shift.

When a client is not making progress with the plan, it is time to reassess. Perhaps the action plan or the goals should be revised. Perhaps the case manager should assume new responsibilities, such as advocating with other service providers on behalf of the client. On the one hand, you don't want a client to change the plan so often that no progress can be made (if this happens, it is important to assess why). And on the other hand, you don't want the case management plan to become so rigid that the client wastes time on actions that are not promoting their health or welfare.

Cristina Arellano: An incident or hospitalization may change a client's care plan goals. They may open up about what happened and begin contemplating making a new behavior change.

I worked with a client who opened up to me about their own struggles with recovery from methamphetamine use after his neighbor passed away from complications related to meth use. The client said, "That could've been me," and talked about the daily temptations that he faced just outside his apartment. I had been working with him for eight to nine months and had never heard him speak about his substance use. During this meeting, he talked to me about how difficult it was for him not to use. He had three years clean and sober. After his neighbor passed away, he decided to reach out for support. I listened and I asked him, "What do you do when you think about using?"

We researched resources and found some local Narcotics Anonymous (NA) meetings and spiritual resources that he can access when he feels the need for additional support. Now we check in about his recovery when we meet.

PREPARING A RELEASE OF INFORMATION

You must never reveal confidential client information to another provider unless they are part of your immediate clinical or case management team, or the client has given you written permission to do so (see Chapter 5). It can be beneficial for case managers to talk with other service providers in order to coordinate care and enhance the quality of services provided to clients. For example, you might refer a client to a physician to treat their cancer, to a drug treatment program, or to an immigration attorney. If you and the client agree that it would be helpful for you to be able to talk with the other service provider, you must all sign a release of information form. These forms clearly identify the client, the service providers, the agency they work for, and the nature of the services that they provide. The form will state that the client authorizes the service providers to share information with each other and why. Most forms will detail what kinds of information can be shared between providers and give a timeline for when the agreement will expire or end. All parties must sign the form. These forms are often integrated into electronic health records or data systems shared among common providers within a geographic region such as a city or county.

PROVIDING HEALTH EDUCATION AND PERSON-CENTERED COUNSELING

Some case managers provide health education and person-centered counseling. For example, a case manager working with a client newly diagnosed with diabetes may assess the client's knowledge about their health condition. Depending on the assessment and the extent of the client's knowledge and interest, the case manager may provide additional health education and information to assist the client in better understanding the condition and knowing how to adhere to treatments, reduce symptoms, and enhance their overall health.

DOCUMENTING PROGRESS

Document or write down each contact you have with the client or other service provider who is working with the client. This will include in-person meetings with the client, phone and online conversations, and correspondence by mail. Document all relevant developments, including accomplishments and challenges to implementing the case management plan.

SELF-ASSESSMENT

As a case manager, remember that your job is to support clients to develop clear goals and a plan to improve the quality of their lives and that of their families. Always keep in mind that *it is the client's plan, not yours*. To make sure that you are doing person-centered work, we recommend that you regularly ask yourself the following questions:

- Am I truly listening to the client (BIG EARS, small mouth)?
- Am I demonstrating my interest in and respect for the client?
- Am I pushing my own beliefs, values or ideas onto the client?
- Does this plan recognize the client's strengths and resources?
- Does it address their priority concerns?
- Did the client establish the goals for their case management plan? Did the client determine the list of actions they will take to reach these goals?
- Does the plan support the client's independence?
- Does the client understand, and are they interested in, the referrals provided?

> **TG:** I can't live my client's life for them ... but sometimes I fight the urge to tell them what to do. It gets so frustrating sometimes watching someone make the same mistake over and over again. When I start to feel this way, it is a sign that I need to take care of myself—and I usually talk with another CHW or my supervisor to get myself back on track. It also helps me to focus on the
>
> *(continues)*

(continued)

positive things, no matter how small they may seem. And every once in a while, you get to focus on the truly big positive things.

I was on the bus going home and this guy kept calling my name, and at first, I couldn't tell who it was. It was a client from way back, someone I never thought would make it 'cause he was so caught up in using, and in and out of jail and prison, and really sick with AIDS. He looked so good. He had gained weight; his eyes were clear. He sat down and told me he was back in college studying to be a drug and alcohol counselor, and he had two years clean and sober. When he was getting off the bus, he grabbed my shoulder and he said: **"You never gave up on me, and that helped me to stop giving up on myself."**

I just sat there and cried—and I'm not someone who really cries—because nothing will ever feel as good as that moment. That's when I know that what I do is worth it.

ENDING CASE MANAGEMENT SERVICES

Ending case management services is sometimes referred to as *discharge* or *termination*. Ideally, the decision about when to end case management services will be made by both the client and the case manager, but clients can always decide whether or not to continue services.

Hopefully, case management ends when clients have successfully implemented key elements of their action plans and enhanced their health or well-being. Case management also strives to assist clients in developing knowledge and skills that will aid them to stay independent and to successfully manage future challenges on their own.

Ending case management, like ending any professional relationship with a client, shouldn't happen suddenly, and should include making plans to support the transition and independence of the client. In preparation for completing or closing case management, the team may talk about the following issues:

- What has been learned and accomplished through case management?
- What are the client's skills and comfort level in managing their health and wellness independently?
- What key resources—including social support and the client's internal resources—will continue to support the client's health?
- Relapse prevention, if relevant. Support clients to learn or enhance skills to prevent relapsing to old behaviors or patterns they want to avoid, such as drug use or relationships characterized by domestic violence. Elements of WRAP Plans described above may be helpful.
- What the client can do in the future if they face challenges or crises. What has helped in the past? Who might they reach out to? What types of services may help them to manage possible challenges?

As a case manager, be sure to thank clients for the opportunity to work together and congratulate them on the accomplishments they have made. Ask them for feedback and any suggestions they have for ways that you and the program/agency you work for can continue to improve the quality of the services you provide.

Ending services can be difficult for both the client and the case manager. If the work has been successful and the team has established a trusting professional relationship, it can be hard to say good-bye. If you find yourself hesitating in bringing your work to a close, reflect on what is happening and seek consultation with your supervisor. You want to be as certain as possible that you are neither prolonging nor rushing to end case management because of your own feelings and needs. Case management should be completed because it is in the best interest of the clients, when they have accomplished key aspects of their plans and gained confidence and skills in promoting their own health and well-being.

Keep in mind that sometimes clients choose to end case management services before you think that they should. Sometimes, clients leave case management abruptly by moving to another city or region, choosing to work with another agency, getting angry with you and/or the agency you work for, or simply by no longer responding to messages from you and your colleagues. Regardless of the circumstances, honor the client's autonomy and their decision. Make time to reflect, as above, on what the client accomplished, on the aspects of case management that seemed to be effective, and on any aspects of the case management relationship and your own work that may have fallen short and could be improved in the future.

- *Have you faced challenges in ending services with clients?*

- *What have you learned about when and how to effectively end services with a client?*

> **TG:** I have terminated [ended] my work with some clients, but then started all over again if things got worse for them—like they relapse and start using drugs or go off their AIDS medications or whatever. Expect this to happen. On the one hand, it can get discouraging because a client who worked really hard to take care of themselves and get their life under control has slipped back—usually because something bad happened to them. On the other hand, I am always happy when a client reaches out to me and asks to work together again.
>
> Sometimes clients terminate working with me. Sometimes they tell me why and sometimes they don't, and I just need to respect that. Sometimes they terminate me because they're mad at something I said, and then they come back and start working with me again. I had one client who fired me five or six times.
>
> I actually get more worried about the clients that don't want to terminate even when they've made good progress on their plan—it's like they get attached at the hip. I always worry—am I doing something to make them dependent on me?

10.4 Other Suggestions for Effective Case Management

KEEPING IN TOUCH WITH CLIENTS

Share your business card with clients, including your phone number and e-mail address, and let them know the best way and time to reach you. Let people know how to leave a message for you and how long, in general, it will take you to return the message.

Protect yourself and the clients you work with by maintaining professional boundaries: don't give out your personal or home telephone number. It is rarely appropriate to extend your accessibility beyond the workplace, no matter how much you may want to support a client. Most organizations will provide clients with guidance for who to contact, and how, for assistance beyond regular work hours (such as 24-hour Health Advice Line).

Ask clients what the best way is to contact them. If they don't have a phone, ask for the number of a neighbor or relative, or the number of the shelter where they're staying, or the number of an agency or program where you may be able to locate them. Document the client's contact information and make sure it gets into their file. Some low-income clients may qualify for a free cell phone (such as a Lifeline Assistance Program phone) to support them with accessing services and managing appointments.

Be as flexible as you can, and as your agency and safety require, in scheduling appointments. You may meet with clients at your agency, in their home, in jail or the hospital, or at a homeless shelter or other agency. If clients are uncomfortable or incapable of coming to you, and your supervisor permits it, ask the client if you can go to them (For more information, see Chapter 11 on Home Visiting).

KEY TIMES TO OFFER GUIDANCE

One of the most important concepts of person-centered practice is to respect the clients' independence and their right to make their own decisions. *However, this doesn't mean that you will or should always agree with or quietly accept a clients' ideas, plans, or actions. There are key moments when it is important to speak up, gently and directly challenge your clients and to offer guidance.* These *may* include moments when:

Clients Establish Unrealistic Goals or Expectations of Themselves

Some clients develop action plans that are overly ambitious. People sometimes feel pressured or motivated to make dramatic changes over a short period of time, and their action plan may not be realistic.

Consider a client who has been living with chronic depression and is socially isolated. The client establishes a goal to join the local YMCA, to church and take classes at a community college as a way of making friends and building a social network. Is it likely that this client will be able to change a longstanding pattern of social isolation overnight? Are they likely to be able to accomplish all three of these goals (YMCA, church and community college) at once? Setting a goal that a client is unable to reach may be harmful to their health and their continued motivation for change.

If you are concerned about whether or not a client's action plan is realistic, speak up and share these concerns. Try using a Readiness or Confidence Ruler (see Chapter 9) to ask them how confident they are—on a scale from 0 to 10—that they will be able to successfully implement their proposed actions. Explain that it is often best to build for success by establishing less ambitious plans at first. Encourage clients to focus on taking one step they feel confident about putting into action in the next few weeks. For example, doing some online research about the YMCA or the community college may be a more realistic first step than making an in-person visit. Let the client know that making changes can be hard and, if they don't reach their immediate goal, you will be there to offer support and help them consider their next steps. If they do reach their first goal, you are there to help them figure out what their next step will be. More information is provided in other chapters about supporting clients to anticipate relapse (Chapter 9) and to revise their action plans (Chapter 16).

Clients Have Unrealistic Expectations of You or Others

Sometimes a client may place their expectations or hopes on you or others to ensure that they succeed in their action plan. Some clients may pin all their hopes on getting access to a particular resource: "When my Section 8 [a housing benefit] comes through and I have a permanent place again, then I'll be able to focus on getting a job." Some clients place high expectations on winning justice through the criminal justice system: *"Once this case is settled, and the judge gives me back custody of my children, then I can think about all this other stuff."*

Your role as a case manager is to support clients to consider possible outcomes and to make plans for continuing to move forward despite disappointments or setbacks. Ask clients to consider how they may be affected if their goal doesn't work out. Help them to establish realistic expectations about providers, programs, and benefits. For example, it can take many months or even years for Section 8 housing to be approved and finally provided. How may the client be affected if it takes a long time for their Section 8 housing to come through? What can they do if their housing application isn't approved? How can they continue to promote their health and wellness while they are waiting for the actions and decisions of others?

These conversations can be difficult, but they help to prepare clients to manage and respond when they face disappointments or setbacks. Supporting clients to enhance their resiliency is a key goal for case management.

Clients Engage in Unsafe or Harmful Behaviors or Choices

People do things that can be harmful to their health, or the health and well-being of others. For example, they may continue smoking after being diagnosed with asthma or chronic obstructive pulmonary disease. They may give up or quit programs or opportunities that hold promise for their health, welfare, or future such as a job training program, new job, or outpatient treatment program. They may continue to fight with their children's other parents or guardians, complicating visitation, custody, or co-parenting arrangements.

While it can be difficult to do so, we encourage you to directly name your concern (see Chapter 6). The client may not want to talk about it right then, or in the future, but we still want to name it. *"Indranil, I know how excited you were about the job training program, can you tell me more about why you decided to drop out?"* or *"I fully support your right to make decisions about your own treatment and medication Indranil, but I'm also concerned that you stopped taking your meds cold turkey rather than tapering off (reducing the dosage slowly over time). I remember last time this happened you ended up going to the Emergency Department. What are your thoughts about this?"*

Sometimes the types of harm that clients disclose must be reported to others with the goal of protecting people from harm. For example, if a client reveals that they have a plan and the means to kill themselves, we have a duty to report that immediately to a supervisor or third party (such as a crisis team or the police). Child and elder abuse must also be reported. Always check with your supervisor if you are uncertain what to do, what to report or two whom. You can also find more information about this topic in Chapters 5 and 18.

- *Have you ever raised concerns with a client about decisions or behaviors that could be harmful to them or others?*

    ◦ *If so, what was this like for you?*

    ◦ *If you haven't done this yet, what are your concerns?*

- *Can you think of other moments when you would consider stepping in to offer more direct guidance to a client?*

Client Scenario: Marcos Bernales (*continued*)

ONE WEEK LATER, MEETING WITH CASE MANAGER, WRAPAROUND HEALTH

Marcos has mostly stayed at the SafeSpace shelter, but also spent a few nights in the doorway of a restaurant. He says, "*I sleep better than I did in the encampment, but I really need to get off the streets and out of the shelter.*"

The Case Manager reminds Marcos that it may take a while before a transitional housing opportunity opens up. "*It's good that you keep bringing up your need for housing. I'm sorry it takes so long. I'll keep checking the waiting list and let you know right away if a housing option opens up. And you can keep reminding me as well. What's the best way for me to reach you? Can I leave a message at SafeSpace for you to call me back?*"

Marcos: You can leave a message for me at SafeSpace. I go by there most days to see if there is a bed.

Case Manager: Is it okay if we spend a few minutes talking more about your goals and your action plan today?

Marcos agrees. He wants to get a job and find safe and secure housing. He talks about his last job as a cook at a local café. "*It's just so loud and crazy all the time in restaurant work. With these headaches, I don't think it's the best plan to work in a restaurant.*"

When the Case Manager asks Marcos what type of work he'd like to do, Marcos says he wants to work outdoors and used to love gardening. "*I worked for a landscaper when I dropped out of high school. He was a friend of my grandmother. I liked the work, and I learned a lot about different kinds of plants, putting up fences, a lot of different things.*"

Marcos never finished high school and expresses an interest in earning his GED (high school degree equivalency). "*I've wanted to finish it for a long time.*"

The Case Manager refers Marcos to The JobStop and explains that they have staff who can help him earn his GED and find work. "*They'll help you search for work and can help with things like your resume and job interviewing skills, if you want.*"

Marcos: Yeah, that sounds good, but I don't know. . .

Case Manager: Would it be helpful if I visited The JobStop with you?

Marcos agrees to visit the job assistance agency with the Case Manager on Friday.

Case Manager: Marcos, you mentioned that you still have headaches. Would you like to schedule an appointment at our clinic? It might be good to have someone check on your eye and your headaches.

Marcos says he'll think about it.

The Case Manager schedules a follow up appointment in two weeks and documents updated information in the InfoHealth system including Marcos's action plan goals and actions, the type of work he wants, the referral to Jobs4Change, Marcos' continuing headaches and light sensitivity, and that Marcos declined a referral to meet with a WrapAround physician but will think about this option for the future.

10.5 Common Case Management Challenges

Some service providers use the phrase "difficult clients" to describe challenges they face on the job. This language can be used to judge, stigmatize and discriminate against people who we don't understand, or know how to work with who deserve our compassion and person-centered skills. Instead of labeling a client as "difficult," try shifting your perspective to view the circumstances that clients experience as difficult. Consider (or remember) what it might be like to lose your job or your home, to be alienated from your family, to be unhoused or to live with a difficult-to-manage health condition.

Keep in mind that clients wouldn't require your assistance if everything was going well in their lives. Remember that anxiety, frustration, and anger are common responses to difficult circumstances. Don't take the client's behavior personally. With time, you may be able to support them in learning more effective ways of handling difficult emotions. Refer to Chapter 12 to review conflict resolution concepts and skills.

> **TG:** Sometimes, when a client is acting out and making a scene or yelling or something, I just get so frustrated. I might have had a really hard day already, or maybe a client died recently, or I had a fight with my boyfriend—whatever—and I worry that I'm going to lose it. Sometimes I just have to remind myself, "This isn't about me. This is their life, not mine." It's not like I don't know this, but sometimes I just have to remind myself so that I can take a step back and find a way to be patient and calm.

MANAGING YOUR CASELOAD

Case managers should be assigned a manageable caseload in order to provide quality services to all clients without facing undue stress and the risk of burnout. Having a blend of clients facing complex and less-complex situations and challenges is helpful for case managers. This means that while some clients will need frequent attention, others are making progress and gaining skills in managing their own needs. When case managers are responsible for serving too many clients who are facing crises or acute challenges, they may be too occupied with these situations to also serve clients facing less immediate concerns. Review your employer's caseload policy to find out the maximum number of clients that you are supposed to be working with at any one time. If you are finding it difficult to manage your caseload, talk with your direct supervisor to ask for support.

WHEN A CLIENT PASSES AWAY

Whether it is anticipated or not, the death of a client often has a significant impact on CHWs and other helping professionals. It is important to take time to process a client's death. Reach out to your colleagues and supervisors to debrief. Spend some time celebrating what you most appreciated about the client, what you learned from them, and what they achieved through your work together. And please take time for some dedicated self-care.

MAINTAINING PROFESSIONAL BOUNDARIES

Clearly communicate with clients about what you can and cannot do to assist them in your role as case manager. Make sure the individual client or family understands your program's guidelines. For example, as a CHW you may be able to assist a family to get groceries from a food bank and refer them to WIC or food stamp programs if they are not already enrolled, but you cannot lend them money for groceries. You can meet or message the client during your work hours, but not outside of your work hours.

> **Lee Jackson:** When it comes to loaning money to clients, no way. I explain my job to them and tell them that I have boundaries. Sometimes they'll ask you to lend them money and say they'll pay you back double or something like that. So, I tell them: "No, I'm not a loan shark. I'm a health worker. I'm here to get you to your appointments and make sure you're okay and get you back on your feet, and if you need housing, we'll help get you housing, but I can't loan you money."

Some clients will find it difficult to understand or accept your professional boundaries. They may test boundaries by asking you personal questions, trying to contact you outside of your work hours, or asking you to provide services that are outside of your scope of practice and job description. Try not to take these attempts to push beyond your boundaries personally; keep in mind that clients are probably just trying to gain access to essential resources and services.

Maintaining healthy professional boundaries protects clients from unrealistic expectations and the disappointments that are inevitable when those expectations aren't met. Clear and consistent boundaries also protect you from exceeding your scope of practice or breaching ethical guidelines. See Chapter 5 for more information about setting and maintaining professional boundaries.

A REMINDER ABOUT SELF-CARE

If you don't learn to take care of yourself with the same dedication you show in working with your clients, you may harm your own health and your ability to provide high-quality, culturally competent services to others. For more information about self-care, see Chapter 12.

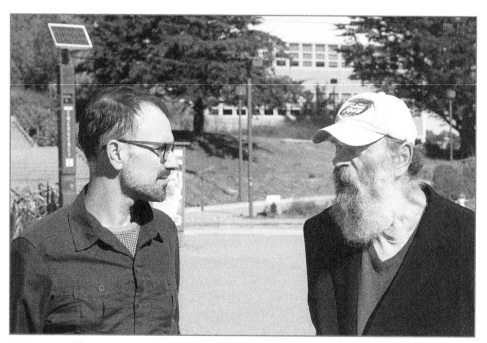

A CHW provide case management in the community.

10.6 Identifying Community Resources and Providing Referrals

A key part of your job as a case manager is to become familiar with local resources including housing, food, legal assistance, employment training, job counseling, education, childcare, health care and mental health care, drug treatment resources, and more. In some cities and counties, local government or private agencies develop and regularly update a list of such resources. Search online to see if you can find a comprehensive and up-to-date resource for the city or county where you work.

If the agency where you work or volunteer doesn't have an up-to-date and comprehensive guide to local resources, you and your colleagues may need to develop one. You might partner with other local agencies to develop a shared resource guide. This should include a plan to regularly update the guide to add new resources and to remove agencies or programs that no longer exist.

Developing an agency or inter-agency referral guide requires time and persistence. It is likely to include conducting research online, looking at examples from other counties or cities that can serve as a model, and talking with colleagues at your own agency and with partner agencies to create a list of the full range of resources that you want to assist your clients to access. Start by creating sub-categories of the types of resources most needed in the communities you serve (such as Housing, Food, Mental Health Services, etc.). Most importantly, don't forget to talk with your clients: they often have extensive knowledge about a wide range of available services, and strong opinions about which ones are the most and least beneficial.

Identifying resources can be particularly challenging when you are working in rural areas or a large county where services may be spread out geographically and difficult for clients to reach, particularly if there isn't a good public transportation system.

Cristina Arellano: The program I work for has developed a "living document" with a list of local resources categorized by type of service. The document is in a shared drive that all case managers can access and edit. Ideally we like to add the resource name, physical address, website, contact person, and contact's direct information. We share responsibility for keeping our resource list updated.

Your up-to-date list of referral resources makes it possible to connect clients to the resources they need. However, *not all referrals are good referrals.* Many people have had the experience of receiving a referral and calling the number only to discover that the line has been disconnected, or they aren't eligible for services. Worse yet is when clients make the effort to visit an agency only to find that the office is closed, that they should have brought certain identification or paperwork, or that they don't meet the eligibility guidelines. To avoid sending your clients or their families on a wild goose chase that wastes their valuable time, provide up-to-date and thorough information about where you're sending them. Visit the agency website or give them a call to find out the best way to refer new clients. If you often refer clients to the resource, build a relationship with a contact person who works for the program. Get to know them by name, so that when you send someone there, you can e-mail or text your contact person and let them know that a client is on their way.

Be aware that some organizations and programs are funded by grants. When the grants end, the program or service may also end or change. Personnel at agencies and organizations also change along with addresses, phone numbers and e-mail addresses. In order to provide clients with quality referrals, try to update your resource list every six months. And remember to reciprocate with other agencies. If your program experiences changes—such as a new address, program, or type of service—get the word out to other agencies so that they can update their resource listings. This way, other agencies will also be able to make effective referrals to your program.

Whether a wonderful guide to local resources already exists or you have to create one, make time to network and establish professional relationships with local organizations and programs. In many cities and counties there are regular meetings (in-person or via video conferencing) of service providers that you can attend often organized by the type of service you provide (job training, housing services, etc.) or the type of community you serve (youth, elders, etc.) Bring your business card, and take time before and after the meeting, and during breaks, to introduce yourself to other providers, talk about your work, and learn about the services that they provide. Collect business cards. If possible, make a time to visit the key resources that you most frequently recommend to clients. While you visit, pick up brochures and other information that will assist you in making effective referrals to the agency in the future.

Consider joining a professional social networking site such as LinkedIn. LinkedIn is free to join and is a great resource for posting job opportunities, searching for and applying to jobs, finding out about professional trainings and conferences, and networking with other professionals and organizations. For more information on LinkedIn and professional networking, please review Chapter 14 on Professional Skills.

Lee Jackson: Since I've been doing this job, I've become friends with people in different agencies. If I need some help or a referral, I can just call these people and say, "Look, I have this client and they need to come in for detox. Do you have any beds?" Then they might say, "Well we have maybe two beds, but we'll hold one for your client."

> **TG**: The longer I do this work, the more I know about the resources that exist out there. I've learned from experience which agencies I can trust to provide good service to my clients. Mostly, it is the same five to six resources that I refer my clients to: places to eat, decent shelters, mental health care, residential or day drug treatment programs, good primary health care—there is a great program at the public hospital, and legal assistance. It has been really hard to find good legal help about immigration issues. My clients have had some horrible experiences. Now I send them to a nonprofit center and let them provide the legal referrals because they are the experts in this area and I'm not. I go to a couple of meetings with different types of service providers so that I can get to know people. I like to know the person that I'm calling—or that my client is calling; it definitely makes a difference in terms of getting a quick response.

What Do YOU Think?

- *What types of services do you think would be most important for clients from your own community?*

- *What types of services or resources do you think will be hardest to find in your community?*

Scarce Resources

It is often difficult to find referral resources for clients. Certain types of services may not exist in your community or nearby. Services may exclude your clients for one reason or another, such as their gender, gender identity, immigration or health insurance status, income, family size, or other factors. Housing, mental health care, legal assistance, and drug and alcohol recovery services are often among the most difficult types of referral resources to locate for clients. Keep building relationships and networking with other health and social services providers to learn about available resources. And be honest with clients about the limited availability of certain resources. *"Darnel, unfortunately there is only one transitional housing program in the city that serves families with young children, and there is a waiting list right now. I can put your family on the waiting list. It may take several months before a place opens up for you."*

CRITERIA FOR REFERRAL RESOURCES

Not all agencies or programs are created equal. Some do an outstanding job at providing culturally responsive, person-centered services. Other organizations, programs and service providers sometimes fall short of this mark and may even treat clients poorly.

In the video referenced below, Ron Sanders talks about his criteria for the best referral sources. Ron is a CHW with the Transitions Clinic in San Francisco and recipient of *Esther M. Holderby Extraordinary CHW Award* in 2014.

Please watch the following video interview with a CHW about *Developing a List of Referrals*.

- *What does Ron Sanders say about how he evaluates the quality of different referral resources?*

- *What are Ron's criteria for whether or not he will share a resource with a client?*

(*Source:* Foundations for Community Health Workers/http://youtu.be/xKJQo6HExq4/ last accessed 21 September 2023.)

PROVIDING EFFECTIVE REFERRALS

Providing an effective referral is more complicated than it may appear. Some providers assume that all they need to do is to pass on information to a client, and the client will quickly and successfully access this new service. But clients may face many obstacles on the way to accessing a new program or service. The referral may not be a priority for the client. The client may not understand the nature of the referral and the services provided. The client or one of their family members may have had a negative experience with the agency (or a similar agency) in the past. The agency you refer them to may or may not provide services that are culturally or linguistically appropriate or accessible to the client.

> **TG:** The thing I always hated when I was a client was when someone would hand me a slip of paper with the name of some organization, I never asked them for and tell me that I should call up such-and-such agency and they could help me with such-and-such problem. Then they would just change the topic or leave and act as if they had done me some kind of favor. First of all, don't tell me to go somewhere without even asking me if I'm interested—that drives me crazy! Second, even if I was interested, do you think some paper with an address or a phone number or even a business card is going to help me down the road if I don't really understand what the place is or what they do or who to talk to or anything? That's not a referral, that's an insult!

Warm hand-offs are more likely to result in a successful referral. A **warm handoff** provides a client with a personal introduction to a service provider who works at the referral agency. You can provide a warm handoff in person, over the phone or via video conference.

Some recommendations for how to provide a successful referral include:

- Check the eligibility requirements of the agencies and their programs to be certain that they still exist and can indeed serve the clients you work with (some programs have requirements based on income, gender, nationality, citizenship, age, language, disability, diagnosis with a specific health condition, length of time in recovery from drug or alcohol addiction, or other eligibility requirements).

- Clearly explain the referral, including the name of the agency or provider, the services they provide, and how these may be relevant to the client's identified priorities and needs. To be absolutely certain that the client understands this information, ask the client to repeat it back to you ("Santos, *I want to make sure that I am communicating clearly. Can you tell me what you understand about this program I am recommending and how it might benefit you?*").

- The referral should be to a service that is of strong interest to the client. Check to see that they are interested in a resource before continuing to provide a referral. *"Tasha, Food4Life offers free healthy cooking classes for individuals and families. Would you be interested in learning more about these classes?"* If Tasha isn't interested, follow their lead and move on to a different topic.

- Provide clear and specific guidance about how, when, and where to access the agency or program. Where is it located? How can the client get there? When is it open? If you know and trust someone who works there and may provide services to a client, give them this professional's name. If you need to make a call to ask for further information, ask the client if they would like to make the call, or if they would like to make the call with you.

- If a client does not speak English (or the dominant language where you work), check to see whether the agency provides services in the client's primary language or will provide language interpretation services.

- Write down, e-mail, or text information about referrals so that clients can remember what you have told them. If you are working with clients who cannot read easily, it is still important to write the information down so that they can show it to family members or friends if they need assistance.

- When referring clients to services that may have a waiting list or be difficult to access, contact the referral agency to let them know you have made the referral.

- Check-in with clients to learn if they followed up with the referrals, if they accessed services, and what their experiences were like. Document this in the client's case files. Following up with clients is particularly important. Taking the initiative to find out what happened allows you to ensure that clients get the services they need. It also provides you with invaluable information about the quality of services that you refer clients to.

● *What else can CHWs do to provide effective referrals?*

Martha Shearer: I explain the program I work for, what clients can expect, and tell them I am there to assist them. I say, "Tell me what you need and let me see how I can help." If I can't do it, I know someone else who can. I know my clients' standard needs are medications, housing, food stamps, clothing, and food. I know all the organizations in and around Birmingham [Alabama] that can provide assistance, so when these issues come up, I am ready to provide a referral to the client. Of course, a lot of the time, with my clients, we go visit the agency or program together the first time. I want to make a personal introduction and make sure I leave them in good hands.

Please watch the following short videos [▶] that show a CHW working with a client and providing a referral.

The first video is a counter role play, highlighting a common mistake that helping professionals may make:

The second video shows a CHW who is applying client-centered skills to provide the referral:

● *What mistake(s) does the CHW make in the counter role play, and how may this impact the client?*

● *What did the CHW do well in the demonstration role play?*

● *What else would you do—or do differently—to provide a client-centered referral in this situation?*

PROVIDING A CLIENT-CENTERED
REFERRAL: ROLE PLAY, COUNTER
(*Source:* Foundations
for Community Health
Workers/http://youtu.be/
SzY0L5tA4DU/last accessed
21 September 2023.)

PROVIDING A CLIENT-CENTERED
REFERRAL: ROLE PLAY, DEMO
(*Source:* Foundations
for Community Health
Workers/http://youtu.be/
2GoI8gJGSZg/last accessed
21 September 2023.)

Client Scenario: Marcos Bernales *(continued)*

THREE WEEKS LATER, MEETING WITH CASE MANAGER AT WRAPAROUND HEALTH

The Case Manager asks Marcos how it's going at the shelter and The JobStop. Marcos says that he's joined a GED class that meets twice a week. *"It's okay, but it goes kind of fast for me. You have to study a lot and the reading is hard for me because of my eye."* He's been assigned a job counselor, Mr. Charles, who is helping him to explore his interest in gardening or landscaping. *"He told me there's a program coming up that I can apply to be a trainee with the city, and they want to train people up to work for Parks and Rec."*

Case Manager: The City Apprenticeship Program?

Marcos: Yeah, I think that's the one.

Case Manager: That's a great opportunity Marcos. How do you feel about it?

Marcos: Trying not get my hopes up. But it would be great to work for the city, outside, helping out. Is there any news about my housing?

(continues)

Client Scenario: Marcos Bernales *(continued)*

Case Manager: Not yet. It looks like some slots did open up this month, so you're moving up the waiting list, but it will still take some time. And remember, when an opening comes up, it doesn't mean that you automatically get it, the program or the landlord will want to interview you first.

Marcos: [Marcos begins to cry] I didn't mean to cry. I'm sorry. [He wipes his face with the sleeve of his jacket.]

Case Manager: I'm here Marcos.

Marcos: [Stands up and turns away. Eventually he sits back down]

Case Manager: Do you want to talk about it?

Marcos: I still have so much pain. My head and my eye hurt a lot of the time. And I have a hard time sleeping at the shelter. I keep waking up worrying about... about everything that happened.

Case Manager: Would you be willing to tell me about it, about your pain?

Marcos reveals that he was assaulted on his day off from work. He was hit in the face with a bat and fell to the ground, hitting his head on the edge of the sidewalk. He was taken to the General Hospital and needed emergency surgery to repair his eye socket. Marcos wasn't able to return to work. He lost his job and couldn't afford rent in a shared apartment. Marcos wears sunglasses because his eyes are sensitive to light, and because he's self-conscious about the big, raised scar over his left eye. He still has headaches, and difficulty sleeping. Sometimes people get into fights at the shelter, *"I can't sleep after that."* Sometimes Marcos wakes up afraid that the man with the bat is looking for him. *"The other day, outside the shelter, I thought I saw him, the man who hit me. I couldn't breathe. But it wasn't him."*

Case Manager: I'm so sorry to hear about the assault Marcos. Thank you for sharing what happened to you. It helps me to better appreciate what you've been going through, including the pain you're experiencing, your difficulty sleeping, and the anxiety and worry that you mentioned. I've learned that these are natural responses to a trauma like being attacked and beaten with a bat.

Marcos: But how long is this all going to last? When will it stop?

Case Manager: Those are such difficult questions to answer Marcos. I've learned that recovering from violence and other trauma is often more complicated and takes longer than we hope for. Can I ask, did you go back to the hospital, or have you had any medical care since the accident? Have you talked to anyone about what happened and what you are going through now?

Marcos: No, I didn't really tell anyone.

Case Manager: We have some wonderful doctors here, at WrapAround. I think it would be a good idea for someone to check on your eye and assess how you're doing since you were attacked. Would you like me to help schedule a medical appointment for you?

Marcos: I don't know. I don't like talking about this stuff.

Case Manager: How does it feel to be talking with me today?

Marcos: Not so bad. [Marcos pauses] Sorry. I mean, it isn't hard to talk to you. But it's difficult to talk about what happened.

Case Manager: Well, you're doing an amazing job of talking about what you've been going through Marcos. I could always go with you for a first medical appointment if that would be helpful. But I also don't want to push you. Take your time in making these decisions.

Marcos: If you go with me, I'll go.

The Case Manager documents the appointment in the InfoHealth database including information about Marcos' assault, his continued headaches, difficulty sleeping, intrusive thoughts and anxiety, and the referral for a medical appointment at WrapAroundHealth.

10.7 Advocacy

Sometimes clients aren't successful in accessing the resources they've been referred to and may benefit from some advocacy from you. For example, you might contact a drug treatment program, domestic violence shelter, or primary care physician and ask them to provide services for a client. A client may ask you to attend a medical appointment with them to help them talk with or advocate with their health care provider. Sometimes clients experience prejudice or discrimination from other providers or programs and you, or another representative from your agency, may step in to inquire further about this and advocate for the client's rights to be respected and supported. If you are uncertain what to do in situations like this, talk it over with your supervisor.

Advocating for clients is a common and important part of the job. However, *keep in mind that the goal of case management is to support the independence of clients and their ability to manage their own lives and health concerns.* If you step in too quickly or too regularly to advocate on behalf of a client, you are likely to increase their dependency on you and other caregivers, and to undermine their own initiative.

To the extent possible, support clients to develop skills and the confidence to advocate for themselves. One way to do this is to ask clients to practice how they will advocate for themselves, and how they might respond if the provider denies their request. You might try making a call to a referral source together and asking the client to do most of the talking. If you decide to step in and talk with the other provider directly, debrief this afterward with the client: ask the client what this experience was like, and if they would like to do it differently the next time. If they make the contact on their own, follow up with them to find out how it went, if they were able to access services, and what their experience was like with the other agency or service provider. As with many aspects of your work as a CHW, the challenge is to strike a balance between supporting the client's independence and autonomy and stepping in as needed to try to prevent unnecessary harm.

- *Can you think of other circumstances when clients may benefit from advocacy?*

- *How have you supported clients to enhance their ability to advocate for themselves?*

What Do YOU Think?

Client Scenario: Marcos Bernales (continued)

TWO WEEKS LATER, MEETING WITH THE CASE MANAGER, WRAPAROUND HEALTH

Marcos and the Case Manager met with a doctor at WrapAroundHealth. The doctor said that Marcos may have some inflammation in his left eye and made a referral to an Ophthalmologist. The doctor also diagnosed Marcos with post-traumatic stress and prescribed some anti-anxiety medications and provided a referral to a therapist.

Marcos refused the medications but did call to schedule an appointment with the Ophthalmologist. The appointment is in three months.

Marcos says he isn't sure about going to therapy: *"My community, we don't do therapy."* He explains that: *"The way I was raised, therapy is for crazy people. I'm not crazy."*

The Case Manager agrees that therapy may not be the right option for everyone, but also explains that many people who are harmed by violence or other types of trauma, are deeply affected. *"They aren't crazy Marcos; they were just hurt."* The Case Manager explains that there other resources that could be helpful, like support groups where people can talk and support each other. *"Going to therapy or taking medications, these are decision that only you can make Marcos. I don't want to push you, but I do want to let you know that I have a colleague here at WrapAround, Mrs. Jenkins. She's a counselor who grew up in this community. She works with a lot of people, a lot of families, who have been harmed by violence, like you have. One option to consider, because this is your decision to make, is to meet with her just one time to talk about the work that she does and how it might benefit you. You could share your concerns about therapy and don't have to share anything personal about what happened to you. Then you could decide if you want to go back or not."*

(continues)

Client Scenario: Marcos Bernales *(continued)*

Marcos: She grew up here? [The Case Manager nods] I probably won't meet with her, but I'll think about it."

When the case manager asks about how it is going at The JobStop, Marcos says that he doesn't like his counselor. *"I mean, I'm happy for being set up for the GED classes and the application for the apprenticeship, but Mr. Charles, he's saying that I need to go back to work right away while I'm waiting for the apprenticeship. I told him I wasn't ready, that I'm still having headaches, but he kept saying I need to show that I'm working. He doesn't know what I'm going through."*

Case Manager: Have you told Mr. Charles all this Marcos? Have you told him that you feel like he's pushing you to do something that you aren't ready to do? Have you talked about your headaches?

Marcos: [Sighs] That guy is hard to talk to.

Marcos and the Case Manager talk about the benefits he's getting through The JobStop, and his right to say that he isn't ready to go to work right now. The Case Manager encourages him to try to talk with Mr. Charles again. Marcos says that he'll try to explain his concerns to Mr. Charles.

Case Manager: Okay. We have about 15 minutes before we need to say goodbye. Is there anything you want to talk about or anything I can support you with before our meeting ends?

The Case Manager documents the appointment in the InfoHealth database including the appointment with the Ophthalmologist, the referral to Mrs. Jenkins (WrapAround Counselor) and his reluctance to consider therapy, Marcos' continued headaches and his participation in GED classes, and his difficulty communicating with Mr. Charles.

10.8 Organizing and Documenting Your Work

KEEP A SCHEDULE

Case management is a challenging job, and no two days are likely to be the same (this also keeps the work interesting). There is no way to accurately predict the times when clients will experience crises, or when your caseload or the number of clients you work with will increase. Time management is key to avoiding burnout as well as maintaining positive professional relationships with your clients.

Create a schedule that shows the time and location of case management sessions, team meetings, case conferences, and other responsibilities each week. Be sure to include time to take a break, eat lunch, and enough time, each day, to carefully document the services you provide. Schedule time for self-care into your week: do something that helps you to relax and renews your energy.

MANAGING CLIENT FILES

Documenting the services you provide and managing case files is an ethical duty and part of your responsibility to clients and your agency. These files may be electronic or paper, or both. Your clear records provide insight into the depth and quality of your work and assist your colleagues in understanding a client's goals, achievements and outstanding needs. Most importantly, these records are useful for understanding a client's progress and provide essential information for improving the quality of services that clients receive.

Basic guidelines for managing case files include:

Explain Note-Taking to Clients

Explain to clients how and why you are taking notes. Let them know that you are documenting essential information they share with you so that you can remember it and provide quality services. You may want to show clients the forms that you use to take notes, so that they can see for themselves the type of information you will be documenting. It can also be helpful to explain to clients that when you are looking down to take notes, you are still listening to them. If you use an electronic health record, it is likely that the client will be able to access this information through their patient portal (their own account).

Keep All Files Confidential

Clients will share personal information with you. In order to maintain your clients' trust, you must protect that information. As a provider, you are also legally required to protect their confidentiality. Don't leave any paper forms or folders where other people might see them. Put any paper records or files in a file cabinet or other location that you can lock at the end of the day. Treat the information with care and respect.

Use Appropriate Forms

Use the forms and data systems that your agency provides to document client information and the delivery of services. Increasingly, you will be asked to document your work and the client's progress in electronic data systems or health records. It will be much easier to keep track of information and share it with other members of your team if everyone is using the same forms. Keep in mind that forms are constantly being updated to remove no longer relevant categories and to add in newly required information. Note that some companies are in the process of developing applications that will support CHWs to take notes easily on their phone or any digital devise, and the data they enter will be synched with commonly used electronic health records.

Write Clearly

Document the services you provide and key information you learn as clearly as possible. If you make handwritten notes, please write so that others can easily read the information. If your handwriting is hard for others to read, print. Keep in mind that you are writing notes not only for yourself, but for others who are currently working with the client as well as for those who will work with the client in the future.

Keep Files Up to Date

Jot down case notes every time you have completed a session with a client. Enter them into the electronic health record if your agency uses one. Be sure to put down the date of the session, what was discussed, referrals you provided, and any agreements on future actions to be taken. Case notes will not help you, the client, or your teammates unless they are clearly written and easy to understand.

> **Lee Jackson:** For documentation I have a client contact sheet, and each time I come into contact with a client, I document it. I make time every day just to do my notes, or I'd never be able to keep up. There's definitely a lot of paperwork with this job. I write down how much time I spend with the client. I document the case management and health education plans we develop, and the client's progress in implementing these plans. At the end of the month, I have to tally up all of my contacts, and we fax a report to the state health department.

ELECTRONIC FORMS AND DATA SYSTEMS

Increasingly, CHWs and case managers enter notes into electronic health records and data systems to document the services that they provide to clients. The electronic data bases vary widely across the country. Some systems are closed or used just by the staff at one agency or program. Other systems are shared between different providers within a city or county, with the permission of clients. Shared data systems allow you as a case manager to review not only your own notes about working with a specific person, but you can also review the types of services that have been provided by colleagues and other agencies and programs. These systems allow providers to review a client's history over time, to learn about past and current health conditions, challenges, or crisis, as well as their goals and accomplishments. When client's give permission for providers to share notes—and clients can always refuse this request—it is with the hope that care and services will be better coordinated among providers and in the client's best interest.

Electronic databases sometimes restrict the type of information that you can enter. Some systems permit you to check off the type of services provided—such as developing or revising a care plan, providing referrals to medical or social services providers or resources for housing or employment—and the date and location where these services were provided. Other systems allow CHWs and other providers to enter more detailed notes about key information that client's share with you, creating a broader and more complete picture of the client's health and life.

The Value of Electronic Health Records and Data Systems

The use of electronic health records (EHR) has grown dramatically since the American Recovery and Reinvestment Act of 2009 was passed into law, requiring private and public health care providers to demonstrate the use of electronic records. They represent a digital version of a traditional patient medical chart and include patient history, diagnosis and allergies, medications, lab results, clinician notes, and other key health information. Electronic records are shared among providers within a practice or team and, with the patient's written permission, can be shared among providers from different agencies, typically within a city or county region. Patients are also able to view their health record—including their action plan—by logging into an online portal on a computer, phone, or other digital device. They can view lab results, ask for medications to be refilled, schedule appointments, and communicate with their providers.

The use of electronic health records has many benefits. They have been shown to:

- Improve communication between patients and providers
- Improve collaboration between providers and agencies
- Improve patient health outcomes
- EHR has been particularly useful for managing ongoing or chronic conditions—such as diabetes, hypertension, and depression—which are the leading causes of illness and hospitalization in the United States.
- Data that is typed into electronic records is more legible or easier to read than hand-written notes, resulting in fewer medical and medication errors.
- Reduce the time that patients or clients spend briefing and repeating information about their health to providers.
- Lab results are reported in a timely fashion and critical values are flagged for clinical staff.
- Reduce duplicate or unnecessary tests and services
- Reduce high administrative costs

Whether you document services on a paper form, on an electronic app, or in an electronic data system, complete documentation as quickly as possible after you provide services in order to maintain a complete and accurate record. Build in time to complete documentation of services into each workday and, if this is difficult to do because of competing priorities and demands on your time, talk to your supervisor for guidance about how, when, and where you can document services in a timelier fashion.

- *How do you document the services that you provide at the agency where you work or volunteer?*

- *If you use electronic records or database, is it shared with other agencies that may work with the same clients? Are there any limitations on the type of documentation you can enter into the electronic data system?*

SYSTEMS AND GUIDELINES FOR TAKING NOTES

There are several different systems and guidelines for taking notes that are widely used in health care and social services settings including SOAP, DAP and APSO notes. Each approach provides a framework for providing accurate documentation of key information about a client's health and social circumstances, their goals and priorities, and any decisions they may make such as goals for an action plan, programs they participate in, and referral resources they plan to access. SOAP notes are the traditional system for documenting patient information in health care settings and are still widely used today. In some settings, APSO notes are replacing SOAP notes. DAP notes are more common in mental health and behavior health care settings.

SOAP, DAP, and APSO are variations for documenting the same type of information. SOAP stands for Subjective, Objective, Assessment, and Plan. APSO uses the same categories but rearranges them as Assessment, Plan, Subjective, and Objective. DAP merges the Subjective and Objective information in a category called Data and includes Assessment and Plan.

The agency you work or volunteer for will orient you to the types of forms and databases they use, the type of information they ask you to gather from the clients you work with, and any systems of note taking that they use.

Subjective information includes a client's reported experiences, beliefs, feelings, behaviors, or accomplishments related to their health.

For Marcos Bernales, the CHW might note: Mr. Bernales reports that he has been unhoused for three years, after losing a job. He used to live with a younger brother but is no longer in touch with him. Mr. Bernales said that he does not want to bother his brother with his own troubles. His expressed priorities are to find safe and stable housing and employment. Mr. Bernales is unhoused and sleeping in the Frost St. encampment and in a doorway on Oak Blvd.

Objective data includes information that you directly observe and hear during your meetings with clients without any interpretation.

For Marcos Bernales, the CHW might note: Marcos wore dark glasses most of the time. He has a large scar over his left eye. Marcos accepted the referral to SafeSpace and completed an application for transitional housing.

Licensed providers will also document Objective information such as blood pressure, physical exam findings, laboratory test results, imaging, and other diagnostic testing data.

Assessment represents a synthesis of both Subjective and Objective data. For CHW case managers, this is where you document your own thoughts and interpretations about what clients have shared with you and what you have observed. You want to be careful about making judgments that the objective evidence does not support, particularly statements that could potentially harm the client.

For Marcos Bernales, a CHW Case Manager might note: Mr. Bernales seems motivated to find safer housing. He seems reluctant to open up and talk about other issues such as where he used to live, his relationship with his brother, and the scar over his eye.

For licensed colleagues, Assessment will include documentation of any possible diagnoses or need for further diagnostic exams or tests. For example, a physician may consider possible diagnoses of depression or post-traumatic stress and make a referral to a licensed mental health provider.

Plan is the place to document what the client and providers plan to do in the future including any actions that the client may take, services and referrals you will provide, and next appointments.

For Marcos Bernales, the CHW might note: Mr. Bernales is on the waiting list for transitional housing. He is attending GED classes on Mondays/Wednesdays at Noon at The JobStop and working with an employment counselor. He is scheduled to meet with Dr. _____, an Ophthalmologist, on 01/07/_____. A follow-up appointment is scheduled in two weeks (11/03/_____).

In the Plan section, licensed colleagues may document additional referrals for services, tests, treatments, or medications.

Client Scenario: Marcos Bernales (*continued*)

THREE WEEKS LATER, MEETING WITH THE CASE MANAGER, WRAPAROUND HEALTH

The Case Manager was able to schedule a drop-in appointment for Marcos with the Ophthalmologist. Marcos was diagnosed with scarring and inflammation in his left eye and prescribed medications. The Ophthalmologist says that the medications may also help with his sensitivity to light and his headaches, and schedules a follow-up visit in two weeks.

Marcos tells the Case Manager that he has some good news to share. *"There's a community garden near SafeSpace, over between 4th and 5th. I know one of the guys there, so I talked to him, and they said they need volunteers, so I started, you know, helping out."*

(continues)

Client Scenario: Marcos Bernales *(continued)*

Case Manager: That's great news Marcos! Can you tell me more about the garden and what you've been doing?

Marcos shares that he's learning a lot and has already helped to build two new raised boxes and to plant some herbs and greens. *"I share responsibility for one of the boxes, so I have to go by there almost every day."*

Marcos is still angry about his last appointment with the job counselor, Mr. Charles at The JobStop. *"I tried to talk to him. He doesn't understand. He just wants to fill his quota and say that I have to get a job, any type of job, and I told him I can't go back to working in restaurants. I'm not going back there if I have to deal with that crap."*

Case Manager: Okay. What is it about the community garden that's different from working in restaurants? You've been working there a lot, right?

Marcos explains that is outside and he finds the work relaxing. He can take breaks when he wants and, *"They don't boss me around. They don't boss anyone around. We work together and we figure it out together."*

Case Manager: I'm disappointed that Mr. Charles isn't listening to you Marcos. But there are several counselors at The JobStop, so one option would be to ask for a different counselor. I think that what they offer—the GED and help with opportunities like the City Apprenticeship—could be worth it in the long run. What if you were able to work with a different counselor, someone who you liked?

Marcos: [thinks] Yeah, I agree, they do have some good programs. I guess if I didn't have to keep working with Mr. Charles, I could go back.

Case Manager: Great. Don't let a bad experience or a disappointing counselor get in the way of your success. [Marcos nods]. I could call The JobStop for you, but you could also talk to them. What could you say to ask for a different counselor?

Marcos: Well, I can't say what I really want to say, but I guess I could just say that I want to try working with a different counselor.

Case Manager: That sounds good. Most places know that not every staff person is the right fit for every client. It can't hurt to ask. And you could be matched with someone who is better able to help you.

Marcos: Okay

Case Manager: Marcos, you're making great progress. I know that you're discouraged about your headaches and the physician and the job counselor, but don't let these things get in the way of your progress. I'm here to help you figure out how to keep moving forward with your goals. Getting a job as a landscaper and having your own place, they're worth it, aren't they?

Marcos: Yeah, I don't want anything else to get in the way. I need to keep moving forward.

Marcos schedules a follow-up appointment in one week. The Case Manager documents the appointment in the InfoHealth database including his prescription from the Ophthalmologist for medication to help with his eyesight and headaches, Marcos' volunteering with the community garden, his challenges at The JobStop, and his intention to ask to switch to a different counselor.

10.9 Team Meetings and Case Conferences

As a CHW, you will always work as part of a team. The number and type of professionals who are part of the team will depend upon the organization you work for. Most teams who work to support the same group of clients or patients meet to share program and agency updates, to review and reinforce protocols and standards of practice, to participate in professional development opportunities, and to discuss challenges and successes.

Case or client conferences bring together members of a team who work with common clients, or colleagues who work with similar clients. The purpose of a case conference is to:

- Improve the quality of services provided to clients
- Improve coordination between service providers and service teams
- Enhance the professional skills of service providers

During a case conference, one team member may be asked to present information about a particular client. If the meeting is taking place only among team members who have permission from the client to share confidential information with each other, then any relevant information may be discussed. If not, then the client's situation is discussed in more general terms, keeping the identity of the client confidential.

Priority is often given to a team member working with a client who is in crisis or facing a notable challenge. If you were presenting, you would share relevant background information (maintaining confidentiality) such as the client's case management goals, progress in meeting their goals, and describes current challenges, questions, or concerns. The team then works together to identify strategies for working with the client, such as identifying referral resources that may promote the client's progress and well-being. Sometimes a colleague will have information about the client that can shed light on their situation. In this way, team members share information and skills with each other, and clients benefit from the identification of new insights, strategies, and resources.

If you have been asked to present at a case conference, make sure to prepare by updating and reviewing the case file including the client's goals, strengths, accomplishments, and outstanding risks, needs, or concerns. Identify the questions or concerns that you want to discuss with your team. Do you have questions about how to address a particular issue with the client? Are you hoping to learn about a particular resource or program that may be of interest to the client?

When others are presenting, provide your colleagues with the same type of support you would most benefit from. For example, share any suggestions that you might have based on your own experiences working with similar clients and challenges. Let them know about the referral resources that have been most beneficial to clients you work with.

Some case conferences include clients and their family members. The goal remains the same: to review how well the team is working to support the client to reach their goals and enhance their health. Key accomplishments will be highlighted and celebrated. Challenges, problems, and mistakes will be addressed with the goal of improving the quality of case management services. Clients will have the chance to ask questions, raise concerns and share feedback, and to propose and set new goals or actions for their case management plans.

10.10 Supervision

Regular communication with supervisors helps to ensure that you provide effective services, remain within your scope of practice, and maintain professional boundaries. Supervision will clarify questions or concerns about topics such as the proper documentation of services and how best to support clients with their action plans. Supervision can also provide CHW case managers with opportunities to reflect on the impact of their work on their own health, to practice self-care and participate in ongoing professional development.

Some case managers benefit from receiving two different types of supervision at work, sometimes referred to as administrative and clinical supervision. They are typically provided by different staff members and serve distinct purposes.

Administrative supervision is provided by a direct supervisor who is responsible for the quality of your day-to-day work. This type of supervision addresses issues such as:

- Scheduling and caseload
- Relationships with co-workers and clients
- Job-related knowledge and skills
- Work habits, performance, and attitude
- Adherence to protocols and standards of care/practice
- Consultation about specific topics such as the need to advocate for a client (or a request to a supervisor to assist with advocacy or other services)
- Annual performance reviews or evaluations

- Opportunities for advancement, pay increases, and promotions
- Opportunities for professional development
- Identification of professional errors or problems and the need to enhance skills and quality of services provided
- Disciplinary action including required steps for improved job performance and termination of employment

<u>Clinical supervision</u> is not provided by a direct line manager or supervisor but typically by a licensed social worker, counselor, psychologist, or other type of professional with the relevant skills. It may be provided in individual and/or group meetings. Clinical supervision provides CHW case managers with the opportunity to talk about the challenges they are facing in their work with clients and to receive guidance and support for providing quality services, for maintaining professional boundaries, for managing ethical challenges, and for maintaining their own physical and mental health.

Case managers work with people who are struggling with health and social issues and who lack access to key resources such as housing, food, employment, social support, and mental health counseling. It can take a toll on the health and well-being of any helping professional to witness clients and community members facing these challenges. As helping professionals, sometimes our own issues, challenges, or past traumas come to the surface. Clinical supervision provides an opportunity to talk about these issues and to receive support and guidance to continue your own healing, recovery, and self-care.

Taking care of yourself is something that many CHWs struggle with because they typically put the needs of others first. Please prioritize your own health and wellness as you would that of a client in need. If you have questions, concerns, or the need for support, please reach out to a clinical supervisor to talk about what you are going through.

- *What type of supervision do you receive at work?*

- *Have you had the chance to participate in clinical supervision provided by someone who is not your direct line manager/supervisor?*

- *How might access to clinical supervision be beneficial for CHWs?*

Client Scenario: Marcos Bernales (*continued*)

ONE WEEK LATER, MEETING WITH THE CASE MANAGER, WRAPAROUND HEALTH

Marcos is sleeping at SafeSpace and is on the waiting list for transitional housing. The medications that Ophthalmologist prescribed have diminished his light sensitivity and headaches. The Associate Director of RootsofChange, the community garden where Marcos has been volunteering, has offered to write a letter of support for his application to the City Apprenticeship. Marcos spoke to one of the staff at The JobStop and they agreed to assign him another counselor. Marcos hasn't met with her yet.

Marcos tells the case manager that he did meet with Mrs. Jenkins, the WrapAround counselor, but he still doesn't want to take the antianxiety medications that the physician prescribed. When the case manager asks what Marcos thinks of Mrs. Jenkins, the WrapAround counselor, he replies, *"She's alright. I'm gonna keep talking with her."*

Marcos: What's up with my housing? How much longer is it going to take?

Case Manager: I hope something opens up soon, but this decision is out of our control.

Marcos: Yeah, I know, but I've been on the streets and in the shelter for so long now. I just want a quiet place, a room that is just mine.

Case Manager: Is there anything you can do that will help you to hang in there while you are waiting?

(continues)

Client Scenario: Marcos Bernales *(continued)*

Marcos: [sighs] I guess I just have to keep gardening, keep seeing you and Mrs. Jenkins, hoping for something to happen, trying not to get too anxious and frustrated about it.

Case Manager: I know that you haven't reached your big goals yet, Marcos, finding a job and getting a safe place to stay. [Marcos nods] But I see that you've been working hard towards these goals and you've made a lot of progress. Can you tell me about what you've accomplished since we first met?

Marcos: Well, I'm not sleeping on the streets anymore, and that is a big improvement. My eye is better. I'm volunteering with the community garden and applied for the City Apprenticeship. And even though I was kind of against it at first, I'm meeting with my counselor, Mrs. Jenkins.

Case Manager: So what do you think about all of that, about what you've accomplished?

Marcos: It's kind of a lot when I say it out loud.

Case Manager: I agree—you've accomplished a lot.

Marcos: Okay [Marcos laughs]

Case Manager: Is there anything else you want to talk about, or to work toward. Any additions to your action plan?

Marcos: My counselor, Mrs. Jenkins, she's asking me to think about calling my brother. She's not pushing me to do it or anything. [Marcos smiles] We're just talking about it.

Case Manager: And how are you feeling about that today?

Marcos: I think if I get the apprenticeship or if I get a place, then ... it would be more comfortable to call my brother. I want them to know that I'm okay, and ... that they don't have to keep worrying about me.

Marcos and the Case Manager schedule a follow-up appointment in four weeks. The Case Manager documents the appointment in the InfoHealth database including the improvement in Marcos' sensitivity to light and headaches, his continued volunteering with the community garden, his successful advocacy to get a new counselor at JobStop, his work with Mrs. Jenkins, and his intention to participate in the WrapAround housing workshop.

Chapter Review

To review case management practices, please do your best to answer the following questions:

- How would you define or explain case management services to a new CHW colleague?
- How might case management services benefit clients? What types of outcomes or achievements are possible with case management?
- What is your scope of practice as a CHW case manager?
  - What types of tasks and services are you able to provide?
  - What types of tasks and services lie outside your scope of practice and should be provided by others?
- How can you work to support a client to develop a realistic case management or action plan to improve or enhance their health and wellness?
- What are the criteria for SMART case management goals and plans?
- When might clients want to revise or change their action plans?

- How can you work with clients in ways that support their independence and honor their experience, identity, knowledge, and skills?
- What types of referral resources are most important for the clients and communities you serve? Which types of resources are harder to find and to gain access to?
- What is your criteria for a good referral resource?
- How can you network with other agencies and providers to share information about local resources?
- What sort of challenges may you experience as a case manager?
- How will you respond if clients don't understand or respect your professional boundaries?
- When might you advocate on behalf of a client? When might you support a client to advocate for themself?
- When might you want to reach out to consult with your supervisor?
- How and when might you end case management services?
- When and how will you document case management services?
- What are some of the benefits of electronic health records or electronic data systems?
- How can you evaluate whether or not you are providing client-centered case management?
  - What questions would you ask to assess your work?
  - What are your criteria or standards for quality case management services?
- If you were a case manager working with Marcos Bernales, what else would you do to support him in implementing his action plan and reaching his key goals?

References

Case Management Society of America. (2022). What is a Case Manager? https://cmsa.org/who-we-are/what-is-a-case-manager/ (accessed 7 November 2022).

Coutinho, M. T., Subzwari, S. S., McQuaid, E. L., & Koinis-Mitchell, D. (2020). Community health workers' role in supporting pediatric asthma management: A review. *Clinical Practice in Pediatric Psychology*, 8(2), 195–210. https://doi.org/10.1037/cpp0000319.

Global Social Service Workforce Alliance. (2022). About Us. https://www.socialserviceworkforce.org/about-us (accessed 7 November 2022).

Global Social Service Workforce Alliance Case Management Interest Group. (2018). Core Concepts and Principles of Effective Case Management: Approaches for the Social Service Workforce. https://bettercarenetwork.org/sites/default/files/Case-Management-Concepts-and-Principles.pdf (accessed 7 November 2022).

National Center for Chronic Disease Prevention and Health Promotion. (2015). *Addressing chronic disease through community health workers: a policy and systems—level approach*. 2nd Edition. Centers for Disease Control and Prevention. www.cdc.gov/dhdsp/docs/chw_brief.pdf. (accessed 7 November 2022).

National Health Service Foundation Trust. (2022). My Wellness Recovery Action Plan (WRAP). Cheshire and Wirral Partnership. https://webstore.cwp.nhs.uk/publications/WRAP2.pdf (accessed 7 November 2022).

Paintain, L. S., Willey, B., Kedenge, S., Sharkey, A., Kim, J., Buj, V., ... Ngongo, N. (2014). Community health workers and stand-alone or integrated case management of malaria: A systematic literature review. *American Journal of Tropical Medicine and Hygiene*, 91(3), 461–470. https://doi.org/10.4269/ajtmh.14-0094.

Smith, W. R., Sop, D., Johnson, S., Lipato, T., Ferlis, M., Mcmanus, C., ... Roberts, J. D. (2019). Case management featuring community health workers reduces inpatient health care utilization in adults with sickle cell disease. *Blood*, 134(Supplement-1), 2104. https://doi.org/10.1182/blood-2019-130441.

Weaver, A. & Lapidos, A. (2018). Mental health interventions with community health workers in the United States: A systematic review. *Journal of Health Care for the Poor and Underserved*, 29(1), 159–180. https://doi.org/10.1353/hpu.2018.0011.

Additional Resources

American Case Management Association. https://www.acmaweb.org/.

Case Management Body of Knowledge. https://cmbodyofknowledge.com/content/introduction-case-management-body-knowledge.

Case Management Society of America. https://cmsa.org/.

Global Social Service Workforce Alliance. https://www.socialserviceworkforce.org/.

National Health Service Foundation Trust. Wellness Recovery Action Plan (WRAP). Cheshire and Wirral Partnership. https://www.cwp.nhs.uk/about-us/our-campaigns/person-centred-framework/recovery-toolbox/wellness-recovery-action-plan-wrap/.

Wellness Recovery Actin Plan. Your Wellness Your Way. https://www.wellnessrecoveryactionplan.com/.

Conducting
Home Visits

Tim Berthold and Francis Julian Montgomery

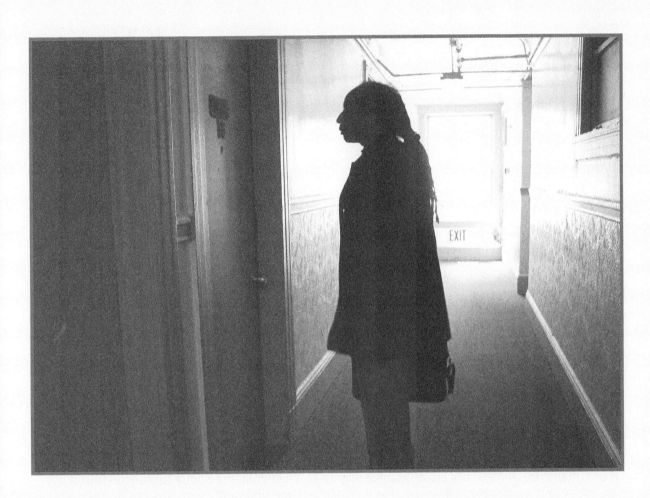

Client Scenario: Burke Turner

Burke Turner is 55 years old and divorced. Burke identifies as African-American and nonbinary and uses he/him pronouns. Burke is a patient at Health4All, a neighborhood health center. He has worked with the same physician, Dr. Fuller, for 20 years. Burke's electronic health record shows that he has been diagnosed with arthritis and high blood pressure. He also received treatment for depression in the past. Burke has done a good job over the years at taking prescribed medications.

Burke has two adult children whom he occasionally visits, and one lifelong friend, Verta, who he is deeply connected to. He has a long history of being unstably housed since childhood. Burke works as an auto mechanic when he is able to do so.

Burke currently lives in a Single Room Occupancy (SRO) unit in a converted downtown hotel. He has his own room with a microwave and minifridge. Down the hall are a shared bathroom and a small kitchen. Burke's room is on the second floor. There is an elevator in the building, but it doesn't always work.

Burke missed his last appointment with Dr. Fuller and did not call to cancel or reschedule. He hasn't picked up his prescribed medication in the past 60 days. Dr. Fuller asks a CHW colleague to reach out to Burke and schedule a home visit.

If you were the CHW assigned to conduct a home visit to Burke Turner, how would you answer the following questions?

- *How will you prepare for this home visit?*
- *What concerns might you have regarding Burke's health status?*
- *What goals will you set for the visit?*
- *What type of assessment can you conduct during the home visit, and how? What information are you hoping to learn from the home visit with Burke?*
- *What will you do to preserve Burke's confidentiality during the home visit?*
- *What guidelines will you keep in mind to help ensure your own safety and that of the client during the home visit?*

Introduction

This chapter provides an introduction to conducting home visits. While not all CHWs will be asked to conduct home visits, many do. Home visits are a valuable way to reach clients, especially those who find it difficult to attend a clinic or office appointment due to illness, disability, family responsibilities, or other reasons. Home visits are often an extension of the kinds of services that you provide in other settings—such as case management or chronic conditions management. The key difference is that you provide these services where someone lives and have a duty to respect their space. Meeting clients in their home can also provide you with an increased understanding of their lives including their strengths, resources, risks, and needs.

WHAT YOU WILL LEARN

By studying the information in this chapter, you will be able to:

- Define home visiting and provide examples of when and why they are conducted
- Prepare for home visits
- Provide person-centered home visits that respect the client's home, their privacy, and promote their independence
- Identify key safety concerns and plan for ways to address them

- Discuss what to do (and what not to do) when you arrive at a client's home
- Conduct a subtle assessment of the home environment and explain why this is important
- Identify and respond to common challenges related to home visiting

C3 Roles and Skills Addressed in Chapter 11

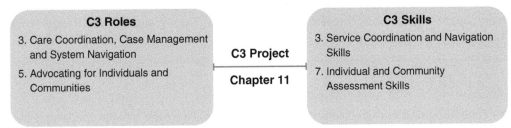

11.1 An Overview of Home Visits

As the name suggests, home visits involve meeting with clients where they live. People live or stay in a wide variety of settings such as:

- A house, apartment, or mobile home
- A car, van, or trailer
- An encampment where several or many unhoused people live
- On the street, in a doorway, a park, or parking lot
- A housing shelter or single-room occupancy (SRO) apartment or hotel
- A nursing home, hospital, rehabilitation, or board-and-care facility
- A residential drug treatment program, sober house, or other residential program

For clients who don't have a regular or consistent place to live, you may also visit them where they spend time or access services. This may include a park, a congregant or community meal site, or at an agency where they receive their monthly disability or social security check.

> **Francis Julian Montgomery:** It's important to know where clients hang out in the community in order to stay in contact, especially if they don't have a phone or an e-mail account. For example, I connect with some clients on the first Monday of the month when they go to pick up a check.

Home visiting is one of the most direct and personal ways to work with clients. You will often learn new information about the clients you visit and discover new opportunities to promote their health. For example, visiting a client with asthma can provide you with an opportunity to assess the home environment and support the client or family to explore options for reducing exposure to risk factors—such as mold, pet dander, and tobacco smoke—that may trigger asthma symptoms.

You may visit people you have never met before to encourage them to come to your agency for testing, health screening, counseling, or other services. You may follow up with existing clients who are unable to come to your agency or clinic because of severe disability, injury, acute health concerns, fear, or other barriers.

Whether you have met the client before or not, visiting them in their homes can enhance your understanding of their living situation, health risks, needs, and strengths. *Visiting clients in their homes requires the utmost respect from you.* They are inviting you into *their* spaces, their lives, and sometimes their families. Remember that you are a guest and be as respectful as you would want a visitor to your home to be.

> **TG:** I worked with clients in all kinds of places, including SROs [single—room occupancy hotels], apartments, shelters, group homes, tents in the park—you name it. No matter what kind of place I was visiting, I always remember that this is where the client lives, this is their space, and I respect that. And I always get a better understanding of my client, of how they live and what they may be up against. Also, I think because I am on their turf and not in my office—sometimes we are able to have the most personal or the deepest conversations. They might talk about experiences and feelings they never shared before.

HOME VISITS IN RURAL, SUBURBAN, AND URBAN SETTINGS

Home visits vary depending on the region or area where you work. There are unique challenges to providing home visits in rural versus suburban or urban areas. Some CHWs work in cities or counties that have a mix of these settings, and others will focus solely on serving rural or urban communities.

Factors that may influence home visiting in different regions include:

- **Transportation:** Transportation can be a barrier in any type of area, especially if there is a lack of reliable and affordable public transportation. The costs of transportation, such as gas and bus fares, are often barriers to services for low-income communities. In rural areas, the traveling time to services may be several hours. As you work with clients, ask them about transportation. How do they travel to visit family or access key services like food and health care? What challenges do they face when traveling? Note that sometimes health insurance, including Medicaid and Medicare, will authorize assistance with transportation such as paratransit for clients with disabilities. Nonemergency medical transportation may also be available for clients with disabilities through a Paratransit service.

- **Isolation and safety:** Safety is always a concern when conducting home visits. In rural areas, CHWs may visit homes that are isolated, without nearby neighbors or businesses, or that have limited cellular service. Approaching a rural home without an invitation can be challenging for reasons that may include protective dogs or relatives. Taking precautions to plan for the visit, in consultation with clients, can help to ensure that visits are safe and productive. Sending a letter to a client's address may be your first type of "outreach."

- **Lack of services:** The areas where your clients live may have limited access to resources such as health care or mental health services, healthy and affordable food, substance use treatment, etc. More than half of all rural counties in the United States lack hospitals with facilities for labor and delivery (PolicyLab, 2019).

- **Telehealth:** Telehealth and videoconferencing visits can connect hard-to-reach clients with health and social services support (see the section below on Telehealth visits).

The Rural Health Information Hub provides resources including model programs and evaluation tools for home visiting programs in rural areas (Rural Health Information Hub, 2022). They highlight programs focused on serving young children, Native American communities, and elders.

TELEHEALTH OR REMOTE VISITS

CHWs also connect with clients via phone or videoconferencing. These types of visits were used extensively during the COVID pandemic and helped people stay connected to vital services.

To participate in telehealth visits, clients must have a cell phone, tablet, laptop, or other digital device with video capability and a phone or WIFI plan. Unfortunately, many clients and communities lack access to digital devices and the internet. Approximately 25% of low-income Americans don't have access to a smartphone, and 40% don't have access to internet or computers (Vogels, 2021).

To help clients access affordable technology and internet service, research available programs and services in your city, county, or state, and check with federal resources such as the federal Office for the Advancement of Telehealth and the Lifeline Program (see Additional Resources posted at the end of this chapter). Keep in mind that some health insurance providers will cover the costs to set patients up with tablets for telehealth visits.

Francis Julian Montgomery: I meet with clients via videoconferencing when it is more convenient for them. I also help clients prepare for how to participate in telehealth appointments because, for some of them, this is new. I help them learn how to schedule telehealth visits on their phones or tablets, and how to minimize and expand the screen on their phone to switch from their text or e-mail to their phone. I help them practice turning on their video and how to hold their phone so that their health care provider can see them. The doctor or the social worker needs to be able to see the client to obtain visual and verbal consent for the visit. Practicing with their technology helps clients feel less stressed about meeting with their providers.

THE PURPOSE OF HOME VISITS

There are many reasons why CHWs conduct home visits, including:

- To visit clients who are unable to come to the agency or clinic where you work
- To follow up with clients who recently received services from your program or who have been discharged from the hospital or other services
- To contact clients who have not kept in touch, to see whether they are all right, and if they are interested in participating in services again
- To check in with clients who have recently experienced a decline in health
- To check in with a client because a family member or friend is concerned and asked you to schedule a home visit
- To encourage clients to come to your agency for important services that cannot be delivered at their homes
- To support new parents, guardians, or caregivers
- To assist clients to assess their home environments and possible health risks, such as fall hazards, exposure to mold, dust, or other allergens that cause asthma
- To provide support and guidance to clients regarding how to take medications properly
- To notify clients that they may have been exposed to an infectious disease and to encourage them to get screened
- To meet with clients who are in the hospital, jail, or other institutions

- *Can you think of other reasons to conduct home visits?*

What Do **YOU?** Think

RESEARCH ON HOME VISITS

Research shows that home visits conducted by CHWs have a positive impact on health outcomes. Home visits conducted by CHWs to high-risk diabetes patients in rural Appalachia demonstrated improvements in blood-glucose levels (Crespo, Christiansen, Tieman, & Wittberg, 2020). Home visits conducted by CHWs to patients with asthma demonstrated positive health outcomes including more days without asthma symptoms, fewer nights when sleep was interrupted by asthma symptoms, and fewer missed work and school days (Stout, Chen, Farquhar, Kramer, & Song, 2021). A review of seven studies of home visits conducted by CHWs in low and middle-income nations showed improved care-seeking by low-income families for ill infants (Tripathi, Kabra, Sachdeve, & Lodha, 2016). Research conducted in Afghanistan shows that home visits provided by CHWs can improve maternal and newborn health. As a result of home visits, both prenatal and postnatal care visits increased, and women were more likely to deliver children in health care facilities (Edmond et al., 2018).

The Home Visiting Evidence of Effectiveness (HomVEE) is a program of the federal Department of Health and Human Services established to assess the impact of early childhood home visits to families from pregnancy through kindergarten or age 5. It provides information about model programs, methods and standards for home visiting programs, and other relevant resources (Home Visiting Evidence of Effectiveness, 2022).

CHW Profile

David Valentine, He/Him/They
CHW and Volunteer Coordinator
Maitri Hospice, San Francisco CA
Hospice/End of Life Care

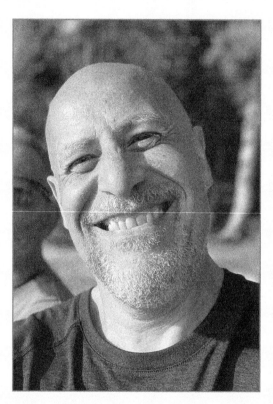

I was living in San Francisco at the height of the HIV/AIDS epidemic and friends were dying. I became active in ACT UP (An HIV advocacy organization). I started volunteering at Maitri, a hospice caring for people at the end of life. At some point, I realized that there was a "professional moniker" for what I was doing, and I thought, "I guess I should just go and get a CHW certificate." And that's what I did.

At Maitri, we offer home-based 24-hour, 7-day-a-week nursing care for people with some kind of chronic illness who are in crisis and need hospice attention or services. We focus on serving folks with HIV/AIDS, marginalized communities and people who are unhoused, people of color, queer, and poor folks. Our population used to be almost exclusively gay men, but we shifted our focus and now it's mixed: men, women, trans, and nonbinary people.

We get people adherent on their medications [taking current medications correctly]. We have a team that looks at their medical history and makes adjustments to whatever their medical needs may be. We have a doctor. We offer shelter, three square meals a day, and a lot of TLC (tender loving care). This can do wonders. We have people who come into hospice care and get stable, housed, and back into the world.

As for me, I wear two hats. I develop and implement the training of volunteers and staff and I also do case management for our aftercare clients. As a Volunteer Coordinator, I train volunteers, doctors, and medical staff on how to be with Maitri clients, including the basics of harm reduction, the use of motivational interviewing, etc. A lot of medical professionals don't have this type of training. I screen potential volunteers and manage them on a daily basis as they're interacting with our residents.

(continues)

CHW Profile

(continued)

Then there's the aftercare program. If folks are stabilized and don't need hospice anymore, we get them into housing. The aftercare program sends volunteers and staff out to do home visits wherever clients are living. We encourage people to become self-sufficient and stable. We also invite them back to Maitri for dinner hangouts, therapy, or case management meetings. We try to build community so that people rely on each other.

I remember a client who came to Maitri and her HIV viral load was extremely high. She was trans and had experienced severe trauma in her life. She had been sex trafficked. At Maitri, we managed to get her viral down to undetectable. She was able to have gender-affirming surgery while she was here. She was stabilized and went back out into the community. She's doing well now. She works in the community. She's a well-respected leader in her field working in the trans community.

In order to do this work properly, you have to be emotionally present. I'm more emotionally vulnerable now than I used to be. Our work also requires maintaining professional boundaries. I'm challenged every day. Finding a way to be with people in a nonjudgmental space has been a benefit for me. It's a spiritual practice to be with somebody with whatever they're going through. To be with them, but not to jump in there with them.

As a CHW or service provider, you're going to mess up. Just know that. That's the biggest challenge. We work every day with resourceful and resilient clients. You are not going to break them. They've seen worse than you. Just find that authentic self and trust that that is going to work. Then you will see that people are growing and thriving.

11.2 Preparing to Conduct a Home Visit

The nature of a home visit that you conduct will be determined by the type of agency and program you work for and the context or situation in which the client lives. Careful preparation will assist you in providing quality services once you reach the client.

PUT YOURSELF IN THE CLIENT'S SHOES

Imagine you are struggling with a challenging health condition and a CHW from a local agency is going to visit you in your home for the first time. How might it feel to have a stranger come into your home? What concerns might you have about the visit? What types of services and support would you want the CHW to provide? How would you want them to behave? What would you *not* want them to do, see, or ask?

Even when a client requests a home visit, it can be stressful to welcome a service provider into their space. They may feel anxious to protect their privacy and worried about revealing certain facts about their identity, health status, behaviors, relationship, or living situation. They may feel embarrassed or ashamed about certain aspects of their home life such as the condition of the place where they live, their lack of access to resources such as running water or food preparation and cooking facilities, or by family or home dynamics.

RESPECTING A CLIENT'S RIGHT TO PRIVACY—DISCREET HOME VISITS

Some clients have concerns about privacy. They may not want others to know that they are working with you or your agency, or that they have a certain health issue such as HIV disease, cancer, or a chronic mental health condition. How can you protect their privacy during home visits?

If you schedule the home visit in advance, ask the client how you can best preserve privacy. For example, will other people be present? If others are present in the home, how should you introduce yourself?

If the visit was not arranged in advance, be cautious and keep concerns about privacy in mind: don't say or do anything that could reveal the client's private information to others. For example, don't introduce yourself by saying: *"Hi, I'm Tranh, and I work for the AIDS Support Center."* If you aren't sure what you can and cannot say in front of others, don't say it! If others are present when you arrive at your client's home, you might say something like: *"Hello Mr. Turner, good to see you today. Is this a good time for a visit?"* Or, if possible, speak with the client in private to ask whether you should continue with the visit or reschedule.

> **TG:** I've worked with clients who didn't share their HIV status with the people they lived with, like their parents, or children, or sometimes their lovers. I need to be careful not to say something that will break this confidentiality. In private, of course, I will ask the client about this. And if they are shooting drugs or having sex with someone, I'll talk to them about taking precautions or disclosing their status. But it is their health, their decision. If I pressure them, or break their trust, my chance to help them is pretty much over.

START THINGS OFF RIGHT

Shadow Another CHW

If you haven't conducted home visits before, spend time learning from an experienced CHW or other colleague, such as a public health nurse. Ask your supervisor if it is possible for you to accompany or shadow a colleague as they conduct one or more home visits. Make sure that the client is notified in advance and has granted permission for more than one provider to participate in the home visit. If you are able to shadow an experienced CHW, closely observe what they do and how they interact with clients and their families.

- How do they introduce themselves?
- How do they build rapport with the client?
- How do they preserve the client's privacy?
- What questions do they ask, and what services do they provide?
- To what extent do they assess the home environment, and how?
- How do they document the home visit?

After the visits are completed, debrief with your colleague, and ask questions about anything you want to learn more about. Incorporate what you have learned into your own work.

Review and Prepare Client Files

Being well prepared and on-time demonstrates respect for the clients you visit.

If you are going to visit a client you already work with, review the client's file and key strengths, risks, needs, and any health conditions. The file may include an action plan (see Chapters 9 and 10). Check to see if referrals were provided in the past. If so, has the client accessed the referral resource(s)? Is the client working with other service providers? Does the file include permissions to release information (or to share information about the client) with other providers? Bring copies of blank release forms in case you need them.

If the client does not have a file at your agency, create a blank one and complete any forms that can be done in advance of your visit. Bring blank copies of any additional forms you may need, such as informed consent forms, referral forms, and home visit assessment forms along with several pens and something for you and the client to write on in case it is needed.

Organize and Pack Resources to Bring on the Visit

Pack everything you may need during the home visit and review it carefully to be sure that you haven't forgotten anything. Develop a standardized checklist of materials (your agency may already have one) to guide you in preparing these resources. Some of the resources you might include are:

- Your identification badge and business card
- Written information (in the appropriate language or languages) about your agency, your program, and key policies and protocols, including confidentiality and its limits (or a HIPAA form as required), and any costs associated with the services provided
- A cell phone and a list of emergency numbers
- The client's address and a map in case you lose cell or internet service
- A tablet, laptop, or other digital devise for reviewing a client's electronic health record with them and documenting key information that you learn and services you provide during the visit. In some locations, you will not be able to access a phone or the internet, so always bring backup paper copies of key forms and information to review with the client, such as any test results that you are authorized to review with the client. Note that some agencies may provide laptops or tablets with portable Wi-Fi access
- Client files, blank new client files, and other forms along with pens for you and the client to use
- Any medications or tests that you are authorized to bring and administer
- Educational materials to explain something more clearly
- Risk-reduction or other health materials such as condoms, lubricants, hygiene kits, nutritional supplements, food or transportation vouchers, phone cards, and so on
- A list of other resources that you may want to share with the client, such as resources for food, housing, health care and mental health services, or legal assistance
- A folding chair or stool to ensure that you have a place to sit during a long visit
- A flashlight, in case you are visiting the client after dark
- Garbage bags in case the client requires help cleaning up their home
- A communication device (cell phone in case of emergency or in case you can't locate the client) and a list of emergency numbers

Organize all of these items into an easy-to-carry bag or backpack. A backpack with several compartments for your resources works well. Backpacks are also one of the most discreet ways to bring items with you to the home visit.

- *What else might be important to bring with you on a home visit?*

Francis Julian Montgomery: I have a folding, portable "travel chair" that I carry with me everywhere I go. I have bad knees, so it is important for me to have a place to sit. But the chair also helps my clients maintain their dignity by allowing me to be respectful while in their home environment.

Many of the homes I visit are small Single-Room Occupancy (SRO) units. There is really not much in each room besides a bed for a person to sit on. But I believe a person's bed is a private and sacred space, just for them, and I wouldn't want to be disrespectful of that by sitting on it. At the same time, it would be odd to stand for 20–30 minutes while I am conducting an assessment. So, I pull out my chair, which makes it more comfortable for both of us. And people get a kick out of seeing me in my chair!

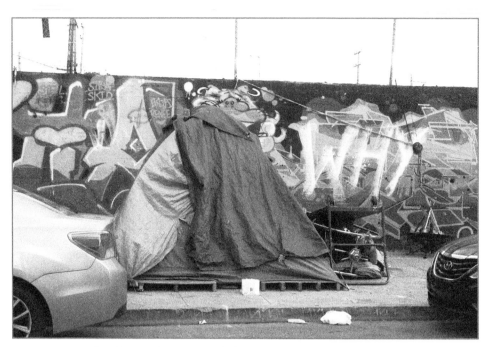

CHWs may conduct home visits to people living in on the streets

PLAN HOW YOU WILL TRAVEL TO THE CLIENT'S HOME

Review the client's contact information. Do you have the proper address? If possible, verify the address by calling the client. You'll want to know *exactly* where you will be going. Look at a map or GPS coordinates if you're unfamiliar with the area, to locate the following information:

- Client's address
- Landmarks nearby. Look up the location online in advance to familiarize yourself with the neighborhood and to plan your travel route and mode of transportation.
- Parking availability or nearby public transportation routes
- For your own comfort, you may want to identify nearby public bathrooms. Not all clients will have a bathroom or feel comfortable with you using theirs.
- Anything you might need to know for your safety (see the section on safety below)

If you have an appointment and can speak with the client in advance, try to determine:

- If there is a clearly marked house, apartment, or room number
- If there is a gate or intercom at the home or building and, if so, what do you need to do to gain access to the home
- If the client has a dog or other pets
- Any possible problems you may encounter when entering the home

Make sure you have the client's phone number with you (if the client has a phone), in case you get lost or have trouble getting into the building. If the client does not have a phone, ask if another household member or neighbor has a phone, and if it is okay to call them if necessary. Be sure to bring this number with you. Remember that low-income clients may qualify for free phones and cell phone plans through the federal Lifeline Program.

REVIEW AVAILABLE CLIENT INFORMATION

Carefully review a client's file before a home visit so that you are prepared to cover current issues, questions, and concerns. Review the most recent notes from your colleagues, clinical team, or other providers. With the use of shared electronic health record (when the client gives permission), you can look at both current and past information about the client's health and social conditions. Make notes for your visit including information such as their housing status, any chronic health conditions they have, and medications that they have been prescribed. You also want to learn as much about their social history as possible such as if they live with other people, if they have children, if they are single, in a relationship, or widowed.

You may be able to review the client's pharmacy records to see what medications are currently prescribed, which have been discontinued, and where the client picks up their medications or if it is mailed to them. Electronic health records will show if the client has picked up their medications in the past 30 or 90 days. If medications were prescribed but they haven't been picked up or sent out, the client may be experiencing a barrier. It could mean that the client forgot about the medication, that they don't intend to take the medication or don't like the side effects, or it could mean that they are having difficulty getting to the pharmacy to pick up their medication. You won't know what is going on until you have an opportunity to talk with the client. Helping clients to access current medications is a very direct way for CHWs to assist them. With authorization from your employer, you may be able to deliver medications to homebound patients or arrange for others to deliver medications to their homes.

IDENTIFY KEY OBJECTIVES

Write down what you hope to accomplish during the home visit. For example, have you been asked to visit a client who has been out of communication to check if they are alright and interested in resuming services? Are you visiting with a client recently released from the hospital to help them with aftercare services? Don't set too many goals for a single visit. While it is important to identify the purpose of your visit, you also want to be flexible and responsive to the client's current concerns and priorities. Talk with the client to learn about their current health status, needs, and priorities.

PREPARING TO CONDUCT A VISIT TO A NEW CLIENT

You may conduct home visits to clients who haven't worked with you or your agency or program before. They may have been referred by another local agency or provider.

If you are visiting someone you have not met before, please review Chapter 8; it provides basic concepts and skills for how to introduce yourself, review the services that your agency provides, and to explain client confidentiality and its limits. Bring any essential forms with you such as a copy of your agency's confidentiality or HIPAA policy.

Your primary goals for a first visit will be to establish a positive connection with the client, to begin to build a small measure to trust, to assess the client's resources and needs, and to determine whether the person is interested in the services that you provide and would like to begin to work together.

PREPARING FOR FOLLOW-UP VISITS

You will also visit clients you have worked with before. Try to prepare yourself for what you may see and learn. It can be difficult to witness a client who is in crisis, whose health is deteriorating, or who is facing the end of life. Keep in mind that these are the times when clients may most require your support, especially if they don't have a strong social support network.

Even if you have worked with the client before and are visiting to follow up on a specific issue you have discussed in the past, don't assume you will both have the same memory or understanding of past visits or conversations. Due to factors such as stress, trauma, dementia, or illness, the client may not remember the nature of your work together, including previous conversations and agreements, or care very much about it at the moment. As always, be patient and compassionate, and take time to reintroduce yourself, to review your previous work together, and, if necessary, to start all over at the beginning. The essence of person-centered work is meeting clients where they are. Don't assume that you know where they will "be" when you conduct a follow-up home visit.

Possible goals for follow-up visits may include to:

- Review any decisions, agreements, or accomplishments that the client previously made
- Assess their current concerns, needs, and priorities—what do they want to accomplish?

- Establish new goals that the client wants to work on and let these guide your work
- Provide health education, person-centered counseling, and referrals, as appropriate
- Bring medications and assist clients with medications management (see Chapter 16)
- Arrange for other services and possible transportation to access other services
- Provide additional supplies as needed (e.g., nutritional supplements, safer sex supplies, bandages, bedding, or clothing, and so forth).
- Set a date and time for your next visit

- *What other goals might you have for these home visits?*

11.3 Common Courtesies and Guidelines

RESPECT THE CLIENT'S TIME

If the client is anticipating your visit, show up for the appointment on time. If something unforeseen happens and you are running late, call or text the client to inform them and to apologize. If you make a practice of being late, you risk losing the client's trust and respect.

If you schedule a home visit in advance, discuss how much time you both have for the visit. If you need an hour, ask for it, but respect the client's limits and needs: *"I'd like to visit for about an hour, will that work for you?"* When you arrive, ask the client if it is still a good time to visit, and how much time the person will be able to spend with you. Stay aware, throughout the visit, of signs that the client may want the visit to end. Be respectful: it is the client's home, the client's time, and the client's life. If you don't accomplish all your goals for the visit, schedule a follow-up appointment in the home, at your agency, or at another location that works for both you and the client.

ANNOUNCE YOURSELF

When you arrive at the client's home, announce yourself. Use your name, but not the name of your agency in order to protect the client's privacy. You might say something like: *"Hello, Mr. Turner? It's Sunil Gupta. We spoke earlier about meeting today. Is this still a good time?"*

> **Francis Julian Montgomery:** For safety, security or other reasons, people may not feel comfortable having a stranger in their home. As a result, when I am trying to conduct a home visit, sometimes I end up talking to someone from outside the door to their room. I might sit in my portable chair in the hallway of the SRO [Single Room Occupancy Hotel], and I make sure I am speaking in a low tone so that no one else can hear. Once a person sees that I am committed to respecting their comfort and their space, they often decide to invite me inside.

INTRODUCE YOURSELF

Once you're inside the client's home, introduce yourself again: *"Hello Mr. Turner. I'm Sunil Gupta. We spoke on the phone earlier. It's nice to meet you/see you."* Be sure you have proper identification with you when you arrive and show it to the client or family if requested.

If you provide services related to sensitive and highly personal issues, and you are not alone with the client, be careful about saying the name of your organization or the issue you address. If other people are around, follow the client's lead. If you aren't sure how to proceed, ask the client: *"Mr. Turner, is this a good time to talk or would you rather reschedule our appointment?"*

IF THE CLIENT IS NOT AT HOME

If no one answers, follow up with the client later. If someone other than the client answers, and the client isn't home, leave a simple message that preserves the client's confidentiality such as: *"Could you tell Mr. Turner that Sunil dropped by to say hello?"*

DRESS FOR THE OCCASION

Make sure to wear clothing that is appropriate for the setting. Consider comfort and what is culturally respectful to the community you are visiting, as well as the safety guidelines discussed below. Some situations call for slightly more professional clothing, and others for more casual wear. If you're visiting someone who is incarcerated, be sure to find out beforehand what the dress code is for visitors to the institution, or you may not be permitted to enter. If you are visiting a family with young children, wear comfortable clothes that will allow you to engage with the children. Ask your colleagues, particularly other CHWs who conduct outreach and home visits, what they would wear, and use your own best judgment.

DEMONSTRATE RESPECT AND ESTABLISH A POSITIVE CONNECTION

Observe common courtesies: introduce yourself to others, ask people how they are doing, and thank them for inviting you into their home.

Be respectful of the client's home regardless of its condition. Anticipate that some of the homes you visit may be cramped, crowded, dirty, smelly, or in need of repair. Clients may be living with challenges such as mental health conditions, substance use, chronic pain, or dementia.

Your warmth, honesty, and kindness will assist in making the visits a success. Let your work be guided by unconditional positive regard, kindness, and respect for your clients' identities, cultures, and right to self-determination.

> **Ramona Benson:** Sometimes the client's family had bad home visits in the past, and based on that experience, they ask me: "Why you want to come to my house?" So, I always say to people, "I don't have to come to your house. I'll meet you anywhere you want me to meet you at." I don't push myself on anybody—that's not going to do anyone any good. Sometimes they want to have the home visit at a McDonald's because home life is not fine, you know? Or they might want to have the home visit at the doctor's office, and so we meet there, but any public place where I'm meeting, I have to make sure that what are we saying is not being heard because of confidentiality.

PRACTICE CULTURAL HUMILITY

Practice cultural humility (see Chapter 7) as you conduct home visits. The cultures, values, and traditions of the clients and families you visit will be reflected in their homes. The furnishings and art, the foods and smells in the homes, the religious symbols or lack of them, the makeup of the families, and their customs may be different from what you are familiar with. View home visiting as an opportunity to learn more about the cultures of others. Abide by the rules in place in their homes, as you would expect in yours, and ask questions if you are unsure about what to do.

SPEAK CLEARLY

Sometimes, people speak quickly or loudly when they are nervous. Your calm voice can help to relax others as well as yourself. If people are living on the streets, in shelters, at the hospital, in SROs or apartments with thin walls, or a large family, your voice may be overheard. Speak loudly enough for the client or clients to hear you, but not so loudly that you broadcast private information to others. If you can't hear or understand what a client tells you, ask them to tell you again: you don't want to miss important information.

Try to determine beforehand if the client is hard of hearing or if they have language requirements that may require culturally appropriate accommodations (such as interpreters or another CHW who can speak their language).

Please watch the following video ▶ interview. In this interview, Francis Julian Montgomery shares tips for conducting successful home visits.

- *What information did the CHW share that you would like to put into practice as you conduct home visits?*

CONDUCTING HOME VISITS: (*Source:* Foundations for Community Health Workers/http://youtu.be/BSgqpdyvZ5w/last accessed 21 September 2023.)

MAINTAIN HEALTHY BOUNDARIES

To assist in preventing potentially dangerous or harmful situations, maintain healthy boundaries with clients. Be cautious about disclosing personal information (home or cell phone number or address) or private details about your life. If a client asks you personal questions that you do not feel comfortable answering, be ready to clarify your role as a CHW and why you won't answer these questions. You might say something like, *"My role is to be here for you, to support you to improve your health. I don't talk about my private life when I'm at work, because that will distract us—this is* <u>your time</u>.*"* Be clear and kind as you assert these boundaries. If a client starts to say things that are not acceptable (such as sexual innuendos or suggestions), interrupt or stop the conversation. If the client continues to push at your boundaries and does not respect the limits that you set, you may have to leave. For more information about boundary setting, see Chapter 5.

STAY ON-TOPIC

Plan for how you will disengage from conversations that are taking too much time and attention away from the primary purpose of your visit. At the same time, be prepared to do some casual visiting. This is a customary part of most visits to another person's home. The client may show you personal belongings, such as family photographs, or want to introduce you to family members who will engage you in discussions about a range of issues, from politics to the latest ball game.

While you hope that clients will feel comfortable enough to open up and talk with you about the personal issues that are influencing their health and well-being, some clients may want to talk with you for a long time about their lives, their families, their hopes, and their dreams. This may be a sign of their isolation and loneliness, or of fears related to their health and mortality. Develop your own polite way to interrupt clients and remind them of the time and main purpose of the visit.

Whenever you are working with a client who talks excessively, figure out a way to calm the person down or slow down the discussion. You might say something to switch the focus of the conversation such as, *"Mr. Turner, I wish I had more time to talk with you. But I want to make sure that we can complete _____. Can I ask you about _____?"*

Client Scenario: Burke Turner (*continued*)

The CHW reaches Burke Turner by phone and schedules a home visit, checking the address carefully. Burke lives in an SRO-unit in a downtown hotel that the CHW is familiar with.

The CHW knocks on Burke's door and introduces themselves. Burke shouts, *"Come on in,"* and the CHW enters his room. Burke is sitting on his bed, propped up with several pillows. There is a small table next to him, with a dozen take-out food containers. Clothes are piled high in front of the bed.

CHW: It's good to see you, Burke. Thank you for meeting with me.

Burke: Thanks for coming here. I know I missed my appointment, but ... I've kind of been stuck over here.

(continues)

Client Scenario: Burke Turner (*continued*)

CHW: It's understandable. When folks aren't feeling well, they don't like to leave the house, even for medical appointments. Can I go ahead and set up my traveling chair over here? [points to space in front of Burke and about eight feet back]

Burke: Yeah, that'll work. [The CHW unfolds a traveling chair and sits down, taking out a clipboard to take notes on, and a cell phone]

CHW: Tell me about what's been going on for you. You say you've been stuck?

Burke: Well, I've got this pain that comes and goes, mostly in my legs. Usually, I manage okay. But my right knee and hip have been pretty bad. It's been harder than usual to get around. I've mostly been staying in bed.

CHW: Are you comfortable right now, sitting up in bed?

Burke: [nods] I'm okay.

CHW: So, you weren't able to come to the clinic for your appointment?

Burke: I couldn't manage it. The elevator was out again and I can't... I can't get down the stairs.

CHW: I'm sorry to hear that you've been in pain and having difficulty getting around. Are you able to get up and go to the bathroom?

Burke: I get up when I really need to go. It's down the hall. And I've also been peeing in a bottle.

CHW: I noticed in your health record that Dr. Fuller diagnosed you with arthritis, is that right?

Burke: Yes, I've had arthritis for... [B. pauses and thinks] It must be at least five years now.

CHW: And you've been managing the pain with Ibuprofen?

Burke: Yeah, it usually works. I didn't want anything stronger. But I ran out of pills. [He looks around the apartment]. I ran out of just about everything.

CHW: Does that include your blood pressure medications?

Burke: [nods] I haven't been able to get to the Walgreens [pharmacy].

CHW: Well, I'm glad I visited then. [Burke smiles]. I can definitely help you with this, getting your medications and such. But I have a few more questions to ask to help me understand what's been going on for you. Is that okay?

Burke: Of course.

The CHW asks Burke if he has a cane or a walker and if he might like a bedside commode for going to the bathroom when he is pain. Burke says that he has always refused getting a walker, but he wishes he had one now. He tells the CHW that he will trying using a commode if he needs it.

The CHW asks how Burke has been getting his meals. Burke says that his youngest son comes by to do laundry and bring him food. He points to the take-out containers on the table next to him.

CHW: I'm glad to hear that your son has been stopping by to help you out. Now, is there anything else that I can help you with? Do you have any other priorities or concerns?

Burke: Well, I guess I need help moving around and something for the pain. I should start back on my blood pressure medications too.

CHW: Okay, we can help you with that. You've done the videoconferencing visits over your phone before, is that right?

Burke: Yeah, I've done that before with Dr. Fuller.

CHW: So, would you be open to scheduling a telehealth visit as soon as possible?

Burke: Yes, that's good with me. I don't know where my phone is just now [Burke looks around]

(continues)

Client Scenario: Burke Turner (*continued*)

The CHW asks for permission to help Burke find his phone. Burke agrees. The CHW finds Burke's cell phone under some food containers. The CHW asks for permission to bag up the take-out food containers and Burke also agrees. The CHW takes some large garbage bags out of his backpack and cleans up the take-out containers. The CHW sets up the cell phone charger and phone on the table so that Burke can reach it from his bed. The CHW asks if Burke is thirsty. Burke asks the CHW for some water and tells them where to find a clean glass. After getting the water, the CHW sits back down on the traveling chair and reviews with Burke how to confirm and log-in to a telehealth visit on his phone.

11.4 Safety Guidelines for Home Visits

Safety concerns for home visiting may include witnessing arguments, domestic violence or other types of violence, observing signs of neglect or abuse, unintentional involvement in police actions, witnessing arguments or encountering an angry, aggressive, or threatening person.

Sometimes our own biases and lack of knowledge about a client or a community may influence our assessment of safety. Try not to let bias guide or distort the way that you assess safety risks or result in discriminating against communities that already experience high rates of prejudice, stigma, and discrimination. Remember that safety issues are present in all work setting and all communities.

Some members of the community may view you as an outsider and with suspicion or fear. This is one of many reasons that it is so essential to take time to get to know the community you will be working in. Knowing as much as possible about the neighborhoods and areas where you do home visits allows you to be prepared, and to keep yourself safe.

When you arrive at the location for the home visit, evaluate the current situation. Your instincts will develop over time. Pay attention to them when you feel particularly ill at ease, anxious, or unsafe—they may be tipping you off to a dangerous situation. If you are concerned that the situation is not safe, consider leaving. Let the client know that you will follow up to reschedule the visit for another time (or, if possible, in a different location).

SAFETY TIPS

Be Prepared

- If possible, contact the client in advance to negotiate a time for the home visit.
- Let your supervisor or another colleague know which client you will visit, where you will be going, and when.
- Find out what type of housing the client lives in and where.
- Find out detailed information about the locations you will be visiting, including the reputation of the areas and recent events such as homicides, assaults, burglaries, or hand-to-hand drug sales.
- Find out as much information as you can about the client you will visit (e.g., have they reported domestic violence, do they live alone, have they made threats to employees in the past, do they have any pets that might be dangerous?).
  - Refer to Oregon's Home Visitor Safety Guide references at the end of this chapter to learn more about how to conduct a preliminary Site Safety Assessment. The Assessment is designed to help staff and agencies determine whether to conduct home visits based on potential safety risks such as the assessed risk of aggression, the presence of weapons, threats have been made against the home visitor or their colleagues, etc. (Oregon Health Authority, 2014)

Lee Jackson: You're going into the trenches. Think about how to mentally prepare for your visits. You may not run into any problems but be prepared in case you do. Be aware of what you're wearing. You want to be sure to wear slacks or jeans and comfortable shoes. Don't wear anything too expensive like nice jewelry or a watch—someone there might really need a fix that day.

- If you are working in areas the community itself considers risky, have a plan, and be prepared. Consider working with a partner. Talk with your supervisor about the situation and what can be done to minimize risks to yourself and to clients.
  - Some organizations assign staff to conduct home visits in teams of two. Working in a team can enhance safety but may be off-putting to some clients. Discuss this option with your team and supervisor.
- Schedule appointments during daylight hours whenever possible. If you are going to be visiting clients after dark, be sure to carry a working flashlight with you.
- Dress appropriately and comfortably. Wear light-colored clothes that are more identifiable at night and sturdy walking shoes. Avoid wearing valuable jewelry or other accessories. Always wear your employee I.D. Carry a whistle or other noise-making item.
- Avoid agency logos or signage on your car, clothing, or anywhere else that might draw attention.
- If you have a cell phone, bring it with you in case you encounter a safety concern or an emergency. If you do not have a cell phone and will be doing home visits, ask if your agency can provide one for safety purposes.
- Take only the items you need for the home visit and leave other valuables at home or in the office.

Pay Attention, and Be Discreet

- Be discreet when visiting a new location. Try not to draw attention to yourself.
- Carry yourself with confident body language.
- The risks to women are different than for men. Be aware of these risks and make decisions that preserve your safety.
- Be aware of your surroundings at all times.
- If you are driving, try to park in a well-lit place close to the client's address. Park on the street if possible rather than in a driveway to avoid being blocked.
- Treat everyone with respect.
- Trust your instincts about the situations you encounter.
- Be ready to think on your feet, to make quick evaluations and decisions about situations as they develop.

If Conflict or Danger Arises

- **Deescalate conflict** and work to calm the person involved. Maintain a calm tone of voice. See Chapter 13 to learn skills for handling conflict effectively.
- **Apologize.** You may have unintentionally done something that provoked the person's anxiety or anger. A sincere apology often helps to reduce or minimize conflict.
- **If you don't feel safe,** *Leave.* Text your supervisor when you can to let them know what happened and where you are.
- **Report and Document** If you witness violence or other reportable incidents related to your clients, report them to your supervisor immediately, and document them in your field notes. Debrief the incidents with someone you trust.
- *Only call the police if it is absolutely required.* Most situations will not require this. If you feel you *must* contact the police in order to preserve your safety, do so. However, consider the effect this might have on your work with this community. Be cautious about calling the police into a community that has a history of tensions with the law; you might lose the community's trust and respect, and hence your ability to continue to work with the community.

- *Can you think of other safety tips?*

- *What are your biggest safety concerns?*

- *How will you address them and keep yourself safe as you work in the community?*

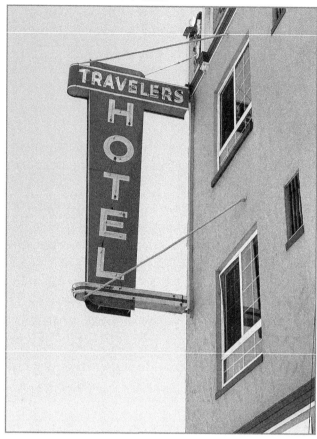

CHWs may conduct home visits to people living in single room occupancy (SRO) hotels.

11.5 How to Conduct a Home Visit

Once you have introduced yourself and been invited into the home, confirm that you are talking to the client (or the primary caregiver in case of a child). If other people such as family members are present, be friendly and patient. Once you are talking with the client or primary caregiver, explain again why you have come and ask for a more private place to meet. Say something like: *"Mr. Turner, it's a pleasure to meet you. I'm Sunil. Is this still a good time for us to visit? Is there a private place where we can sit down together to talk?"*

Clearly explain why you are conducting the home visit and ask what the client would like to accomplish.

> **LaTonya Rogers:** On my first home visit, I tell the families, I'm here to help you get what you need to handle your child's asthma. What would you like to talk about today?

CONDUCT AN ASSESSMENT

During each home visit, you will conduct some type of assessment. Topics that you may assess include:

- A client's strengths, risks, and goals in order to develop a case management or action plan
- A client's current health status and need for additional services such as access to food, transportation, or in-home support services.

- A client's knowledge about and interest in a particular service
- Adherence to specific treatments such as taking daily medications
- A client's progress with their case management or action plan
- Exposure to environmental health risks

> **Francis Julian Montgomery:** I know I'm asking for a lot of personal information during an intake or assessment, so I try to make it a conversation instead of an interrogation. I don't just read questions off of an intake list. And I make sure to really listen because clients will often tell me things in response to one question that fills in answers to other questions as well.

CHWs often conduct home visits to clients who are living with chronic health conditions. In these circumstances, the assessment may also address:

- The client's current understanding of their health condition. For example, what does the client understand about type 2 diabetes and how to manage it?
- Current signs and symptoms. While CHWs are not clinicians and must not work outside of their scope of practice (see Chapter 5), they are often trained and authorized to check and report on specific symptoms and to communicate their findings to their colleagues. This may include current asthma symptoms or complications from HIV disease.
- Recent test results. Occasionally CHWs will be trained, certified, and authorized to perform certain tests, such as COVID or HIV antibody tests, or to teach clients how to understand the meaning of recent tests, such as blood pressure readings.
- Support with self-management (see Chapter 16) and implementation of a personalized Action Plan
- Medication management (see Chapter 16).
- Scheduling and reminders about upcoming appointments, such as well-baby exams, and showing clients how to plan to keep the appointment.

CONDUCTING AN ENVIRONMENTAL ASSESSMENT

During a visit, you will observe the home environment. What you observe may provide you with a better understanding of the client's strengths, risks, and needs. For example, you may observe:

- Basic living conditions, including access to clean sheets, clothing, and resources for hygiene (running water, soap, shampoo, toothpaste, and so on)
- Availability of food, food storage, and cooking facilities
- Environmental risks such as mold, dust, insect or rodent issues, or safety hazards for young children or seniors (clutter and tripping hazards are significant risks for seniors)
- The presence or absence of friends, family, roommates, and the quality of those relationships
- The client's level of stress at home
- Challenges with mobility within or outside of the home
- Possible abuse or neglect

- *What else might you observe during a home visit that could inform you about a client's health and well-being?*

What Do **YOU?** Think

CHWS Assist Elders with Injury Prevention: The Community and Home Injury Prevention Program for Seniors (Chipps)

Falls are the leading cause of death for older adults, and the most likely place for a fall is in their own home, yet falls are preventable with minor behavior and environmental changes. Each year, on average, 1800 older adults die from falls and 1.5 million are treated in emergency departments for injuries (Centers for Disease Control and Prevention, 2022).

Falls are a threat to the health of older adults and can reduce their ability to remain independent; however, falls in the home are preventable with evidence-based practices to reduce falls and other injuries and ensure the safety of older adults in their homes.

Multi-lingual and multi-cultural CHWs trained in injury prevention are important educators as part of The San Francisco Department of Public Health's *Community and Home Injury Prevention Program for Seniors* (CHIPPS).

CHIPPS's CHWs provide outreach and engage low-income older adults impacted by health disparities such as social isolation, food and housing insecurity, economic instability, and language barriers. In addition to community presentations on injury prevention for older adults, CHWs meet directly with older adults and people with disabilities in their homes to help themselves prevent falls and injuries so they can live safely and independently at home. CHWs provide one-on-one education and conduct a home safety assessment to suggest simple behavior changes such as removing throw rugs as well as recommending minor home modifications such as installing grab bars to increase safety in the home. Simple items CHWs distribute, such as bathmats, night lights, kitchen timers, grab bars, and shower chairs have a significant impact on reducing falls and injuries.

CHWs find that many older adults do not have the social support needed to thrive, nor do they know where to find such support. When CHIPPS CHWs are in the home, they notice and listen to the individual's needs and even provide resources beyond home safety, such as food support, help to communicate with landlords and property managers, facilitate linkages to case managers, and more. CHWs become a resource to the older adult as well as the family to keep our aging population in San Francisco safe, connected, and healthy in their own homes.

The CHIPPS CHW's express personal pleasure in being able to do this work, as well as learn about other issues facing older adults. Older adults regularly share the value and impact the CHWs on their lives.

Comments Shared by Older Adults with CHWs

- *"I do not know where to buy a bathmat and I've fallen in the bathtub many times. I asked my friends and they do not know where to buy it as well. No young people help me, I am all by myself and I am old."*

- *"My husband had spine surgery last year and we need a wheelchair, cane, and a commode to help him. However, none of these are covered by the insurance, and I felt some burden if we pay out of pocket for these items. Your program helps us so much, at least now, we have grab bars and handrails installed in the house and provide good support for him."*

- *"Your program is amazing. Nowadays, it's really difficult to find a Chinese-speaking handyman to do small jobs like installing grab bars. I am so grateful your program provides the Chinese interpretation and helps us with installation. We've been thinking to install grab bars and handrails because I cannot walk well. We do not know where to start since we do not live with our children, one lives in Canada, and one lives out of the state. Thank you for caring for seniors."*

For more information about the CHIPPS Program, please go to https://www.sfdph.org/dph/comupg/oprograms/CHEP/Injury/CHIPPS.asp

Occasionally, you will be asked to conduct a more thorough environmental assessment during a home visit—with the client's participation and permission. For example, if you are working with a client living with asthma, diabetes, depression, cancer, or other chronic health conditions, you may assess:

- Exposure to environmental factors that may trigger illness. In the case of asthma, this might include assessing exposure to excessive dust, mold, animals, second-hand smoke, and diesel emissions from a nearby street or highway.

- Access to food. Is there food in the house? Is it nutritious and in keeping with the diet prescribed by the person's health care provider? What did the client eat this morning or last night?

- Access to clean sheets and clothes, or a laundry

- Exposure to safety risks such as physical threats or abuse

- Signs of alcohol and/or drug use. Has the client relapsed? Do they understand how street drugs and alcohol may interact with their medications and impact their health condition?

- The status of medications. Are they up to date? Does the client have enough medication for the next few days, week, or month? Is the client taking the medications? Are the medications clearly labeled and organized? If the client takes multiple medications in a day, is there a schedule or system to remind the person to do this?

- Needs for immediate assistance or referral to a medical provider

You can conduct an environmental assessment by observing what is in sight and asking the client's permission to look at other parts of the home. For example, you might ask: *"Burke, can you show me where you keep your medications? Is it alright with you if I check to see that your medications are up to date?"* Never start to look around a client's home without the person's knowledge or permission. Be sensitive in the way that you ask, the way that you look, and the comments you make as you learn more about the home: this type of assessment can be difficult for clients who may be acutely embarrassed by the current state of their living conditions.

Your goal is always to assist clients to identify any barriers or risks to their health, and to work with them to identify realistic changes that they want to make to their environment to reduce these risks. This may mean assisting clients to organize their medications, to report mold to the landlord or housing authority, or to arrange for home delivery of healthy meals.

PROVIDING CASE MANAGEMENT, PERSON-CENTERED COUNSELING, AND HEALTH EDUCATION

Depending on the client's needs, your skills, and your existing relationship, you may provide additional services such as person-centered counseling, health education, or case management. Please note that these topics are addressed in depth in other chapters of the *Foundations* book.

Francis Julian Montgomery: CHWs are sometimes asked to visit a client while they are in the emergency department or when they become admitted as a patient into the hospital. It is always important to notify your clinical team about this, and to communicate clearly with the hospital staff. I always go to the nursing station first and introduce myself and the agency I represent. I tell them who I am there to visit. Sometimes you can visit with the patient at their bedside, but sometimes that isn't possible. I do avoid visiting a client if they are in the Intensive Care Unit (ICU) because you may just be in the way of the hospital staff.

With regular inpatient units, you can visit with the client and provide support and encouragement. If I can, I try to bring a card or flowers or something of that nature because, with some clients, they may not have any other visitors. This helps to brighten up their day. Usually, clients are grateful to see you, and this can create an opportunity for them to share new information with you. The client can tell you if they are facing any difficulties or would like any help communicating with hospital staff or family. I always try to ask clients what led up to their hospitalization. This information that can help the client to improve their health in the future and could prevent future hospitalizations.

(continues)

(continued)

You may also help with discharge planning, arranging for necessary services to be continued when the patient returns home or if they are transferred to another facility like a rehabilitation hospital. Sometimes you work with the hospital staff, the nurses, and social worker to prepare a client for discharge. This is always a gentle dance because you don't want to step on the toes of the hospital staff, but you do want to advocate for the client, and you probably know more about the client's home situation. I help to make sure that they get any durable medical equipment that they might need, or access to physical or occupational therapy if they need it, or in-home supportive services.

After the client returns home, I try to visit them to check how they are doing and if they need any assistance with things like meal or grocery delivery, medications, or in-home support services.

EXPLAIN THE NEXT STEPS

Take time to clarify and document the next steps you and client plan to take. This plan should clearly address the concerns and priorities the client discussed with you. Confirm the date and location of your next appointment. Write down the plan and leave it for the client. Follow-up with a text or e-mail if the client has access to electronic communications. If the client can't read, ask if there is someone who can review the plan with them.

GOOD-BYE AND THANK-YOU

Tell the client (and other family members) good-bye. Thank them again for their time and hospitality. If you need directions or assistance getting out of the building, ask before you leave.

Client Scenario: Burke Turner *(continued)*

Burke's electronic health record shows that he has been diagnosed and treated for depression in the past. In accordance with their training and scope of practice, the CHW asks Burke a few questions about his emotional health based on a commonly used depression assessment tool.

Burke: Not being able to get around and being in pain, it kind of makes the depression come back, you know? I've had it—depression—before.

CHW: Well, depression can kind of creep back in there when we're not doing well. Especially when we've experienced depression before.

Burke: Yeah.

CHW: I'm wondering if you're open to talking with someone about your depression. They will conduct a more thorough assessment and they might even recommend some treatments. How does this idea sound to you Burke?

Burke: I trust doctor Fuller. I want to talk to him.

CHW: Well, it sounds like you and Dr. Fuller have a good partnership. [Burke nods] It seems like connecting with Dr. Fuller is the appropriate thing for you in this moment, not only for your medical health but for your emotional health as well.

Burke: We go way back. He's helped me with my depression before.

CHW: Okay. Burke, we've talked about a number of things this morning and I just want to make sure that I didn't miss anything. I'm going to request a telehealth visit with Dr. Fuller right away. If Dr. Fuller isn't available in the next 24-hours, are you open to talking with another provider so that we can get you set back up with your medications, maybe getting you a cane or a walker, and possibly a bedside commode?

(continues)

Client Scenario: Burke Turner (continued)

Burke: I'll meet with whoever is available, but I'd also like to meet with Dr. Fuller again as soon as I can. I missed my last appointment.

CHW: Okay, given that the elevator is out, and you're having difficulty with pain and mobility, a telehealth visit with Dr. Fuller might be best. When you and Dr. Fuller agree to meet in person, we can arrange some assistance with transportation to get you to the clinic. Is there anything else that we can help you with right away?

Burke: The only other thing is, at least for now, I can't really get out, but I don't like to keep asking my son for help. He can still come by and do the laundry, but can you help me with food?

CHW: Yes, while you're doing that Telehealth visit, make sure you mention that you need help with food, and they'll make a referral for home-delivered meals. I'm not sure if you've ever had meals delivered before [Burke shakes his head "no"]. Well, I just want you to know how it works. Someone from the Meals2Home agency will bring the meals here and knock on your door. And if you're able to get up, you can answer the door and accept the meal. If you're not able to get to the door, they'll hang the meal on your doorknob and go about making that next delivery.

Burke: I've seen them in the building. Some of the other residents, they get the meals. I would appreciate that. I don't want to keep asking my son.

The CHW calls the clinic and is able to schedule a drop-in telehealth visit for Burke in two days with Dr. Fuller. Together, Burke and the CHW review what he wants to communicate to Dr Fuller. The CHW helps Burke write down his top three priorities in an Appointment Plan. The CHW schedules a visit for the following week to follow-up with Burke.

Burke: That's good. In case I forgot anything, I can let you know.

CHW: I'll do my best to help you out.

Burke: Before you came, I was starting to get a little worried.

CHW: You're juggling a lot right now, especially when you're not feeling well right. I'm glad that we connected.

Burke: Yeah, I've only seen you in the clinic before and I didn't know you came out here. But I'm glad you came.

CHW: Yeah, I come out to visit folks – me and my chair visit everybody!

11.6 After the Visit

After a home visit, there are several key tasks to complete.

- Take time to reflect on the visit and assess the quality and effectiveness of your work. Did you reach your goals? Did you remain person-centered? Did you listen patiently to the client? Did you demonstrate cultural humility? Did you support the client's independence or autonomy? Did you face any new challenges? What aspect of your work was most successful? What lesson did you learn that may help you to enhance the quality of services in future home visits?

- Complete required documentation of the visit including services and referrals provided, agreements made, any assessment you conducted, and any new information you learned. The longer you wait to document your work, the less you will remember.

- Write down future appointments or visits in your planner, calendar, and/or electronic data system.

- Research any referral resources or other information that needs to be followed up on, such as the name of an agency that delivers hot meals to people unable to leave their homes.

- Check in with the client by phone, text, or e-mail to thank them and to schedule or confirm a follow-up visit, or an appointment at another location. Check to see if the client has followed through or faced challenges in completing the action steps that you discussed together, such as a plan to see the doctor.

- Talk with your supervisor or another colleague about any remaining questions or concerns that you may have.

  - *What else would you want to do to follow up on a home visit?*

What Do YOU Think?

Client Scenario: Burke Turner *(continued)*

The CHW scheduled a follow-up home visit with Burke one week after his telehealth meeting with Dr. Fuller. Burke and the CHW greet each other and the CHW sets up a traveling chair about eight feet in front of where Burke is resting on his bed.

CHW: Hey Burke, I'm back again. How are you?

Burke: I think I'm doing better, actually. I did get to talk to Dr. Fuller, so I appreciate that.

CHW: I'm glad to hear that. Were you able to talk to Dr. Fuller about everything on your Appointment Plan?

Burke: Yes, I had my plan with me.

CHW: Great. So, what is the status of the referrals that Dr. Fuller set up? Have you received your medications? And what is the status of your meal delivery?

Burke explains that his medications were delivered the day after his appointment with Dr. Fuller and meal delivery started two days ago. "The guy who delivers the meals, he says that I'll get seven meals a week, but they come by five days a week. It's pretty good."

CHW: I'm so glad to learn that the meal delivery has started. Burke, do you need any assistance, setting up a Medi set or pill organizer, or do you take your tablets straight out of the bottle?

Burke: I'm just taking the one high blood pressure pill in the morning, so that's pretty easy. I have them next to the bed. [Burke points to table beside his bed] And I just take the Ibuprofen when the pain in my leg acts up. It helps.

CHW: I'm glad to hear that you have a set routine with your meds. Now, did you and Dr. Fuller talk about your mobility? Is he going to order a walker or any other medical equipment to help you get around?

Burke reports that Dr. Fuller said he would order a walker to be delivered, but it hasn't come yet. He's looking forward to receiving it because it will make it easier to get to the bathroom down the hall and, when the elevator is working again, to go outside.

CHW: Okay. It seems like the referrals that Dr. Fuller put in are being filled quickly. If you haven't received the walker or a call from the durable medical equipment by this Monday, is it okay for me to follow up to see what the status is?

Burke: Yes, I'd appreciate that. I wouldn't know who to call.

CHW: Did you and Dr. Fuller have a chance to talk about your depression or mental health?

Burke: Yeah, we talked about it. He reminded me that I used antidepressants in the past and asked me if I wanted to try them again. I said I wanted to wait and see because, you know, I think having you visit and help me out with all stuff makes me feel less trapped.

CHW: I'm glad to hear it Burke.

Burke: Dr. Fuller, he encouraged me to reach out to my friend Verta. We grew up together. I haven't seen her in a while because when I am in pain ... I just kind of forget to be in touch.

(continues)

Client Scenario: Burke Turner (continued)

CHW: Yes, that's natural and normal with pain and depression. I'm glad that you made a plan to contact Verta. And there are some other sources of telephonic support out there for people who are struggling in the moment or stuck in their home. Would you be interested in learning about some of these resources?

Burke: Can you tell me a little bit more about what they do and how that would work?

The CHW describes two services. One is a warm line that Burke can call 24 hours a day to talk to a volunteer about what is going on with him. The other is an organized drop-in group that Burke can join by videoconferencing one a week.

CHW: You can join the drop-in group just like you did for your meeting with Dr. Fuller. People call in to something like Zoom and meet for an, and they provide encouragement and support.

Burke: Yeah, I might be interested. But, for me, talking to people one-on-one is more comfortable. Being nonbinary, I sometimes feel like people are looking at me funny or talking to me funny, so I'm more . . . hesitant with groups.

CHW: There are a couple of support groups around that are inclusive of nonbinary people. This organization called REACH has a number of in-person and video meetings for people who are lesbian, gay, bisexual, transgender, queer, questioning, and intersex, and they provide community and cultural support.

Burke: For me, part of what gets me isolated or depressed is, well, I've had kind of a rocky road with my family around my transition and my identity. So, a group where there are other nonbinary people—that sounds good. If you send me that information then I'll think about trying it.

CHW: Definitely. I'll text you the numbers and the websites for the individual support and for the groups at REACH. For the individual support you just call in whenever you want, and you decide what you want to talk about, and the counselor will just follow your lead and offer encouragement and support. For the groups at REACH, they will want to talk to you first to tell you about their groups. Then they will e-mail you the schedule and the topics for each group, and it's up to you to decide when and how you want to participate.

Burke: Okay.

CHW: It seems like you have accomplished a great deal this past week. I want to commend you on your follow-through and your perseverance, and of course, I'm very happy to hear that you are feeling somewhat better. Before I go, let's review what we've covered today and talk about the next steps.

11.7 Common Challenges

Home visits can be challenging for several reasons:

- Clients may not want you to visit or may not want to talk with you when you visit.
- Your clients may be very ill or facing the end-of-life.
- Clients may be difficult to communicate with due to factors such as dementia, depression, or substance use.
- Clients may be embarrassed about their living conditions.
- Clients may be concerned about their privacy.
- Clients may worry that you will judge them if they live in nontraditional families, or they may have other cultural concerns.
- Clients may worry that you will learn about or expose their immigration status or worry that they could lose certain health, housing, or social benefits.
- Clients may have had bad experiences with home visits from child welfare, social workers, the police, or other authorities.

- Clients may become upset, angry, or nonresponsive.
- You may witness or learn about drug use, neglect, or abuse.
- You may face risks to your personal safety.

- *Can you think of other challenges that you may face when conducting home visits?*

VISITS TO PEOPLE WITHOUT TRADITIONAL HOMES

When you conduct a home visit to someone who is unhoused, it may take place on the street, in a doorway, under a highway overpass, in a shelter or nursing home, or in a park or parking lot where they spend time or sleep. Be as respectful of this space as you would of any other home. All the same rules apply. If clients express that they don't want you there through words or actions, leave. Do your utmost to keep your communication confidential. Keep your voice low. If others are nearby and may be listening, don't discuss confidential matters, and follow your client's lead.

> **Lee Jackson:** To work with clients who are homeless, I'll ask them for three locations where they tend to hang out. This is a big help when I am trying to check in with them later on.

OVERCOMING OBSTACLES

You will encounter a wide range of obstacles and distractions that may get in the way of your work with a client. The telephone may ring. People may be sharing a meal, watching television, or playing video games. Other people or pets may make it difficult to focus on the purpose of the visit. This goes with the territory when conducting a home visit—unexpected things will happen. As you become more accustomed to doing home visits, you will learn how to handle different experiences. Allow yourself time to adjust and learn.

Media: To handle distractions such as the television, radio, phones, or video games, ask the client if it would be possible to turn these off or to turn down the volume so that you can focus on assisting them. Be patient and polite. Always keep in mind that this is the client's home, not your office, and it is up to the client to make these decisions.

Pets: If there is a pet such as a large dog that makes you uncomfortable, ask if it would be possible to put it in another room or area of the room. Describe this as *your* need. Explain that it will help you to better focus on supporting the clients with their concerns and priorities. But keep in mind that for many people, pets are family: they may not understand your request or may be most at ease with the animal beside them.

Other People: If other people prove to be a distraction, find an opportunity to ask the primary client if it would be possible to talk privately. Perhaps you can move to another place, or the client could ask people to move or leave for the duration of the meeting.

Drug and alcohol use: You may visit a client who is drinking or using drugs. Clarify your agency's policy about this. Some programs may limit your ability to work with people who are currently altered by substance use. A key concern is the ability of people to give informed consent when they are using substances. However, you may work with clients who are often or usually using substances, and it may not be realistic to wait until they are sober to provide services. Do your best to talk with the client, to provide the services you are authorized to provide. Be sensitive to informed consent issues, and don't ask a client to make big life-changing decisions when drunk or high. Evaluate if, how, and when you may be able to meet with the client when the person is not using. If the client has a history of being abusive or violent while high, don't attempt to work under these circumstances: this is a safety issue for you and the client, and leaving is probably the best policy.

Cluttering or hoarding: You may enter a home or space that is filled with items that take over or block the space. You may find it difficult to walk or move in these areas, and this may get in the way of your ability to work with the client in this space. Furthermore, the clutter or hoarding sometimes creates health hazards from factors such as mold, shifting piles of contents, or structural damage.

Hoarding Disorder is a recognized mental health condition and should be addressed with great sensitivity. CHWs don't want to offend or stigmatize clients by making critical or negative comments about the clutter, or attempt to move anything, as this could be severely disruptive and upsetting to the client. Unless you are trained and authorized to do so, don't try to negotiate with the client to move or dispose of their belongings. If a client is interested, however, you may provide and set up a referral to an organization that specializes in assisting people with hoarding.

We recommend bringing a portable chair or stool to sit on when you conduct home visits and to find a less-cluttered area where you can talk with the client. If the clutter creates a safety issue (such as mentioned above), you may express your concerns to the client, provide education about the safety issue, and explore finding a different and mutually convenient location to meet. This could be a local park or public library, for example.

When a client becomes Ill during a visit: During a home visit, you may notice that a client appears to be very ill or that their health condition suddenly declines. Watch for signs that a client may start to look droopy or drowsy or that they have difficulty breathing. A client may be dizzy, unsteady on their feet, or experience a fall. They may begin to slur their speech or become unable to communicate. Don't take any chances in these situations. If you witness clients with what appear to be serious health issues or rapidly declining health, call 911. The 911 Dispatcher will ask you questions to clarify the situation including any signs or symptoms that you observe, any diagnosed medical conditions that the client may have and medications they are taking, and their name and address. If the client doesn't recover immediately, 911 may arrange for an ambulance to transport them to a hospital for an assessment and any necessary treatment.

If you conduct home visits, talk with your supervisor in advance about how to handle situations like potential health emergencies.

When a client's mental health status changes or declines: A client's mental health condition may change or decline during the course of a home visit. This could be due to a mental health condition, substance use, or other factors. The client may have difficulty communicating or participating in a conversation. They may become anxious or agitated. If a client is unable to participate in a home visit actively and productively, or if you begin to feel unsafe, end the visit. Tell the client you will be leaving and will contact them later to follow up and to reschedule the visit. If the client lives in a residential setting, such as a building with supportive services on-site, talk with a staff member at the front desk and ask them to check in with the client after you leave.

Follow up with a call or text to the client in the next few days. If and when they are ready, talk with them and ask to schedule another visit at your clinic or office or, if appropriate, at their home. As always, if you have questions or concerns about what to do, consult with your supervisor.

If there is a conflict with another party: Sometimes a home visit may be interrupted by a conflict between the client and another person, or by a conflict between other people who live in or are visiting the home. If you start to hear escalating voices, shouting, threats, or fighting, it is time to end the home visit. If you are able to get the attention of the client—and they are not part of the conflict—let them know that you need to leave and that you will call them later to check and see if they are okay. Leave as quickly and quietly as possible.

As always, document the incident. Debrief it with a colleague or supervisor. With each home visiting challenge that you face, you will gain knowledge, awareness, and confidence for handling future situations.

- *What are some other challenges that you might encounter when conducting a home visit?*

- *Which types of challenges may be most challenging for you?*

What Do
YOU?
Think **!**

If a Client's Conduct Is Inappropriate

Francis Julian Montgomery: A couple of times, during home visits, a client has become undressed. Either their bathrobe falls open or they take off their shirt or they excuse themselves to the bathroom and they come back not wearing trousers. They don't have to be fully clothed, but anything between the shoulders and the thighs should be covered if I'm going to visit with you.

I'm a guest in their home and they get to do what they want, but I can't stay if they are uncovered. I let them know that it is not a good time for the visit. I tell them that I'm going and suggest we continue the appointment over the phone. I can't stay in the home if someone is naked or undressed, or if they are using substances in front of me.

Sometimes clients engage in a level of flirtation that crosses the line. It goes beyond complimenting your shoes and becomes sexual comments or innuendo. It may be happening due to a mental health condition or substance use, but whatever the reason, you need to protect yourself. You don't want to get yourself into a situation that could escalate and end up with a complaint that you did something inappropriate. You want to avoid those situations and those risks. If a client doesn't stop flirting with me or making sexual comments, then I remove myself from the situation.

WHEN CLIENTS ARE ANGRY

Expect to work with clients who are upset, frustrated, or angry. You might experience the same emotions if you were walking in their shoes. While their anger may sometimes be about you—related to something you or someone else from your agency said or did—it is more often about other issues they are confronting such as experiences of discrimination, separation or conflict with family members, the loss of jobs, homes, or relationships; the deterioration of their health; or confronting the possibility of their own death.

As discussed in Chapter 13 on Conflict Resolution, do your best to stay calm and remain patient. Take a few deep breaths. Keep in mind that you don't want to do anything that will harm the client or your professional relationship and reputation. Stay respectful, professional, and polite. Don't raise your voice or respond in anger. However, if the client is acting in ways that are threatening or physically aggressive, and you are unable to de-escalate their anger, leave the situation.

Lee Jackson: Lots of times, a client will be upset. Sometimes they'll be verbally aggressive. If you treat everyone like a human being and don't act judgmental, they'll usually come around. Always remember it's not personal. I will talk with them calmly and see if that helps. I might explain: "I'm here today to escort you to your appointment. If we need to, we can schedule you for a different time." If the client refuses to go, then rescheduling is a good way to go. If they can, maybe we go for coffee or a pastry. If I can't calm them down, I leave. I don't argue.

Chapter Review

Review the Client Scenario presented at the beginning of this chapter about Burke Turner. Do your best to answer the following questions about conducting a home visit with Burke:

- What are your goals for the home visit?
- What challenges might you face?
- What safety concerns might you have, and how will you address these?
- How will you greet Burke?

- What do you want to assess during the home visit? What questions will you ask?
- How might you conduct an environmental assessment? What might you learn that would be helpful in guiding your work with Burke?
- How will you follow up with Burke about actions that he can take to improve his health?
- What referral resources will you provide?
- How and when will you document the services you provide?
- What questions will you ask yourself to evaluate the quality and effectiveness of your work with Burke Turner?
- What topics or questions might you want to discuss with your clinical team or supervisor?

References

Centers for Disease Control and Prevention. (2022). Keep on Your Feet—Preventing Older Adult Falls. https://www.cdc.gov/injury/features/older-adult-falls/index.html (accessed 23 March 2023).

Crespo, R., Christiansen, M., Tieman, K., & Wittberg, R. (2020). An emerging model for community health worker–based chronic care management for patients with high health care costs in rural Appalachia. *Preventing Chronic Disease*, 17, 190316. https://dx.doi.org/10.5888/pcd17.190316.

Edmond, K. M., Yousufi, K., Anwari, Z., Sadat S. M., Staniczai, S. M., Higgens-Steele, A., Bellows, A. L., Smith, E. R. (2018). Can community health worker home visiting improve care-seeking and maternal and newborn care practices in fragile states such as Afghanistan? A population-based intervention study *BMC Medicine*, 16, 106. https://doi.org/10.1186/s12916-018-1092-9.

Home Visiting Evidence of Effectiveness. U.S. Department of Health & Human Services, Administration for Children & Families. https://homvee.acf.hhs.gov/ (accessed 7 November 2022).

Oregon Health Authority. Public Health Division. (2014). Oregon's Home Visitor Safety Guide. https://www.oregon.gov/oha/ph/HealthyPeopleFamilies/Babies/HealthScreening/BabiesFirst/Documents/home-visiting-safety-guide.pdf (accessed 7 November 2022).

PolicyLab. Children's Hospital of Philadelphia. (2019). Home Visiting Programs Address Rural Health Challenges Head On. https://policylab.chop.edu/blog/home-visiting-programs-address-rural-health-challenges-head (accessed 7 November 2022).

Rural Health Information Hub. (2022). Home Visiting Programs. https://www.ruralhealthinfo.org/toolkits/transportation/2/models-to-overcome-barriers/home-visiting-programs (accessed 7 November 2022)

Stout, J., Chen, R., Farquhar, S., Kramer, B., & Song, L. (2021). *Examining home visits from community health workers to help patients manage asthma symptoms*. Patient-Centered Outcomes Research Institute (PCORI). https://doi.org/10.25302/12.2020.AS.130705498.

Tripathi, A., Kabra, S. K., Sachdeve, H. P. S., & Lodha, R. (2016). Home visits by community health workers improve identification of serious illness and care seeking in newborns and young infants from low- and middle-income countries. *Journal of Perinatology*. https://www.nature.com/articles/jp201634.pdf?origin=ppub (accessed 7 November 2022).

Vogels, E. A. (2021). Digital divide persists even as Americans with lower incomes make gains in adoption. Pew Research Center. https://www.pewresearch.org/fact-tank/2021/06/22/digital-divide-persists-even-as-americans-with-lower-incomes-make-gains-in-tech-adoption/ (accessed 7 November 2022).

Additional Resources

Early Head Start, Southern Oregon. (2011). Home Visit Guidelines. https://www.socfc.org/SOHS/EHS/Home%20Visit%20Guidelines%208-12.pdf (accessed 7 November 2022).

National Home Visiting Resource Center. Resources about early childhood home visiting. https://nhvrc.org/ (accessed 7 November 2022).

Lifeline Program for Low-Income Consumers. (2023). https://www.fcc.gov/general/lifeline-program-low-income-consumers.

Office for the Advancement of Telehealth. (2023). Health Resources & Services Administration. https://www.hrsa.gov/rural-health/topics/telehealth.

ENHANCING PROFESSIONAL SKILLS

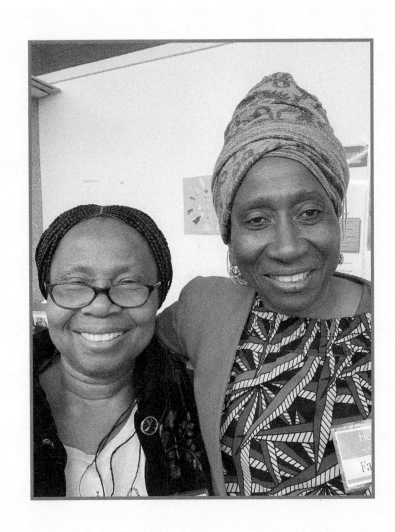

Stress, Health and Self-Care

Tim Berthold

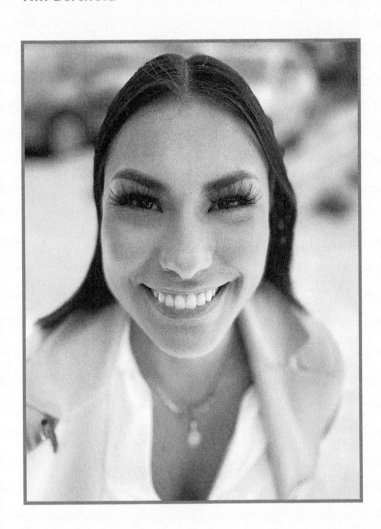

Foundations for Community Health Workers, Third Edition. Edited by Tim Berthold and Darouny Somsanith.
© 2024 John Wiley & Sons, Inc. Published 2024 by John Wiley & Sons, Inc.
Companion website: http://www.wiley.com/go/communityhealthworkers3E

CHW Scenario: Vivian Chapman

Vivian Chapman is a Community Health Worker with the Perinatal Health Program at the River City Native American Health Center. For the past seven years, Vivian has conducted outreach to encourage families to access early prenatal care. Vivian facilitates a 5-week educational group for expecting families, and a 6-week support group for new parents and their families. As part of her duties, Vivian conducts home visits to assess the health of newborns and the needs of their families, providing encouragement, education, and linkages to local services.

Vivian loves her job, but it is becoming increasingly difficult to juggle on top of family responsibilities. Two years ago, Vivian's mother-in-law moved into her family home. Vivian and her husband are now sleeping in the living room so that their two school-aged children, and her mother-in-law, can occupy two small bedrooms. Initially, Vivian's mother-in-law was a great help in taking care of the home and her grandchildren, but then she began to experience significant memory loss and confusion. Now diagnosed with early onset dementia, Vivian drops her mother-in-law off each morning at a program for seniors and picks her up at the end of the day.

Last month, as Vivian was picking up medications for her daughter at the drug store, a man behind her in line yelled at her to hurry up and called her a racist slur. The clerk who was helping Vivian didn't say or do anything. Vivian was so shocked that she just took the medication and ran out to her car. These types of racist incidents are happening more frequently to members of her community. One of her patients was recently assaulted by a stranger who also called her racist names.

Vivian is having difficulty sleeping because she is so anxious. She used to be eager to go to work, but lately, she feels overwhelmed. Last week, Vivian snapped at a young mother during an educational group session; she had never spoken in such an angry tone to a client before. Vivian is also increasingly worried about what will happen with her mother-in-law. Should she quit work to take care of her full-time?

While Vivian is a gifted CHW who is highly skilled in supporting others; she is less skilled at promoting her own health and wellness. She questions why she is becoming so stressed out and blames herself for not being stronger.

Please take a moment to reflect on the following questions:

- What type of stressors is Vivian Chapman experiencing?
- How is stress affecting Vivian's life?
- What might happen to Vivian if she doesn't find a way to reduce stress and enhance self-care?
- What types of self-care strategies might support Vivian with stress reduction and improved well-being?
- What are the key sources of stress that you face in your life and at work?
- What happens to you when you are feeling "stressed out?"
- What skills have you learned for coping with or managing stress?

Introduction

Stress is an inevitable and common part of life. We face it at home, in the community, and at work. Community Health Workers often face a high degree of stress on the job, and witness firsthand how stress impacts the health of the clients and communities they work with.

Stress has a broad and significant impact on all aspects of our health. It increases our risks for physical and mental health conditions and, when it is chronic, can even reduce life expectancy.

This chapter will identify common sources of stress. It also examines the ways in which the social determinants of health, including systemic racism and other forms of discrimination, can lead to chronic stress and illness.

Over time, job-related stress can lead to burnout. Learning how to assess your risks for stress and burnout and to take action to enhance self-care is critical for your health, your professional success, and for the welfare of the clients and communities you work with. The organizations that employ CHWs can also take action to promote their health and wellness.

WHAT YOU WILL LEARN

By studying the information presented in this chapter, you will be able to

- Define stress, chronic stress, and burnout
- Recognize common sources of stress and stress responses
- Identify unique sources of stress that CHWs may experience on the job
- Identify internal and external resources that can influence stress responses
- Discuss how the social determinants of health, including racism and other forms of discrimination, contribute to illness, premature death, and health inequities
- Assess your own risks for stress and burnout
- Identify organizational practices that help to prevent burnout and promote well-being among CHWs and other helping professionals
- Develop and implement a realistic action plan for stress management and self-care
- Support a client with stress reduction planning

C3 Roles and Skills Addressed in Chapter 12

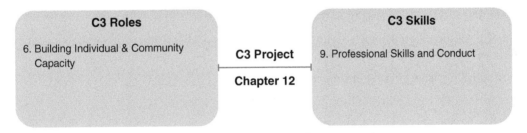

WORDS TO KNOW

Allostatic Load	Secondary Resilience
Burnout	Secondary Trauma
Chronic Stress	Supportive Supervision
External Resources	Stress
Internal Resources	Stressor
Post-Traumatic Stress	Weathering

12.1 Defining Stress

Stress is the way that we respond to and are affected by life events and circumstances that pose a risk, a change, or a challenge. These events and experiences are known as **stressors**. They result in a wide range of physical, emotional, social, and spiritual stress responses and can impact all aspects of our lives and our health. Stress may be acute (temporary) or chronic (ongoing exposure to stressors). How deeply we are affected by stress is influenced by our internal and external resources.

STRESSORS

Stressors include events that may be characterized as positive, such as competing in sports, graduating from school, or falling in love. Stressors also include more negative events or dynamics such as meeting deadlines at work or at school, the loss of a job or a home, incarceration, divorce or separation from family, or exposure to war or armed conflict.

Stressors include the social determinants of health. The lack of equitable access to resources and rights that promote health—such as housing, food, clean water, employment, health care, and civil rights—are common and significant stressors in the United States.

Other common stressors include:

- Moving
- Starting a new job
- Rushing to meet deadlines
- Conflicts or disagreements with co-workers
- Illness and disability
- Joining a new community or social group
- Family conflicts
- Parenting or taking care of children
- Being a caregiver for an adult living with a disability or chronic health condition
- Loss of a job or home
- Financial difficulties
- Lacking a safe place to live or access to sufficient food
- Experiences of prejudice, harassment, assault, or other forms of discrimination such as racism or homophobia
- Incarceration in jail, prison, or a detention center
- Immigration or leaving your home behind to resettle in a new nation

- *What are the most common stressors in your life?*

What Do YOU? Think

CHWs also encounter stressors as part of their work or volunteer positions, such as:

- A heavy caseload (too many clients to serve and not enough time to provide quality services to all of them)
- Witnessing a client:
  - With declining health
  - Facing the end of life
  - Struggling with depression or suicidal thoughts
  - Facing criminal justice charges or incarceration
  - Continuing to engage in harmful behaviors
  - Experiencing prejudice and discrimination based on their real or perceived identity, health condition, or history
- Living in the same community where you work.
  - While other colleagues may go "home" to different neighborhoods after work, many CHWs remain in the same neighborhood, encountering the same economic, political, social, and health challenges as the

clients they serve. Living in the same community, it is harder to take a break from work and to create protective professional boundaries. CHWs may frequently encounter clients/patients in the areas where they live, shop, go to church or temple, and so on.

- Managing paperwork and meeting deadlines
- Public speaking (such as presenting to your organization or in the community)
- Managing professional boundaries
- Ending a successful professional relationship with an ongoing client
- Lack of local resources for your clients such as housing, drug treatment, or health care
- Supervising others
- Conflict with a coworker or supervisor
- Starting a new job or earning a promotion
- Lack of opportunities for career advancement or promotion within your organization
- Insufficient training and skills to perform a particular duty, such as facilitating a training or support group
- Ethical challenges
- Lack of status and recognition for the role and contributions of CHWs
- Lack of understanding from other providers or colleagues of the value of CHW skills and contributions
- Lack of stable and sufficient funding to support CHW positions
- Low rates of pay and benefits (such as professional development, vacation, sick time, or paid time off (PTO)

- *Can you think of other on-the-job stressors for CHWs?*

- *What types of client situations might be particularly stressful for you as a CHW?*

What Do YOU? Think

Estela Munoz de Cardenas: For me, the greatest stress is not having enough resources for the clients when they need it. Right now, so many families need housing. I see families with little ones, and they have to go to a shelter. They don't know how their kids will get to school. They worry about getting the next meal. As a CHW and a parent, it breaks my heart. We live in California, the richest state in the United States, and we still have these disparities and we let families live without housing.

DISCRIMINATION AND STRESS

One of the most destructive forms of stress arises from living in a society that does not fully respect your identity or protect your life. Millions of Americans face prejudice and discrimination based on their real or perceived ethnicity, race, nationality, immigration status, language, religion, gender identity, sexual orientation, size, disability, and other factors.

Discrimination comes in many forms, including interpersonal (discrimination by one or more other people) and institutional or structural discrimination (discrimination by organizations, the government, policies, and practices). Discrimination encompasses a wide range of actions and behaviors including verbal remarks and threats, harassment, assault, and homicide. It includes unequal treatment and access to resources such as housing, employment, financial benefits, education, voting, and other civil rights.

Research evidence shows that exposure to chronic or ongoing stress such as discrimination has a significant and harmful impact on our bodies and minds (American Psychological Association, 2012; Davis, 2020; Sternthal,

Slopen, & Williams, 2011). Even anticipating prejudice in interpersonal interactions can result in increased psychological and cardiovascular stress responses (Sawyer, Major, Casad, Townsend, & Mendes, 2012). Chronic stress increases our risks for chronic disease and other health conditions and shortens our life expectancy. More information about the consequences of chronic stress is presented later in this chapter.

Too often when the topic of stress is discussed, the conversation focuses on why individuals are so "stressed out" and what they should do to reduce or better manage their stress. While we can certainly take action to better manage our own stress, we can also organize for collective action to address the root causes of stress in our society such as persistent racism and other forms of discrimination. The organizations that employ CHWs can also implement workplace policies and practices that help to prevent stress and provide CHWs and other employees with access to resources to help manage the effects of stress.

To read more about the link between discrimination, stress, and health status, please look for the resources posted at the end of this chapter.

- *Has exposure to prejudice and discrimination affected you or your family?*

- *How has exposure to prejudice and discrimination impacted clients and communities that you work with or belong to?*

CHW Profile

Porshay Taylor (She/Her/First Lady)

Case Manager

St. James Infirmary and The Taimon Booton Navigation Center, San Francisco, CA

Serving transgender, gender nonconforming, and intersex women who are unhoused

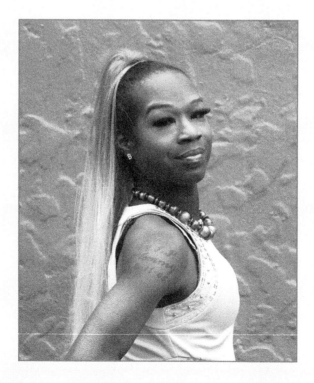

(continues)

CHW Profile

(continued)

I am transgender, born and raised in San Francisco. My transition to becoming transgender was a relentless journey filled with extreme challenges. It was difficult to find stable housing. I lived in a tent, on the streets, with family and strangers, in hotels. You face a lot of stigma and degradation when you are homeless, African American, and transgender. Being all three is like a triple negative in our society. But despite all the adversity, there is always hope.

Things started getting better when I joined the Transgender Gender-variant and Intersex Justice Project and was able to exhibit my capabilities as a mature, responsible, and diligent transgender woman. Ms. Janetta Johnson was an influential woman in my life who encouraged me. She became an Auntie to me and believed in me when others didn't. She showed me that we are sisters, aunties and uncles, sisters and brothers — and we are in this fight together.

Now I'm the Auntie, and I'm not going to give up on nobody. I'm a Case Manager with the Taimon Booton Navigation Center, part of St. James Infirmary. We have a shelter for transgender, gender nonconforming, and intersex people to find sanctuary and support. We offer meals, laundry and shower facilities, health care, and case management services. I work with participants who are unhoused to find a more stable situation. I help them get 'document ready.' People need proper documents to qualify for services and benefits right? They need a form of I.D. like a birth certificate or driver's license or social security number. I help them get food stamps and connect them to other agencies and services. I tell them not to be discouraged because of what they've gone through. I tell them it's going to take a while before everything changes. When you finally see a sister doing better, getting stable, finding housing, getting a job — it's a beautiful thing.

When I started working at the Navigation Center I met this young lady. She came from Sacramento to get health care and didn't want to go back. She needed help making a start in San Francisco, which isn't easy. So I got her a place at the Navigation Center. She participated in all the activities and didn't get distracted. Eventually, I got her a place in the Bobbie Jean Baker House which is a transitional housing program for our community. She's been texting me every day to say good morning and to let me know that she's okay. She's so thankful and happy and that's what this work is all about, isn't it?

I have this lived experience. I guess that's the difference between me and people working in the field who have a degree. When I meet someone living in a tent who is really scared, I know something about that. I just feel really honored now to be on the other side, helping my community. But I want better services. It shouldn't be so hard to connect people who need housing with a safe place to live. Why can't it be one straightforward process? Why are so many people left behind?

For people who are starting out doing this work. Just know that you're gonna get frustrated. You're gonna get triggered by people's stories and situations. You're going to make mistakes and call the wrong person and not be able to find resources and you're gonna watch people that don't make it or who give up on themselves. Encourage yourself. Day by day it's gonna get better. Reach out to your mentors. Keep asking them for support. Learn all you can.

12.2 Internal and External Resources

People respond to stressors in different ways. To a great extent, our response to stress depends on our access to internal and external resources.

INTERNAL RESOURCES

Internal resources reside within us and may include:

- Patience
- Our cultural and social identities and values

- The ability to put events in perspective
- A sense of humor
- Good health, particularly a healthy immune system
- The ability to achieve a calm and relaxed state of mind and body
- The ability to connect in meaningful ways with other people
- A sense of pride in your professional contributions
- An understanding that facing stress is a natural part of life
- Healthy self-esteem (what you think and how you feel about yourself)
- Past personal and professional achievements
- Confidence in your ability to face adversity
- History of successfully coping with stressful life events
- Knowledge of stress management techniques
- Love of music, reading, writing, or other pastimes
- The ability to reach out and ask for support when you need it
- Engaging in regular exercise
- Faith, including religious or spiritual faith

- *What are your most important internal resources?*

EXTERNAL RESOURCES

External resources are located outside of us and may include:

- Close and supportive relationships with family
- Strong friendships
- A sense of connection and belonging to a particular community or communities
- Safety (including home, neighborhood, and society free from violence)
- Cultural histories, traditions, and values
- Supportive coworkers
- A skilled and respectful supervisor at work or a mentor
- Pets
- Access to quality education, stable housing, good nutrition
- Connection to organizations or movements such as religious, cultural, social, sports, or political organizations
- Access to parks and other recreational facilities
- Employment benefits including health care, sick pay, and vacation leave
- Government-provided disability benefits
- Respect for and enforcement of your civil and human rights

- *What are your most important external resources?*

12.3 Stress Responses

Stress can impact all aspects of our health and our lives. It can provoke physical, emotional, social, cognitive (brain/mind), behavioral, and spiritual responses. There is no way to predict how any individual will respond to a specific stressor. Please note that the following lists do not include every possible response to stress.

COMMON PHYSICAL RESPONSES

Stress is sometimes thought of primarily as a physical phenomenon. When confronted with a crisis or a significant challenge, our body responds by releasing hormones, such as adrenaline and cortisol, which speed up our heart and respiration rates (breathing), blood pressure, and metabolism. These hormones deliver more oxygen and blood sugar to our large muscles and dilate our pupils to improve vision. This physical stress response is sometimes referred to as the "fight-or-flight" response, as it prepares us to take action during emergencies to avoid harm.

While this type of stress response helps us to take action during an emergency, having our body on high alert for long periods is harmful to our health.

Other physical responses to stress may include:

- Freezing or the inability to move or take physical action
- A surge of energy
- Quick reactions in moments of crisis
- Fatigue
- Changes in sleeping patterns, including insomnia and nightmares
- Chest pain, palpitations, or tightness
- Breathlessness
- Pain, including headaches, stomachaches, backaches, muscle tension, or pain
- Impairment to concentration and memory
- Changes in menstrual cycles
- Increased risk of preterm delivery (before 37 weeks of pregnancy)
- Nausea, digestive tract problems, ulcers
- Increased risks for developing a wide range of chronic health conditions including cardiovascular disease, cancers, diabetes, anxiety, depression, and other mental health conditions.

- *Can you think of other physical stress responses to add to the list?*

What Do
YOU?
Think

COMMON EMOTIONAL RESPONSES

- Embarrassment or shame
- Guilt
- Anxiety or fear
- Sadness, sorrow, or despair
- Numbness or lack of emotion
- A feeling of hopelessness
- Frustration and anger, including anger directed at yourself
- Elation, joy, satisfaction (particularly when we respond to crisis in effective ways)

COMMON COGNITIVE RESPONSES (THOUGHTS)

- Difficulty concentrating
- Trying to avoid thinking about the stressful situation

- Thinking about stressful experiences over and over again
- Memories of other similar stressful experiences
- Doubting your own abilities and value
- Thoughts about escaping your current situation by quitting your job, dropping out of school, ending a relationship, or moving
- Thoughts that life is no longer worth living, or thoughts of suicide
- Reflecting upon your own strengths and ability to withstand challenging situations

COMMON BEHAVIORAL RESPONSES

- Withdrawing from family, friends, or community
- Avoiding locations or activities that are stressful, including work, school, and home
- Snapping at or yelling at others, including people who have not had a part in causing the stress
- Changing patterns of eating, drinking, smoking, drug use, sexual behavior, hygiene, or dress
- Engaging in behaviors that may seem to relieve or escape the stress, but that are harmful, especially smoking, drinking alcohol, overspending, or using drugs
- Stopping behaviors that used to give you pleasure
- Developing behaviors that enable you to better manage stress, including exercise, meditation, talking with friends, reading or writing, going to support groups, spiritual practices, playing an instrument or making music
- Building community by working with others to confront common challenges or stressors.

COMMON SPIRITUAL RESPONSES

- Loss or weakening of religious, spiritual, or metaphysical faith or beliefs
- Loss of a sense of meaning or purpose
- A sense of hopelessness or despair
- A sense of alienation from others
- Anger at God, creator, humankind, fate, or luck
- Finding or strengthening religious, spiritual, or metaphysical faith, beliefs, and practices
- A sense of connectedness to others, the world, to God or creator

The Impacts of Chronic Stress

Stress may be acute (a single episode) or chronic (ongoing exposure to stressors). **Chronic stress** occurs when people are exposed for a long time to stressors such as living in poverty, being unhoused or incarcerated, experiencing discrimination and the threat of discrimination, and living in on-going situations of violence such as war or domestic violence. CHWs typically work with clients and communities that experience high rates of chronic stress and may themselves experience chronic stress.

The term **allostatic load** refers to the cumulative impact, over time, of stress on our bodies including our cardiovascular, metabolic, and immune systems. Individuals and communities with a high allostatic load have higher risks for physical and mental health conditions, and premature aging and death (Zsoldos, Filippini, Mahmood, Mackay, Singh-Manoux, Kivimaki, Jenkinson, & Ebmeier, 2018; Greenberg, 2020; Guidi, Lucente, Sonino, & Fava, 2021).

Weathering refers to the inequities in physical and psychological health that result from greater exposure to chronic stress and allostatic load among communities of color and other communities facing adversity and discrimination in our society (Sandoiu, 2021; Forrester, Jacobs, Zmora, Schreiner, Roger, & Kiefe, 2019; Geronimus, Hicken, Keene, & Bound, 2006). *Just as a wooden fence is worn down over time by exposure to wind and rain, human beings are also worn down over time by exposure to systemic racism and other forms of discrimination.*

12.4 Burnout and Post Traumatic Stress

Burnout is a state of physical, emotional, psychological, and spiritual exhaustion that a person reaches after exposure to chronic stress. It is usually thought of with respect to workplace burnout.

The Stage Theory of Burnout (International Training and Education Center on HIV, 2005) shows how it can develop over time:

First stage: The initial stage includes physical warning signs, such as the inability to shake off a lingering cold or fever, frequent headaches, and sleeplessness. The thought of going to work loses its appeal.

Second stage: The middle stage involves such emotional and behavioral signs as angry outbursts, obvious impatience, or irritability, or treating people with contempt. An attitude of suspicion often intensifies at this stage.

Third stage: The last stage is critical and severe, and it occurs when we sour on ourselves, others, and humanity. Intense feelings of loneliness and alienation are characteristic.

For CHWs, when commitment to clients is combined with stress on the job and the lack of adequate professional support, it can lead to burnout. Situations that CHWs commonly witness on the job and in the communities they serve can aggravate and increase the likelihood of burnout.

Because burnout tends to happen gradually, or over a series of stages, it can be difficult to recognize in ourselves or in others. When we are burned out, we are often incapable of providing quality services. In the worst circumstances, we may actually harm clients. A CHW – or other helping professional—who is "burned out" may:

- Not show up to work on time or keep appointments with clients
- Fail to listen deeply to clients
- Act as if they don't particularly care about the client's situation
- Bring their own issues and feelings into their work with clients
- Act out their frustration on clients or coworkers
- Fail to pay attention to details and miss opportunities to make effective referrals that could prevent poor health outcomes for clients
- Not complete necessary paperwork accurately or in a timely fashion

- *Have you ever received services from a CHW, nurse, social worker, teacher, or another professional who may have been burned out?*

  - *What did you observe?*

  - *What was this experience like for you?*

- *Have you ever experienced any of these stages of burnout? What signs did you experience and when did you recognize them?*

POST-TRAUMATIC STRESS

Post-traumatic stress may occur when people are exposed to war, torture, child abuse, sexual assault, incarceration, natural disasters, and other traumatic experiences characterized by intense fear, horror, or a sense of helplessness (for more information about post-traumatic stress, please read Chapter 18). These events often involve the loss of control and a threat of bodily harm or death. The impact of traumatic experiences on survivors can be similar to the list of stress responses provided above.

Exposure to traumatic events is very common and affects both CHWs and the clients and communities they work with.

CHWs are also at risk for a phenomenon known as **secondary or vicarious trauma**. As a consequence of working with survivors of trauma, helping professionals may develop their own symptoms of traumatic stress. Developing strong skills in self-care is essential to preventing secondary trauma among CHWs.

We encourage you to seek out opportunities for additional training on issues related to trauma. Workshops, courses, and trainings are available online and at local colleges and public health, mental health, or social services agencies. For example, many cities and counties have rape crisis centers, suicide prevention centers, and domestic violence agencies that provide outstanding training in exchange for a volunteer commitment. These trainings will enhance your knowledge and skills as a CHW.

12.5 Assessing Risks for Stress and Burnout

Sometimes we become used to living with stress; it becomes our 'new normal.' Because we are not always aware of how we are affected by stress, and may not notice early signs of burnout, it is important to periodically assess our status.

1. **Reflect upon your exposure to stress and its impact on your life:** The following questions may guide your reflection.

   - What types of stressors have the greatest impact on your health and your life?

   - What event or circumstance was particularly stressful for you today, this week, and in the past year?

   - In general, how do you know when you are under stress?

     How does stress impact your body? Your thoughts? Your emotions? Your behavior? Your spirituality or beliefs?

     - How do these stress responses impact your personal life, relationships, work, or experience in school?

   - What have you done when you experience stress that has heightened your stress responses or made the situation worse?

   - What have you learned that helps you to better manage stress?

2. Because we don't always have a clear picture of how stress affects us, **ask someone who knows you well to share their observations about how you are affected by stress:** Be sure to ask for this feedback at a time when you are prepared to listen to what your friend, family member, or colleague may have to share with you. Be prepared to learn something new about yourself. Ask questions that will assist you in clarifying the feedback you receive (e.g., "Can you share a couple of examples with me? Do you notice anything about the type of situation when I may be more likely to respond in this way?").

   Continue to reflect on what you hear from others. What else would you like to know? How might this information be useful in your life?

3. **Take a stress or burnout self-assessment:** You can find a wide range of free self-assessments for stress and burnout online. These assessments generally use surveys to gather information about your exposure to stressors and your stress responses or signs of burnout. Typically, the assessments provide you with a score or rating that is designed to help you assess your level of stress/burnout.

For example, the **Professional Quality of Life Scale (ProQOL)** is a 30-question survey designed for helping professionals—like CHWs—to assess their job satisfaction, stress, and risk for burnout (Professional Quality of Life, 2022). It incorporates questions regarding risks for secondary trauma. Each question—such as #7. "I find it difficult to separate my personal life from my life as a helper"—are rated on a 5-point scale from 1 (Never) to 5 (Very Often). Your scores are used to assess Compassion Satisfaction, Burnout, and Secondary Traumatic Stress.

After taking a self-assessment, if the results indicate that you are experiencing a lot of stress or are at risk of burnout, please take action to promote your wellness. Reach out for support at work, at home, or in your community. Redouble your efforts to practice meaningful self-care.

12.6 Stress Management Strategies and Resources

Researchers have found high rates of stress, burnout, and turnover among CHWs (Aryal & D'mello, 2020; Brinkley, 2018; Nkonki, Cliff, & Sanders, 2011). These findings should raise an alarm among organizations that employ CHWs and a call to action to address these challenges.

ORGANIZATIONAL STRATEGIES FOR PROMOTING CHW HEALTH AND WELLNESS

While some organizations do very little to support employees with the risks of stress and burnout, others establish policies and programs designed to enhance the well-being of staff and volunteers and promote job satisfaction and retention.

What Do YOU Think?

- *Should employers take an active role in preventing stress and enhancing the wellness of CHWs?*
- *How does the organization you work/volunteer for promote staff well-being?*
- *If you were an employer, what one policy or action would you implement to promote the well-being of CHW employees?*

Factors that contribute to burnout and high rates of turnover among CHWs include work overload, lack of care team integration, lack of proper supervision, lack of autonomy, and the lack of consistent training (Health Leads, 2019). To address these risks CHW employers are encouraged (Ibid) to:

- Increase awareness about burnout and self-care
- Provide adequate training for CHW supervisors
- Increase the visibility of CHWs within the organization
- Provide adequate training to CHWs
- Adopt effective and inclusive interdisciplinary team-based care delivery

Many organizations that employ CHWs are not prepared to support their success. These organizations may lack skilled supervisors who fully understand the roles, contributions, and values of CHWs, and the unique stressors they face on the job. These supervisors may not be well prepared to provide effective support and guidance for professional development.

Traditional approaches to supervision often emphasize fault finding or focus on what individual employees are not doing or not doing well enough, and the use of disciplinary action to promote change. This 'autocratic style' of supervision often fails to motivate employees to improve their skills or advance in their careers.

In contrast, **supportive supervision** is a strength-based approach. Supportive supervisors identify areas for improvement and work with employees to develop a clear plan of action to enhance skills and services, they highlight what employees are already doing well, their key contributions, and their value to the organization. This type of supervision is better designed to promote a positive sense of connection to the organizations we work for and to provide support for the professional growth and career success of individual employees. Supportive supervision benefits individual employees and the workplace overall, increasing the quality of services provided, creating a more positive work environment, and reducing turnover among staff (Brown, Kangovi, Wiggins, & Alvarado, 2020).

Other strategies for reducing stress and promoting the health of CHWs in the workplace include:

- Living wages and benefits for CHWs
- Self-assessments of stress and burnout
- Work-based wellness activities and programs
- Clinical supervision – provided by someone other than a direct supervisor—to provide a safe place to talk about challenges with clients and related personal issues (for more information on clinical supervision see Chapter 10)

- Access to ongoing professional development workshops and resources
- Release time and tuition support for educational advancement
- Visible and practical pathways to promotion and increased pay
- Hiring senior CHWs to serve as program managers and supervisors of other CHWs

THE ROLE OF LOCAL, STATE, AND NATIONAL CHW NETWORKS AND ASSOCIATIONS

Some cities, counties, and states have a CHW network or association. There is also a National Association for CHWs (see the link under Additional Resources at the end of the chapter) with resources on mental health and self-care (click on the 'Resources' tab on their website). These networks and associations are established to promote the CHW profession, to connect CHWs, and to provide access to research, trainings, and other resources. Many CHW networks host workshops and provide other resources on the topics of stress reduction and self-care.

- *Is there a local or state CHW Association where you work?*

- *Have you joined or considered joining the National Association of CHWs?*

What Do
YOU ?
Think **!**

ADDRESSING THE ROOT CAUSES OF STRESS

Stress is a leading social determinant of health. Chronic stress—such as living in poverty and facing on-going prejudice and discrimination—contributes to health inequities and increased risks for illness and early death.

Public health approaches to preventing chronic stress include working to challenge and dismantle discriminatory policies and practices that are so destructive to the health and well-being of communities that continue to be the focus of prejudice, harassment, assault, and structural discrimination. Racism and other forms of systemic discrimination should be identified and addressed as critical public health priorities (Villarosa, 2022). Across the country, individual activists and organizations continue a long history of advocating for social change and equity.

Cultural histories, traditions, and organizations are vital for reducing the impacts of discrimination and chronic stress. A sense of pride in one's cultural identity can provide resilience and protection from stress responses (Iturbide, Raffaelli, & Carlo, 2009). Collective action taken by communities that face systemic discrimination can prevent or reduce discriminatory practices and can also provide a sense of shared identity, pride, and resilience.

As we write this revised edition of *Foundations*, political actions are being taken in the United States to limit accessibility to voting and reproductive rights; to ban teaching about slavery, Jim Crow and racism in American schools; to limit the rights of lesbian, gay, bisexual, transgender, queer, questioning, intersex, asexual (LGBTQIA+) people; and to ban books in schools and libraries that teach about civil rights movements and that represent the identities and lives of LGBTQIA+ people. These actions reinforce our nation's history of bigotry and discrimination.

- *How are organizations and communities working to challenge discrimination and advocate for equity in the city or state where you live and work?*

- *What types of policy changes could reduce chronic stress and promote health equity for the communities you work with?*

What Do
YOU ?
Think **!**

12.7 Enhancing Stress Management Skills

Many CHWs place their own needs behind those of their clients, co-workers, and families. Please don't wait until you are overwhelmed with stress or on the verge of burnout to take action.

The *good news* is that we can cultivate positive, life-affirming, and health-sustaining activities that help us to better manage stress and reduce harm. When we develop skills and habits for caring for ourselves, we are better able to manage future challenges.

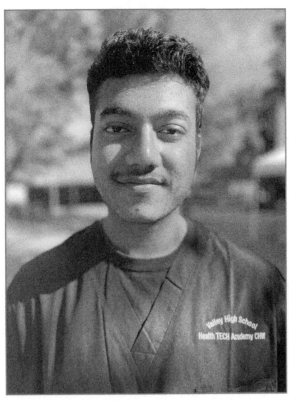

CHWs need to learn how to manage stress.

As you consider activities and resources to enhance your self-care, please keep the following criteria in mind:

- **Accessible:** For example, is the resource easy to get to (or is it far away)? Is it something that you can do at home or in your neighborhood? Is it something that you can do given your body, age, and any physical limitations? Does it take a lot of time?

- **Affordable:** Can you afford this type of stress reduction? Keep in mind that many forms of stress reduction and self-care are free.

- **Culturally relevant:** Sometimes you may wish to engage in activities that are grounded in or connected to your cultural identity or traditions. At other times, you may want to learn about and participate in different traditions of wellness and self-care.

- **Welcoming:** If the activity involves other people or is organized by others, are they welcoming and supportive of you? Do you feel comfortable participating in the program or activity?

- **Pleasurable:** Does the activity bring you pleasure? Does it leave you feeling better when you have completed it?

How Do You Relax?

Many of us already participate in practices that are relaxing and stress-relieving. Many activities can alleviate or reduce stress, such as

- Talking with a trusted friend or family member
- Listening to or playing music, or singing
- Playing games
- Physical activities including walking, dancing, swimming and playing sports

(continues)

How Do You Relax?

(continued)

- Journaling, writing, poetry
- Painting, drawing, sculpting
- Praying or meditating or going to church, temple, mosque or other place of worship
- Gardening
- Taking a hot bath
- Walking or sitting in parks or on the beach or in other natural settings
- Participating in activities such as tai chi or yoga including chair yoga and stretching activities that people can do sitting or lying down
- Spending meaningful time with family, friends, and pets
- Getting adequate rest and sleep
- Preparing and eating a well-balanced and nutritious diet

- *What are you already doing to relax and alleviate stress?*

What Do YOU ? Think

Estela Munoz de Cardenas: *When I feel really stressed, I just go by myself to church. I go to church a lot! Not to mass or a regular service, I just walk in by myself and sit down and talk to God. I talk about a client who is going through a difficult time, and I ask for guidance so that I can figure out what to do. I pray for the families I work with. And as I talk to God, I feel relaxed. My heart feels happy.*

Please watch the following video interview about stress management:

STRESS MANAGEMENT. (*Source:* http://youtu. be/YH2na2xuuuo.)

12.8 Self-Care

There are many approaches to self-care. We highlight a few resources below and in the Additional Resources listed at the end of the chapter. Keep in mind that the best self-care strategies are the ones that work for you!

PHYSICAL ACTIVITY

Engaging in physical activity can reduce stress. A regular program of physical activity such as walking, riding a bicycle, playing sports, running, swimming, dancing, doing tai chi, yoga, or any activity that gets the body moving benefits our health (see Chapter 17) and can help us to better manage stress.

Walking is a great form of physical activity. It has the advantage of being free, something that you can do alone or with others, and is relatively accessible to people of all ages and fitness levels. In some workplaces, people hold walking meetings or have created groups for walking during the lunch hour or during breaks.

There are also many forms of physical activities that are accessible to us as we age and if we are living with disabilities. For example, there are forms of sitting yoga and other activities for people who may be unstable or unable to stand up. A growing diversity of physical activity programs are available that take people's age, health status, and cultural identity into consideration. Look for programs in your community or search for them online. You can also find more information in Chapter 17 on Healthy Eating and Active Living.

- *Do you engage in physical activity that helps you to relax?*

- *Can you make time to engage in physical activity, even briefly, in the next week?*

CHW

> **Jerry Smart:** I am not exempt from stress. I am a working, single father who is also in school. It's important for me to have quiet times when I can turn off the TV or take a walk. I like to take really long walks, to be by myself, and to stay away from drama or negative environments. Doing this helps me to get myself back; I can be restored.

DEEP BREATHING

A simple and effective relaxation method is diaphragmatic or deep breathing (the diaphragm is a dome-shaped muscle located between the lungs and abdominal cavity). It involves taking a deep breath while flexing the diaphragm and is marked by the expansion of the abdomen (belly) rather than the chest. Usually, individuals inhale slowly through the nose until the lungs are filled and then slowly exhale through pursed lips to regulate the release of air. Practicing diaphragmatic breathing for a few minutes every day—or when you can—may significantly reduce your level of stress.

A Deep Breathing Activity

Try this simple deep-breathing activity.

Place the tip of your tongue against the roof of your mouth just behind your front teeth and keep it there throughout this activity. Exhale through your mouth (feel free to make noise when you do this).

1. Close your mouth and breathe in through your nose, letting your belly expand, for a count of 1-2-3

2. Hold your breath for a count of 1-2-3

3. Exhale and push all your breath out through your mouth to a count of 1-2-3

Repeat this breathing rhythm 3-5 times. If you continue to do this activity, try to hold your breath for longer counts—as long as it is comfortable for you to do so.

- What was this activity like for you?

- What changes, if any, do you notice in your body, your thoughts or feelings, and your level of stress?

- Will you try this activity again?

PRAYER, FAITH, AND SPIRITUALITY

Religious or spiritual faith and prayer can also provide relief from stress. Religious or spiritual practices vary significantly. Some individuals attend a church, temple, mosque, or other center. Others practice their faith independently, on their own, or with others.

- *Is prayer, faith, or spirituality an important resource in your life?*

- *How can you enhance your ability to access these resources in ways that relieve stress?*

> **Lee Jackson:** I'm spiritually grounded. To me that's number one. That's the key in my life. I don't push it off on anyone else, but that's what works for me: a firm belief in a supreme being or a force greater than me that's a power unseen. That's God to me.

MEDITATION

Meditation is a term that covers a wide range of practices that generally involve awareness or contemplation. It includes religious, spiritual, and secular or nonreligious practices. There are many forms of meditation practice including relaxation, visualization, concentration, chanting, and prayer. Yoga and Tai Chi are often considered examples of movement-based meditation.

You can practice meditation wherever you are. It's free and doesn't require special equipment. Meditation involves learning how to focus your mind and calm the body. It eases some of the symptoms of stress, such as a racing heart or repeated thoughts about a stressful event. It can create an opportunity to gain a fresh perspective on the situations and challenges we face.

How to Practice Meditation

While there are many different forms of meditation and ways to practice, learning a basic meditation for beginners (Cherry, 2020) is a great place to begin:

1. **Choose a quiet spot that is free of distractions:** Turn off your phone, television, and other distractions. If you choose to play quiet music, select something calm and repetitive.

2. **Set a time limit:** If you are just getting started, you might want to stick to shorter sessions of about 5 to 10 minutes in length.

3. **Pay attention to your body and get comfortable:** You can sit cross-legged on the floor or in a chair as long as you feel that you can sit comfortably for several minutes at a time.

4. **Focus on your breathing:** Try taking deep breaths that expand your belly and then slowly exhale. Pay attention to how each breath feels.

5. **Notice your thoughts:** The purpose of meditation is not to clear your mind—your mind is inevitably going to wander. Instead, focus on gently bringing your attention back to your breath whenever you notice your thoughts drifting. Don't judge your thoughts or try to analyze them; simply direct your mind back to your deep breathing.

MINDFULNESS

Mindfulness practice has been growing in popularity in the United States and is often used to reduce or better manage stress and promote wellness. Jon Kabat-Zinn defines mindfulness as "awareness that arises from paying attention, on purpose, in the present moment, non-judgmentally" (Mindful Staff, 2017). There are many different forms of mindfulness including those that are connected to religious and spiritual traditions and practices. It can also be practiced as a way to reduce and better manage stress and can be done while sitting, lying down, walking, or even gardening. Like meditation, mindfulness has been shown to reduce stress and improve health conditions including depression and high blood pressure (Mayo Clinic, 2021).

A Walking Meditation

The Mayo Clinic shares a simple form of mindfulness practice as a walking meditation:

Find a quiet place 10–20 feet in length and begin to walk slowly. Focus on the experience of walking, being aware of the sensations of standing and the subtle movements that keep your balance. When you reach the end of your path, turn and continue walking, maintaining awareness of your sensations. (The Mayo Clinic, 2022)

HEALTHY EATING

What we eat and drink impacts our health and wellness. Chapter 17 provides guidelines for healthy eating that are grounded in research. These guidelines encourage us to develop a daily diet that honors our cultural traditions and identities and features vegetables, fruits, and whole grains. Try to reduce your consumption of processed foods that often include saturated and trans fats, cholesterol, corn syrup or other added sugars, salts, or alcohol. Take time to review to consider what steps you can take to improve the quality of your diet.

- *Do you have a favorite healthy meal?*

- *Can you make time this week to prepare and savor a healthy meal (on your own or with family or friends)?*

- *What one thing can you do to improve the quality of your daily diet?*

STRESS REDUCTION BY PROFESSIONALS

There is a wide range of professional services that can be helpful in managing stress and preventing burnout. These include:

Coaching and Therapy are overlapping models. Coaching generally focuses on the here and now, problem-solving, and assisting individuals in developing new skills to cope and adjust to present life situations. Therapy focuses on evaluating, diagnosing, and treating emotional problems and psychological conditions, and may address experiences rooted in the past. Although talking about your sense of distress with a friend, family member, or peer may be effective, seeking professional support is recommended if the level of stress is high and interfering with your sleep, life, or work. Professional support is particularly valuable if you are experiencing post-traumatic stress.

Massage is the systematic and intentional manipulation of the body and may include joint movements and stretching. The goal is to assist the body to achieve well-being while alleviating distress and specific disease-related symptoms. There are many different traditions and types of massage. Practitioners usually use their hands to apply fixed and movable pressure to the body.

Acupuncture works by correcting the balance of energy. It involves inserting hair-fine needles into specific anatomic points in the body to stimulate the flow of energy. Practitioners also apply pressure, suction, electromagnetic stimulation, or heat to the acupuncture points.

Sweat lodges and temexcales are sacred and spiritual healing spaces created and utilized by the indigenous peoples of North and South America, respectively. The lodge or *temexcal* is often seen as a womb that gives birth and life and also serves for communing with the Creator. The sweat lodge ceremony is complex and traditionally led by an experienced elder. The etiquette varies according to the lodge leader and may include singing, chanting, and drumming, all of which are considered prayer. The lodge ceremony provides cleansing of the spirit, heart, mind, and body, and has been successful in treating certain conditions.

- *Can you think of other professional services and traditions that may be helpful in reducing stress?*

- *What healing traditions and professional services are most common in the communities where you live and work?*

CHW Peer Support for Self-Care

At City College of San Francisco, CHWs in training work in teams of two to support each other in developing a practical self-care plan. While CHWs aren't always great at promoting their own wellness, they are wonderful at supporting others.

Reach out to a fellow CHW to ask if they are willing to provide mutual support for stress management and self-care. Schedule a time to meet and take turns using person-centered skills to support each other in developing a personalized and realistic plan for self-care.

Schedule a future meeting to check in with each other to assess how you are each doing. What challenges are you facing? What success have you experienced? How could you revise your self-care plan to be more realistic? What have you learned from your colleague?

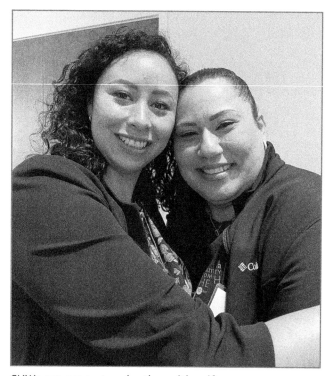

CHWs can support each other with self-care.

- *What other forms of stress reduction and self-care are you familiar with?*

- *What types of stress reduction/self-care are practiced by the clients and communities you work with?*

- *Would it be possible to incorporate stress reduction activities into the organization or program that you work or volunteer for? How could this be done?*

12.9 Talking with Clients about Stress Reduction

As a CHW, you have an important role to play in supporting clients to enhance stress management skills. Start by listening to your client. Facilitate dialogue using person-centered concepts and skills such as Motivational Interviewing (see Chapter 9) and provide clients with an opportunity to talk about the stress they face in their life, how it affects them, and the skills they already have for stress management. As you support clients to enhance their skills for stress management, keep the following principles in mind:

1. **Maintain a neutral stance:** Keep an open mind as you listen to the client's experience. Keep any thoughts or judgments about the client to yourself (or better yet, try to let any judging thoughts or assumptions go altogether). *You probably know from your own personal experience how it feels when you sense that you are being judged and how it is not useful in developing trust or encouraging you to make any changes.*

2. **Be person-centered:** Let the client's experience, culture, knowledge, skills, and beliefs guide the discussion, and form the basis of any plan for stress management.

3. **Use a strength-based approach:** Focus on the strengths that the client already possesses. Sometimes clients doubt or have a difficult time noticing their own strengths. Ask them if they have had success with managing stress in the past, and what strategies and resources they have used to reduce stress and enhance self-care. Encourage them to build on the knowledge and skills they already have.

4. **Apply harm reduction:** Keep the principles of Harm Reduction in mind: any actions that reduce potential harm to the client or their loved ones are a positive step toward promoting their health and wellness.

5. **Support realistic action plans:** Support clients to develop a practical action plan for stress management that they have a good chance of implementing. Remember that behavior change is hard, and often begins with a small step forward. Check-in regularly, if possible, to support clients to implement their Action Plan and to revise it over time.

6. **Provide positive re-enforcement:** Provide positive feedback and encouragement for the actions and decisions that clients take to better manage stress and promote their own wellness.

7. **Provide referrals:** Some clients may benefit from a referral to a colleague or a community resource to support them with stress management. Be sure to ask the client if they are interested in learning more about a particular resource or service before describing it in detail. If the client is interested in the service, provide a detailed and person-centered referral (see Chapter 9), and don't forget to follow up to learn if they accessed the service, what their experience was like, and how they are doing.

Please watch the following video of a CHW supporting a client to better manage her stress:

- *How did the CHW use the principles addressed in this chapter to support the client to better manager her stress?*

- *What did the CHW do well in supporting this client with stress management?*

- *What else would you do as a CHW to support this client with stress management?*

ACTION PLANNING AND STRESS MANAGEMENT: ROLE PLAY, DEMO. (*Source:* Foundations for Community Health Workers/http:// youtu.be/H_ 62Cbm5W_c/ last accessed 21 September 2023.)

Chapter Review

To review the concepts covered in this chapter, please consider your responses to the following questions:

1. What stressors have the greatest impact on your health?
2. What types of workplace stressors do CHWs face on the job?
3. What types of stressors have the greatest impact on the health of the clients and communities you work with?
4. How does exposure to stress impact our health?
5. What forms of systemic discrimination are most common in the communities where you live and work?

6. What is burnout? How does it affect us? What are some of the early warning signs that we may be at risk for burnout?

7. How can you assess your risks for stress and burnout?

8. What can you do to better manage and reduce the impact of stress in your life? What types of self-care practices have you put into action this week?

9. What can CHWs do to support each other with stress prevention and management?

10. What can the organizations that employ CHWs do to help prevent and minimize the impact of stress?

11. What types of social change are necessary in our society to reduce or end chronic sources of stress arising from inequity and systemic discrimination? What organizations are leading the types of social change that you want for our nation?

References

American Psychological Association. (2012). Fact Sheet: Health Disparities and Stress. https://www.apa.org/topics/racism-bias-discrimination/health-disparities-stress (accessed 9 November 2022)

Aryal, S., D'mello, M. K. (2020). Occupational stress and coping strategy among community health workers of Mangalore Taluk, Karnataka. *Indian Journal of Public Health*, 64(4), 351–356. https://doi.org/10.4103/ijph.IJPH_549_19.

Brinkley, A. (2018). Knowledge is Not Enough: Work Stress in Community Health Workers. Doctoral Dissertation, University of Connecticut. https://opencommons.uconn.edu/dissertations/1818.

Brown, O., Kangovi, S., Wiggins, N., & Alvarado, C. S. (2020). Supervision strategies and community health worker effectiveness in health care settings. *National Academy of Medicine Perspectives*. https://doi.org/10.31478/202003c.

Cherry, K. (2020). What is Meditation? Verywellmind. https://www.verywellmind.com/what-is-meditation-2795927 (accessed 9 November 2022).

Davis, B. A. (2020). Discrimination: a social determinant of health inequities. *Health Affairs Blog*. http://doi.org/10.1377/hblog20200220.518458.

Forrester, S., Jacobs, D., Zmora, R., Schreiner, P., Roger, V., Kiefe. C. I. (2019). Racial differences in weathering and its associations with psychosocial stress: the CARDIA study. *SSM – Population Health, Science Direct*, 7, 003. https://doi.org/10.1016/j.ssmph.2018.11.003.

Geronimus, A. T., Hicken, M., Keene, D., & Bound, J. (2006). "Weathering" and age patterns of allostatic load scores among blacks and whites in the United States. *American Journal of Public Health*, 96(5), 826–833. https://doi.org/10.2105/AJPH.2004.060749.

Greenberg, A. (2020). *How the stress of racism can harm your health – and what that has to do with Covid-19*, NOVA, Public Broadcasting Service. https://www.pbs.org/wgbh/nova/article/racism-stress-covid-allostatic-load/ (accessed 9 November 2022).

Guidi, J., Lucente, M., Sonino, N., & Fava, G. A. (2021). Allostatic load and its impact on health: A systematic review. *Psychotherapy and Psychosomatics*, 90(1), 11–27. https://doi.org/10.1159/000510696.

Health Leads. (2019). Battling burnout: Self-care and organizational tools to increase community health worker retention and satisfaction. *Resource Library*. https://healthleadsusa.org/resources/battling-burnout-self-care-and-organizational-tools-to-increase-community-health-worker-retention-and-satisfaction/ (accessed 9 November 2022).

International Training and Education Center on HIV (I-TECH) and the Ministry of Health and Child Welfare, Zimbabwe. (2005). *Integrated counselling for HIV and AIDS prevention and care: Training for HIV primary care counsellors*. Unpublished training manual.

Iturbide M. I., Raffaelli M., Carlo G. (2009). Protective effects of ethnic identity on Mexican American college students' psychological well-being. *Hispanic Journal of Behavioral Sciences*, 31(4), 536–552. https://doi.org/10.1177/0739986309345992.

Mayo Clinic. (2021). Stress Management. https://www.mayoclinic.org/healthy-lifestyle/stress-management/in-depth/stress-symptoms/art-20050987 (accessed 9 November 2022).

Mayo Clinic. (2022). Meditation: A Simple, Fast Way to Reduce Stress. https://www.mayoclinic.org/tests-procedures/meditation/in-depth/meditation/art-20045858 (accessed 9 November 2022).

Mindful Staff. (2017). Jon Kabat-Zinn: Defining mindfulness. *Mindful*. https://www.mindful.org/jon-kabat-zinn-defining-mindfulness/ (accessed 9 November 2022).

Nkonki, L., Cliff, J., & Sanders, D. (2011). Lay health worker attrition: important but often ignored. *Bulletin of the World Health Organization*, 89(12), 919–923. https://doi.org/10.2471/BLT.11.087825.

Professional Quality of Life (ProQOL). (2022). https://proqol.org/ (accessed 9 November 2022).

Sandoiu, A. (2021). 'Weathering': What are the Health Effects of Stress and Discrimination? *Medical News Today*. https://www.medicalnewstoday.com/articles/weathering-what-are-the-health-effects-of-stress-and-discrimination (accessed 9 November 2022).

Sawyer, P. J., Major, B., Casad, B. J., Townsend, S. S., & Mendes, W. B. (2012). Discrimination and the stress response: psychological and physiological consequences of anticipating prejudice in interethnic interactions. *American Journal of Public Health*, 102(5), 1020–1026. https://doi.org/10.2105/AJPH.2011.300620.

Sternthal, M., Slopen, N., & Williams, D. (2011). Racial disparities in health: How much does stress really matter? *Du Bois Review: Social Science Research on Race*, 8(1), 95–113. https://doi.org/10.1017/S1742058X11000087.

Villarosa, L. (2022). *Under the skin: The hidden toll of racism on American lives and on the health of our nation*. New York: Doubleday.

Zsoldos, E., Filippini, N. Mahmood, A., Mackay, C. E., Singh-Manoux, A., Kivimaki, M., Jenkinson, M., & Ebmeier, K. P. (2018). Allostatic load as a predictor of grey matter volume and white matter integrity in old age: The Whitehall II MRI study. *Nature Scientific Reports*, 8, article 6411. https://doi.org/10.1038/s41598-018-24398-9.

Additional Resources

American Public Health Association. (2022). Racism: A public health crisis. *National Public Health Week*. https://nphw.org/Themes-and-Facts/2022-Racism (accessed 9 November 2022).

California Community Health Worker Community of Practice. (2022). https://cachw.org/ (accessed 9 November 2022).

Lick, D. J., Durso, L. E., Johnson, K. L. (2013). Minority stress and physical health among sexual minorities. *Perspectives on Psychological Science*. 8(5), 521–48. https://doi.org/10.1177/1745691613497965. PMID: 26173210.

National Association of Community Health Workers. (2022). https://nachw.org/ (accessed 9 November 2022).

National Resource Center for Refugees, Immigrants, and Migrants (NRC-RIM). (2022). Self-care for community health workers: A curriculum for those working in refugee, immigrant and migrant communities during the COVID-19 pandemic. *CHW Solutions*. https://nrcrim.org/self-care-community-health-workers (accessed 9 November 2022).

Smith, M., Segal, J., & Robinson, L. (2021). Burnout prevention and treatment. *HelpGuide*. https://www.helpguide.org/articles/stress/burnout-prevention-and-recovery.htm (accessed 9 November 2022).

University of California, Los Angeles. Behavioral Wellness Center. (2022). Self-Assessments: Take Your Temperature. https://medschool.ucla.edu/bwc/self-assessments (accessed 9 November 2022).

Williams D. R. (2018). Stress and the mental health of populations of color: Advancing our understanding of race-related stressors. *Journal of Health and Social Behavior*, 59(4), 466–485. https://doi.org/10.1177/0022146518814251.

World Health Organization. (2020). Doing What Matters in Times of Stress: An Illustrated Guide. License: CC BY-NC-SA 3.0 GO. https://www.who.int/publications/i/item/9789240003927 (accessed 9 November 2022).

Conflict Resolution

Tim Berthold

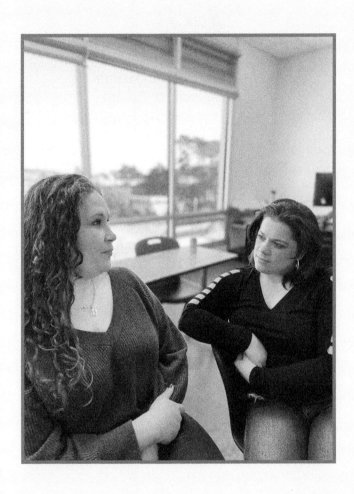

Foundations for Community Health Workers, Third Edition. Edited by Tim Berthold and Darouny Somsanith.
© 2024 John Wiley & Sons, Inc. Published 2024 by John Wiley & Sons, Inc.
Companion website: http://www.wiley.com/go/communityhealthworkers3E

CHW Scenario: Cindy and Stephanie

Cindy and Stephanie are Community Health Workers at a busy neighborhood health center. Their supervisor asked them to complete a program report, and the deadline is coming up soon. Cindy takes the lead and asks Stephanie for her contribution to the report. Stephanie responds that she has been too busy to work on the report, and their interaction escalates.

Please watch this short video depicting a conflict between Cindy and Stephanie

Stephanie: Cindy, did you ever get a chance to finish the report?

Cindy: What report are you talking about, because I know there were a few reports … so can you tell me?

Stephanie: The one that's due tomorrow.

Cindy: You know what, I didn't. It's been really hard for me. I have been in the field a lot, doing a lot of outreach.

Stephanie: I mean, I understand but this deadline is tomorrow!

Cindy: I haven't even had no time to do it … I'm barely touching base here!

Stephanie: It's been on your desk for two weeks!

Cindy: Wait, hold on, who put you in charge?

Stephanie: The deadline that's due tomorrow made me in charge.

Cindy: You're my equal!

Stephanie: I understand that, but we have a deadline, and I've been …

Cindy: But who made you in charge?

Stephanie: But I have to keep us on task and stay focused on deadlines. Deadlines can't be pushed back.

Cindy: Then why don't you do some of the outreach? I'm dealing with this guy, one of our patients, that just had a stroke … and I've been working with him every day.

(*Source:* Foundations for Community Health Workers/http://youtu.be/8wHwNAnhC1Y/last accessed 21 September 2023.)

Answer the following questions about the conflict between Cindy and Stephanie:

- *What is the conflict between Cindy and Stephanie really about?*
- *Have you ever experienced a similar workplace conflict?*
- *How might this conflict impact both Cindy and Stephanie and their work?*
- *What conflict management styles are Cindy and Stephanie using?*
- *If you were Cindy, how would you deal with the issue of Stephanie's missing report?*
- *If you were Stephanie, how would you respond to Cindy?*
- *How would you work to resolve this conflict? Which conflict resolution concepts and skills would you use?*

Introduction

Conflict is common and impacts our personal and professional lives. Community health workers (CHWs) are likely to experience workplace conflict. This may include conflicts with clients, community members or co-workers.

Learning how to respond effectively to conflict is essential for your own career success. The inability to handle conflict on the job is a key reason for termination or loss of employment as well as missed opportunities for advancement and promotion. Gaining skills and confidence to resolve conflict is also important for the success of your colleagues, the organization you work for, and the clients and communities you support.

This chapter provides an introduction to the topic of conflict resolution. We strongly encourage you to look for additional resources and opportunities to continue your training in conflict resolution. These skills will support your long-term career success.

WHAT YOU WILL LEARN

By studying the material in this chapter, you should be able to

- Define and discuss workplace conflict
- Identify common types and causes of conflict in the workplace
- Analyze potential consequences of workplace conflict
- Discuss common conflict management styles
- Explain approaches for resolving workplace conflict
- Negotiate a common framework and process for resolving conflict
- Analyze how status, power, discrimination, and anger can affect conflict resolution
- Describe techniques for de-escalating anger and conflict
- Identify resources for resolving conflicts while promoting equity

C3 Roles and Skills Addressed in Chapter 13

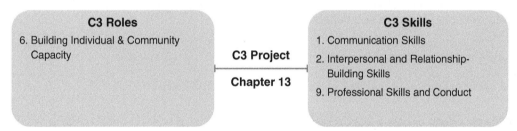

WORDS TO KNOW

Conflict

Restorative justice

13.1 Defining Workplace Conflict

One commonly cited definition of **conflict** is "a struggle between at least two interdependent parties who perceive incompatible goals, scare resources, and interference form the other party in achieving their goals" (Hocker & Wilmot, 1985, p. 23).

Workplace conflicts include:

- Conflicts with a co-worker
- Conflicts with a supervisor or agency leader
- Conflicts with a client or patient
- Witnessing conflicts between clients and community members

Workplace conflict is commonplace (Pollack Peacebuilding Systems, 2022):

- An estimated 85% of employees experience conflict of some type
- Workers in the United States spend an average of 2.8 hours a week engaged in some type of conflict

Because workplace conflict is so common, it is helpful to anticipate and prepare for how to manage conflicts.

TYPES OF WORKPLACE CONFLICT

Common types of workplace conflict include task, relationship, and value conflicts (Shonk, 2022).

Task conflict: These types of conflicts are about work assignments and issues such as workload, teamwork, division of work, policies and procedures for conducting work tasks, and employee expectations.

For example, CHWs may face conflicts about the assignment or division of work duties or their work schedule. Team members may disagree or argue about the best way to approach their work, or how to interpret and implement workplace policies and procedures. Colleagues may have different expectations about work culture and assignments.

Relationship conflict: These conflicts are often characterized by clashes of personality types, work, and communication styles. They may involve conflicts between two individuals, two groups, or a larger constellation of people.

CHWs may experience difficulty creating or sustaining positive working relationships with co-workers, supervisors, other administrators, or with people working for other agencies in the community. Difficult relationships sometimes include repeated avoidance, competition for assignments and recognition, arguments, hazing, bullying, and the spreading of rumors.

Value conflict: These conflicts arise from differences in values and identities, which may include differences in political, social or cultural beliefs.

For CHWs, these conflicts may involve different views of the community served, the nature of the relationship between clients and the organization, approaches to specific issues such as drug and alcohol use and treatment, harm reduction, incarceration, gun violence, immunizations, support for people who are unhoused, returning home from prison, and people who are lesbian, gay, bisexual, transgender, and non-binary. These conflicts often touch upon our core identities and beliefs.

- *Have you ever experienced task, relationship, or value conflicts in the workplace?*

- *What other types of workplace conflicts have you witnessed or experienced?*

What Do
YOU ?
Think

SOURCES OR CAUSES OF WORKPLACE CONFLICT

Understanding the factors that cause and contribute to workplace conflict is often essential to finding resolution and preventing future conflicts. Common causes of workplace conflict include:

- **Inadequate training:** Organizations sometimes fail to properly train and prepare employees for the tasks and services they provide, the technology and systems used to document work, and the types of challenges they may face.

- **Lack of understanding of workplace policies and procedures:** Some organizations fail to adequately post and explain key workplace policies and protocols.

- **Unclear job roles and expectations:** Some workers lack a job description, or their job duties are vague or frequently changing.

- **Workloads:** This may include unrealistic workloads, unequal workloads, and the perception of unequal workloads.

- **Limited resources:** Organizations often lack sufficient resources necessary for providing quality services including staffing, professional development, qualified managers, technology, pay, and benefits.

- **Resistance to change:** Organizational change is often accompanied by anxiety, stress, and fear of losing status or employment. Some people react to changes in the workplace with denial, confusion, anger, and resistance.

- **Poor communication:** This may include failure to communicate about key issues, tasks or deadlines, or communication styles that are perceived as disrespectful or unprofessional.

- **Lack of supervision and poor supervision:** Some workers lack regular supervision, guidance, and feedback. Some supervisors lack skills in how to effectively encourage and support the people they manage.

- **Personality differences and clashes.**

- **Differences regarding workplace values and goals.**

- **Prejudice and discrimination:** Perceived bias, prejudice, and discrimination are common in the American workplace. Over 61,000 workplace discrimination charges were filed in 2021 (Pollack Peacebuilding Systems, 2022).
- **Bullying and harassment:** Workplace harassment is common, including sexual and racially motivated harassment, and may be perpetrated by anyone associated with a workplace including frontline employees, leadership, volunteers, customers or patients, and vendor or subcontracting agencies.
- **Toxic workplace environments:** Toxic workplace environments are the result of chronic and significant conflicts that are unaddressed and unresolved, such as ongoing harassment.

Of course, many workplace conflicts are the result of a combination of the factors identified above.

- *What additional factors contribute to workplace conflict?*
- *How could an understanding of the causes of a workplace conflict assist you in addressing it?*

CONFLICTS INVOLVING CLIENTS AND COMMUNITY MEMBERS

Some of the most challenging workplace conflicts are those that involve clients or community members. You may witness a conflict between participants of a training, meeting, or support group that you are facilitating. You may be working at a community event and observe a conflict among people who you do or don't already know. Finally, you are likely to experience conflicts—large and small—with individual clients and families that you provide services to.

Conflicts with clients and community members arise from factors such as:

- **Lack of Resources:** Inability to provide a client with a service or resource they want such as housing or other difficult-to-find resources.
- **Setting limits and professional boundaries:** Clients may respond negatively when CHWs set limits such as the length of a meeting, how many times they communicate with clients in a week or a month, limiting or denying access to specific benefits or services such as food or transportation vouchers or housing referrals.
- **Respect:** People who have often been disrespected are highly sensitive to the way that others treat them. Clients may feel insulted, put-down or disrespected by your tone of voice or body language, by what you say or fail to say, and by decisions you make or fail to make.
- **Treatment by Service Providers:** Perceptions that a client is being treated differently than others, or provided with less or lesser quality services ("Why can't I get a transportation voucher? I know that _____ got one!")
- **Bias or Discrimination:** Perceptions or allegations of bias, prejudice, or discrimination including accusations of racism, transphobia, and other types of discriminatory treatment.
- **Differences of Opinion and Understanding:** Disagreements about topics such as COVID-19, immunizations, drug treatments, harm reduction, etc.
- **Anger:** Acting out in anger that is about other challenges, losses, or crisis such as the loss of employment, benefits or housing, being unhoused or experiencing domestic violence, involvement in the criminal justice system.

- *Can you think of other common sources of conflict for clients?*

Your Experience

What types of conflicts have you experienced with clients, patients, customers, or program participants?

- What factors caused or contributed to these conflicts?
- How did you respond to these conflicts?
- What did you do well that you hope to apply in the future?
- What do you hope to change or do differently?

It can be helpful to look at the issues that may lie beneath the surface of a conflict with a client or a member of the community. When people are in pain, scared, or suffering in some way, they may be impatient, frustrated, anxious, or angry. Most of us have experienced moments when we acted out in anger or disappointment in ways weren't healthy or productive. This is a time to channel your unconditional positive regard.

> **Anonymous:** Sometimes I've wanted to snap back at a client who went off on me. Sometimes I need to walk away from the situation because I am just too triggered. Over time, it has gotten easier for me to deal with clients who are angry. I try to remember that they are probably deeply frustrated with the process of trying to get help for their circumstances. In my city, there are few resources for people who are unhoused. Some people have been living on the streets for years, decades even. So, if a client is upset or angry, I try to remember why I became CHW in the first place and it wasn't to judge or fight with people. It was because I wanted to offer the patience and kindness that me and my family didn't always receive when I was growing up. Keeping perspective helps me to stay grounded and humble in these moments.

13.2 Consequences of Workplace Conflict

Conflict can be productive or counter-productive, beneficial, or harmful.

When conflicts stay at the level of a debate or disagreement about a work question, problem, or strategy, they can result in new perspectives and solutions. Conflict may even result in improved relationships among co-workers, increased participation, and creativity.

When conflicts about substantive issues are ignored or unresolved, they can cause significant harm. Potential consequences of workplace conflict include:

- Increased stress, burnout, anxiety, depression.
- Reduced work satisfaction and morale. When we face an ongoing conflict at work, it can influence all aspects of our work experience and make us reluctant to go to work, cause us to avoid certain colleagues or meetings, and even diminish a sense of pride or satisfaction that we previously experienced related to our work.
- Reduced productivity.
- A decline in the quality of services provided.
- Increased staff absenteeism and turnover.
- Continued or increased bias, harassment, or other forms of discrimination.
- Rumors about colleagues, programs, or community members.
- A climate of mistrust that harms teamwork and cooperation.
- Negative perspectives or opinions about a program or an agency within the community and by clients or patients.
- A decline in referrals from other clients and agencies and the possible loss of clients.

Workplace conflict can be widespread and may impact:

- The individual or "parties" directly involved in the conflict.
- Co-workers, managers, and supervisors.
- The program or organization where the conflict takes place.
- The clients and communities served by the organization.

- *Can you think of other ways that workplace conflict may be beneficial or harmful?*

What Do YOU Think?

> **Anonymous:** I ended up leaving what was possibly my best job ever. My boss got a promotion, and a new supervisor was hired from outside the agency. We never really got along. I don't think he really understood what we did. I felt like all he did was point out my mistakes. He even did this in team meetings—he kind of scolded us in front of our colleagues. He didn't talk about the things that I did well. I tried to talk with him, but it just made things worse. I started looking for a new job. In the end, a bunch of us quit. But I still miss the way it was before we got a new supervisor.

13.3 Common Responses to Conflict

Five types or styles of managing conflict are commonly referenced in the literature on conflict resolution. Thomas-Kilmann rank each of the five styles based on their level of assertiveness and cooperativeness (Kilmann Diagnostics, 2022):

Avoidance: This style of conflict management is low in both assertiveness and cooperativeness. People may try to avoid the other parties in a conflict, deny that there is a conflict, postpone, or reschedule meetings or decisions related to the conflict and, in some cases, hope that by avoiding the situation the conflict may "go away." Avoidance is sometimes a wise response, especially if the conflict is particularly heated or the issue in question is less significant or unlikely to occur again. However, avoidance can quickly escalate a conflict that is chronic or ongoing and which involves important work tasks, deadlines, or values.

Accommodation: This style of conflict management is low in assertiveness and high in cooperativeness. This conflict management style involves agreeing to or giving in to what the other party(ies) to the conflict want in order to avoid continued conflict. This can be an effective style if the conflict isn't significant or if accommodation doesn't require the sacrifice or abandonment of an important value or goal.

Compromise: This style of conflict management is moderate in both assertiveness and cooperativeness. It seeks to find a solution that is acceptable to all parties. Compromising typically involves giving up some of what you want with the trade-off of preventing the continuation or escalation of conflict. Compromise can be an effective way to resolve conflict, especially when other parties also compromise. However, giving up one's own goals or values can be harmful when repeated over time.

Competition: This style of conflict management is high in assertiveness and low in cooperativeness. It is characterized by asserting your own goals, needs, and solutions, and sometimes pushing these priorities over the ideas, needs, or solutions of others. This style is more concerned about the outcome of the conflict rather than the process of resolution or the quality of relationships with the others involved in the conflict. Maintaining a competition style to workplace conflicts tends to result in the deterioration of teamwork, relationships with colleagues, and productivity over time, and can lead to escalating or worsening conflict.

Collaboration: This style of conflict management is high in both assertiveness and cooperativeness. It involves actively participating with others to find a solution that satisfies the concerns of all parties. It typically requires discussing the nature of the conflict including underlying concerns and needs. Collaboration takes time and a commitment to engage. It has the benefit of contributing to more robust and lasting solutions to conflict and to improving professional relationships and teamwork.

Note that we may use different styles or approaches to resolving different types of conflicts. Depending upon the nature of the conflict, each of these conflict resolution styles has value.

A survey of professionals from over 36 countries (Niagara Institute, 2022) highlighted the following information:

- 87.8% said that they are willing to compromise if it will break a deadlock or impasse
- Collaboration was identified as the most common conflict style (59.8%)
- 55.7% of respondents said that they prioritize restoring harmony when faced with conflicts
- When asked what their greatest strength was, 24.8% of respondents indicated "finding a middle ground" and 28% said "suggesting creative solutions."

- *What are the pros and cons of each of these five conflict resolution styles?*
- *Can you identify situations where it might be valuable to use each of these different styles?*
- *What problems can arise from using each style?*
- *What do you think is your dominant or primary style of managing conflict?*

THE VALUE OF COMPROMISE

Many people approach conflicts with a win/lose mentality. They may feel that they are mostly (or completely) in the right, and other parties are mostly (or completely) in the wrong. They seek a resolution to the conflict that will affirm their own position and compel others to concede and make changes.

Unwillingness to compromise is problematic for many reasons:

1. Conflicts are rarely so simplistic that one party is 100% correct and the other party is 100% wrong.

2. Even if you are completely right, holding out for a "win/lose" solution where only the other party has to give in is likely to become a "lose/lose" solution in the long run. This mentality often leads to resentment and continued conflict that undermines your sense of comfort at work, and it is likely to create an environment that negatively affects clients and co-workers.

3. Being right is not the most important thing. Ultimately, it is much more important to find a way to work peacefully, professionally, and respectfully with co-workers and clients so that you can effectively promote community health.

4. Holding on to the need to be right is likely to create a lasting perception that you are rigid, controlling, or worse. It may undermine your career advancement.

5. Always needing to be right is stressful and likely to be harmful to your physical and mental health. Learning to accept responsibility for your own contributions to conflict, and to compromise, can be deeply rewarding in and of itself and promote your well-being. These skills are likely to be useful in your personal and family relationships as well, especially if you are a parent.

- *Have you ever interacted with someone who had a compelling need to be right?*
- *Would you like to be in an ongoing professional relationship with someone who had difficulty compromising?*
- *What gets in the way of your ability to compromise?*
- *What assists you in seeking a win/win solution to a conflict?*

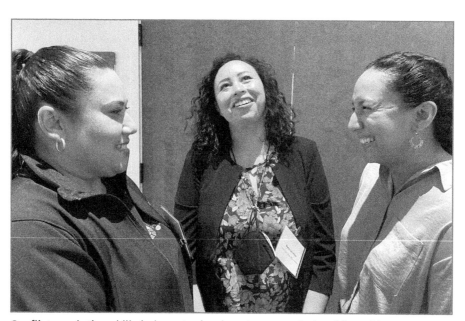

Conflict resolution skills help us to develop stronger relationships with our colleagues.

THE INFLUENCE OF CULTURE

Our cultural identities influence how we understand, communicate about, and react to conflict. For example, some cultures are more likely to value the needs of the group over the needs of the individual. They may emphasize harmony and compromise in the face of conflict in contrast to cultures that encourage people to stand up for their individual rights.

Continue to develop and practice cultural humility (see Chapter 7) as you face conflict in the workplace. Keep in mind that *your way* of dealing with conflict, informed by your own culture or cultures, is just one way, not *The Way* of responding to conflict. Don't make assumptions about the conflict styles of co-workers or clients.

- *Have you experienced conflicts that were influenced by cultural differences?*

- *How do your cultural identities and values influence your approach to conflict?*

CHW Profile

Monica Rico, She/Her

Community Health Worker

VIDA (Virus Integrated Distribution of Aid), and the City of Gonzalez, CA

Community Health Engagement and Resources

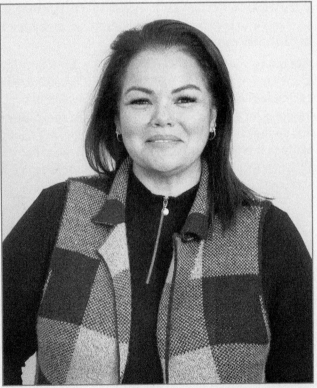

I come from an underserved background, and I saw a need in my community, especially among non-English speakers. They hesitate to visit a clinic to see a doctor and to reach out to any government office because of their immigration status or language barriers. I feel a need to help my community empower themselves. I want them to know that they still have a voice to express themselves. They can speak in Spanish and have someone to support them.

(continues)

CHW Profile

(continued)

I work primarily with first-generation Mexican American families and agricultural workers who came to United States for a better life. We conduct door-to-door outreach to meet people at their home because they may not reach out to us if they need help. We let them know who we are, and we talk to them about a wide range of resources. We inform them about COVID-19, about vaccinations, and how to get help at the health clinic. Once they get to know us, and we gain their trust, other things start coming up. We help them with tenants' rights, substance abuse, employment, and other resources that families need. We've been doing demonstrations about healthy eating to help people with their chronic diseases.

When COVID-19 started, a woman came in and she wanted to be vaccinated but she was scared, and she put it off. Then she got very sick with COVID. She was in the hospital for several weeks, so I kept in constant contact with her family members to see how she was doing. I was so concerned for her. Finally, she came out of the hospital and a few weeks later she came to find me at my work. I was so overwhelmed because not everyone came back from the hospital. She got vaccinated and she took her husband and her kids to be vaccinated too. I've been helping her with her diabetes. I help her set up appointments at the clinic, and I help her plan for what she wants to tell them and what questions she wants to ask. Now that she's been going to the clinic, her health is much better.

Everybody goes through something. Sometimes it is easier for people to look away and ignore it, because they don't want to deal with it. As a CHW, I am more understanding about the people around me and their needs. I am passionate about my work. Sometimes families talk to me, but they aren't speaking up to ask for what they want. So, I have learned to read between the lines, to observe their body language, to let them know that I am here for them, that they can tell me anything.

If somebody comes and reaches out to you for help, don't let them leave your office without giving them a little bit of hope. If you don't, they might leave and never come back because they'll think: "I reached out and you didn't help me." So, listen to them and try to support them even if it is just one thing. You might have some information or a resource, or you can call another agency to see if they have resources. Sometimes if I don't have an answer, I pick up the phone and call someone who might. I call right in front of the client so they can see that I am making that effort, that I want to help them, and that I don't want to leave them empty handed. And you know, when they leave with a little hope, I also leave my office with a little hope.

13.4 Common Challenges to Resolving Conflict

Responding to workplace conflicts is complicated when the conflict is characterized by or influenced by additional factors such as differences in power or authority, and the emotion of anger.

POWER AND AUTHORITY

Over the course of your career, you are likely to experience conflict with a co-worker who has equal status within the organization, with a supervisor who has power over you, and with a client whom you have power over. How will these differences in power affect your approach to conflict resolution?

Conflict with a supervisor can be particularly challenging. People often worry that addressing these conflicts will place their job at risk. Ideally, we want supervisors to invite and encourage us to speak freely about our professional concerns and challenges. However, supervisors often face competing pressures and may neither have the time nor the ability to listen or communicate well.

If you are experiencing a conflict with a supervisor, take time to reflect before you speak with them. Not all supervisors are skilled in conflict resolution. Sometimes silence and avoidance are prudent choices. Based on prior experience, do you trust that your supervisor will be able to work constructively and respectfully with you to resolve the conflict? If not, consider what the possible consequences of keeping silent or speaking up may be for yourself, your program, and your clients.

If you decide to address the conflict directly, be sure to follow your organization's "chain of command" and speak first to your supervisor rather than going above their head to speak to *their* supervisor. If your supervisor discovers that you have spoken to others about a mutual conflict before speaking directly with them, it may undermine your working relationship and your job. There are very few exceptions to this rule. However, if the conflict involves issues that are as serious as allegations of corruption or sexual or racial harassment, it is often best to speak to someone who is higher up in the chain of command at the agency you work for.

When you have a conflict with someone you have power over—whether that is someone you supervise, someone who volunteers with your program, or a client—you have a responsibility to take leadership in resolving the conflict. Recognize that by reaching out to communicate with you about a conflict, the other person is taking a risk. Volunteers and staff may be concerned about risking their position. Clients may be afraid of harming their ability to access services with you or your agency. You may need to take the lead in assuring others who you have power over that you welcome their input and encourage them to talk with you about their concerns.

Know Your Workplace Policies and Procedures

By law, all employers have workplace policies and procedures for reporting and managing grievances including complaints related to conflicts, bullying, harassment, or discrimination. Workplace harassment—sometimes based on factors such as sex, gender-identity, sexual orientation, nationality, ethnicity, and religion—is illegal, and employers have an obligation to prevent and resolve it.

It is helpful to know your workplace policies for handling complaints or grievances—including grievances that reports of harassment or conflict have not been handled properly. Find out if your human resource manual outlines a grievance procedure. Do you have an employee assistance program in place that will allow you to talk to a counselor? Do you have a union representative who can advise you?

In most workplaces, employees are expected to work through a conflict the other person or people involved first. If this isn't successful or if it isn't possible or safe to do so (e.g., in situations of sexual or racial harassment or assault), you should speak with your direct supervisor next. If the conflict persists and your direct supervisor is not helpful in resolving it, then you can speak to someone with greater authority in your organization such as someone in the Human Resources department, if available.

THE INFLUENCE OF ANGER

Conflicts are often accompanied by strong emotions including anger. Anger is a natural and powerful emotion with the potential to be beneficial or harmful. Anger can mobilize an individual, a team of workers, or a community to make positive changes. Anger becomes a problem when it is expressed in ways that are insulting, demeaning, or threatening to others.

Learning how to better manage your anger starts with being aware of what pushes your buttons. *What activates or provokes your resentment, defensiveness, or anger?*

HOW TO HANDLE YOUR ANGER PROFESSIONALLY

Knowing how to manage our anger without causing harm to ourselves or others is an essential life skill and crucial for professional success. The following recommendations for managing anger come from the federal Substance Abuse and Mental Health Services Administration (SAMHSA, 2022):

Self-management: Pay attention to cues that you are getting very angry, and when you notice them, take a break. You may want to count to 10, take a quick walk, or try some of the relaxation techniques listed below.

Assertive communication: If you are angry with a person, it may make sense to talk with him or her directly about it when your anger is at a manageable level to do this. When you're ready, try to use "I" statements and avoid the words "always," "never," and "should."

Problem-solving approach: If you find you are often becoming angry in a specific situation, you may want to consider ways you can change the situation. If changes are not possible, it may help to focus on areas of life you can control.

Forgiveness: Use forgiveness as you can and as it makes sense. Forgiveness may take time, but if you can experience it, it may enhance your relationship with the person you forgive.

Additional tips (Mayo Clinic, 2022) include:

Get some exercise: Physical activity can help reduce stress that can cause you to become angry. If you feel your anger escalating, go for a brisk walk or run. Or spend some time doing other enjoyable physical activities.

Take a time-out: Time-outs aren't just for kids. Give yourself short breaks during times of the day that tend to be stressful. A few moments of quiet time might help you feel better prepared to handle what's ahead without getting irritated or angry.

Stick with "I" statements: Criticizing or placing blame might only increase tension. Instead, use "I" statements to describe the problem. Be respectful and specific. For example, say, "I'm upset that you left the table without offering to help with the dishes" instead of "You never do any housework."

Don't hold a grudge: Forgiveness is a powerful tool. If you allow anger and other negative feelings to crowd out positive feelings, you might find yourself swallowed up by your own bitterness or sense of injustice. Forgiving someone who angered you might help you both learn from the situation and strengthen your relationship.

Use humor to release tension: Lightening up can help diffuse tension. Use humor to help you face what's making you angry and, possibly, any unrealistic expectations you have for how things should go. Avoid sarcasm, though it can hurt feelings and make things worse.

Practice relaxation skills: When your temper flares, put relaxation skills to work. Practice deep-breathing exercises, imagine a relaxing scene, or repeat a calming word or phrase, such as "Take it easy." You might also listen to music, write in a journal, or do a few yoga poses—whatever it takes to encourage relaxation.

Know when to seek help: Learning to control anger can be a challenge at times. Seek help for anger issues if your anger seems out of control causes you to do things you regret or hurts those around you.

> *What types of workplace situations or dynamics provoke your anger?*
>
> *How do you typically respond when you are angry?*
>
> *What have you learned that helps you to manage your anger and to respond in ways that are productive?*

What Do YOU ? Think

Please watch the following videos ▶ that show a CHW who, at first, does not respond well when a client expresses her anger (Counter Role Play). The second role play (Demonstration) shows the same scenario, but this time the CHW does a much better job of responding to the client's anger.

- *What mistakes did the CHW make in the Counter role play? How might these mistakes impact the relationship between the CHW and the client?*
- *What did the CHW do differently in the Demonstration role play?*
- *What did the CHW do well in this role play, and what else could she have done or said in responding to the client's anger?*

RESPONDING TO ANGER: ROLE PLAY, COUNTER. (*Source:* Foundations for Community Health Workers/http://youtu.be/kOZWxisLm5s/last accessed 21 September 2023.)

RESPONDING TO ANGER, ROLE PLAY, DEMONSTRATION. (*Source:* Foundations for Community Health Workers/http://youtu.be/lMxXFufpHFc/last accessed 21 September 2023.)

SUGGESTIONS FOR DE-ESCALATING THE ANGER OF OTHERS

Here are some recommendations for de-escalating anger in others while keeping safety in mind:

- Try to remember that, *given the types of challenges that clients and community members face, it is no wonder that they sometimes act out of frustration, anxiety, or anger.*

- **Breathe and calm your own emotions:** Your emotions—including your own anger—may be activated by the conflict. Breathe and try to regroup. If necessary, take a break and return to the conversation after your heart rate and your anger have lessened.
  - Deep breathing is highly effective at calming our anxiety and anger. Take a deep breath in through your nose. Hold it. Wait. Breathe out a long breath through your mouth. Repeat.
  - Depending upon the circumstances and the extent of your prior relationship with the other party, you might try asking them to join you in doing a few minutes of deep breathing. This can help to settle both of your emotions and thoughts and is a positive first step to take together.

- **Control your body language and tone of voice:** We communicate a lot through our body language. When someone is angry, don't roll your eyes, check your watch or phone, cross your arms, or sigh in frustration. Strive to find your best self, the CHW who knows how to respond with patience and kindness. Lower the one of your voice. Speaking in a softer tone can sometimes prompt others to stop raising their own voice.

- **Respect personal space:** Don't stand or lean in too close to the other party of the conflict. Take a step back.

- **Express your desire to listen to the client's concerns:** Use your calm tone of voice to communicate your desire to listen to what the other party has to say.

- **Listen:** Don't consider what you want to say or how you will respond as you listen. As some CHWs say, "listen with your mind and your heart and your spirit."

- *Use your Motivational Interviewing skills*, including your OARS to help the client to reflect on the situation and the factors that are prompting their anger.

- **Allow for silence and reflection:** Allow time for yourself and the client to find the words for what you wish to communicate.

- **Acknowledge emotions:** This might include frustration, anxiety, fear, or anger. These are common and natural emotions. When they are acknowledged calmly and directly, it can help them to become more manageable.

- *Apologize* for your contribution to the conflict. You may have interrupted the client, made an assumption about their life or the meaning of their words, you may have let them down or failed to follow through with a task or service. Reflect on what you may have said or done that contributed to the conflict between you and, if you are able, offer a genuine apology (See the section on the Power of Apology).

- **Set limits:** Ask for what you need in order to maintain a respectful and professional relationship and to resolve the conflict. Remind the other person of relevant agency or program policies. This may include taking a break, lowering the tone of your voices, or rescheduling a time to continue the conversation. For example, you might say something such as: "Let's keep our program policies in mind, including not to yell at one another. It can be difficult to hear each other if we raise our voices. Can we take a step back and lower our voices? Would it be helpful to take a break?" or "Let's take a 15-minute break and see if we can find a way to communicate more effectively. I really want to try to work this out together."

- **Focus on the future:** Sometimes it is difficult or impossible to resolve a conflict about a past incident. Sometimes it can be helpful to focus on the future and how you can contribute to building an improved relationship.

- *Watch for signs of escalation, safety concerns*, and the need to disengage. Sometimes, despite our best efforts, conflicts continue to escalate with anger, raised voices, pointed fingers, and disrespectful words or statements. Continuing to engage is only likely to do more harm to the professional relationship. If you are unable to de-escalate the tone of the conflict or disagreement or if you feel threatened or unsafe, it is best to calmly and politely disengage. If you are in a private setting such as a closed office or exam room, open the door and step out into a public space where others can serve as witnesses and provide support.

- **Maintain your own integrity:** No matter what the other person may do or say, walk away from the conflict knowing that you handled it to the best of your ability. Don't let a conflict draw you away from your code of ethics as a CHW or your best self. Stay patient and kind.

If you are unsuccessful in de-escalating the situation and are still concerned about your own safety or the safety of others, you may need to leave the situation or to ask the other party to leave. If you ask the other party to leave, do so in a calm manner. The agency you work for should have a policy for responding to safety concerns. If possible, request assistance from a colleague, make an excuse and leave, or (if necessary) call a crisis response program for assistance.

Make time to debrief the situation with your colleagues. Discuss what you and others did well to manage the conflict and how you can improve your response in the future.

- *Have you ever had to de-escalate conflict or anger?*

- *What did you do in the situation, and what was the outcome?*

- *What recommendations do you have for others who face similar challenges?*

13.5 Communication Skills for Conflict Resolution

Resolving conflicts requires strong communication skills. The following three concepts come from *Difficult Conversations* (Stone, Patton, & Heen, 2010), a widely used resource for conflict resolution authored by a team from The Harvard Negotiation Project.

MOVING FROM CERTAINTY TO CURIOSITY

We have a tendency to make assumptions and judgments about conflicts, including what *really* happened and what the other parties did, thought, and felt. When we bring these assumptions to a conversation designed to resolve the conflict, we are likely to undermine our efforts and the outcome.

Try shifting your perspective from one of certainty about the situation ("I know what really happened") to one of curiosity ("What happened? What was going on for _____ [the other party to the conflict]?").

When you can set aside your prejudices and assumptions, you are likely to discover new ways of understanding yourself, the other party, the conflict itself, and possibilities for its successful resolution.

DISENTANGLING INTENT FROM IMPACT

During conflicts, we often make assumptions about the intentions of others. When we are hurt or by a conflict, we may assume that the other party intended this result. Once again, these assumptions can keep us from seeing the true nature of the conflict and moving forward toward its resolution.

For example, Jason and Manuel get into a conflict. Jason says or does something that offends Manuel.

- Just because Manuel is offended, that does not mean that Jason intended to offend him.
- Just because Jason didn't intend to offend him doesn't mean that Manuel is not offended.

Give the benefit of the doubt to the other party. When we are able to separate the impact of actions from their intentions, we often diminish the emotional charge of the conflict and reduce its potential for escalation.

DISTINGUISHING BLAME FROM CONTRIBUTION

When in conflict, people are often caught up in making accusations and assigning blame. Trying to prove who is to blame can easily derail us from being able to listen, to learn, to find solutions, and to build new working relationships and alliances.

Rather than focusing on what the other did wrong, focus on understanding the contributions that each party made to the conflict, *with an emphasis on trying to understand your own contributions first*. You are likely to find that both or all parties did or said something that contributed to the conflict. Understanding this can support you in identifying solutions and preventing similar conflicts in the future.

The shift in focus from blame to contribution may seem subtle, but it can powerfully transform your efforts to resolve the conflict.

For example, in the CHW Scenario between Cindy and Stephanie (continued below), Stephanie shares several ways that she contributed to the conflict: "I'm sorry how I spoke to you," and, "I'm sorry I didn't really listen when you were telling me about the client who just had a stroke." Cindy also acknowledges her own contribution: "I snapped back, didn't I? Not my best moment. I'm sorry Stephanie," and "I know I should have worked on the report or gotten back to you sooner."

ESSENTIAL CHW SKILLS

Foundational CHW concepts and skills can be applied to help you navigate, respond to, and resolve conflicts in the workplace:

Cultural humility: Cultural humility (Chapter 7) prevents us from imposing our own assumptions, beliefs, and standards on others. It reminds of us who we are, and who we are not, of where we have power and privilege, and where we lack it. It guides us in working with clients in ways that recognize their expertise and transfer power or authority from us (providers) to them (clients). It can also be helpful during moments of conflict. Observe any tendencies you may have to impose your own understanding or values on the other parties to the conflict. Accept that there are different experiences, stories, emotions, and beliefs about the conflict.

Unconditional positive regard: Chapters 6 and 9 discuss the concept of unconditional positive regard or showing acceptance and support for everyone you work with. In the midst of conflict, it is even more important to embody this concept.

Big Eyes, Big Ears, small mouth (Chapter 6): In the midst of conflict, step back to observe and listen to what others are saying. Listening can be particularly difficult when your emotions are triggered and you may be feeling defensive or angry. Slowing down to listen is essential to resolving conflict. What can you learn from the other parties to the conflict? What is their experience? What are they feeling? What do they want?

> **Anonymous:** I think one of the most helpful ideas for me—in terms of handling conflicts better—is that one about moving from certainty to curiosity. I can easily get stuck thinking that I know something about other people's actions or their feelings about me. But instead of leading with my own—usually stupid—assumptions, I just need to back up and ask and listen. It is really just about using my Big Eyes and Ears and my motivational interviewing skills. If I can ask open-ended questions, I usually learn a lot about what the other person's experience is, and it is usually different from what I thought.

Motivational interviewing: Your motivational interviewing knowledge and skills (Chapter 9) will guide most of your work as a CHW and are vital resources in responding to conflict. When in doubt about how to respond, try using your OARS. Ask **O**pen-ended questions that invite others to share more of their experience. Provide **A**ffirmations that demonstrate your respect for others. Use **R**eflective statements to help everyone in the conflict to reflect more deeply on their own feelings and concerns and the factors that may be contributing to the current conflict. From time to time, **S**ummarize what you have discussed and especially anything that you have agreed on, such as ground rules for negotiating the conflict, or next steps that you will take toward resolving the conflict.

Ecological models: Ecological models (Chapter 3) encourage us to look beyond the immediate issues or problems we are facing to consider broader social factors that may be influencing the conflict. For example, Are current community challenges or crisis influencing this conflict? Are local social or political conflicts influencing interactions in your workplace?

A commitment to equity: The CHW profession is committed to promoting equity and social justice. Are factors of fairness, status, power, privilege, or prejudice influencing the conflict? What types of solutions may be found to the conflict that also promotes your organization's broader goals of promoting equity?

THE POWER OF APOLOGY

We strongly believe in the power of an apology to transform relationships. This is true with co-workers, supervisors, and clients. We view making an apology, like compromising, as a demonstration of generosity, humility, and strength of character. Be prepared to take responsibility for actions that may have contributed to the conflict and unintentionally hurt or harmed the situation or the other party.

Some examples are:

- "I forgot to text you about the support group. I'm really sorry."

- "I apologize. I didn't communicate very well. I know that I can't understand your experience and I shouldn't have said that. What I mean to say is that I want to learn as much as I can about what you are going through."

Unfortunately, some people seem to think that making an apology is the same thing as saying, "I am a bad person who is 100 percent wrong and deserve to be punished for the rest of my life!" However, if you don't learn to take responsibility for your own mistakes and to provide an honest apology when appropriate, you will undermine your professional relationships and career advancement.

- *Have you ever received a meaningful apology from a service provider that had a positive impact?*

- *Is it hard for you to apologize to others? If so, why?*

- *How can you enhance your skills for offering an authentic apology?*

What Do
YOU ?
Think ⦁

Please watch the following video interview addresses the importance of learning to provide a timely and authentic apology to a client or co-worker.

THE ART OF APOLOGY.

(*Source:* Foundations for Community Health Workers/http://youtu.be/ obtQn3fdGOY/last accessed 21 September 2023.)

13.6 Approaches to Prevention and Resolving Workplace Conflict

Here are some resources for resolving workplace conflicts.

DEVELOPING A COMMON FRAMEWORK AND PROCESS FOR RESOLVING CONFLICT

We strongly recommend that you talk about the process you will use to resolve the conflict before you start to talk about the conflict itself.

Attempts to resolve conflicts are often undermined because people don't take time to develop a set of ground rules to guide their conversation. They jump right into the heart of the conflict, making accusations and stirring up strong emotions. This can escalate the conflict and make it more difficult for parties to communicate effectively in the future.

Take time for a pre-conversation to discuss how you will work together to resolve the conflict. Consider the following guidelines for initiating a conversation designed to resolve a conflict:

1. Express your commitment to resolving the conflict.

2. Express your desire to establish a positive working relationship.

3. Acknowledge the value of the other party or parties. Find something positive to say about who they are, the work that they do, and a time when you worked well together.

4. Identify and acknowledge your common values, such as your commitment to providing quality services to clients or to advocating for social justice.

5. Be prepared to move from certainty to curiosity. Express your desire to listen and learn about their experience and perspective.

6. Negotiate common ground rules for your discussion that use the active listening skills described later on in this chapter. Ground rules may include, for example:

   a. Agree to take a break if the discussion seems to be escalating the conflict. Stepping away for a few minutes or a few days can help strong emotions to settle and provide an opportunity for deeper reflection about the conflict and how to resolve it.

   b. Take turns talking and listening to each other's personal experience of the conflict. After each party speaks, ask the other(s) to repeat or reflect back what they have said to check for understanding. It is amazing how deeply listening, without interrupting or making judgments, can often transform our understanding of the other party's intentions and feelings, and of the conflict itself.

   c. Agree not to raise your voices, insult each other, use disrespectful words, or otherwise escalate the conflict.

7. Don't focus on assigning blame (discovering who was wrong), but instead on understanding what contributed to the conflict and identifying how you can transform your relationship to avoid similar problems in the future.

8. If you mean it, apologize and take responsibility for something you said or did that may have contributed to the conflict or been hurtful to the other party.

9. After you have talked about what contributed to the conflict, agree to focus on what you can do now to improve the situation and your ability to work well together in the future.

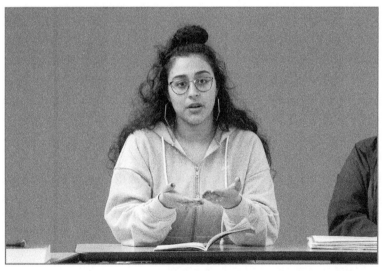

Learning how to communicate about workplace conflict is essential for your professional success.

CHW Scenario: Cindy and Stephanie *(continued)*

Cindy and Stephanie meet to talk about how to resolve their conflict.

Stephanie: I don't want to fight with you Cindy. You trained me when I started, and I've always looked up to you. I really want to work this out and find a way to move forward.

(continues)

CHW Scenario: Cindy and Stephanie *(continued)*

Cindy: Oh [pauses] I don't want to fight either. I miss the times when we were working closer together. It seems like now I only see you in meetings or when we have to do these reports.

Stephanie: I know. I'm really sorry how I spoke to you. I've just been so anxious about the report.

Cindy: Well, I snapped right back, didn't I? Not my best moment. I'm sorry too.

Stephanie: Let's figure out how to get the report done. But I know that you're also dealing with a difficult client situation. I'm sorry I didn't really listen when you were telling me about the client who just had a stroke. I'm wondering if there is anything I can do to help out there?

Cindy: Oh [thinking] Well, I've been visiting him in the hospital, and I told his wife I'd drop off a bag of groceries, but I don't know when I can do it.

Stephanie: Where do they live?

Cindy: Southside, between 5th and Oak.

Stephanie: Okay, I'm heading that way tomorrow, so maybe I could drop off the supplies?

Cindy: That would be a big help. [smiles] Thank you Stephanie.

A PROCESS FOR CONFLICT RESOLUTION

The following process for conflict resolution is adapted from the University of California, Berkeley (2022). Recommended steps for conflict resolution include:

- **Acknowledge that a difficult situation exists:** Honest communication is essential to resolving conflicts. Acknowledge that a conflict exists, and that workplace conflicts are very common.
- **Let individuals express their feelings:** Feelings of anger or hurt usually accompany conflict situations. Before any kind of problem-solving can take place, these emotions should be expressed and acknowledged.
- **Define the problem**: What is the stated problem? What is the negative impact on the work or relationships? What factors seem to be contributing to the current conflict?
- **Determine underlying needs:** The goal of conflict resolution is not to decide which person is right or wrong; the goal is to reach a solution that everyone can live with. Looking first for needs, rather than solutions, is a powerful tool for generating win/win options. To discover needs, you must try to identify why people want the solutions they have proposed. Through discussing the advantages of proposed solutions, you can often undercover people's needs.
- **Find common areas of agreement, no matter how small**:
  - Agree on the problem
  - Agree on the procedure to follow
  - Agree on worst fears
  - Agree on some small change to give an experience of success
- **Find solutions to satisfy needs**:
  - Problem-solve by generating multiple alternatives
  - Determine which actions will be taken
  - Make sure everyone involved in the conflict buys into or agrees to the proposed actions to be taken.
- **Determine how you will follow up to ensure that the conflict is resolved:** For example, you may want to schedule a follow-up meeting in a week or two to discuss how things are going if the proposed resolution is working and if any new actions need to be taken.

- **Identify opportunities to prevent similar conflicts in the future:** When the time is right, reflect on what lessons can be learned from the conflict. What opportunities exist for your organization to prevent similar conflicts in the future. Can this type of conflict be addressed in part through training? Can it be addressed through changes to program policies or protocols?

CHW Scenario: Cindy and Stephanie *(continued)*

Stephanie: What can we do to finish our part of the report?

Cindy: [sighs] I don't know. I know I should have worked on the report, or at least returned your messages. I was overwhelmed and . . . well, I just didn't know how to manage it all.

Stephanie: What if we go over the report questions right now, and I can take notes and draft up a report for Dr. Allen? If we sit at your computer I think we can get your program data pretty quickly, right?

Cindy: Thank you. That would be such a big help.

Stephanie: That's okay. You've always helped me when I needed it. That's what we're supposed to do, right?

Cindy: Right. And maybe we can talk with Dr. Allen to find a better way to do these reports in the future.

Stephanie: Yeah, it would be so helpful if they could not schedule us for any client or clinic appointments for at least a half day a week or so before the report is due.

Cindy: That's a great suggestion. Do you think Dr. Allen will approve it?

Stephanie: Well, I think if we ask together there is a better chance she will say yes.

13.7 Equity and Conflict Resolution

Many workplace conflicts stem from bias, prejudice, and discrimination. Racism and other forms of discrimination are common in our society and in the American workplace (Fekedulegn et al., 2019). A study conducted in 2019 showed that 61% of employees in the United States have witnessed or experienced discrimination in the workplace based on age, race, gender, or LGBTQ identity (Glassdoor, 2019).

Organizations frequently struggle to prevent and manage prejudice, discrimination, and related conflicts. Many organizations attempt to avoid, deny, or ignore incidents and patterns of prejudice and discrimination. Others address bias and prejudice in an incomplete way such as by holding diversity workshops or trainings which do not, on their own, adequately address or resolve these complex issues (Coleman, Chen-Carrel, & Regan, 2022).

Emerging models call for conflict resolution strategies that are based on equity principles. Coleman and his colleagues (Ibid) call for "an approach that blends conflict resolution tactics with a social justice mindset is needed to support constructive, genuine change." Their model includes a range of strategies for reducing conflict that include surveying the status of intergroup relationships and bolstering constructive diversity, equity, and inclusion practices at all levels of an organization. They caution that success requires "altering underlying enduring patterns" and sustained commitment from formal organizational leaders.

Robert Livingston writes on "How to Promote Racial Equity in the Workplace." He states: "The real challenge for organizations is not figuring out 'What can we do?' but rather 'Are we willing to do it?'" (Livingston, 2020). His **PRESS model** calls for:

Problem awareness. Many organizations deny the existence of prejudice, discrimination, and conflict.

Root-cause analysis. Organizations are often reluctant to study the nature of the problems they face.

Empathy or expressed concern about the problem and the people it afflicts.

Strategies for addressing the problem.

Sacrifice. It take.s commitment, time, and resources to effectively address workplace prejudice and discrimination.

Courageous Conversation is a model for "effectively engaging, sustaining and deepening interaction dialogue." Their resources are used by organizations to promote equity and prevent conflict (Courageous Conversation, 2022).

Some educational institutions use an equity-based conflict resolution model known as restorative justice. While **restorative justice** is primarily implemented in k-12 schools, the principles may be applied more widely to other types of organizations. The approach was developed to replace traditional models of discipline that were often discriminatory and harmful to the students who broke rules or acted out in school. Restorative justice brings together the person who was harmed with the person who caused the harm and consulting community members. The goal isn't discipline or punishment, but "reintegrating the person who caused harm back into the community with the skills and awareness to make better decisions in the future." (Capstick, 2022). For more information about restorative justice, please see the resources provided at the end of the chapter.

Many communities have dispute or conflict resolution programs that offer free mediation and arbitration services to the parties or people involved in a conflict. They aim to seek solutions that prevent further conflict, litigation, and other harmful outcomes. For example, see the reference to New Justice Conflict Resolution Services provide at the end of the chapter.

13.8 CHW Leadership

Leadership can come from any level of an organization. It can come from clients and the community, from volunteers and frontline providers as well as people who hold formal leadership positions such as managers, directors, or boards of directors. While sustained organizational change must eventually engage the commitment of formal institutional leaders, *the impetus or initial starting point for change may come from you.*

Consider how you can contribute to creating a workplace culture that welcomes and supports all clients and employees and that is effective in resolving conflict. How can you work to establish healthy and respectful professional relationships with your colleagues? How can you respond in the moments when you witness or are involved in conflict?

You may have (currently or in the future) a formal leadership role in an organization. How will you work to prevent conflict in ways that advance equity goals across your program or agency? How will you work to develop policies and practices that promote the timely resolution of workplace conflict?

Chapter Review

Apply conflict resolution knowledge and skills to the scenario between Cindy and Stephanie introduced at the beginning of the chapter. Answer the following questions:

- What type(s) of conflict are Cindy and Stephanie experiencing?
- What may be some of the sources of this conflict?
- What conflict management styles are they using?
- What are some of the possible consequences of this conflict, and for whom?

If you were Cindy or Stephanie, how might you answer the following questions?

- How can you shift the way that you view this conflict, using the suggestions from the Harvard Negotiation Project?
- How would hold a pre-conversation to establish clear guidelines for resolving the conflict?

- What do you want to communicate to your colleague at the very start of your conversation?
- What ground rules do you want to negotiate?
- What type of compromise are you willing to make?
- What will you do to follow up after you reach an initial resolution to the conflict?
- What other resources might be helpful to you in resolving this conflict?
- In your current role as an employee, volunteer, or student, how can you contribute to creating a workplace that works to prevent and resolve conflict?

References

Capstick, L. (2022). The 5 R's of Restorative Justice. The Conflict Center. https://conflictcenter.org/the-5-rs-of-restorative-justice/ https://conflictcenter.org/the-5-rs-of-restorative-justice/ (accessed 12 December 2022).

Coleman, P., Chen-Carrel, A., & Regan, B. M. (2022). A New Conflict-Resolution Model to Advance DEI. https://sloanreview.mit.edu/article/a-new-conflict-resolution-model-to-advance-dei/ MIT Sloan Management Review. (accessed 11 December 2022).

Courageous Conversation. https://courageousconversation.com/about/ (accessed 13 December 2022).

Fekedulegn, D., Alterman, T., Charles, L. E., Kershaw, K. N., Safford, M. M., Howard, V. J., & MacDonald, L. A. (2019). Prevalence of workplace discrimination and mistreatment in a national sample of older U.S. workers: The REGARDS cohort study. *SSM-Population Health*. https://doi: 10.1016/j.ssmph.2019.100444.

Glassdoor. (2019). Diversity & Inclusion Study 2019. https://about-content.glassdoor.com/app/uploads/sites/2/2019/10/Glassdoor-Diversity-Survey-Supplement-1.pdf (accessed 13 December 2022).

Hocker, J. L. & Wilmot, W. W. (1985). Interpersonal Conflict. Dubuque, Iowa: University of Michigan. 23.

Kilmann Diagnostics. (2022). An Overview of the TKI Assessment Tool. https://kilmanndiagnostics.com/overview-thomas-kilmann-conflict-mode-instrument-tki/ (accessed 12 December 2022).

Livingston, R. (2020). How to Promote Racial Equity in the Workplace. Harvard Business Review. https://hbr.org/2020/09/how-to-promote-racial-equity-in-the-workplace. (accessed 12 December 2022).

Mayo Clinic. (2022). Anger Management: 10 Tips to Tame Your Temper. https://www.mayoclinic.org/healthy-lifestyle/adult-health/in-depth/anger-management/art-20045434 (accessed 9 December 2022).

Niagara Institute. (2022). Workplace Conflict Statistics: How We Approach Conflict at Work. https://www.niagarainstitute.com/blog/workplace-conflict-statistics (accessed 9 December 2022).

Pollack Peacebuilding Systems. (2022). Workplace Conflict Statistics 2022. https://pollackpeacebuilding.com/workplace-conflict-statistics/ (accessed 12 December 2022).

Shonk, K. 2022. 3 Types of Conflict and How to Address Them. Harvard Law School: Program on Negotiation. https://www.pon.harvard.edu/daily/conflict-resolution/types-conflict/ (accessed 11 December 2022).

Stone, D., Patton, B., & Heen, S. (2010). *Difficult conversations: How to discuss what matters most*. New York, NY: Penguin Books.

Substance Abuse and Mental Health Services Administration. (2022). Coping with Anger. https://www.samhsa.gov/dtac/disaster-survivors/coping-anger-after-disaster (accessed 9 December 2022).

University of California, Berkeley. Guide to Managing Human Resources. (2022). Berkeley People & Culture. https://hr.berkeley.edu/hr-network/central-guide-managing-hr/managing-hr/interaction/conflict/resolving (accessed 11 December 2022).

Additional Resources

Bowland, S. Y., Batts, H., Roy, B, & Trujillo, M. A. (2022). *Beyond equity and inclusion in conflict resolution: Recentering the profession (The ACR practitioner's guide series)*. New York, NY: Rowman & Littlefield.

Colorado Department of Regulatory Agencies. (2020). De-Escalation Tips for Conflict Resolution. https://dre.colorado.gov/division-notifications/de-escalation-tips-conflict-resolution (accessed 12 December 2022).

New Justice Services. https://www.newjusticeservices.org/home.aspx (accessed 11 December 2022).

Professional Skills: Getting a Job, Keeping a Job, and Growing on the Job

14

Jimmy Ly and Thelma Gamboa-Maldonado

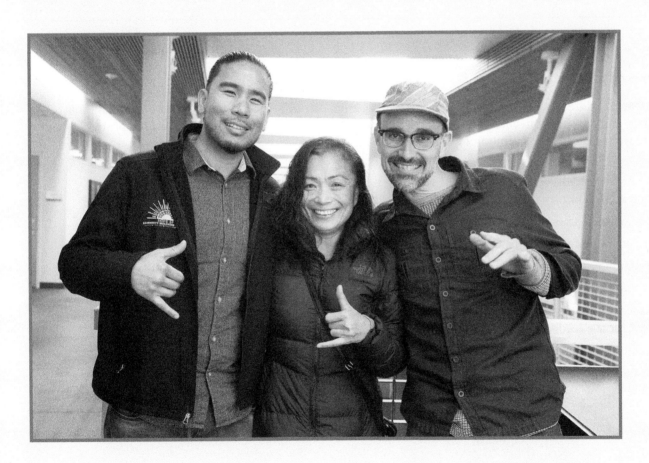

Foundations for Community Health Workers, Third Edition. Edited by Tim Berthold and Darouny Somsanith.
© 2024 John Wiley & Sons, Inc. Published 2024 by John Wiley & Sons, Inc.
Companion website: http://www.wiley.com/go/communityhealthworkers3E

CHW Scenario: Priyadarshi Mehta

Priyadarshi Mehta has worked as a community health worker (CHW) for five years at a large non-profit agency that provides outreach and case management services to people who are unhoused. Priyadarshi is highly respected by co-workers and the clients and communities he serves.

Recently, Priyadarshi applied for a promotion to be the supervisor of a team of six CHWs.

Priyadarshi was not offered the position. Priyadarshi met the other candidate on the day of their interviews. Priyadarshi dressed casually—as he usually does for work—and made a presentation to the hiring committee using flip chart paper. The candidate who was hired wore a suit and brought a laptop computer and made a presentation using PowerPoint slides.

When Priyadarshi asked the executive director why he wasn't offered the position as supervisor, he was told that he needs to improve his professional skills, including the way that he presents himself, and his technology and written communication skills.

Introduction

This chapter addresses professional skills for securing a job or volunteer position as a CHW, keeping that position, and advancing in your career. These skills will also assist you to be more effective in promoting the health of the clients and communities you work with.

WHAT YOU WILL LEARN

By studying the information in this chapter, you will be able to:

- Explain the challenge of code switching and the imposter syndrome
- Develop a professional résumé
- Prepare for a job interview
- Identify dress codes at your internship site or workplace
- Discuss verbal and written communication skills relevant for CHWs, including how to provide and receive constructive feedback in a professional manner
- Apply time management skills to your life, study, and work
- Develop a professional development plan for career advancement

C3 Roles and Skills Addressed in Chapter 14

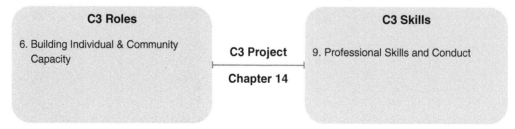

WORDS TO KNOW

Code Switching

Résumé

Supportive and Corrective Feedback

14.1 The Challenges of Code Switching and the Imposter Syndrome

All workplaces have written and unwritten codes of conduct that guide standards for dress, time management, professional boundaries, written and spoken communication, and giving and receiving constructive feedback. Adapting to professional environments and codes of conduct can be challenging. This challenge is sometimes called **code switching** (or moving between one or more sets of expectations and guidelines for conduct or behavior).

There are different codes of conduct for different contexts, communities, cultures, and employment settings. The codes that we learn from our families and in our communities may be different from the codes that guide employment settings. When we move from our family to the community and to the workplace, we may not understand the new codes of conduct and why they matter. As a consequence, like Priyadarshi, we may miss out on opportunities for employment or promotion.

Most of us have experience with code switching, though we probably didn't think of it in these terms. We act or speak differently with our family and friends, at school, at work, or in church or other religious or spiritual places.

- *Can you think of places where you switch codes?*

- *Have you ever been in a new environment and not known what the codes of conduct were? What was this like?*

- *How did you begin to identify and adapt to the new codes of conduct?*

Code switching is a valuable skill for CHWs. The ability to adapt to different settings and to build positive working relationships with diverse communities is a tremendous asset for building a long and successful career.

However, it is also important to note that institutional codes can be biased and may represent and promote a particular cultural standard for dress, speech, and conduct. At their worst, professional codes may discriminate against people from different educational or cultural backgrounds or identities, such as people who look, dress, and speak differently from those in authority.

Consider the following quotes from City College of San Francisco (CCSF) students who encountered bias in an educational or workplace setting:

A graduate of the CCSF CHW program reports: *"I finally made it to graduate school, but it wasn't always a very supportive place. I was the only Black woman in my cohort. During my first week, the only Black female professor at the school pulled me aside to tell me that I needed to straighten my hair and buy a suit if I wanted to succeed. It may have been meant kindly, but it didn't come across that way. It made me feel like I didn't belong. Even if I had the money, I wasn't going to straighten my hair. But on top of working full-time and raising my family, I made sure that no one ever had a reason to challenge the quality of my work. And I want people to know that I did earn my master's degree!"*

A student who was completing his internship with a local agency reports: *"You know that I read, write and speak English very well. It's my third language. At a staff meeting [at the agency where the student is doing their internship], I spoke up a couple of times, and it felt good to be participating, you know? After the meeting, one of the managers thanked me for participating, but he also told me that I needed to work harder to "lose my accent." I don't know if that is even possible. And is it okay for them to say that to me? If I work well with the clients, and they accept me, isn't that good enough?"*

- *What comes up for you as you read these testimonies?*

- *Have you or your ever encountered challenges like this in the workplace (or at school)?*

- *How can you adapt to new codes while retaining your own identity, language, and culture?*

While the codes that guide conduct in employment settings should be clearly presented to all employees and volunteers, often they are not. The codes should be used to promote the organization's mission and goals, as well as respectful communication among colleagues and between the staff and the clients and communities they serve. The codes of conduct in workplace settings shouldn't require us to abandon our own cultures or identities, including identities that are related to ethnicity, nationality, religion or faith, disability, sexual orientation, or gender identity.

Some additional drawbacks or potential harms of code switching include (Kang, DeCelles, Tilscik, & Jun, 2016):

1. Downplaying one's racial group can generate hostility from in-group members, increasing the likelihood that those who code-switch will be accused of "acting white."

2. Seeking to avoid stereotypes is hard work and can deplete cognitive resources and hinder performance.

3. Faking commonality with co-workers also reduces authentic self-expression and contributes to burnout.

The decision about whether or not you will switch codes to adapt to a professional setting is up to you. We would rather that you had an opportunity to make an informed choice about code switching, however, instead of losing job opportunities for failing to meet a professional standard that you didn't know existed.

Code switching is also a relevant concept for the clients you work with. They may not know about or want to follow the codes of conduct at the various agencies and institutions they turn to for assistance with legal, medical, public benefits, housing, or social services. Unfortunately, the professionals in these agencies may sometimes judge or discriminate against clients who do not adapt to their codes of conduct. We hope that as CHWs, you will always do your best to make clients feel welcomed and respected regardless of their identity, background, desire, or ability to "switch codes."

IMPOSTER SYNDROME

Imposter syndrome is a psychological pattern in which people doubt their skills, talents, or accomplishments, and are afraid of being exposed as a "fraud" (Langford & Clance, 1993). Research suggests an estimated 70% of people experience at least one episode of imposter syndrome at some point in their lives (Sakulku & Alexander, 2011). People who experience imposter syndrome believe that they are undeserving of their achievements and the high esteem in which they are, in fact, generally held. As a result, they assign guilt to those feelings of ineptitude and often attribute their accomplishments to external causes and factors such as luck, good timing, or a high level of effort that they cannot maintain over time. Those with imposter syndrome are often well accomplished; they may hold high office or have numerous academic degrees. Imposter syndrome may feel like nervousness and manifest as negative self-talk. Symptoms of anxiety and depression often accompany imposter syndrome.

Impostor feelings and a sense of being an outsider may also be fueled by factors outside of a person, such as their environment or institutionalized discrimination. A sense of belonging fosters confidence. "The more people who look or sound like you, the more confident you feel. And conversely, the fewer people who look or sound like you, it can and does for many people impact their confidence" (Young, 2011). This is especially true "whenever you belong to a group for whom there are stereotypes about competence" (Ibid) including racial or ethnic minorities, immigrants, English language learners, women in science, technology, engineering, and mathematics (STEM) fields or international students at American universities (Ibid).

- *Have you ever experienced imposter syndrome or doubted your professionals skills and abilities?*

What Do YOU? Think

Being caught between wanting to thrive and fear of achieving success can be painful and paralyzing. Imposter syndrome can stifle the potential for growth by preventing people from pursuing new opportunities to learn, develop, and make meaningful connections with others.

Overcoming imposter syndrome requires changing your mindset about your own abilities. While you may sometimes feel that you do not belong, remind yourself that you earned your place in the professional, academic, or personal environment. Here are some suggestions for how to overcome imposter syndrome (Cuncic, 2022):

1. **Acknowledge and share your feelings:** Acknowledge your feelings and invest time in understanding the core beliefs that fuel your insecurities. Talk to friends or mentors about how you are feeling. Don't isolate yourself and allow irrational thoughts to circulate through your mind. People who have more experience can reassure you that what you're feeling is normal.

2. **Question your thoughts:** Question whether your thoughts are rational. Does it make sense to believe that you are a fraud given everything that you have accomplished?

3. **Stop comparing:** Instead of comparing yourself to others, focus on listening to what others are saying. Be genuinely interested in learning more. Use social media moderately to reduce the opportunities for comparing yourself to others or portraying a false image of yourself.

4. **Assess your abilities:** Self-assess your abilities. Do your accomplishments match up with your abilities?

5. **Take baby steps:** Do not strive for perfection. Instead, do things reasonably well and reward yourself for taking action.

6. **Focus on others:** Help others who may also struggle with imposter syndrome.

7. **Refuse to let it hold you back:** Don't let your negative self-talk stop you from pursuing and reaching your goals. Do not self-sabotage.

14.2 Career Readiness

Career readiness is the process of developing the skills we need to acquire, maintain, and grow within a job (Hummel, 2022). Before starting your job search, assess your level of readiness for your desired career.

The following eight professional Career Readiness Competencies have been identified by the National Association of Colleges and Employers (NACE, 2021) to help you prepare and succeed in the workplace. Employers want to hire job seekers who can demonstrate these skills, talents, and strengths. Mastering these competencies will make you a competitive candidate for future employment.

1. **Career and self-development:** Take action to enhance your personal and professional knowledge, awareness of your strengths and weaknesses, navigation of career opportunities, and develop professional networks within and outside of your organization.

2. **Critical thinking:** Identify and respond to needs based upon an understanding of situational context and logical analysis of relevant information.

3. **Communication:** Clearly and effectively exchange information, ideas, facts, and perspectives with persons inside and outside of an organization.

4. **Equity and inclusion:** Demonstrate the awareness, attitude, knowledge, and skills required to equitably engage and include people from different local and global cultures. Engage in anti-racist practices that actively challenge the systems, structures, and policies of racism.

5. **Leadership:** Recognize and capitalize on personal and team strengths to achieve organizational goals.

6. **Teamwork:** Build and maintain collaborative relationships to work effectively toward common goals while appreciating diverse viewpoints and shared responsibilities.

7. **Technology:** Understand and leverage technologies ethically to enhance efficiencies, complete tasks, and accomplish goals.

8. **Professionalism:** Knowing work environments differs greatly, understands and demonstrates effective work habits, and acts in the interest of the larger community and workplace.

CHW Profile

Dante Casuga, He/Him

Site Manager, Community Health Ambassador Program

YMCA of San Francisco and HOPE SF

Residents of public housing sites in San Francisco

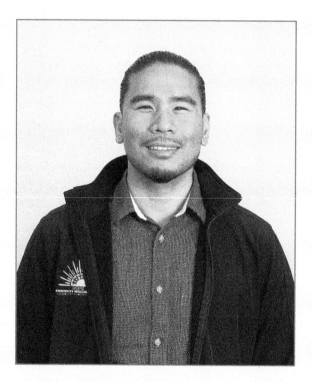

Growing up, my family and elders were present in my life. I was fortunate to have positive role models who gave me consistent support and kept me on the right path. I started working with youth part time while in college. Many of the youth had bad experiences in school from educators and other people that put them down, especially the youth of color. I wanted to be a positive influence in their lives. I learned that working with youth is refreshing for the heart and the spirit.

After receiving my CHW Certificate I started working with families from public housing sites with an intention to promote health closer to home. I work with HOPE SF, a public housing revitalization initiative for communities that have been historically ignored by the City and lack access to health care, mental health services, healthy foods, etc. The residents we serve live well below the poverty line and experience trauma from all kinds of violence including gun violence, police violence, and domestic violence. Through my work with HOPE SF residents, I have observed what true resilience is.

I work as a site manager for one of the Hope SF communities (Alice Griffith) with the Community Health Ambassador Program (CHAMPS). We train residents and hire them to promote health within their community. I train them to do community outreach, health education, program planning, creating groups, and organizing community events. One of my favorite times is participating in our Healthy Eating classes. We take traditional recipes and slightly adjust them to make them healthier. We also provide health education information and tools during our groups to help the clients we serve to build lasting healthy habits.

(continues)

CHW Profile

(continued)

I help the Ambassadors manage their boundaries at work. They live on site so sometimes they get called on for help 24-7. A resident may knock on their door and ask for food. Sometimes it's hard for the Ambassadors to explain that it is their day off or they are off the clock. Together, we role-play how to handle someone coming to your door after works hours and how to set boundaries to prevent burnout. We make sure the Ambassadors get some well-earned rest!

There was a senior in our community who was over 80 years old. Everyone knew him. He was at every meeting and every group, walking around and engaging with everyone. Then he disappeared. We were worried, so one of the Ambassadors checked on him. He was having a lot of problems with balance and couldn't walk anymore. I worked with the Ambassador. She advocated and got him an electric scooter. It seems like a small thing, but now he's back in the community. He got his independence back.

Since I've been working as a CHW, I'm more gentle with myself. I'm better with having healthy boundaries. I'm more able to help with sensitive issues come up for my own family and friends. I see a lot of people just working for a paycheck, but, for me, my work is rewarding. It gives me more purpose, you know?

For new CHWs just starting out, I'd say get organized; it will save you a lot of stress! And remember that self-care and resilience sometimes show up as saying "No." You can't take everything on. Prioritize making time for your own self-care and self-preservation. And remember to celebrate the little victories that clients have. You want to fill up your cup and honor the work you do for your community. You've got to have gratitude for this work, and faith that things can get better, little by little.

GETTING A JOB

Getting a job often requires these key steps:

1. Finding out about available jobs
2. Applying for jobs
3. Interviewing for jobs

FINDING JOB OPPORTUNITIES

There are many ways to find out about jobs in your community:

- Search online job sites on your own or with the help of a career or employment counselor (generally available for free at a community-based or community college career center)
- Review the web sites of local employers to look for job openings
- Call or visit agencies that you are interested in working for to learn about potential job opportunities
- Network and talk with CHWs and other public health providers to see if they are aware of any job openings with their own agencies or other organizations

Once you find a job you want to apply for, carefully read the job description. If you are interested in the position, use the information to guide you in writing your application.

Sample Job Description

Community Health Worker with the Central City Health Center. This position will conduct outreach and provide health education and case management services to patients living with chronic health conditions. Duties include supporting patients with the self-management of health conditions such as cardiovascular disease, depression, diabetes, and asthma. CHWs provide services at the clinic and in community settings and provide home visits as necessary. Qualified candidates will have skills for providing person-centered health education and case management services, strong oral and written communication skills, and the ability to work effectively with people from diverse backgrounds.

Additional Qualifications

High school diploma or GED required.

How to Apply

Email cover letter, résumé, and the names and contact information of three professional references to Audra Laing. Email: ALaing@centralcityhealthcenter.org.

- *If you were interested in the job as a CHW with the Central City Health Center, which of your personal or work experiences and skills would you highlight in your application?*

What Do
YOU?
Think

NETWORKING AND APPLYING FOR JOBS: APPLICATIONS, COVER LETTERS, RÉSUMÉS, AND REFERENCES

Networking

You've heard the saying before, "It's not what you know, it's who you know." This is true in every aspect of career development. Studies have shown that more than 80% of people are in their current job as a result of networking (Ton, 2020). Has someone you know ever helped you get an interview or a job? Whether you are looking to jumpstart or advance your career, networking is a valuable skill.

Networking is about establishing and nurturing long-term, mutually beneficial relationships with personal and professional contacts. Whether you're in line to order coffee, attending a career fair, or in a college classroom, networking opportunities are all around you.

LinkedIn is the world's largest online professional network and is commonly used by employers and professionals in the fields of public health, healthcare, and social services. You can use LinkedIn to search for a job or internship, connect and strengthen professional relationships, and learn the skills you need to succeed in your career. Most of all, it is a powerful networking platform for job seekers. One of the features, LinkedIn Groups, provides a space for professionals in the same industry or who have similar interests to share their insights and experiences, ask for guidance, and build valuable connections. By joining a LinkedIn Group, you can engage in conversations, discover employment opportunities, and send message requests to individual group members.

Applications

It is critical to understand how the job application and selection process works from an employer's point of view. Having some basic knowledge and knowing what tricks and tools recruiters and hiring managers use can give you an edge before you even begin your job search.

For most jobs, you will be asked to fill out an application. The employer will review all applications received. You want your application to stand out in a positive way. If possible, type the application, or fill it out on a computer. If the application can only be filled out by hand, use a black or blue pen, and fill out the application clearly and neatly. Check your résumé to correct any spelling or grammatical errors.

Some job applications ask you if you are a U.S. citizen and if you have ever been convicted of a crime (Chapter 15 discusses Ban the Box initiatives that aim to prevent employment discrimination against people with histories of incarceration). It is important to answer these questions truthfully. Citizenship or permanent resident status may not be a requirement, and the agency may distinguish between misdemeanor and felony convictions, between long-past and recent convictions, and understand concepts of recovery and rehabilitation.

Cover Letter

If the employer requires a cover letter, include your contact information at the top, the date, the person to whom you are submitting the application (by name if possible), and a formal salutation (Dear Ms. Laing). In a couple of brief sentences, identify the job you are applying for (the exact title and job number if there is one), how you learned about the job, and why you are qualified for the position.

Sample Cover Letter

Cassie Adanya
P.O. Box 14567
Philadelphia, PA, 19876
November 9, 2023

Audra Laing, NP
Center City Clinic
3000 Hamilton St., Suite 505
Philadelphia, PA 19130

Dear Ms. Laing:

Attached please find my résumé and application for the job of Community Health Worker with the Central City Health Center.

I am a certified Community Health Worker. I have two years' experience working as CHW in urban settings and several years' experience as a volunteer with community-based social service organizations.

I am dedicated to promoting the health of vulnerable communities. I am interested in working in a primary healthcare setting and supporting patients who are living with chronic health conditions. I have skills in providing health outreach and case management services and would love the opportunity to apply these skills in working with the patients at Central City Health Center.

Thank you for your consideration of my application.

Sincerely,

Jane Q. Doe

Attached: application; résumé

Résumés

When you apply for a job, employers will usually ask for a résumé, a formal document listing your work experience and education. The goal of a résumé is to engage a potential employer's interest at a glance. Please note that these documents are sometimes called a CV or a curriculum vitae.

Your local library, community college, or employment development department may hold free résumé writing classes. You can also review sample résumés on the internet.

Résumés follow standard style guidelines, although there are a variety of accepted styles. Take a look at the sample résumé below. Notice the order of the words, the type of information the applicant provides, and how easy it is for potential employers to:

- Find the applicant's experience
- Review the applicant's skills
- Know exactly where to call or email the applicant to discuss the job

Writing a résumé: One example of a résumé is shown in Figure 14.1. Regardless of how you organize your résumé, it should always include the information on one to two pages and be organized in a way that is easy to read.

Name and contact information: Your name and up-to-date contact information should be at the top of the résumé. Make sure that your contact information is current, including your email address and phone number. Including your mailing address is not necessary, but listing your city and state is recommended as some employers may prefer to hire locally.

Education: List your education and training, beginning with your current or most recent educational experiences. Be sure to include any certificates, degrees, scholarships, or honors.

Work and volunteer experience: Clearly present information about your employment history, starting with your most recent job and going back in time. Include the name of the company or organization, the city where it is located, your job title, and the dates you worked. Don't use any acronyms in your résumé, such as the initials used for an agency or coalition instead of the full name of that agency or coalition. List your professional responsibilities, the skills you used on the job, and your key accomplishments. Use action words as described in the text box below. Do the same for any volunteer experiences that highlight relevant skills and accomplishments.

Always be 100% truthful about the information you include on your résumé. Any inaccurate statements may be cause for termination and could seriously damage your reputation in the community.

> **Action Words:** When you list your experiences, use action words to explain your responsibilities and accomplishments. These words show an employer the skills you have to offer. Be sure to use the past tense for past experiences and the present tense for your current work. Describe briefly how you Led, Demonstrated, Coordinated, Accomplished, Created, Provided, Managed, Organized, Repaired . . . you get the idea.

"I don't have any work experience! What do I put on my résumé?"

Even if you have never had a full-time job, you have accomplishments and skills that are relevant for employment. Focus on what you have learned by helping out in your family, school, or community, and use action words to present your skills to employers.

References

As you near the end of the hiring process you will be asked to provide references who can tell a potential employer about your qualifications for the job. Be sure to ask each person in advance if they are willing to be listed as a reference so they are not caught-off guard when a prospective employer contacts them. Current and former supervisors and co-workers are the strongest references. Teachers or community leaders can also be references. Avoid using family members or friends when possible. Tell your references about the job you are applying for and mention a few of your strengths and skills that they can highlight. You can also ask them if

Cassie Adanya
409 Andover Street
New Orleans, LA 70183
(614) 222-5555
cassieadanya@email.com

PROFESSIONAL EXPERIENCE

Counselor and Program Coordinator   **New Orleans Safe House, New Orleans, LA**

October 2014–Present. Work with developmentally disabled children ages 6–12.   Facilitate small group activities and provide individual counseling as required. Coordinate the Safe House Summer Camp Program.   Organize daily activi- ties, manage work assignments, and supervise 3 staff and 8 volunteers.

Assistant Teacher   **Jubilee Camp, Elbert, LA**

January 2011–September 2014. Provided daycare services for infants and children ages 0–36 months.   Responsible for creating and implementing a daily activity plan, and facilitating small groups of three to six children.

VOLUNTEER EXPERIENCE

Food Pantry   **First Methodist Church, New Orleans Parish, LA**

2010–Present. Assist staff with the inventory of food items, packaging food and delivering food to shut-in clients twice each month.

Youth Summer Camp   **New Orleans Regional YMCA, New Orleans, LA**

Summer 2008 to 2010.   Assisted with managing activities for youth with special needs, ages 8–12. Designed and facilitated arts and sports projects, and group trips to local   New Orleans attractions.

EDUCATION

Carlton Community College, New Orleans, LA

Community Health Worker Certificate, 2013

Associates of Science Degree, 2015

Ceder Cliff High School, New Orleans, LA

Graduated, 2010

TRAINING AND ACHIEVEMENTS

- First Aid and CP R certification. American Heart Association. Renewed June, 2016
- Awarded Gabriela Munoz Family Scholarship, Carlton Community College, September 2014
- Recognized by the New Orleans Regional YMCA with the Youth Leadership Award, August 2009

REFERENCES

Precious Mamphele, Director, New Orleans Safe House

(123) 456-7890

Dr. Alberto Reyes, Director, Jubilee Camp

(234) 567-8901

Lucky Martinez, Instructor, CHW Certificate Program, Carlton Community College

(345) 678-9012

Figure 14.1 Sample Résumé

they will write you a letter of reference for CHW jobs. You can include copies of these letters of reference with your résumé and application or bring them with you to interviews.

- *Who will you ask to be your references?*

- *Which of your skills, personal qualities, and experience will your references be able to discuss with potential employers?*

INTERVIEWING, NEGOTIATING AND ACCEPTING A JOB, INTERNSHIP, OR VOLUNTEER POSITION

What's the secret to doing well in job interviews? The answer is simple—practice and preparation! Don't wait until you hear from the employer to start preparing for an interview. If you wait until you've been called for an interview, you may only have a few days to prepare.

Job interviews are about finding out whether there is a good "fit" between the interviewee, the job, and the agency. The interviewer asks questions to learn whether you would be the best candidate for the position they are trying to fill. You can also ask questions to determine whether the organization is one you would like to work for. In other words, they are interviewing you, but you are also interviewing them.

What Employers Want

- Skills and knowledge related to the job
- Cultural humility
- Strong communication skills. The ability to provide structured and organized answers
- Interest in the agency and the position
- The ability to manage time efficiently
- Personal qualities: Enthusiasm and confidence

Preparing for the Interview

Know the agency: Review the organization's website to help you determine if this is an agency you want to work for. Your research can help you identify questions to ask the employer at the end of the interview. Research the following information:

- What is the agency's mission?
- Which communities do they serve?
- What services do they provide?
- What have they accomplished?

Think about how you can connect the information you learn about the organization to your experience, knowledge, and skills. This can strengthen your answers to common interview questions.

Practice interviewing: We encourage you to practice or rehearse what you will say in the interview. Practice with a trusted friend or family member, a colleague or classmate, or a professional at a local employment or career counseling center. You can also practice on your own. You can create an audio or video recording of your rehearsal and review it to identify strengths and areas for improvement.

Practice responding to common interview questions such as:

- Why are you interested in this position?
- Please describe your qualifications for this position.
- What are your professional goals?
- What experiences have prepared you for this position?

- Why are you considering changing jobs?
- Please describe your educational background and accomplishments.
- Please briefly describe your skills in (topics and areas such as outreach, case management, group facilitation, or health education)
- Why are you the best candidate for this position?
- What are your greatest accomplishments or successes?
- What are your greatest strengths and your greatest weaknesses?

Do your best to stay on topic when answering interview questions. It is important to respond to each question *briefly*, prioritizing the most important points only. A common mistake is to spend 10 or even 15 minutes answering a question when speaking for 2–3 minutes would have provided sufficient information to the employer.

Ask for honest feedback and how you might improve or clarify your responses. Be prepared to address or explain gaps in your employment history and reasons for leaving previous jobs.

Pro tip: Practice does not mean memorize! Avoid sounding overly rehearsed. Instead of writing a script for your answers, jot down important key talking points you want to include in your answer. This will allow you to weave in those points and pivot your answer to adapt to questions more easily and be more genuine.

Familiarize yourself with virtual interviewing technology. Increasingly, employers conduct job interviews on videoconferencing platforms such as Zoom. Practice using the technology as you rehearse for an interview. Below are tips to help you prepare for virtual interviews.

- Test technology to ensure audio and video capabilities are working.
- Choose a place that is quiet with stable internet connection.
- Eliminate distractions. Make sure that the background that appears behind you is appropriate for the interview. Clean up any clutter that an interviewer may see or blur or use a virtual background.
- Dress as if you are interviewing in-person.
- Prepare for unexpected technical issues. Communicate with the interviewer about what to do if technical issues occur such as losing internet connection.
- Keep notes handy in case you need to refer to them.
- Look at the camera and not at yourself. Turn off video mirroring if you're tempted to look at yourself.

Dressing for the interview: Dress in a professional manner and more formally than you would on the job. Conservative business casual attire with neutral colors (gray, black, brown, tan, and blue) and dress shoes are often best. Wearing a suit or suit jacket over dress pants or a skirt is almost always considered appropriate for an interview, even for places with a much more casual daily work culture. Don't wear jeans, T-shirts, shorts, or other casual clothes. Prepare what you will wear in advance and not the night before your interview.

What to Take with You to the Interview:

- Copies of your résumé, a list of professional references, or letters of recommendation.
- Documents to verify identification and employment authorization.
- Transcripts and/or certificates, if necessary.
- Samples of your professional work, such as flyers, brochures, reports, or articles that you personally developed.
- Notes to study as you arrive early.

During the Interview: Greet each of the people who are interviewing you. Speak slowly and clearly and make eye contact with your interviewer(s) often. Use the interview to find out how you could fit into the organization and as an opportunity to share your skills with a potential employer.

The interviewer will generally break the ice and make an introduction. They may ask for general information about you, your background, or your goals, such as:

- "Please tell us about yourself."
- "Why are you interested in our organization?"
- "What are your goals for the next year? Next five years?"
- "Why did you enter this field?"

The interviewer will probably share general information about the organization and the job position before asking you more specific questions.

Strategies for Responding Effectively to Interview Questions:

1. Listen carefully to the question and answer it as specifically as possible.
2. Honesty is always the best policy—don't exaggerate or provide false information to the employer.
3. Ask clarifying questions when necessary.
4. Speak clearly and concisely. Try not to repeat yourself or ramble.
5. Use examples from your professional, academic, and life experiences to support your skills, abilities, and qualifications.
6. Focus on your accomplishments and successes.
7. Clearly demonstrate why you are interest in the position and why you are the best fit for the position.
8. Don't forget to be yourself. Let your authentic voice and personality to shine through.
9. Believe in yourself and the qualities, values, knowledge, and skills you have to offer.

Engage the interviewer. Instead of seeing the interview as an exam you must pass, try to view it as a conversation in which you have valuable information to share with the employer, and they have valuable information to share with you. Prepare to ask the interviewer one or more questions during or after the interview process such as: "How does your agency support ongoing training or professional development for employees to stay current in their fields?" "What do you think is the greatest opportunity or challenge facing the organization in the near future?" "What do you like best about working here?" Be careful not to ask questions if the answers can be found on the job description or company website such as, "What communities does your agency serve?" Wait to ask questions regarding pay and benefits until after the employer has offered you the job.

Closing

This is a time to ask any remaining questions you may have *but, again, be conscious of time and don't ask too many questions*. These questions might include, for example: "Is there anything else I can tell you about my qualifications or experience?" "I have copies of my letters of recommendation. May I leave them with you?" "When may I expect to hear from you?"

After the Interview

Reflect upon your performance. What did you do well? How might you improve your performance in future interviews?

Thank the interviewer for the opportunity to meet with them by sending a brief thank you email within 48 hours of your interview:

- Reference specific moment(s) from your conversation.
- Fix any missteps or rephrase anything you communicated poorly during the interview or forget to mention.
- Reaffirm your candidacy: "After interviewing for this position, my interest for this position grown and I am so grateful for. . . ."
- Create an opportunity for the interviewer to ask follow-up questions: "Please contact me if you have any further questions about my experience/qualifications."

Accepting and Negotiating a Job Offer

Most people who receive a job offer accept the job right away. This may be your best option. However, depending on your situation, take time to evaluate the job offer and determine if the job and the employer are right for you. Are the salary and benefits reasonable?

Negotiating your salary is highly recommended. Most employers expect it and respect job seekers who advocate for themselves, but 58% job seekers don't feel comfortable negotiating and often accept the employer's initial offer (Fox, 2023). Successful negotiation begins with researching the compensation for your job, field, and location. Job market and wage information are available through the US Bureau of Labor Statistics (See Additional Resources at the end of the chapter). This online resource also provides state and area data. In addition, a simple job search on popular websites such as glassdoor.com, salary.com, payscale.com, and indeed.com will allow you to see the wages of similar jobs you are targeting. Your desired dollar amount should be supported by facts and details to demonstrate your value as a future employee. Knowing your strengths and what makes you unique from other applicants can be leveraged to negotiate a higher starting salary. Factors that can influence your compensation include years of experience, leadership roles, skills, education level, and license and certifications. Studies show that job seekers who negotiate are successful in receiving a counteroffer 85% of the time (Fox, 2023).

It is also important to know when to stop negotiating and either accept the job offer or move on. Pushing too hard leaves a bad impression and can cause the employer to offer the job to another candidate.

14.3 Keeping the Job

Keeping your position as a CHW will depend to a great extent on your interpersonal skills. A critical part of your job is how well you build and maintain positive relationships with clients, co-workers, and your supervisor. The ability to get along well with colleagues in other agencies, and with the communities you serve, is also key to your long-term success.

DRESS CODE: WHAT YOU WEAR MATTERS

What you wear is often the first information that someone has about who you are. The doctor's white coat, the mechanic's overalls, and the team uniform are obvious examples of clothing that communicate to others something important about who someone is or what they do. You dress up for a job interview as a signal to a potential employer that you understand the codes of the professional world. Before getting dressed for an interview or workday, consider where you are going and who you will be meeting with, and the message that you hope to convey with what you are wearing.

Phuong An Doan Billings: For the Vietnamese community, our culture is very formal. I have to wear my best clothes when I go out to the community. To me it's very natural. That's the way we are. As a teacher in Vietnam, I had to stand in front of a few hundred students every day. Before I left the house, I always had to dress up, even going to the market, because I might meet my students there.

When you work with the community, you have to know how to present yourself. I don't dare to go out to do presentations if I don't have on good clothes. If I didn't dress formally, they wouldn't listen to me. I have to be formal and in a style appropriate to my age and my status.

If I have some staff that I feel do not dress appropriately, we talk about it. I say to them, "You know, this is how our community is. We are formal. That's the reality we have to accept."

The dress code at your job may be different from the dress codes for the clients and communities you work with. When you work in the community, consider these questions about what you wear:

- Will it put my clients at ease? Will it alienate them?
- Will it show respect to the community I'm working with?
- Will it give people the confidence that I have the skills and knowledge to assist them?

In most situations, a helpful guideline is to dress a half to one step above how your clients dress. Wearing jeans and T-shirts may not be appropriate, but if your clients typically dress in jeans and T-shirts, dressing a half to one step above their clothing may translate into wearing khakis and a button-down shirt, polo-style shirt, or a jacket. As we saw above, however, some communities may expect you to dress much more formally as a sign of respect or to gain their confidence.

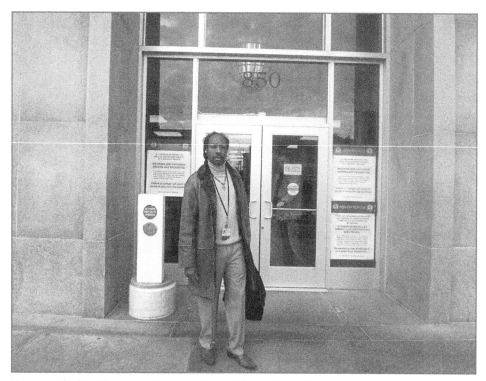

Some work situations require more formal dress. Lee Jackson prepares to attend a court hearing with a client.

As a CHW, how would you dress to meet with the following groups?

- People who are unhoused
- Your agency's board of directors
- A leadership group at the local mosque, temple, or church

In order for you to be welcomed and respected, you may need to alter your appearance to fit the context (e.g., wearing a jacket, dress, or tie to talk with the local health commission). These adjustments can help people to focus on your message, rather than getting distracted by what they think about your appearance.

VERBAL COMMUNICATION AND BODY LANGUAGE

How you present yourself verbally and through body language makes a difference in how people perceive you and your message.

Do you stay focused on the topic when others are speaking? Is your voice friendly, assertive, and clear? How loudly are you speaking?

Do you stand or sit very close or far away from others? Do you fail to engage in eye contact or insist upon it? When others speak, do you cross your arms, frown, or roll your eyes? How might these or other types of body language be perceived by others?

Some types of communication are not welcome in the workplace:

- Sexist, racist, homophobic, and other types of prejudicial language are never appropriate. It is illegal and could get you fired.

- Profane language. Don't use curse words at work. Some words might not be curse words but are still rude or distasteful.

- Gossiping or talking negatively about your co-workers or supervisors is unacceptable. Use the appropriate outlets to communicate your concerns. See the section of giving and receiving constructive feedback below.

- Repeating the same information over and over, constantly interrupting others, or taking time away from a common agenda to talk about other topics can be perceived by others as rude or disrespectful.

Talking on the Telephone

You are likely to spend a lot of time on the phone, contacting clients about their appointments, talking with representatives from other agencies who can provide services for your clients, or contacting local businesses to ask for donations or support for events in your community.

Here are some tips for professional phone calls:

1. Start with a friendly, time-appropriate greeting such as "Good morning."
2. Identify yourself and your agency.
3. State the reason for your call and ask whether it is a good time to talk, giving an indication of how long the call might be.
4. Write down any key information that other callers provide you, such as names and phone numbers, and read them back to make sure they are accurate.
5. If you will need to call again, say so and ask when you might do so.
6. End the call with "thank you" and "good-bye."

If you leave a message:

1. Begin with a greeting such as "Good morning" or "Good afternoon" followed by the person's name. Deliver these words in a friendly voice.
2. Follow the greeting by identifying yourself and your agency.
3. Briefly state the reason for your call.
4. Repeat your name and give your phone number again.
5. End the call with "thank you" and "good-bye."

Preserve confidentiality: Do not leave any sensitive or confidential information in a message.

Keep up with technology: Our jobs change to accommodate advancements in technology. It is important to have basic to proficient skills with computers and other technology. Virtual meetings with clients, supervisors, colleagues, and other health professionals are becoming the norm. Other duties may involve using case management software, navigating online resources, documenting the services you provide in an electronic heath record, and utilizing design tools to create flyers for outreach. Keeping up with technology plays a vital role in keeping your position, while being flexible and willing to learn new technology can help advance your career.

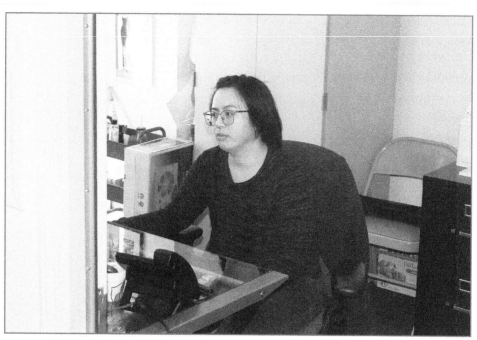

A CHW documenting their work with clients.

Written Communication

How well you write makes a lasting impression on the people who receive your communications. Written communications pose particular code-switching challenges. The emphasis in school on spelling, punctuation, and grammar was basically teaching you a "professional" (white, middle-class, English-speaking) code. The way we were taught, and the way that we were judged, can leave us feeling inadequate and intimidated when we have to write letters, memos, emails, and reports.

If writing in English is a challenge for you, consider an adult education class at your high school or community college. Here are some commonsense tips to make your written communications reflect your skills as a successful CHW.

Why are you writing? Depending upon the length and scope of what you write, you may want to jot down a brief outline of what you really want to say before writing. What are your main points? Think of questions your reader may have and answer them.

Use a simple structure: Start with an introduction. Give the details. Summarize or conclude.

Put yourself in your reader's place: Read your message aloud. How would you feel reading this letter or email? Remember: once it has been sent, you cannot take it back. Is your message short, clear, and easy to read? Is there any slang that may not be understood by everyone or may not be appropriate? Is the information accurate? Did you double-check your facts? Is your tone professional and courteous?

Use clear language: Don't use too many abbreviations, acronyms, or jargon used only at your agency or only in your profession. Keep the language simple and at a level you know all people will understand.

Use spell-check and grammar check: When you have completed the message, use spell-check and grammar check before you send it.

Email

Increasingly, professional communication is conducted through email. Because it is so easy to write and send, we can be tempted to think of email as less formal or less important than mail that's printed out on paper. Email is professional communication just like any other forms of written communication. Everything about written communication above applies to email, and there are a few tips that apply to email in particular.

Subject line: The subject line is like the headline of a news story. Be sure that what you write in the subject line is short and accurate. Some busy people will not open email if the subject line doesn't grab their attention.

Replying: Sometimes you will get an email that is addressed to an entire group of people. Be careful about who you reply to. Don't "Reply All" unless you want your message to be sent to everyone who received the original email.

Don't hit the send button when you're mad!: We've all done it; someone sends you an email message that upsets you, and you respond from your anger. If you're upset, don't send the email: wait until you are in a calmer state and can think more clearly about the potential impact. You might want to check out some of the conflict resolution tips in Chapter 13.

Texting and Calls

Similar to email, texting in the workplace has become increasingly popular due to accessibility and quicker response times. Although this is viewed as a more casual method of communication, it is important to still conduct yourself professionally when texting clients, colleagues, and supervisors.

Depending upon the time and place, receiving cell phone calls or text messages can be distracting in the workplace. Be sure that your digital technology is turned off during meetings and do not check digital technology while talking to others. Checking text messages makes you seem distracted and uninterested. If you must respond to urgent text messages or calls, be courteous and politely excuse yourself. Overall, avoid using your cell phone if it is not work related.

Always be aware of your surroundings. If you are working in the community and need to make a call concerning a client, find an appropriate place to speak quietly on the phone without disclosing confidential information in public.

GIVING AND RECEIVING CONSTRUCTIVE FEEDBACK

Part of being a CHW is learning to receive constructive feedback about the quality of your work from clients and community members, co-workers, and supervisors. You will also provide feedback to others.

Your ability to provide and receive feedback in a respectful and professional manner is key to the long-term success of your career. The inability to handle feedback is a common reason why employees miss out on opportunities for promotion, face disciplinary action, or lose their jobs.

The purpose of constructive feedback is to improve the quality of the services provided to clients and communities. For CHWs, the purpose of constructive feedback is to enhance your knowledge and skills, and the quality of your professional relationships with co-workers and clients alike.

Constructive feedback may be supportive or corrective. **Supportive feedback** reinforces knowledge, skills, and conduct by identifying what is being done well or right. **Corrective feedback** indicates desired changes in behavior, by explaining what didn't work, is unacceptable in the workplace, or needs improvement. In both cases, the goal should be to improve performance and effectiveness.

Challenges with Receiving or Providing Feedback

Many of us have had difficulty with receiving or providing feedback in a calm and productive manner. Some of the factors that get in our way include:

- Past negative experiences with feedback
- Learning from poor role models that the way to provide feedback is through conflict or accusation, with anger or sarcasm
- Bias, prejudice, or discriminatory treatment or policies
- Anxiety or fear, such as the fear of losing your job
- Emotions such as anger or frustration that may result in defensiveness
- The desire to be right, and related difficulties accepting accountability or negotiating compromise

- A lack of self-awareness and ability to acknowledge our own limitations and areas for personal and professional growth and development
- Difficulty providing a sincere apology

- *Have you faced challenges in providing or receiving feedback in the workplace?*
- *What lessons have you learned that help you in providing and receiving feedback?*

Guidelines for Giving and Receiving Feedback

We encourage you to re-frame the way that you view feedback. Try to consider it as an opportunity to learn and improve your skills, especially when the nature of the feedback provided is difficult to hear.

We will share brief guidelines for giving and receiving constructive feedback. We also encourage you to seek out professional development opportunities to enhance your skills and to learn from experienced and respected colleagues. The information provided in Chapter 13 on conflict resolution may also be helpful.

Giving feedback: When providing others with feedback, we recommend sandwiching corrective feedback between substantive supportive feedback. In other words, start and end your conversation by sharing positive feedback with your colleague. Everyone we work with has strengths. Let them know what you appreciate about their attitude, knowledge, skills, and contributions.

Other guidelines include:

- **Feedback should be timely**: Share it in the moment it occurs or as soon afterward as possible.
- Express what you value about the other person and your working relationship.
- Don't provide feedback when you are feeling angry or unable to focus on supporting your colleague.
- Speak in a respectful tone of voice. Don't raise the level of your voice.
- Provide detailed feedback (what, where, when) about the person's behavior or conduct. Provide your colleague with specific examples. What did they do—or not do—that you want to draw to their attention to?
- Explain what you think the impact of a specific decision, behavior, or policy may be on others such as yourself, your colleagues, or on the clients and community you serve.
- Provide *practical and realistic* suggestions for what your colleague could do differently the next time they face a similar situation. If relevant, refer to your agency or program standards, goals, or policies.
- Don't hold back on sharing important corrective feedback. When we do this, we deprive a colleague of the opportunity to learn how to enhance their skills and performance.
- Invite the person or group to ask questions to clarify the feedback you provide and to respond.
- Invite your colleague to talk with you and to identify concrete steps they can take to improve their skills and performance.

- *What else do you want to do when providing constructive feedback to a colleague?*

Receiving Feedback: Suggested guidelines include:

- Breathe! Try to remain calm and strive to listen and understand the information that is being shared with you.
- Assume the person who is providing you with feedback is doing so with a positive intention (such as improving the quality of services and working relationships).
- Listen for key content such as feedback about specific behaviors or decisions, and any suggestions for what you could do differently.
- Ask questions to clarify the information your colleague (or a client or community member) is providing. If the feedback is vague or unclear, ask them to provide you with a specific example.

- Maintain a conversational tone and voice level.

- Paraphrase or summarize the feedback to make sure you have heard it correctly.

- Notice if you are feeling defensive. Don't react in the moment with anger, or try to defend yourself, especially if the person providing the feedback is a client, your supervisor, or another leader at your agency or in the community.

- Ask for a break if you need one, and only return to the conversation when you are truly prepared to listen to what your colleague has to say. Vent any strong emotions later, away from the workplace. You can always respond to your colleague at a later date, when you are prepared for a respectful and productive conversation.

- Reflect on the feedback provided and decide if and how you wish to incorporate what you have learned into your future work. What did you learn that might help you to improve your skills and performance?

- Clearly and respectfully communicate any specific requests you have for the other party to make changes to their own conduct (or to policies).

- Regardless of how you feel in the moment, express your appreciation to the other party for taking time to provide you with feedback.

- If it is relevant and desirable, schedule a future meeting to follow up on the issues discussed at this meeting.

- *What else would you want to do when receiving constructive feedback from a colleague?*

What Do YOU? Think

Please watch this video interview ▶️ with CCSF Faculty about the challenge of providing and receiving constructive feedback in the classroom and beyond:

PROVIDING & RECEIVING CONSTRUCTIVE FEEDBACK.
(*Source:* Foundations for Community Health Workers/http:// youtu.be/7NqVU0-foEw/last accessed 21 September 2023).

COMMUNICATING WITH YOUR SUPERVISOR

In an ideal work situation, communication with your supervisor is frequent, clear, straightforward, and respectful. Unfortunately, most of us are likely to face challenges in working with supervisors over the course of our careers. Some supervisors lack leadership skills and may not be effective in communicating workplace expectations and protocols, or in motivating and supporting staff.

Supervisors are responsible for helping you and the program you work for to be successful. They are looking for employees who are reliable, consistent, and who can learn and grow on the job. Do your utmost to forge and sustain a positive working relationship with your supervisor, especially during times when you have different perspectives, needs, or values. Try to find common ground. Look for opportunities, or create them, to work together in a focused way on a common task in which you each have valuable expertise to offer.

Express Your Concerns

If you face difficulties or challenges in your relationship with your supervisor, consider taking the initiative and ask to talk about your concerns. Keep in mind that your supervisor may not already be aware of your concerns or perspectives. *Draw upon your person-centered skills!* Be respectful and patient. Ask open-ended questions to help clarify your understanding of the supervisor's perspective and position. Summarize key information that they share with you in order to confirm that you have understood it correctly. Listen calmly. Don't do or say anything in the heat of moment (if you are frustrated, angry or hurt) that might undermine your employment status or career. And don't talk negatively about your supervisor—or other colleagues—behind their back. This is a powerful way to damage trust and the quality of professional relationships.

Accept Limitations

Keep in mind that it may not be possible to work out every difference of opinion or conflict with your supervisor. *Part of work is accepting constraints or conditions determined by our employers and supervisors.* This includes accepting policies and protocols that we don't like or agree with. Try to distinguish between differences or disagreements that you are able to accept and live with, and those that you feel so strongly about that you are willing to take a risk to advocate for.

Speak Directly to Your Supervisor

Always try to speak directly with your supervisor about any complaint that you have about their performance. Going around your supervisor to speak to another administrator may be perceived as "going behind their back," and further damage your working relationship (note that there are a few exceptions to this rule, such as complaints of sexual harassment or other charges of illegal conduct). If you have difficulties with a supervisor that you cannot resolve, you may need to turn to your union or human resources department for assistance.

Weigh Your Options

Despite the problems you encounter, continue to bring your best self to your interactions with your supervisor. Work to improve the relationship. At some point, if the changes you desire do not occur, you may need to reconsider your strategy. You may decide to seek employment elsewhere, either within the organization you currently work for or with a different agency. If you decide to stay in your current position, find a way to focus on the aspects of your job where you have greater autonomy, as well as those that bring you satisfaction and meaning.

And please remember to take care of yourself along the way. Disharmony or conflicts with supervisors take a significant toll on our professional life and on our physical, mental, and spiritual health. Apply your skills for stress management and self-care and engage in life affirming activities outside of work.

MANAGE YOUR TIME

As a CHW, you will have a lot of tasks and deadlines to manage, as well as the challenge of balancing work with your personal life. Time management can make the difference between success and failure at work and in life. It provides resources to make conscious decisions about how to address competing demands.

Some people resist the idea of time management because they like the idea of being spontaneous. But having a plan for each day can free you from the stress of remembering what to do or being backed into a corner when a deadline is fast approaching. Managing your time also helps you to free up time for the things you most want to do.

Plan Your Week

If you don't use one already, start to use a portable print or electronic calendar or planner. Write down your appointments, meetings, deadlines, family obligations and activities, and so forth.

Make a "to-do list" of all the other tasks you need to accomplish that don't have a specific date and time commitment. Mark those tasks that are the highest priority for the upcoming week.

Don't schedule every minute of each day: leave room for new tasks and for ongoing activities that always take time, such completing case notes and other forms of documentation. Review your calendar and your to-do list to make sure that you have scheduled all key tasks and obligations.

Review Tomorrow's Schedule

At the end of each day, take 10 minutes to review tomorrow's schedule. Identify one or two priorities and make sure you have set aside enough time to complete them. Look at appointments already scheduled and consider if you need to prepare anything in advance. Review your personal and family needs for the day to see if you need to do errands on the way to or home from work, if you need to make phone calls, or complete any urgent tasks at home. This one simple habit, if you do it each evening at the end of the workday, or at home before you go to bed, will help you feel prepared to manage your responsibilities at work and at home.

Set Priorities

Most of us have more things to do than we can actually accomplish. Part of managing your time involves making conscious decisions about what your priorities are—what you will do right now, what you will postpone, and what you won't be able to accomplish. There will be times when you have to say "No" to certain activities and responsibilities and stick to your original plan in order to complete your tasks. At work, your commitment to your clients should always be your number one priority. Don't fill up your calendar with other activities that make it difficult for you to fulfill your commitment to the community.

When you start managing your time, you may find yourself frustrated or feeling as though keeping a planner and maintaining a daily to-do list is taking up too much time. Don't give up! In the long run, this kind of planning will give you more control over your busy days. It will help you make sure you get the most important tasks done. And it will help you balance your work demands with taking care of yourself and your family.

14.4 Professional Development and Career Advancement

Let's assume that you've settled into your current position as a CHW and are doing a great job. Now is the time to think about professional development to enhance knowledge and skills for your present job and future career advancement. Whether you aspire to create change in your community or want to earn more money, professional development opportunities will help you to achieve your goals.

PROFESSIONAL DEVELOPMENT

Professional development is seeking out opportunities to enhance your knowledge and skills in key areas related to your work as a CHW. This might include knowledge about:

- Specific health issues such as chronic conditions management, depression, post-traumatic stress, or harm reduction
- Local resources such as mental health services
- The history, resources, and health concerns of specific populations or communities
- Statistics or epidemiology

It may also include skills in areas such as:

- Public speaking
- Crisis intervention and suicide prevention
- Program planning and evaluation
- Research or program evaluation
- Grant writing
- Community organizing and advocacy
- Conflict resolution
- Cultural humility
- Supervising and managing others
- Leadership
- *What other skills or knowledge do you think would assist you to advance in your career as a CHW?*

Professional development opportunities include participating in free or low-cost trainings at a nonprofit agency or the local health department; enrolling in a class or webinar; attending a lecture at a local college or university; conducting research; and reading articles and books or watching a documentary by yourself or with others.

Case Conferences

If you work in a team setting, you may have the opportunity to participate in case conferences (see Chapter 10) and to discuss your work with colleagues. This is a wonderful opportunity for professional development: you receive immediate feedback from peers and other professionals on an urgent problem such as working with a client in crisis. Whether you're receiving the advice or assisting a colleague, case conferences are a great opportunity for continuing education.

Support and Mentoring

Mentoring by an experienced CHW may be the best form of professional development you can hope for. You may work surrounded by doctors, nurses, or social workers who want to know, or think they know, what it takes to be a great CHW: but only an experienced CHW really understands this. Ask to meet regularly with an experienced CHW. Share your questions and concerns and listen to their guidance. Consider joining a local or statewide CHW network. You can also join the National Association of Community Health Workers (see Chapters 1 and 2 for more information about NACHW).

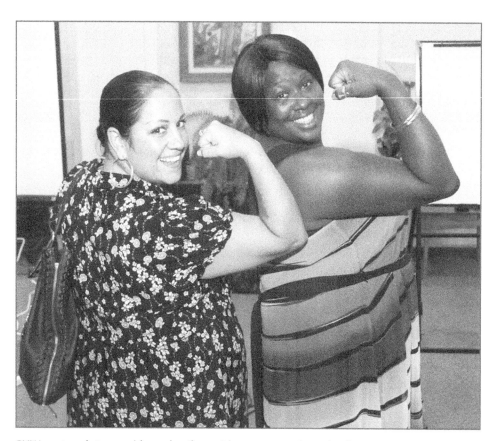

CHWs network to provide each other with support and motivation.

Informational Interviewing

If you are unable to find a mentor, an alternative strategy is to conduct an informational interview. This one-on-one meeting with a professional employed in your field of interest. Informational interviews give you the opportunity to ask an expert questions to learn more about a position/career path. Sample Questions:

- What kinds of challenges do you deal with?
- What steps would you recommend I take to prepare for/advance in this field?
- What skills, abilities, and personal attributes are essential to success in this job/field?
- What professional organizations do people in this field belong to?
- What current issues and trends in the field should I know about/be aware of?

After the interview, write down what you learned, what you'd like to know more about, and your reactions in terms of how this field or position aligns with your lifestyle, interests, skills, and future career plans. This is also an opportunity to network with experienced CHWs and other public health professionals. Keep in touch with the person, especially if you had a particularly nice interaction. If you followed up on their suggestions and advice, let them know as this relationship could become an important part of your network.

Pro tip: Send the person you interviewed a request to connect on LinkedIn

It's safe to say that most people enjoy talking about themselves and are happy to share information about their career or line of work

Chapter Review

Please review the information covered in this chapter by responding to the following questions and suggestions:

- What advice might you share with Priyadarshi Mehta, the CHW from the CHW Scenario presented at the beginning of this chapter? What else might Priyadarshi do—if anything—to adapt to the codes of his workplace and advance his career?
- How can you enhance your own skills for code switching while maintaining your own identity and culture?
- Develop or update your résumé
- Rehearse what you might say in a job interview about your experience, knowledge, and skills as a CHW
- Create a prioritized to-do list—including professional and personal responsibilities—for next week, and schedule these activities in a planner
- In the next month, practice giving or receiving professional feedback. Reflect on your performance using the guidelines presented in this chapter.
- Identify two or more skills or areas of knowledge that you would like to learn or enhance that will assist in advancing your career. Identify professional development opportunities to enhance your knowledge and skills.
- Identify a CHW Association or an experienced CHW who might serve as a source of support or a mentor to you. How do you feel about contacting these resources? What type of support will you ask for? What questions do you have?

References

Cuncic, A. (2022). What is Imposter Syndrome? VeryWellMind. https://www.verywellmind.com/imposter-syndrome-and-social-anxiety-disorder-4156469 (accessed 8 December 2022).

Fox, M. (2023). Negotiating a Job Offer Works: 85% of Americans Who Counteroffered were Successful Here's How to Do it. CNBC. https://www.cnbc.com/2022/05/13/85-percent-of-americans-who-negtiated-a-job-offer-were-successful.html (accessed 5 January 2023).

Hummel, B. (2022). What is Career Readiness and How Do You Teach It? Applied-Educational-Systems. https://www.aeseducation.com/blog/what-is-career-readiness (accessed 5 January 2023).

Kang, S. K., DeCelles, K. A., Tilscik, A., & Jun, S. (2016). Whitened resumes: Race and self-presentation in the labor market. *Administrative Science Quarterly*, 61(3). https://doi.org/10.1177/0001839216639.

Langford, J. & Clance, P, P. (1993). The imposter phenomenon: Recent research findings regarding dynamics, personality, and family patterns and their implications for treatment. *Psychotherapy*, 30 (3), 495–501.

National Association of Colleges and Employers. (2021). What is Career Readiness? https://www.naceweb.org/career-readiness/competencies/career-readiness-defined/ (accessed 5 January 2022).

Sakulku, J. & Alexander, J. (2011). The imposter phenomenon. *International Journal of Behavioral Science*, 6(1), 73–92. doi:10.14456/IJBS.2011.6.

Ton, J. (2020). Networking: It's Not What You Think. Forbes. https://www.forbes.com/sites/forbestechcouncil/2020/10/15/networking-its-not-what-you-think/?sh=33ba29217985 (accessed 5 January 2023).

Young, V. (2011). *The secret thoughts of successful women: Why capable people suffer from the impostor syndrome and how to thrive in spite of it.* New York: Random House, Inc.

Additional Resources

LinkedIn. https://linkedin.com.

National Association of Community Health Workers. (2023). https://nachw.org/.

The U.S. Bureau of Labor Statistics. (2023). https://www.bls.gov/ooh/community-and-social-service/health-educators.htm.

APPLYING CORE COMPETENCIES TO KEY HEALTH ISSUES

PART
4

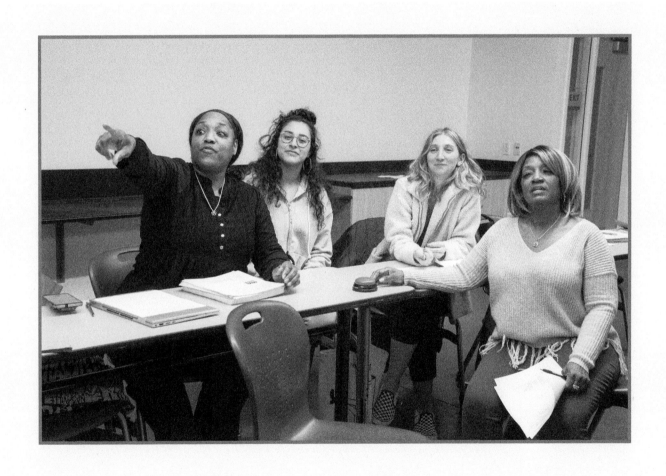

Health Care Is Reentry: Promoting the Health of People Who Have Experienced Incarceration

15

Amie Fishman and Joe Calderon

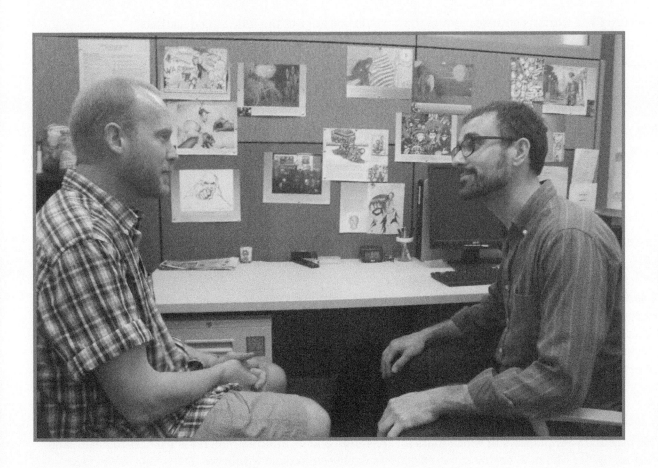

Foundations for Community Health Workers, Third Edition. Edited by Tim Berthold and Darouny Somsanith.
© 2024 John Wiley & Sons, Inc. Published 2024 by John Wiley & Sons, Inc.
Companion website: http://www.wiley.com/go/communityhealthworkers3E

Client Scenario: Sean Jones

You meet Sean Jones, a 57-year-old man, while doing outreach at a transitional home for people recently released from prison. Sean was released after serving 25 years for a nonviolent crime with prior convictions. While in prison, Sean burned bridges and lost contact with all of his family members.

In your meeting, Sean lists his known medical issues as anxiety, Hepatitis C, and a history of substance use. Sean shares that he doesn't like the room he's in (a full room with bunk beds) and opens up about the violence and trauma he witnessed and experienced in prison and as a child growing up. Sean tells you his parents were both violent and that is one of the reasons he started drinking when he was so young. He tells you that the only friend that never hurt him was drugs. Sean shares with you that he has never had a real job, never paid a bill, and doesn't know how to read.

The day before his first clinic visit, Sean calls you. He is anxious about how he'll get to his appointment, afraid that he'll get on the wrong bus, or get lost and won't be able to read the names of the bus stops. Sean explains that he's run out of his diabetes medication (he forgot to mention his diabetes when he first met with you). He doesn't feel well and thinks it may be due to missing his medications.

If you were a CHW working with Sean Jones, how would you answer the following questions:

- How might Sean have been impacted by his experience of incarceration? How might his family have been impacted?

- What obstacles and challenges is Sean likely to face as he re-enters society after being incarcerated?

- What concepts and techniques will guide your work with Sean?

- How will you work to establish a supportive working relationship with Sean and to build trust?

- Based on what you have learned so far, what may be some of Sean's priority concerns?

- What can you do right now to support Sean?

Introduction

The United States has the highest incarceration rate in the world (629 per 100,000) and, with over 2 million people in jails and prisons across the country, represents 25% of the entire world's prison population (Pew Research Center, 2021; World Prison Brief, 2021).

Why is the United States the global leader in incarceration? Incarceration has long been used in the United States as a means of social, political, and economic control. The roots of our current policies can be traced back to the end of slavery and subsequent "Jim Crow" laws targeting Black people, immigrants of color, and other historically excluded communities. Decades of "tough on crime" policies such as mandatory minimum sentencing laws, harsh immigration laws, and the "War on Drugs" resulted in huge increases in jail and prison sentences, especially for low-income communities of color, who have been the targets of these approaches and those most affected by their outcomes. People of color, particularly Black and Indigenous people, are subjected to many forms of police and incarceration abuse, including excessive use of force, overpolicing, arrests, and detentions (Human Rights Watch, 2021).

This chapter analyzes the ways in which mass incarceration and its aftermath increase barriers to health and well-being. People who have been incarcerated are severely stigmatized within our society and often face fractured relationships and a sense of dislocation when returning home. You will learn about the many laws and regulations that make it more difficult for your clients returning home and the stigma and discrimination they face. This chapter draws on the experience of some of the country's first CHWs whose practice is focused on post-prison health and wellness.

As a CHW working with marginalized communities, you are likely to have clients who have been incarcerated themselves, or who have a family member or loved one who has been incarcerated. Your knowledge about the realities of incarceration and its health and social impacts will allow you to serve your clients returning home with compassion, empathy, and respect. Understanding these realities will also better prepare you to advocate for your clients' needs and rights as they encounter barriers to their health and reentry. By approaching clients in a nonjudgmental way, linking them with appropriate resources, fostering social support, challenging stigma and discrimination, advocating for your clients, and promoting social change, you will be in a position to challenge some of the worst collateral effects of incarceration and contribute to building healthier communities.

WHAT YOU WILL LEARN

By studying the information in this chapter, you will be able to:

- Analyze the ways that incarceration influences the health of individuals, families, and communities
- Identify common health issues faced by people returning home from prison
- Explain the stigma and the systemic barriers to reintegration faced by people recently released from prison
- Discuss the role of CHWs in promoting the health and well-being of clients who have experienced incarceration
- Examine best practices and emerging models for promoting the health of people who have experienced incarceration
- Identify areas of potential policy change and the role of CHWs as advocates for change
- Identify trauma-informed reasons why those affected by incarceration and systemic discrimination may distrust health care systems and providers
- Learn about resources for successful reentry

C3 Roles and Skills Addressed in Chapter 15

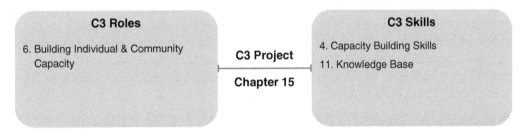

WORDS TO KNOW

Prison Industrial Complex

Recidivism

Stigma

15.1 Basic Terms and a Note on Language

JAILS VERSUS PRISONS

While people sometimes use these terms interchangeably, jails and prisons are different. Jails are run by the county sheriff's department and detain people who are awaiting trial and people who are sentenced for a short term, usually less than a year. Prisons are run either by a state or federal correctional department; they hold people who have been convicted of a crime, and usually those sentenced for more than a year.

DETENTION CENTERS

Detention facilities hold people suspected of a crime, awaiting trial or sentencing, or found to be undocumented immigrants. Young people are often held in juvenile detention centers while awaiting court hearings and/or placement in long-term care facilities and programs. Immigrants who are in custody for more than 72 hours are held in detention centers overseen by the Department of Homeland Security (DHS).

PROBATION AND PAROLE

People do not have to be physically incarcerated in order to have their lives monitored and affected by the criminal justice system. In fact, in 2020, almost 4 million adults were on probation or parole (Kaeble, 2021). **Both probation and parole involve the supervision of people who have been convicted of crimes, but the systems are distinct.**

Many people are placed on probation instead of being sent to prison, allowing them to serve their sentence in the community. While on probation, a person must avoid further contact with the law and must fulfill certain requirements, such as restrictions on travel, periodic drug testing, or attendance in specific classes or programs. People on probation are monitored by a probation officer and must report on a regular basis. If someone violates a condition of probation, the court may place additional restrictions on that person or order them to serve a term of imprisonment. A judge can also sentence someone to probation following a period of incarceration. Probation is generally reserved for persons sentenced to short terms in jail: it is not combined with a long prison sentence.

A person subjected to supervision after prison is placed on parole and monitored by a parole officer. Parole is granted by a parole board and signifies early release from prison.

THE SIGNIFICANCE OF THE LANGUAGE WE USE

The language we use for people who are in or have been in jail or prison is critically important because of the **stigma**—or negative label—that our society places on incarceration and the risk of alienating the very clients and communities we are pledged to serve. Societies often label groups of people by their actions or circumstances, and in the process, undermine their identity and status as human beings. When we refer to people as convicted felons (or as addicts or mentally ill or illegal aliens or homeless), we set them apart from others in ways that diminish their value.

In reality, people who use drugs, break the law, and experience hardship or mental illness are not "those other people"—they are our family members, friends, neighbors, and even ourselves. One of the quickest ways to undermine your ability to work with any client is to diminish their humanity by assigning them an unwelcome label such as those referenced above. These labels can demonstrate disrespect and lack of understanding to those we are trying to support, creating real barriers to developing trusting relationships. They also reveal our own internalized beliefs and biases, which we must constantly reflect on and work to undo in order to promote the well-being and healing of our clients.

Many institutions, the media, and even helping professionals use highly stigmatizing language to refer to people who have been incarcerated, creating barriers to developing effective professional relationships based on respect. This includes the use of terms such as "offenders," "convicts," "felons," "convicted criminals," "cons/ex-cons," or "inmates."

In this chapter and in our work, we put the person and their humanity first by using the terms such as *"returning community member"*, *"person who has experienced incarceration,"* or *"person who has been incarcerated,"* language that many people use to self-identify. How people choose to refer to themselves is always changing and will continue to change, which makes it even more important to listen to and honor the terms people use to describe their own experiences. Respecting a person's self-identification *is* practicing cultural humility, helping to create space for healing and understanding.

15.2 The Roots of U.S. Incarceration Policies

Many in the United States do not question the high numbers of people in jails and prisons, on probation or parole, or the massive expansion of prisons that occurred over the last 30 years, even as rates of violent crime consistently declined (Federal Bureau of Investigation, 2023). While the U.S. prison population has declined in the last few years, it remains the highest in the world (Wisconsin Poverty Center, 2023). Currently, over 5.5 million adults—1 out of every 47 people—in the United States are under the control of the criminal justice system through incarceration, probation, or parole (Bureau of Justice Statistics, 2022). That is roughly the population of the entire state of Colorado or Minnesota, and the entire country of Norway or Singapore. As a CHW, you are likely to encounter a client who has been personally affected by or experienced incarceration themselves.

How did the United States come to use imprisonment more than any other society, and what are the lasting impacts today? To answer these questions, we need to look into the history of our oldest institutions: slavery and colonization.

Michelle Alexander, author of The New Jim Crow, begins her book with this paragraph:

> *Jarvious Cotton cannot vote. Like his father, grandfather, great-grandfather, and great-great-grandfather, he has been denied the right to participate in our electoral democracy. Cotton's family tree tells the story of several generations of black men who were born in the United States but who were denied the most basic freedom that democracy promises—the freedom to vote for those who will make the rules and laws that govern one's life. Cotton's great-great-grandfather could not vote as a slave. His great-grandfather was beaten to death by the Ku Klux Klan for attempting to vote. His grandfather was prevented from voting by Klan intimidation. His father was barred from voting by poll taxes and literacy tests. Today, Jarvious Cotton cannot vote because he, like many black men in the United States, has been labeled a felon and is currently on parole. (Alexander, 2010, p. 1)*

Jarvious Cotton's family history shines a powerful light on the legacy of slavery in this country and how this history continues to affect its descendants today.

Approximately 12 million Africans were enslaved and brought to the Americas and the Caribbean between 1525 and 1866, the year *after* the 13th Amendment officially abolished slavery (Pacific Broadcasting Network, 2023a). Following the trauma of being forcibly stolen from their families and communities, enslaved Africans endured horrifying conditions of confinement, and over two million did not survive the journey. Of those that survived, roughly 338,000 landed in the United States, where they were sold into chattel slavery, meaning that they and their offspring were considered legal property and could be bought, sold, and owned forever (Ibid).

Colonies established in what would become the United States, in search of gold and other valuable resources and to expand the reach of the Spanish empire. The Indigenous people they encountered represented a problem in need of a solution. Through the rapid introduction and spread of diseases such as smallpox that Indigenous communities lacked immunity to, to outright conflict and war, many Indigenous people were killed and their land and other possessions were taken by colonizers. Those who survived were forcibly moved to reservations in order to free up desired land for colonizers.

Starting in the 1800s, tens of thousands of Indigenous children were removed from their families and sent to boarding schools to be "re-educated," a process of stripping away language, familial roots, history, and cultural heritage. This cultural erasure and intergenerational trauma continued for 125 years, and included abuses and deaths of thousands of children, many of whom were buried in unmarked graves (Bureau of Indian Affairs, 2022, pp. 35–36, 39, 52–56).

Chain of Destruction

Both slavery and colonization utilized principles of dehumanization to justify and codify into law the theft and destruction of people's lives, land, and communities. These principles—known as the "Chain of Destruction"—are powerfully described in the 2012 documentary about the war on drugs in the United States called *The House I Live In*. The five links in this chain are explained as follows:

1. **Identification:** a particular group of people is identified as the cause of the problems in that society, causing people to perceive them as bad or evil. Their lives are therefore seen as less valuable or worthless.

2. **Ostracism:** we are taught to hate and fear that group, so we take their jobs away or make it otherwise harder for them to survive. People lose their homes and are often forced into ghettoized communities where they are physically isolated and separated from the rest of society.

3. **Confiscation:** people lose their rights and civil or human liberties. The laws change, so it becomes easier for this group to be searched and for their property to be confiscated. Taking people's property away makes it easier to start taking them away too.

(continues)

Chain of Destruction
(continued)

4. **Concentration:** the government begins to concentrate people in prisons and camps, where they lose their rights. They can't vote or participate in society. Their labor is often exploited.

5. **Annihilation:** this may be indirect, by withholding medical care or food, or by preventing future births through forced sterilization or confinement. Or it may be direct, where people are deliberately killed.

Throughout history, these tactics have justified oppression and exploitation, often through racialized dehumanization of specific groups. Indigenous communities in the United States were portrayed as lazy, stupid, dangerous, or savage, enabling land theft, displacement, and cultural genocide. Enslaved Africans were similarly depicted as savage, dangerous, and inferior, justifying the denial of their rights, freedom, and lives. There were also many examples of powerful resistance to colonization and enslavement, the most famous being Nat Turner's Rebellion in Virginia in 1831, where slaves killed 60 people during an uprising. (American Anthropological Association, 2023).

Efforts to control the growing population of slaves and stop resistance took many forms, including militia-style attacks and the implementation of increasingly restrictive and punitive laws called the **Slave Codes**. Slave Codes varied by state and included:

- Virginia's 1659 law barring slaves from owning or carrying weapons
- Maryland's 1664 law prohibiting marriage between slaves and nonslaves
- South Carolina's 1724 law stating that a slave who hits or bruises his/her master or their family will be killed

Property and slave owners who failed to comply were subject to fines or having their slaves taken away. People who employed slaves, gave them alcohol, or taught them to read and write were also fined (American Anthropological Association, 2023). On the other hand, the Slave Codes meant that slave owners could inflict harsh punishments, and even death, on enslaved people without risk of being punished themselves.

Slave patrols, which began in the early 1700s, essentially functioned as the first police in the U.S. Militias of white male citizens formed a "government-sponsored force [of about 10 people] that was well organized and paid to patrol specific areas to prevent crimes and insurrection by slaves against the white community" in the antebellum South (Turner, Giacopassi, & Vandiver, 2006).

After the Civil War and the passage of the 13th Amendment, slavery was abolished "except as punishment for a crime" (Vera Institute of Justice, 2023). Some of these same slave patrols transitioned to become the first police departments in the Southern U.S. To deal with freed slaves who broke the rules designed to control Black people, many states adopted **convict or vagrancy laws that these groups enforced.** Alexander explains:

> *Nine Southern states adopted vagrancy laws—which essentially made it a criminal offense not to work and were applied selectively to blacks—and eight of those states enacted convict laws allowing for the hiring-out of county prisoners to plantation owners and private companies. Prisoners were forced to work for little or no pay....* (Alexander, 2010, p. 28)

This history reflects the deep-seated racism and social control at the core of our present-day incarceration system. While slavery officially ended in 1863, the introduction of "Black Codes" followed from 1865 to 1866, aimed at enforcing segregation, criminalizing Black people, and curtailing their rights. Black Codes impacted all aspects of Black people's lives, including work, property ownership, drinking, preaching, marriage, and residential location. The enforcement of these codes led to a significant increase and change in the prison population, which became 95% Black by the 1870s.

These laws were eventually overturned, making way for the **Reconstruction Era** (1865–1877), a period in which many Black people began to vote, own property and businesses, hold office, and generally experience growth and prosperity as a community.

The social, economic, and political gains made by Black people during the Reconstruction Era were met with a fierce backlash. Racial segregation continued to be a prominent feature of U.S. culture, encouraged by efforts to discourage "race-mixing" and maintain racial hierarchy. Along with the fact that the nation never addressed the underlying racism and white supremacy that supported slavery and colonialism, these factors set the stage for, as Alexander describes it, "a new racial caste system as stunningly comprehensive and repressive as the one that came to be known simply as **Jim Crow**" (Alexander, 2010, pp. 30).

Led by Southern conservatives who wanted to reverse Reconstruction and dismantle the agencies that promoted it and supported by the emerging Ku Klux Klan who terrorized those who participated in Reconstruction, the Jim Crow era (1877–1954) saw the gains made by Black people quickly unravel. The federal government stopped enforcing civil rights legislation and funding for the Freedman's Bureau, a federal agency designed to help formerly enslaved people, was slashed to the degree that the agency essentially folded.

Alexander explains what happened next:

> *Once again, vagrancy laws and other laws defining activities such as 'mischief' and 'insulting gestures' as crimes were enforced vigorously against blacks. The aggressive enforcement of these criminal offenses opened up an enormous market for convict leasing, in which prisoners were contracted out as laborers to the highest bidder. Douglas Blackmon, in Slavery by Another Name, describes how tens of thousands of black people were arbitrarily arrested during this period, many of them hit with court costs and fines, which had to be worked off in order to secure their release. With no means to pay off their 'debts' prisoners were sold as forced laborers to lumber camps, brickyards, railroads, farms, plantations, and dozens of corporations throughout the South. (Ibid, p. 31)*

These laborers suffered horrible conditions, beatings, and often death, as "private contractors had no interest in the health and well-being of their laborers." And as convicted people, these laborers had no rights and were understood to be "slaves of the state" (Ibid, p. 31).

The **Civil Rights Era** (1954–1968) marked the first significant legal gains toward true equity, in which laws were passed that "guaranteed Black people the rights they should have always had" (Hannah-Jones, Roper, Silverman, & Silversteing, 2021, p. 467). With landmark legislation such as Brown versus Board of Education, which desegregated schools, and the Civil Rights Act of 1957, which made it illegal to prevent people from voting, Black people in the United States saw the hope of more equitable participation in civil society. However, these laws did not repair the harm done, and they were again met with resistance from white communities (Ibid). The laws also required enforcement, something that police forces, many of which continued to espouse racist beliefs, were often reluctant or unwilling to do. You can learn more about the experiences of Black Americans from the 1619 Project (The 1619 Project, 2023).

Civil rights activists organized sit-ins, marches, boycotts, and other means of fighting for equal protection under the law. Again, the backlash was fierce, with many leaders arrested, incarcerated, or assassinated. More people behind bars meant more prison building, prison industry, and ultimately, more prison profits. Critical Resistance, a national organization founded by Civil Rights leader Angela Davis that works to challenge incarceration practices and imprisonment as a whole, uses the term **the Prison Industrial Complex** to describe "the overlapping interests of government and industry that use surveillance, policing, and imprisonment as solutions to economic, social, and political problems" (Critical Resistance, 2023).

What Do
YOU?
Think

- *In what ways has prison and incarceration been used as a means of social control?*

- *What impacts has that had on communities?*

In the 1980s, cities in the United States were undergoing an economic collapse due to a number of factors. The bold changes brought by the Civil Rights and other social movements of the 1960s were met with a backlash of new law-and-order rhetoric that appealed to racial fears. Ronald Reagan's highly racialized appeals to poor and working-class whites are exemplified in his false but often repeated story of a "Chicago welfare queen with 80 names, 30 addresses, and a tax-free income of $150,000" (Alexander, 2010, p. 48). At the top of his agenda was the "War on Drugs," a war "that had little to do with public concern about drugs and everything to do with public concern about race" (Ibid, p. 49). Under Reagan's tenure, the Anti-Drug Abuse Act was signed, instituting harsh penalties and "mandatory minimums" resulted in longer required sentences for drug possession.

George Bush Sr.'s political victory ushered in a tough-on-crime agenda, with the War on Drugs moved to center stage. Under his leadership, law enforcement budgets were higher than ever, and the prison population exploded.

Bill Clinton escalated what his Republican predecessors began, with a $30 billion crime bill that "resulted in the largest increase in federal and state prison inmates of any president in American history" (Guard, 2008). The bill mandated life sentences for some three-time offenders ("three strikes" laws) and created a number of new federal crimes that carried the death penalty. While false and racist (the "welfare queen" was almost always depicted as a Black woman, even though many poor whites relied heavily on welfare and social services to make ends meet), the rhetoric was extremely effective at generating the political will to effectively end social and welfare programs by imposing a five-year lifetime limit on welfare assistance. Meant to be a safety net to be used during difficult economic times, welfare became a much more restricted resource under Clinton. This approach led to skyrocketing incarceration rates in the 1990s through the early 2000s, with the vast majority of the new admissions to state prisons having been convicted of nonviolent, primarily drug-related offenses.

After decades of these policies and millions incarcerated, the United States finally started to address drug law reform. Laws such as the Fair Sentencing Act in 2010, which reduced sentencing disparity between crack and cocaine, started to address some of the drivers of mass incarceration. In 2014, Barak Obama launched a federal drug policy reform approach focused on prevention, treatment, and training, signaling a shift away from law enforcement and incarceration.

This shift started to align the United States more closely with many other countries across the world that promote access to treatment, counseling, and employment rather than punishment for what is broadly understood to be a medical and health issue. In the 1990s, Portugal stopped actively prosecuting drug use to focus on other criminal justice issues and provided community-based access to clean syringes and works, drug treatment, and other services (Szalavitz, 2009). As a result, incarceration rates fell dramatically. For many decades in Great Britain, heroin was dispensed to users under legal supervision; this model was adopted in other countries, and nowhere was there any indication that these policies led to higher rates of addiction (Maté, 2008, p. 322). More recently, Canada has implemented harm reduction strategies, such as safe injection sites and naloxone distribution centers, to decriminalize substance use and reduce overdoses and deaths (Health Canada, 2023).

More U.S. states are decriminalizing marijuana and other drugs, and in 2022, the House of Representatives introduced legislation that would have decriminalized marijuana at the federal level. While it has not yet passed, these moves do indicate a growing shift away from the War on Drugs, with a recognition that incarceration as a strategy for public safety has not been effective.

Despite the fact that the rates of drug use do not differ significantly by race, the burden of incarceration continues to fall disproportionately on members of racial and ethnic minorities, a disparity that cannot be accounted for solely by differences in criminal conduct. Black people constitute roughly 29% of drug arrests, 44% of persons convicted of drug felonies in state court, and 38% of people sent to state prison on drug charges, even though they make up only 13% of the U.S. population, and Blacks and whites engage in drug offenses at equivalent rates (Drug Policy Alliance, 2023; The Sentencing Project, 2021a).

In 2018, Black males were 3.6 times more likely to be arrested for marijuana possession than white males overall. Depending on the state, that number is even higher. In Montana, Black men are 9.6 times more likely to be arrested for marijuana possession than white males (American Civil Liberties Union, 2023). In 2019, the total prison rate in the United States was 419 per 100,000, but more than double (1096 per 100,000) for Black people incarcerated, 547 per 100,000 for Indigenous/Native Americans, and 525 per 100,000 for Latine/a/os. White people were incarcerated at a rate of only 214 per 100,000, well below the average overall and disproportionately low considering that white people make up approximately 75% of the U.S. population (U.S. Census, 2023).

The American prison system has developed into a system of social control unparalleled in history (Alexander, 2010). People of color face systematic discrimination across the criminal justice spectrum and are more likely to be searched, prosecuted, convicted, and sentenced to longer periods of incarceration (The Sentencing Project, 2021a). While Black people represent 13% of the U.S. population, they still comprise more than 38% of the overall prison population (Prison Policy Initiative, 2023). The lifetime chance of incarceration for Black men is 1 in 3, for Latino men, it is 1 in 6, and for white men, it is 1 in 23 (Ibid, 2021a). This pattern of systematic discrimination is similar to patterns discussed in Chapter 4 that highlight the ways in which people of color are denied equal access to safe housing, quality education, employment, civil rights, and other essential resources and rights.

While women of all races use drugs at approximately the same rate, Black women are incarcerated at twice the rate of white women and Indigenous women at three times the rate. In comparison, Latina women are incarcerated at 1.4 times the rate of white women and Asian women at 0.5 times the rate (The Sentencing Project, 2021b). The War on Drugs and its collateral consequences for people of color is far from over.

- *How has the War on Drugs affected communities that you belong to and/or work with?*

- *What percentage of people who are incarcerated in your city, county, or state are serving time for a drug-related crime?*

Age is a factor as well. Of all age groups, people under the age of 26 are most likely to be incarcerated (Smith, 2018). Like adults, youth of color experience what is known as "disproportionate minority contact," which means they are more likely than white youth to be surveilled and in contact with police, arrested and incarcerated due to racial, bias, sentenced to longer terms, and experience more punitive policies (Campaign for Youth Justice, 2023). This includes higher rates of disciplinary action taken in schools toward youth of color. Lack of knowledge about mental health, post-traumatic stress, and its symptoms can lead to labeling adolescents who are struggling as "delinquent" or "troublemakers." Some researchers and activists use the term "cradle to prison pipeline" or "school to prison pipeline" to describe ways that low-income youth and youth of color are funneled toward the prison system (American Civil Liberties Union, 2023).

While incarceration rates overall declined dramatically in the last 10 years, these reductions were largely the result of pandemic-related delays and practices, rather than significant long-term policy changes (Prison Policy Initiative, 2023).

Imprisonment on this scale is creating an under-caste of people who are locked up, and then locked out of mainstream society upon their return. Incarceration is widely accepted as a natural and normal part of society, and even promoted as a tool for public safety. But despite our beliefs, increased incarceration does not actually reduce crime. Addressing the social determinants of health does more to create safety and a reduction in crime (Stemen, 2017). In the next section, we will discuss the many health, social, and economic impacts of incarceration, on the individual, their families, and our communities and society as a whole. As we do, it is important to question the persistent societal belief that reliance on incarceration makes us safer.

15.3 The Health Impacts of Incarceration

Incarceration is recognized as a social determinant of health. In fact, incarceration operates as *both* a social determinant of health, and as a consequence of other social determinants including poverty, systemic racism, exclusion from access to education and health care, creating what is known as the "pipeline to prison" for low-income communities of color (Hemez, Brent, & Mowen, 2020; National Research Council, 2013).

As much as prisons are designed to create a literal wall between people in prison and the rest of society, those inside are nevertheless part of the broader community. More than 9 million people are released from jails and prisons each year, and just as their absence profoundly affects those left behind, their return affects the community as well (Pacific Broadcasting Network, 2023b). This is a population that had a higher rate of chronic disease than the general population before going to prison. Substandard medical care while incarcerated means that people often return home with deteriorated health (National Research Council, 2013). Approximately 80% of those returning home have a mental health, chronic disease, or substance abuse issue, and the vast majority have little access to primary care (National Alliance on Mental Illness, 2023; National Institute on Drug Abuse, 2020).

In many states, people are released from prison without medication prescriptions or adequate referrals, making it difficult to access medical care and continue to take necessary medications. Experiences of discrimination and substandard care while incarcerated also lead many to have an understandable mistrust of the health care system, creating yet another barrier to accessing care. Most importantly, they come home to a society which, through social stigma and policy, creates nearly insurmountable barriers to a safe return. This reality challenges a commonly held belief in our society—we are taught that incarceration is a means of repaying a debt to society. In reality, people who experience incarceration continue to be impacted and punished for years through the collateral effects on their health, well-being, and ability to be employed, housed, and receive care.

Please watch the following video interview ▶ with Donna Willmott, a contributor to this chapter. She talks about the importance of understanding mass incarceration as a public health issue:

INCARCERATION AS A PUBLIC HEALTH ISSUE.

(*Source:* Foundations for Community Health Workers/ http://youtu.be/ o7AdDUAyu54)

HEALTH CONDITIONS IN JAILS AND PRISONS

People in prison have higher rates of chronic illness, including mental health conditions, than the general population. Lack of proper diet, fresh air, and exercise can exacerbate many chronic illnesses. People who are incarcerated live with a fairly constant level of stress from the prison environment itself, and the emotional stress of separation from loved ones takes an additional toll on their health. As discussed in Chapters 12 and 16, research evidence demonstrates that prolonged exposure to stress is a key cause of chronic disease and of inequities in rates of illness and death among populations. Additionally, it is estimated that at least 10% of the prison population is 55 years or older (Prison Policy Initiative, 2023). As people in prison age, their health problems worsen, leading to increased disease and premature death. People with physical and/ or developmental disabilities, whether they came into the prison disabled or became disabled while incarcerated, also experience barriers to accessible and quality care.

Rates of human immunodeficiency virus (HIV) disease and hepatitis C virus (HCV) are significantly higher among incarcerated populations (Spaulding, 2023; Centers for Disease Control and Prevention, 2022). Although risks for HIV and HCV infection occur in prison through the reuse of needles in injection drug use and tattooing, and consensual and nonconsensual sex, the vast majority of men in prison living with HIV disease were infected in community settings (Ibid). The high rates of infection in incarcerated populations reflect the fact that the majority of people inside come from impoverished and disenfranchised communities with limited access to prevention, screening, and treatment services. These same communities have the highest rates of HIV, HCV, sexually transmitted infections (STIs), and other infections on the outside. Most recently, COVID-19 transmission inside jails and prisons was more than four times higher than in the general population, and people experiencing incarceration were more than twice as likely to die from COVID-19 (COVID Prison Project, 2021; National Commission on COVID-19 and Criminal Justice, 2021).

In prison and jail settings drug use, tattooing, and sexual activity are all punishable offenses in most facilities. Harm reduction practices such as provision of condoms, clean needles, and even masks are rarely sanctioned, thus thwarting attempts to further prevent infection by people themselves inside prison and jails.

Prison medical care is generally far below the community standard; treatment is often delayed and inadequate, there is very little follow-up, and preventative care is almost nonexistent. Prison health care is further compromised by inadequate staffing, lack of resources, and insufficient training for medical staff (National Research Council, 2013). Even though people who are incarcerated have a long-established Constitutional right to health care, many institutions are not in compliance with the law. For example, the California Department of Corrections and Rehabilitation was under court-ordered receivership from 2005 to 2013 because of "an unconscionable degree of suffering and death" resulting in an average of one needless death per week in its prisons (California Correctional Health Care Services, 2021; Plata v. Schwarzenegger, 2005). The privatization of medical care in nearly half of U.S. facilities has also contributed to poor quality health care that leaves people who experience incarceration with compromised health.

In addition to a lack of access to quality medical care, people in prison often experience long delays in receiving treatment and prescribed medications. People who require regular medication for seizures, high blood pressure, heart disease, diabetes, Hepatitis C, HIV, and other conditions can find their chronic condition becoming unmanageable.

Sam's Story (Told by CHW Joe Calderon)

Sam was a man who we all watched on the [prison] yard get sicker and sicker day by day. As we saw Sam get sicker, many of us asked our electronics teacher (where Sam was also a student) and Sam's cellmate (cellie) how he was doing. Sam's cellie told us he could hear Sam struggling to breathe at night. Sam had pleaded for medical treatment a multitude of times without receiving care. Sam's cellie and electronics teacher also advocated for Sam to receive medical attention.

Sam died. In some ways, Sam was killed by medical indifference, drowning in his own fluids. He was so weak he couldn't call out for help as his lungs filled and he could no longer breathe.

While Sam's name has been changed, I saw this unfold with my own eyes. Why is a story like this so important when we think about medical incarceration and reentry?

Stories like this explain what is often a healthy mistrust of systems that returning community members experience. It's important for CHWs to understand the healthy mistrust of systems that some of the clients they work with will have.

- *How would you approach a client who told you such a story and shared that they were afraid to go to the doctor?*

Experience with substandard medical care in prison often makes it more difficult for people to access health care services after they have been released. People who have been incarcerated may expect to be treated poorly by health care professionals in any setting, and this may lead to delaying or avoiding medical attention when in need. A key role of CHWs and other frontline providers is to help ensure that formerly incarcerated clients are supported in their efforts to access quality health.

Charisse Shumate, a co-founder of the California Coalition for Women Prisoners who was sentenced to 16 years in prison, helped to organize a legislative hearing in 2011 on health care conditions and access for incarcerated women. Despite the risk of retaliation, these courageous women spoke directly to California lawmakers about the conditions they experienced in prison. The footage, available through the Freedom Archives, provides harrowing and powerful testimony about the medical neglect and cruelty they experienced (Freedom Archives, 2023).

IMMIGRATION DETENTION

Migration has always been a part of the human experience—people have migrated with and without permission (or documentation) for survival, food, opportunity, freedom, safety, and other reasons. Ellis Island and the Statue of Liberty are visible symbols of a United States that welcomes immigrants, but the reality is much different. As borders were created and solidified, the question of who belongs and who does not has shifted due in large part to racism. Activists have drawn attention to this reality with slogans such as "No Human is Illegal" and "We didn't cross the border, the border crossed us." Yet every day, low-income people of color are detained and confined in facilities for the crime of being undocumented.

Over 230,000 people were booked into immigration detention facilities in 2021 in highly restrictive conditions, even though most have no criminal records (U.S. Immigration and Customs Enforcement, 2021). Of the almost 2 million people detained in crowded, often freezing-cold immigration detention facilities from February 2017 through June 2021, more than 650,000 were under the age of 18 (Flagg & Preston, 2022).

People are confined with little access to their families or outside legal support, and often receive substandard medical and mental health care. As a result, their health can deteriorate very quickly (Physicians for Human Rights, 2021). Sexual and physical abuse often goes unreported, and people detained in immigration facilities are frequently abused and threatened with not being able to see their family members again if they complain or report. Because many of these facilities are private, there is a lack of oversight or accountability for abuses occurring there.

People in immigration detention centers also encounter language barriers (no access to guards who speak their language), limited access to legal assistance, law libraries, and the criminalization of their families who cannot visit because of their own immigration status.

MENTAL HEALTH

As social services have been cut across the United States, and mental illness and homelessness have become increasingly criminalized and jails and prisons have become the primary psychiatric facilities in the United States. More than 383,000 people with severe mental illnesses are admitted to U.S. jails and prisons every year (Torrey, Kennard, Eslinger, Lamb, & Pavle, 2010). Approximately three out of four people who are incarcerated have a history of substance abuse (Bronson, Stroop, & Zimmer, 2020). Mass incarceration is directly linked to our failure to develop sound public policies that provide access to quality and affordable mental health and drug treatment services to those in need. Moreover, traumas experienced from the conditions of confinement and prison are likely to exacerbate pre-existing traumatic experiences and post-traumatic stress, leading to worsening mental health and long-lasting negative impacts.

Survivors of trauma often suffer from traumatic stress (see Chapter 18) and increased risks for suicide. Solitary confinement units often induce psychosis, especially in those who have histories of mental illness or a predisposition to psychiatric breakdown. Those in solitary confinement are eight times more likely to commit suicide than those housed in the general prison population, and the risk of suicide remains even after they are released from solitary confinement (Haney, 2018).

When treatment services are available in jails and prisons, their quality is often questionable. A community standard of psychological counseling and therapy is virtually unheard of in most jails and prisons, and most people with serious mental health problems who are incarcerated leave prison more damaged than when they entered. Additionally, confinement is inherently traumatic, involving loss of connection to family and community, loss of control over even one's most basic functions, and exposure to violence, sexual abuse, and other factors. Punishment is inherently at odds with healing, and in an environment where punishment remains the dominant frame, the efficacy of any program's healing ability is limited by the constant traumatic nature of the conditions in which it exists.

SOCIAL CONDITIONS IN PRISON

Contrary to the commonly promoted notion that prison is a place of rehabilitation, the culture of prison is designed to diminish a person's self-worth. All privacy is denied, as is any control over the most mundane aspects of life: when and what to eat, when to make a phone call or take a shower, when to read a book, when to have a conversation with another person. Budget crisis and extremely overcrowded prison facilities have led to the dismantling of most meaningful educational and vocational programs, as well as drug treatment programs.

In many prisons, fear defines day-to-day existence, leading to a kind of hyper-vigilance that is carried over once released to the community. Many people in prison work hard to develop a "prison mask," cultivating an ability to hide their feelings, sometimes at risk of extreme alienation, from themselves and others. People have to face isolation, literally and psychologically, from family, friends, and community as part of incarceration. The fracturing of these bonds contributes to depression and makes reintegration into the community a significant challenge.

Women are one of the fastest-growing groups of incarcerated people in the United States—as of 2021, there were approximately 231,000 women in jails and prisons throughout the United States (The Sentencing Project, 2021b). These women face additional problems. A government study revealed that a majority of women in state prison (59%) reported a history of physical or sexual abuse (Noonan, Rohloff, & Ginder, 2013). The environment of most women's prisons extends that history of abuse. Women in prison are subject to strip searches, pat searches by male guards, and degrading and sexually explicit language from guards on a daily basis. This sexualized environment contributes to worsening mental health and post-traumatic stress disorder (PTSD) for many women, especially those who are survivors of violence and abuse. In the words of one woman, "the prison just took up where my abusive boyfriend left off" (Ibid). Very few prisons offer support or treatment for survivors of trauma.

Dorel Clayton (North Carolina Transitions Clinic): Prison isn't somewhere to get sick: bad care, and people who don't care!

Transgender, gender-nonconforming, and intersex people in prison are visible targets for homophobic and transphobic discrimination and abuse within prisons by the administration, guards, and others incarcerated there. Prisons are sex-segregated; authorities typically house people according to their birth-assigned sex and/or genitalia, and often refuse to recognize their gender identities. While some transgender people in prisons may choose to be isolated in protective custody, many are isolated against their will. Regardless of placement, transgender people who are incarcerated report being subjected to humiliation, verbal harassment, sexual and physical assault, and rape: 23% reported being physically assaulted, and 20% reported sexual assault (James et al., 2016). In addition to being subjected to the inadequate medical care suffered by most people in prison, transgender people are often denied hormones and other related treatments that affirm their gender identity (McCauley et al., 2018).

15.4 The Impact of Incarceration on Families and Communities

The multi-generational impacts of mass incarceration reverberate in our communities. The war on drugs has taken a particular toll on the health and well-being of whole families as more and more women are removed from the community. While incarceration rates for men have started to decline, the number of incarcerated women has increased by 450% in the last 40 years, and women are the fastest-growing group of people experiencing incarceration (Dholakia, 2021).

As of 2020, 2.7 million children in the United States had a parent in prison, leaving them at risk for entering the foster care system; 70% were children of color and two-thirds of the parents were incarcerated for nonviolent offenses (Annie E. Casey Foundation, 2016; The Pew Charitable Trust, 2021). The human cost of the War on Drugs is beyond calculation: families are torn apart, human potential is wasted, and whole communities are permanently marginalized and excluded from participation in society.

Families are affected financially and emotionally when someone is in prison. As a society, we recognize that children who grow up with safety and stability have a better chance to become healthy adults, but we fail to recognize that the criminal justice system often undermines this likelihood. Children of incarcerated parents suffer humiliation and shame. They often experience feelings of loss, abandonment, and extreme anxiety, and these feelings are more prominent when incarcerated parents are not able to see their children—a situation that holds true for many women in prison (Annie E. Casey Foundation, 2016).

Maintaining family ties through phone calls and visiting makes it much less likely that the parent will return to prison and in most cases is a benefit to the children's sense of well-being.

Testimonial: Jessica Calderon-Mitchell

Electric gates, barbed wire, and high towers making their appearance in my line of vision. Prisons are ominous.

I remember being a child walking into a visitation center: demanding correctional officers, scuffed linoleum, anxiety-riddled families, and the loud clanging of change machines. Everything in me would be shaking but I had to be calm, collected, and aware. I would be scared the outfit my Mom and I put together would not fit the bill to make it into my visit despite it being meticulously planned out the night before. I would feel paranoia as I walked through the metal detector, scared something prohibited would magically appear in my pockets even though I knew there was nothing. It felt like I was a prisoner too. A child shouldn't have to feel that way to see their parent; it is unnatural and unnecessary. Children and families are casualties to the Prison Industrial Complex.

While everyone else is scared of who resides in prisons, I was scared of the actual prison System. The way grips, grabs, rips, and tears through families.

All we want is to feel the hug of our loved one in the visiting room (preferably in the outside world). All I wanted was to play board games with my Mom and Dad to roleplay some sense of normalcy. I could pretend to be the nuclear family from the confines of a visiting room. It was pure magic for as long as we were allowed. It is precious, precious time. The long excited wait for my Dad to enter the room, the laughs, and good bye hugs will forever be imprinted in my brain.

Many children in Jessica Calderon-Mitchell's situation lose the relationship to their parents forever. The Federal Adoption and Safe Families Act mandates that any parent who has not had custody of their child for 15 out of the previous 22 months can have their parental rights automatically terminated, forever breaking family bonds. The children are subject to placement in foster care if no relative who is judged suitable is able to take custody of them while their parent is imprisoned.

These policies mean that Black and Latine/a/o children are much more likely to lose family ties and become wards of the state. It also means that many Black and Latino men are physically removed from their communities—their relationships, connections to family, ability to earn, and income are all stripped away. The intergenerational ability of families then to develop wealth and stability is deeply impacted, all while perpetuating racist stereotypes about these men and their absence from their families and communities.

"By taking children from their imprisoned parents on a permanent basis, simply because they are imprisoned, we have effectively transformed parental incarceration into a mechanism for permanent family disintegration and dissolution" (Drucker, 2011). The failure of child protective agencies to actually protect children whose parents are caught in the system is well publicized. Individuals who are in foster care experience higher rates of physical and mental health problems than the general population and suffer from not being able to trust (Greeson et al., 2011). This cycle puts children at an increased risk of incarceration themselves as they are more at risk for adverse childhood experiences including exposure to trauma, school suspension and discipline, and more (Martin, 2017).

Antonio's Story

When I was four years old, my mother started doing drugs. She used to be in and out of jail, and then she started going to prison when I was seven years old. That's when I first got taken from her. Her friends took me to social services, dropped me off, and left me there.

I've been in about 18 different group homes since then, and three or four foster homes. I don't care how bad whatever we were going through, I still wanted to be with my mom … One foster home I was in, I called the lady my grandmother, "cause she took care of me. She always made sure that I got in touch with my mom. Even if my mom was locked up and tryin" to call collect, she could call there. My grandmother knew that mattered in my life.

The other places, they didn't care. There were only a couple of people that I lived with that actually took me to see my mom.

In the group homes, they knew my mom was in jail and they would just tell me, "Oh, it's gonna be alright." But they don't know how I feel because they're not going through it.

(San Francisco Children of Incarcerated Parents Partnership, 2005)

More and more grandparents are raising grandchildren while their own children are incarcerated, straining their finances and taxing their own health. Relative caregivers often receive less financial support than foster parents who are unrelated; sometimes they receive no support at all. Many seniors live on the edge financially, and assuming full responsibility for their grandchildren can drive the entire family deeper into poverty.

Client Scenario: Eddy

You are in the process of getting to know a new client, Eddy. Over the course of several meetings, he has gradually opened up to you. In a previous meeting, Eddy told you about the challenge of controlling his high blood pressure and about recent difficulties with his longtime girlfriend, Brigitte, and alienation from his family.

(continues)

Client Scenario: Eddy

(continued)

You feel good about the rapport you are building with this new client. You appreciate his sense of humor, his ability to discuss relationship challenges, and his determination to better manage his high blood pressure and to take care of his health in general.

Today, Eddy tells you that he is transgender. *"I figured I should tell you cuz it's kind of related to the stuff we've been talking about."* Eddy has been taking testosterone for about six months and is happy with the results. He explains, *"I just feel more like me. I look more like me and I just don't have the same problems with passing [being perceived as his true gender identity] any more—I think, I may be wrong, that people just see me as a man now."*

However, Eddy's physician is worried about the link between taking Testosterone and his high blood pressure: *"I mean, yeah, it's getting worse I guess, the blood pressure. But even if the testosterone is causing it to go up, I've read different things about this, and, basically, using testosterone is still so worth it to me. I tried to explain and maybe I didn't do too well, but I don't think she (the physician) understands where I'm coming from."*

Eddy also tells you: *"My girlfriend—she's been having a real hard time with the transition. You know, she says I've changed, and I have, and it's confusing for her. We've just been fighting more and more, and I'm scared she's gonna leave me...."*

Eddy has also lost contact with most of his family: *"My mom will still talk on the phone, but only if my Dad's not home. To him, I guess, I don't exist anymore."*

- *What strengths or health resources does Eddy have?*
- *How might you approach working with Eddy to promote his health and wellness?*
- *How will cultural humility influence your work?*
- *How will you approach working with Eddy's doctor?*

Most people coming home from jail or prison return to communities that suffer the impacts of racism and poverty. They experience the lack of affordable housing, inadequate educational opportunities, and high unemployment rates. While all people living in poverty suffer these conditions, people who have experienced incarceration face additional challenges including the stigma of incarceration and the many legal barriers to reentry. These interlocking barriers have a profound impact on the family and the community at large. They create instability, homelessness, and unemployment; they make family reunification difficult and increase the likelihood that families will remain fractured. For immigrant families, parental incarceration may mean permanent separation with no possibility of direct contact between parents and children in the future. These policies make it harder for people to stay clean and sober, and to resist returning to illegal activity to support themselves. Parents who want to reunify with their children often find themselves caught in a vicious cycle, defeated in their efforts to rebuild their families.

Incarceration impacts the entire community in the form of broad-scale economic hardships and destabilization, increased risk of exposure to disease, and weakened social networks. High incarceration rates take an economic toll on the whole community, a phenomenon referred to as the collateral consequences. Imprisonment means a loss of income to the family left behind and reduces the future earnings of people newly released from prison whose prospects for employment are diminished. Even a short stay in jail can lead to loss of a job or home. For many years, incarceration was regarded first and foremost as a criminal justice issue. But as the negative social effects of increasingly harsh sentencing policies become more evident, mass incarceration is also recognized as a public health issue, and a significant social determinant of health. Policies that were supposed to create public safety have in fact brought extreme economic hardship and social instability to communities most affected. These policies have dramatically increased the existing health inequities based on race, gender, and socio-economic status.

In this way, the costs or consequences of incarceration continue well beyond the sentence itself and perpetuate discrimination and inequity not just for the person who was incarcerated but for their families and communities as well.

- *Can you think of other ways that incarceration harms families and communities?*

- *How has incarceration impacted the communities that you belong to and/or work with?*

What Do YOU? Think

15.5 The Challenges of Reentry or Coming Home

Once you are labeled a felon, the old forms of discrimination—employment discrimination, housing discrimination, denial of the right to vote, denial of educational opportunity, denial of food stamps and other public benefits, and exclusion from jury service are suddenly legal. As a criminal, you have scarcely more rights ... than a black man living in Alabama at the height of Jim Crow. We have not ended racial caste in America, we have merely redesigned it. (Alexander, 2011, pp. 2)

As people return home from prison with the intention of rebuilding their lives and reuniting with their families and communities, they face systemic legal barriers. Accessing basic needs such as stable housing, employment, and benefits becomes a major hurdle once a person has been convicted, especially of a drug-related offense. These post-conviction penalties are not part of anyone's original sentence; they are additional, enduring discriminatory punishments that often contribute to **recidivism** or return to jail or prison. On the one hand, policy makers urge people who have experienced incarceration to reintegrate themselves into society, and on the other hand, public policies create significant barriers to successful reintegration.

HOUSING

People who are released from jail or prison, especially those returning to their communities after a lengthy sentence, face a very basic challenge of where to live. There are few programs and services that connect those recently released from jail or prison to housing. Many people on parole are sent to transitional homes located in communities that are also struggling with substance use, poverty, and lack of stable and affordable housing, creating more challenges for those recently released.

Public policies discriminate against people who have experienced incarceration, making it more difficult for them to find and maintain a stable home. The federal "one strike" housing policy bans anyone with a drug-related or violent offense from living in Section 8 or other federally assisted housing, and the entire family can be evicted if a family member with a history of incarceration is found living there. In reality, this means that some people are forced to abandon their children or partners or risk eviction and becoming homeless. While public housing authorities can make case-by-case decisions, the threat of losing housing is devastating to families. Many landlords now ask about incarceration history on housing applications and, because of social stigma, are more likely to choose tenants without prior convictions. Often, homeless shelters will not allow someone with certain types of offenses to stay, leaving them no option but to live on the streets. Without the possibility of stable housing, it's very difficult for people returning home to rebuild their lives.

> ### Client Scenario: Ahn
>
> Consider the case of Ahn, who is coming home from prison after seven years. His family lives in Section 8 housing, so he can't stay with them. As a condition of his parole, he is not allowed to associate with other parolees or people with felony convictions. So he can't live at home, and he can't stay with many of his friends.
>
> *(continues)*

Client Scenario: Ahn

(continued)

Ahn stays in shelters and couch surfs here and there, but has no stable housing. Without stable housing, he has nowhere to receive mail or phone calls, so he is having trouble getting calls back from potential employers. Because he doesn't have stable housing, he has nowhere to keep his clothes, so they are wrinkled and he shows up for job interviews and parole meetings disheveled. Keeping track of appointments is more difficult, and he has a hard time staying connected with his family, who are scared to even have him over since they fear it will put their housing at risk.

- *What other factors in Ahn's life and reentry are affected by this discriminatory housing policy?*

EMPLOYMENT

People with a history of incarceration often have difficulty finding work, sometimes because there are legal prohibitions against their employment and sometimes because employers are reluctant to hire someone with a criminal record. Many states will not allow someone with a conviction to work in certain jobs; this is especially true in the areas of health care, education, and childcare. With diminished access to employment opportunities, people's ability to earn a living wage is diminished, creating another significant barrier to building a stable and secure life.

The Fair Chance to Compete for Jobs Act of 2019 is a federal "ban the box" initiative that aims to remove the "box" on a job application form that asks if you've ever been convicted of a felony. This box has been a major barrier to employment for those with a prior conviction (National Employment Law Project, 2021). Additionally, in large part due to the organizing efforts of people who have experienced incarceration, 150 cities and 37 states have taken steps to remove this barrier. While this initiative is an important step toward addressing employment discrimination, barriers to licensing and other certifications still exist, limiting people with conviction histories from many types of employment.

PUBLIC BENEFITS AND AID

In 1998, Congress passed a law banning Federal loans to students who were convicted of selling or possessing illegal drugs, further restricting access to education. For people newly released from prison who are trying to further their education after their release, this is yet another barrier to creating a stable and productive life. Given the disproportionate number of people of color in prisons, this policy had a significant and adverse impact on educational opportunities for low-income students and students of color. Thankfully, this ban was lifted in 2020, reinstating access to Pell grants for people in prison.

In 1996, the federal government passed a lifetime ban on Temporary Assistance to Needy Families (TANF) and food stamps for people with felony drug convictions regardless of their rehabilitation and recovery. States were permitted to opt out of the ban, and by 2020, all U.S. states had either modified or removed the ban entirely.

DISENFRANCHISEMENT

While there has been a recent trend toward reinstating voting rights for some people convicted of felonies, the practice of stripping people indefinitely of these rights is still practiced in 11 states, and in 14 states, people with a felony conviction still lose their right to vote for an extended period of time (National Conference of State Legislatures, 2023). This is far from the norm in other countries, like Germany, that actively encourage people returning home to vote as an important factor for promoting successful reintegration into society.

Michelle Alexander writes:

> *If shackling former prisoners with a lifetime of debt and authorizing discrimination against them in employment, housing, education and public benefits is not enough to send the message that they are not wanted and not considered full citizens, then stripping voting rights from those labeled criminals surely gets the point across. (Alexander, 2010, pp. 153)*

FAMILY REUNIFICATION

One of the most common and important goals for people who have experienced incarceration is to rebuild relationships with their families. While many are successful, others struggle to reconnect. The children of incarcerated parents are often deeply affected by the experience and may wrestle with feelings of confusion, anger, fear, and distrust. Formerly incarcerated parents may be affected by lasting guilt and doubts about how to reconnect and rebuild trust with their children.

Parents who go to prison are at risk of losing their children permanently because of the Adoption and Safe Families Act. It's important to remember that children and parents are both harmed when families are torn apart, and that most children want to maintain a relationship with their parents, even under difficult circumstances.

Many parents owe child support to the government for the period of time when their children are in foster care, and newly released parents can find themselves in overwhelming debt. On average, about 25% of parents leaving prison in debt, owing back child support payments. Since their wages will be garnished when they find a job, this policy drives many people into the underground economy (Prison Policy Initiative, 2023).

There is a need for community-based services and programs that support families scarred by incarceration to build and sustain healthier relationships.

Please watch the following digital story ▶ about the journey that one man took from prison to establishing a career as a CHW:

- *What did you learn from Emory's story?*
- *How may Emory's story inform or influence your work as a CHW?*

EMORY'S STORY. (*Source:* Foundations for Community Health Workers/ http://youtu.be/ oSx1OPt6r8M)

STIGMA AND DISCRIMINATION

In some ways, the systemic barriers to reentry after incarceration are not the worst part of coming home from prison. For many, it's the social stigma and discrimination that comes with being labeled "criminal"—a kind of social exile that can become a permanent exclusion from the rest of the community. As a society, we are bombarded with negative, highly racialized images of incarcerated people that create a pervasive sense of suspicion and automatic distrust of someone who has done prison time. Michelle Alexander describes this with painful accuracy:

> *Criminals, it turns out, are the one social group in America we have permission to hate. In 'colorblind' America, criminals are the new whipping boys. They are entitled to no respect and little moral concern … criminals today are deemed a characterless and purposeless people, deserving of our collective scorn and contempt … Hundreds of years ago our nation put those considered less than human in shackles; less than a hundred years ago, we relegated them to the other side of town; today we put them in cages. Once released, they find that a heavy and cruel hand has been laid upon them. (Alexander, 2010, pp. 138)*

People who have experienced incarceration often report profound isolation. This feeling of being permanently exiled by housing officials, employers, neighbors, and sometimes family members is described this way:

> *The shame and stigma that follows you for the rest of your life—that is the worst. It is not just the job denial but the look that flashes across the face of a potential employer when he notices that 'the box' has been checked—the way he suddenly refuses to look you in the eye. It is not merely the denial of the housing application but the shame of being a grown man who has to beg his grandmother for a place to sleep at night. It is not simply the denial of the right to vote but the shame one feels when a co-worker innocently asks, 'Who you gonna vote for on Tuesday?' (Alexander, 2010, pp. 157)*

The stigma and social isolation attached to imprisonment often create a deep sense of shame and self-hatred that is experienced not only by the person returning home, but by their family as well. Fear of negative stereotypes and judgments can lead to silence and the denial of prison experience. Family members sometimes feel they have to lie about the whereabouts of an incarcerated loved one to avoid the negative judgments of teachers, ministers, friends, and neighbors. This collective silence makes true reintegration and healing nearly impossible.

In this context, the role of a culturally sensitive CHW becomes critical. By refusing to reinforce such stigma, by providing nondiscriminatory care to people who have experienced incarceration, CHWs can be part of creating a different, more inclusive culture that does not demonize an entire population and reaffirms the humanity of people who have been to prison.

CHW Profile

Lorena Carmona, She/Her
Community Health Worker and Program Manager
Roots Community Health Center, Oakland, California
Low-Income Communities of Color

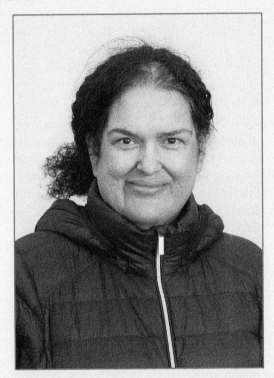

My biggest motivation for becoming a CHW is the time in my life when I faced a lot of barriers, especially returning home from a 10-and-a-half year sentence in prison. I didn't know how to navigate my reentry into society. I didn't have a job or a resume. I didn't know how to interview for a job. There was no one to guide me. I don't want people returning home or anybody to go through what I went through. I want to be a person who supports others, who welcomes them, shows them the ropes, and connects them to services.

I work for Roots Community Health Center in Oakland, California. I'm a navigation manager and I supervise a team of CHWs. We provide comprehensive primary health care, behavioral health, and social services including workforce enterprise and training. We also provide street medicine with a mobile health van.

I serve predominantly African Americans and Latinx communities, people who are unhoused, displaced, and marginalized. I am bilingual and work with English and Spanish-speaking clients. I work with folks who are using drugs and alcohol, who have diabetes, hypertension, and other chronic illnesses. I help clients access primary health care and to learn how to manage their chronic health conditions. I provide ongoing case management services and referrals to other service providers.

(continues)

CHW Profile

(continued)

As a Program Manager, I supervise a team of 12 CHWs. I help them enroll in local CHW certificate programs and provide on-the-job training. I support them to ensure that their work with clients is grounded in cultural humility.

I worked with a client just out of prison. He was paroled and confined to a wheelchair. He had hypertension, diabetes, and was on oxygen. His biggest fear was public transportation. We worked with him and created a health action plan to improve his health and get out of his wheelchair. After two years, he's mobile, he's walking. He went through health education classes to help with his diabetes and hypertension, and his health conditions are under control. He was able to get his driver's license, a car, and a job. Today, he's in the process of getting permanent housing, which was his end goal. He even got involved doing community advocacy work and is paid a stipend for interpreting for the Spanish-speaking community. When I look at him today, it warms my heart knowing that he fought the odds. He always thanks us, and I tell him: "It wasn't us, it was YOU- you did the work."

Even though my life is great now, when I sit in front of someone who needs housing or food, it makes me humble and reminds me of where I come from. It inspires me to do this work with my whole heart. You don't know how far a person can go. Everybody just needs a little help. If I can provide that help, it moves me 100%.

For CHWs just starting out, don't forget to ask questions. Remember that you have a team behind you. Don't feel like you have to solve all the problems on your own; that's not what a CHW does. Some of the CHWs in my program get frustrated with themselves because they can't help someone find housing. But I tell them that's okay, you're filling out the housing application and putting them on a waiting list is one step closer to getting housing. There's so much stress in this job and the risk for burnout is so real. I remind other CHWs to consider their self-care. With my team, I tell them if it's getting overwhelming, walk away from the computer, take a break, and do something to take care of yourself.

15.6 The Role of CHWs

Being released from prison is a highly vulnerable time. People newly released from prison are much more likely to die than members of the general public in the first two weeks after release. The principal causes of death include drug overdose, cardiovascular disease, homicide, and suicide. A recent study in North Carolina found that people recently released from prison are 40 times more likely to die from opiate overdoses than the general public (Ranapurwala et al., 2018).

> **Ron Sanders:** Basically, it's scary getting out. You have nowhere to go; you have $200 if you have that. It's scary. And if they make it to us [The San Francisco Transitions Clinic], we make sure we take care of them. It's a long road between San Quentin and San Francisco; there's a lot in between here and there.

Unemployment, lack of education, poverty, unstable housing, substance abuse, PTSD, depression, and other chronic health conditions are some of the challenges faced by people released from jail or prison. The transition from prison to community can be emotionally overwhelming as people begin to readjust and rebuild relationships, especially with family members. To compound the situation, people who have been incarcerated face stigma as well as the multiple systemic barriers to rebuilding their lives. The immediate struggle for survival often takes precedence over other concerns.

For many people, these competing priorities mean accessing health care falls to the bottom of the list. Because they are trusted members of local communities, CHWs play an important role in creating a supportive reentry process, as well as advocating for policy and health care reform to support the health and well-being of people who have been incarcerated. Many CHWs have first-hand knowledge of the impacts of incarceration, and many are already serving people who have experienced incarceration and their families. This experience puts them in a unique position to help someone transitioning from prison to the community and is a strength and an asset. People who have experienced incarceration can relate to CHWs as people who have "been there, done that," whose similar life experiences and roots in the community help to establish a trust that may not be there otherwise.

FIRST MEETING BETWEEN A PATIENT AND CHW. (*Source:* Foundations for Community Health Workers/ http://youtu.be/ OrfXKN8lgxA)

Ideally, this work starts even before a client leaves the prison: CHWs can support discharge planning and help smooth the transition from prison to the community. As a CHW, you will play a key role in your clients' reentry, by providing a bridge to services and support, informal counseling and social support, direct services and referrals, culturally relevant health education, advocacy, assurance, and capacity-building.

Please watch the following video ▶ of a CHW talking with a client about the first time they met, shortly after she was released from prison:

Ron Sanders: We know where they come from; we've been there, done that. We also know the barriers, the doors closing on you ... We've faced those same barriers, and we've overcome them. [Our clients] respect the realness, they respect the dignity, they're not a number.

Juanita Alvarado: Having that connection [inside and outside prison] is important. We write our patients [before they get out]; we have somebody who works inside San Quentin. Just seeing that friendly face inside the prison, then seeing us here, in the field, that's comforting to them. They see our faces all over the place. They know that we're going to make that appointment for them when they get out and help them take steps to be successful ... it makes them feel like they're cared about, truly cared about. They're not just a number, not just another parolee coming out. People make mistakes; it's OK to make mistakes ... we're not here to judge.

As a CHW, you are likely to be one of the strongest bridges between a client and the social support necessary to rebuild a life after prison. For example, many people returning home come to the health care system with a great deal of distrust and anxiety. By working with a client respectfully and treating them with dignity, you can lay the basis for a relationship of trust with new health care and other service providers.

A CHW WITH A HISTORY OF INCARCERATION. (*Source:* Foundations for Community Health Workers/ http://youtu.be/ PfBJ9GCvkKk)

Please watch the following video ▶ interview with a CHW who has a history of incarceration talking about his work with clients who are coming home from prison:

A culturally humble CHW who approaches a person coming home with respect, compassion, and a nonjudgmental stance can make a significant difference. One formerly incarcerated person described their positive experience with a health provider:

Just to have someone who wasn't afraid to be in the same room with me, who wasn't afraid to touch me, who didn't judge me, made me feel like I wanted to come back. The doctor I saw in prison wore a mask and gloves the whole time, even though I wasn't contagious. He sat behind his desk and refused to touch me, even though I had a lump on my breast Anonymous. (Willmott, personal communication.)

> **Juanita Alvarado:** One [patient] was in the hospital, and we were right there. They didn't have any family, they didn't have anybody. We were there. And we're right there when they go back to jail; we're there visiting them. We're the ones they can call.
>
> **Ron Sanders:** I have two words [for CHWs working with people returning home from prison]: passion and genuine. If you're not genuine, they'll read you in a heartbeat and turn straight off on you. They won't even deal with you if they feel you're not genuine and you don't care and it's just a job to you. You have to really care, and you have to have passion.

UNDERSTANDING YOUR OWN VALUES AND BELIEFS

Our values and beliefs influence our interactions with others and the services we provide. In order to effectively serve formerly incarcerated clients, it is essential to reflect on your own beliefs about people experiencing incarceration and the prison system. This is particularly important because we are all constantly exposed to negative, racialized images of people in prison that paint a biased picture of crime and the criminal justice system. Sometimes we fail to notice when we are making biased assumptions that are based on our own experiences and values. Learning to practice cultural humility means identifying our own challenges in working with people who have experienced incarceration and addressing the negative stereotypes and beliefs we have internalized.

Take a few minutes to consider the following questions and to reflect upon your answers:

- *What images and thoughts come to mind when you think about people who have been to prison?*
- *Do you have certain expectations about the behavior of people who have been in prison? Where do those expectations come from?*
- *How do you feel about the idea of working with formerly incarcerated clients? If you knew what your client was in prison for, would that influence your ability to provide compassionate and unbiased service? Would it vary according to the offense they were convicted of? If so, why?*
- *Do you have personal experience with the prison system (yourself, a friend, or family member)? If so, how did this experience impact the person who was incarcerated? How did it impact their family?*
- *What are your beliefs about the ability of a formerly incarcerated person to create a positive and meaningful life? What are your beliefs about the types of contributions that people who have experienced incarceration can make to their community?*
- *What can you do to increase your knowledge and skills in order to work effectively with formerly incarcerated clients?*

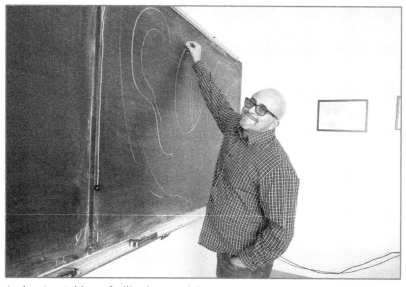

Author Joe Calderon facilitating a training on Reentry.

MAKE CONSCIOUS CHOICES ABOUT THE LANGUAGE YOU USE

Many formerly incarcerated clients expect you to be just one more person who judges them as somehow less worthy of respect than people who have not been incarcerated. They may expect you to use the same stigmatizing language that they hear from others on a daily basis: convict, felon, ex-offender, criminal, or perp. Your use of these terms may present a significant and lasting barrier to developing a positive working relationship with a formerly incarcerated client and may even keep them from accessing essential programs and services.

All of your clients deserve the same respect, including the right not to be called out of their name or referred to with language that they find offensive. Ask your client how they would like to be called (such as Sean, SJ, or Mr. Jones) and honor this request. If it is appropriate to refer to their history of incarceration, we recommend that you use language such as "formerly incarcerated" or "person experiencing incarceration." Most importantly, if you make a mistake and use a term that you suspect or can tell is uncomfortable or offensive to your client, apologize in a sincere fashion and do your best not to repeat the mistake.

- *Have you or your family members ever been called names that you find offensive?*

- *Have services providers (physicians, social workers, teachers, outreach workers, etc.) ever used such language with you?*

- *What would it be like for an important service provider to constantly refer to you by a name or label that you found offensive?*

RECOGNIZING THE CHALLENGES OF COMING HOME

The vast majority of people who go to prison are eventually released, and they come home with the same health issues that developed or worsened in prison. Many people lose their benefits and housing while in prison and may have difficulty accessing those things upon release. Many have lost their connection to family and community.

Keep in mind that the first few weeks after release are the most risky for people coming home from prison. A CHW who understands the tremendous legal barriers for those coming home from prison will be in a position to view her patients' lives in a holistic way. They will recognize the social aspects of the person's situation (keep the ecological model in mind!), be able to offer appropriate resources and, most importantly, will remain patient and compassionate during the process of the client's long journey home.

Some people returning home, and their families, may be reluctant to access government agencies for assistance. Using a harm reduction approach, CHWs can effectively support formerly incarcerated clients to address multiple issues, both medical and social, and to navigate complex and sometimes overwhelming systems of services.

> **Ron Sanders:** I didn't put so much emphasis on the health aspect in the beginning, when I was a drug counselor... then I started to see that if I got them housing, employment, education, that their health outcomes will be better.

A PERSON-CENTERED APPROACH

Person-centered concepts and skills, including motivational interviewing, should guide your work *with all clients*. Keep in mind that people who have been incarcerated have had personal freedom and control taken away, often for a prolonged period of time. Do your best not to replicate this dynamic by taking control away from your client through your practice. Watch out for any tendencies to undermine a client's control by directing conversations or sessions toward a specific question, topic, or outcome or, for example, by trying to influence an Action Plan, or telling a client what you think their priorities and choices should be.

> **Joe Calderon:** CHWs are advocates, warriors, bridges over barriers and biases, and healers of communities empowering people around autonomy and their rights. Let people be people, and self-care is a must.

Remember that person-centered practice aims to enhance the autonomy and capacity of all clients to better manage their lives and promote their own health and welfare. Use your OARS and other motivational interviewing skills (see Chapter 9) to support clients to explore their own experience, ideas, values, and feeling; to choose what to talk about during your time together and what to keep private; to determine their own health goals and the steps they want to take to reach those goals. Remember the Big Ears, Big Eyes, and small mouth of the effective CHW (Chapter 6). Don't dominate conversations and interactions with clients. Listen deeply to what the client chooses to share with you and build from there.

Try to be aware of your own desire to know certain information about the lives of your clients. Remember that we don't have a right to know why someone was incarcerated, how many times they were incarcerated, or for how long they have been incarcerated. Prying into any aspect of a client's life, especially when they have indicated that they wish to keep it private, is only likely to push them away, and has the potential to do them harm.

- *What other aspects of person-centered practice are important when working with formerly incarcerated clients?*

What Do YOU Think?

Please watch the following video role-play of a CHW working with a client who is coming home from prison. In this role play, the CHW does not do a good job in demonstrating person-centered practice:

- *What mistakes does the CHW make in this role-play?*
- *How might the CHW's action impact this client?*
- *What would you do differently to demonstrate person-centered skills in working with this client?*

LISTENING TO A CLIENT'S PRIORITIES. (*Source:* Foundations for Community Health Workers/ http://youtu.be/ n96TZKnnhec)

ETHICAL DILEMMAS

Being a formerly incarcerated person can be a real asset for a CHW serving people who have been incarcerated, but it can also present some particular ethical challenges. Ron and Juanita, CHWs at Transitions Clinic (introduced in Section 15.7 below), describe their experiences this way:

> **Ron Sanders:** A lot of times, you have to watch the ethical things. I have a few clients I've known from way back. I did time with, I got high with them ... I had to break away from that "prison thing" and focus on what I'm doing now. They'll try to tie me to that, like "You owe me." But I don't owe you. A lot of them have seen me at my worst, so this [seeing me as a professional health worker] is inspiring for them, too.
>
> **Juanita Alvarado:** A lot of our patients are people I did drugs with, or people I bought drugs from. They'll ask, "you got a couple extra dollars" or "will you do a UA (urine analysis) for me?" ... that's a big no-no, we won't go there. I'm not willing to sacrifice my job; I have children and I'm not willing to lose everything I worked hard for to do a favor. Those are some of the things we run into.

PROMOTING PARTNERSHIPS, ADVOCATING FOR CHANGE

In addition to assisting individual clients, CHWs are well positioned to shape reentry programs and promote partnerships that build stronger, safer communities. Communities that are dramatically impacted by mass incarceration may feel an increased sense of powerlessness in the face of so much loss and instability. CHWs can play a positive, empowering role by bringing people together to challenge the systemic factors that create ill health and encourage community organizing to promote health and safety. For example, CHWs from the Transitions Clinic in San Francisco have served on city-wide Reentry Councils and advocated for the rights of their clients on the state-wide level.

Community health workers can become powerful agents for social change. The crisis of mass incarceration presents an opportunity for major policy changes, and frontline health workers have the potential to make a real difference in this movement toward social justice and equity. Again, the CHWs from Transitions offer us examples of the powerful role of frontline health workers in advocating for systems change. They have been vocal advocates for treatment over incarceration, challenging discriminatory policies and laws that create barriers to successful reentry and health.

> **Ron Sanders:** Watching people turn their lives around, being productive, seeing people working, going to school ... those are the biggest rewards. When they're housed, taking good care of their health, making their appointments, they're an asset to the community, instead of being against the community.
>
> **Juanita Alvarado:** Being this role model for this population helps with my personal growth, to stay sober, to stay on track. Everybody around me wants to do the same thing, like "what did you do?" Because I was the person who was the addict, who tried to kill myself, who didn't give a damn about anybody. For people who know me, it's "wow, she's doing it, she's a professional." It brings tears and it warms my heart.

15.7 Best Practices and Emerging Models

The Transitions Clinic Network (TCN) is an innovative response to the complex needs of individuals returning from incarceration with more chronic health conditions than the general population and diminished employment opportunities due to the collateral consequences of conviction (Transitions Clinic Network, 2023). TCN is committed to reversing the harms of mass incarceration by eliminating racial health and economic disparities. TCN transforms health systems to serve impacted communities by building capacity in community-based primary care programs to improve the health and social determinants of health of individuals returning from incarceration and training formerly incarcerated individuals to work as CHWs embedded into primary care teams. TCN partners with existing primary care clinics to implement their evidence-based model nationally. As of 2023, there are 42 TCN sites in 10 states and Puerto Rico, including 21 sites throughout California.

Central to the TCN model are CHWs with lived experience of incarceration working within the health system. TCN has a specialized, 12-week in-house training that focuses on working within a primary care system and supporting individuals recently released from incarceration. TCN CHWs are embedded into the primary care team to support returning community members and serve as liaisons to primary care services. CHWs meet newly released individuals where they are, such as at the parole office, homes or halfway houses, community centers, and faith-based organizations; when possible and permitted by facilities, CHWs perform in-reach to jails and prisons to begin building a rapport with clients even prior to release. CHWs link returning community members to primary health care early in the reentry process, avoiding unnecessary emergency department utilization. CHWs are trained to identify the highest-risk individuals and provide case management, culturally appropriate health education, referrals to specialists, and connections to social services (such as housing, transportation, employment, and food support providers) to ensure patients have what they need to thrive. For a patient population that is often mistrustful of health systems due to prior negative experiences, stigma, and discrimination, the shared history of incarceration helps build trusting relationship between patients and CHWs, leading to better outcomes. CHWs with lived experience of incarceration are uniquely qualified to get returning community members in the door to medical appointments; provide mentorship, emotional support, and teach chronic disease self-management; and advocate for their needs with the clinical team while advocating to transform the system.

In addition to training CHWs, TCN trains health systems' clinicians and staff to effectively collaborate with and utilize CHWs as integral members of the care team. TCN provides a yearlong comprehensive training to transform health systems to integrate and best support CHWs with lived experience of incarceration. The TCN model addresses a critical employment issue by providing formerly incarcerated individuals opportunities to work in health care, a field that individuals with conviction histories have traditionally been excluded from despite a national shortage of health care workers. TCN prioritizes hiring CHWs with significant incarceration history who often have larger obstacles to employment due to felony conviction, as well as a deeper understanding of the impacts of incarceration on health. This model helps ensure the representation of Black and brown people in the health care profession and strengthens under-resourced communities in need of health care workers. TCN programs have served over 20,000 returning community members and created jobs for over 100 CHWs with lived experience of incarceration.

Studies of the TCN model have found:

- Increased engagement in medical care (Santa Clara Valley Medical Center, unpublished report).
- 51% reduction in emergency room utilization (Wang et al., 2012).
- Reduced quantity and duration of preventable hospitalizations (Wang et al., 2019).
- Reduced technical violations of parole and probation (Ibid).
- Reduced incarceration days(Ibid).
- Lower criminal justice system costs (Harvey et al., 2022).

TCN's model improves health and legal system outcomes for patients while creating employment opportunities for CHWs living and working in communities harmed by systemic racism. The power of lived experience is at the heart of this innovative model, transforming the barrier of a criminal record into a strength.

> When Ron Sanders, our CHW sits down with a new patient, the patient trusts him and opens up about what's going on in their life because Ron has been through it too, he understands. The shared lived experience between our CHWs and patients is the secret sauce that makes this model so effective. Healthcare access is important, but engagement is critical too, particularly for a patient population that has had so many negative prior experiences and has every reason not to trust the healthcare system" (Shira Shavit, MD, Executive Director of TCN.)

> When I interviewed for this position, it wasn't a factor about my criminal history. My past was my past...I fit right in. (Ron, TCN CHW)

> Knowing I was interviewing for a position where my history of incarceration was beneficial, it allowed me to be me—a person who had made an awful decision decades earlier, but today is not defined by my past action; today I am defined by who I am, not who I was. (Joe, TCN CHW)

> Don't judge what you see on paper. Don't let the black and white be your decision. We need a chance. We need to be heard and we need to be able to help." (Charlezetta, TCN CHW)

> I knew that I was able to bring something to the table that some other employer might find not beneficial and not an asset, but this position did. I believe it's a confidence builder. It's a self-esteem builder. I've received so many things from having this position as a community health worker. (MaDonna, TCN CHW)

All TCN CHWs have lived experience of incarceration. These videos share their stories and how they came to be CHWs:

RON'S STORY:
(*Source:* Foundations for Community Health Workers/http://youtu. be/ePDOB5OtjzM)

JUANITA'S STORY:
(*Source:* Foundations for Community Health Workers/http://youtu. be/_AfVE1DCEVc)

TRACY'S STORY:
(*Source:* Foundations for Community Health Workers/http://youtu. be/KEVRnTTGQlw)

The following videos highlight the impacts of incarceration on health and the value for patients of being able to access quality health care services at a program that truly supports their return from prison:

ERNEST'S STORY:
(*Source:* Foundations for Community Health Workers/http://youtu. be/2HVB_ZDRs1s)

LEE'S STORY:
(*Source:* Foundations for Community Health Workers/http://youtu. be/VElbOb7BkmQ)

As you watch any of these short digital stories, consider the following questions:

- *What did you learn from the story?*
- *How may these stories influence your work as a CHW?*

CASE STUDY — Because Black Is Still Beautiful

Because Black Is Still Beautiful is a nonprofit organization based in the San Francisco Bay Area. Their mission is *"building pathways to liberation for Black women and girls **Because Black is Still Beautiful.**"*

BBISB was founded by Dr. Marilyn Jones while she was a student at the City College of San Francisco (CCSF). Two years post-incarceration, Marilyn decided to change her life and began taking classes at CCSF to pursue a career as an HIV counselor. However, she became extremely concerned by what she learned about health disparities that existed in the Black community, particularly the fact that Black women were the fastest-growing group for HIV infection. As a result, Marilyn became active in her community to create change, and BBISB was born. She decided to continue her education, and today Dr. Jones holds a Doctorate in Educational Leadership from San Francisco State University.

(continues)

CASE STUDY   # Because Black Is Still Beautiful (*continued*)

The work of BBISB encompasses three areas (BBISB, 20:

- **Academic engagement and retention:** *Just Say Know* is a culturally affirming program designed to promote academic engagement and retention among criminal justice-impacted Black women. Efforts were centralized at CCSF, but due to COVID, school closure, and Zoom meetings, the scope of the program has grown. BBISB now offers online support groups to women with histories of incarceration who are pursuing education without boundaries. Hundreds of incarcerated and formerly incarcerated women have been reached through BBSIB's *Just Say Know* program.

- **Araminta approach training:** The Araminta Approach is a culturally affirming, theoretical model designed to improve outcomes in the lives of Black women with histories of incarceration and is based on Dr. Jones' research and life experience. The Araminta Approach was named after Harriet Tubman; her birthname was Araminta Ross. BBISB has provided training to community-based organizations, community thought leaders, academic faculty, and public health professionals. The Approach is currently being piloted at Young Women's Freedom Center in the San Francisco Bay Area to document best practices for systems-involved Black youth.

- **Intergenerational work:** *The Missing Link* is an intergenerational program in collaboration with Young Women's Freedom Center, a nonprofit that develops leadership skills among systems-involved youth. Over a six-week period, Black women and girls with histories of incarceration from two generations (ages 16–24 and 50+) met together. The program was documented in a video entitled *Bridging the Gap*. BBISB understands the importance of intergenerational activities and has found that each generation is equally important. *It takes a village* is more than a slogan. The video was well received by the community. BBISB has begun another cohort of Black women and girls and is committed to creating more opportunities for intergenerational work nationwide.

To learn more about BBISB, their programs, success stories, and other resources, visit their website at www.bbisb.org.

15.8 Continued Professional Development

Do you want to learn more about incarceration and its effect on our communities? Do you want to increase your knowledge and skills for working with formerly incarcerated clients and their families? Here are some suggestions for how to enhance your professional skills:

- Become informed about conditions of confinement and the movement challenging mass incarceration.

- Continue to develop and reflect upon your person-centered practice skills including cultural humility, the strength-based approach, and Motivational Interviewing.

- Learn about the effects of trauma and how to include trauma-informed practices in your work (see Chapter 18).

- Invite a prisoners' rights activist to speak at your organization's function. A comprehensive list of organizations is available from the Prison Activist Resource Center.

- Volunteer with a prisoners' rights organization.

- Read and respond to newspaper stories. Write letters of encouragement for sympathetic editorials and challenge tough-on-crime op-eds.

- Keep informed about relevant bills/laws and contact your representative to voice your opinion.

- Challenge those around you who subscribe to stereotypes about people who have experienced incarceration.
- If you are an employer, consider hiring people with incarceration histories for job vacancies.
- Understand and advocate for the rights of people who are incarcerated. You can learn more about how to do that from Legal Services for Prisoners with Children's manual: Fighting for our Rights (LSPC, 2023)

And please remember always to listen deeply and learn from what your formerly incarcerated clients tell you. They will be your most important teachers.

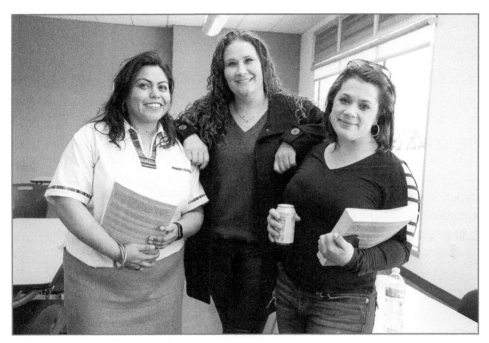

CHWs continue to develop their professional skills.

- *What else could you do to increase your capacity to provide quality services to formerly incarcerated clients and communities?*

Please see the list of Additional Resources included at the end of this chapter.

Chapter Review

Please review the two case studies presented in this chapter featuring *Sean* and *Eddy*. Consider what your goals would be for working with each client. Do your best to answer the questions that accompany each case study.

In addition, please do your best to answer the following questions:

- How does incarceration influence the health of formerly incarcerated individuals? How does it influence the health of their families?
- Why do some professionals say that mass incarceration is a public health issue?
- What health conditions are most common among people who have experienced incarceration?
- Why do some formerly incarcerated clients feel distrustful of the medical system? What risks does this pose for their health? How might you work to build the trust of such a client?
- How does stigma influence the health of people returning home from prison?
- What legal barriers to reentry do people returning home from prison commonly face?
- Describe a best practice model for providing quality health care services to formerly incarcerated clients.

- What language will you use when working with clients returning home from prison? What type of language will you avoid using, and why?
- Identify at least three changes to public policy that could better promote the health of people who have experienced incarceration.
- What types of mistakes might CHWs make that could get in the way of establishing and maintaining an effective professional relationship with formerly incarcerated clients?

References

Alexander, M. (2010). *The new Jim Crow*. New York, NY: New Press.

American Anthropological Association. (2023). Understanding Race. Retrieved from www.understandingrace.org/history/ (accessed 31 May 2023).

American Civil Liberties Union. (2023). The War on Marijuana in Black and White: Billions of Dollars Wasted on Racially Biased Arrests. Retrieved from www.graphics.aclu.org/marijuana-arrest-report/ (accessed 31 May 2023).

Annie E. Casey Foundation. (2016). A Shared Sentence: The Devastating Toll of Parental Incarceration on Kids, Families and Communities. Retrieved from www.aecf.org/resources/a-shared-sentence (accessed 31 May 20023).

Because Black is Still Beautiful. (2023). www.bbisb.org/ (accessed 14 May 2023).

Bronson, J., Stroop, J., & Zimmer, S. (2020). *Drug use, dependence, and abuse among state prisoners and jail inmates, 2007-2016*. Bureau of Justice Statistics.

Bureau of Indian Affairs. (2022). Federal Indian Boarding School Initiative Investigative Report—May 2022. Retrieved from www.bia.gov/sites/default/files/dup/inline-files/bsi_investigative_report_may_2022_508.pdf. (accessed 31 May 2023).

Bureau of Justice Statistics. (2020). Crime, arrest, and release trends, 1990-2019. Retrieved from bjs.ojp.gov/content/pub/pdf/cpus20st.pdf (accessed 31 May 2023).

California Correctional Health Care Services. (2021). History of Receivership. Retrieved from www.cchcs.ca.gov/history-of-receivership/ (accessed 30 May 2023).

Campaign for Youth Justice. (2023). Disproportionate Minority Contact (DMC). Retrieved from www.juvjustice.org/our-work/safety-opportunity-and-success-project/issue-areas/dmc (Accessed 31 May 2023).

Centers for Disease Control and Prevention (CDC). (2022). HIV Group. Retrieved from www.cdc.gov/ (accessed 31 May 2023).

COVID Prison Project. (2021). Our Data. https://covidprisonproject.com/data/ (accessed 31 May 2023).

Critical Resistance. (2023). Not-So-Common Language. Retrieved from https://criticalresistance.org/mission-vision/not-so-common-language/ (accessed 29 May 2023).

Dholakia, N. (2021). Women's Incarceration Rates are Skyrocketing. These Advocates are Trying to Change that. Vera Institute of Justice. www.vera.org/news/womens-incarceration-rates-are-skyrocketing (accessed 31 May 2023).

Drucker, E. (2011). *A Plague of Prisons: the Epidemiology of Mass Incarceration in America*. New York, NY: New Press.

Drug Policy Alliance. (2023. Race and the Drug War. Retrieved from www.drugpolicy.org/issues/race-and-drug-war. (accessed 31 May 2023).

Federal Bureau of Investigation. (2023). UCR Data Tool Crime Trend Explorer. Retrieved from www.de.ucr.cjis.gov (accessed 31 May 2023).

Flagg, A., & Preston, J. (2022). The 'Out of Sight' Crisis: Migrant Children Are Still Being Detained. Politico Magazine. Retrieved from www.politico.com/news/magazine/2022/06/16/border-patrol-migrant-children-detention-00039291 (accessed 31 May 2023).

Freedom Archives. (2023). Charisse Shumate: Fighting for Our Lives. Retrieved from www.freedomarchives.org/ publications/charisse-shumate-fighting-for-our-lives/ (accessed 31 May 2023).

Greeson, J. K. P., Briggs, E. C., Kisiel, C. L., Layne, C. M., Ake III, G. S., Ko, S. J., & Fairbank, J. A. (2011). Complex trauma and mental health in children and adolescents placed in foster care: Findings from the National Child Traumatic Stress Network. *Child Welfare*, 90(6), 91–108.

Guard, D. (2008). Clinton crime agenda shortsighted; May hurt poor and minorities, advocates say. www. stopthedrugwar.org/trenches/2008/apr/15/clinton_crime_agenda_shortsighte (accessed 31 May 2023).

Haney, C. (2018). The psychological effects of solitary confinement: A systematic review and meta-analysis. *The Journal of the American Academy of Psychiatry and the Law*, 46(4), 490–505.

Hannah-Jones, N., Roper, C., Silverman, I., Silversteing, J. (2021). *The 1619 project*. New York: One World, Randomhouse.

Harvey, T. D., Busch, S. H., Lin, H.-J., Aminawung, J. A., Puglisi, L., Shavit, S., & Wang, E. A. (2022). Cost savings of a primary care program for individuals recently released from prison: A propensity- matched study. *BMC Health Services Research*, 22(1). https://doi.org/10.1186/s12913-022-07985-5.

Health Canada. (2023). Supervised Consumption Sites: Explained. Retrieved from www.canada.ca/en/health-canada/services/substance-use/supervised-consumption-sites/explained.html (accessed 31 May 2023).

Hemez, P., Brent, J. J., & Mowen, T. J. (2020). Exploring the school-to-prison pipeline: How school suspensions influence incarceration during young adulthood. *Youth Violence and Juvenile Justice*, 18(3), 235–255. doi: 10.1177/1541204019880945.

Human Rights Watch. (2021). World Report. www.hrw.org/world-report/2021/country-chapters/united-states (accessed 31 May 2023).

James, S. E., Herman, J. L., Rankin, S., Keisling, M., Mottet, L., & Anafi, M. (2016). *The report of the 2015 U.S. transgender survey*. Washington, DC: National Center for Transgender Equality. Retrieved from www.transe-quality.org/sites/default/files/docs/usts/USTS-Full-Report-Dec17.pdf.

Kaeble, D. (2021). Probation and Parole in the United States, 2020. Retrieved from www.bjs.ojp.gov/library/publications/probation-and-parole-united-states-2020 (accessed 30 May 2023).

Legal Services for Prisoners with Children. (2023). Fighting for our Rights. https://prisonerswithchildren.org/wp-content/uploads/2020/04/Fighting-for-Our-Rights_New.pdf (accessed 14 May 2023).

Martin, S. S. (2017). The Hidden Consequences of the Impact of Incarceration on Dependent Children. National Institute of Justice. Retrieved from www.nij.ojp.gov/topics/articles/hidden-consequences-impact-incarceration-dependent-children#noteReference13 (accessed 29 May 2023).

Maté, G. (2008). *In the realm of hungry ghosts*. Berkeley, CA: North Atlantic Books.

McCauley, E., Eckstrand, K., Desta, B., Bouvier, B., Brockmann, B., & Brinkley-Rubinstein, L. (2018). Exploring healthcare experiences for incarcerated individuals who identify as transgender in a southern jail. *Transgender Health*, 3:34–41. doi: 10.1089/trgh.2017.0046.

National Alliance on Mental Illness (NAMI). (2023). Re-entry & Post-Incarceration. Supporting Community Inclusion and Non-Discrimination. Retrieved from www.nami.org/Advocacy/Policy-Priorities/Supporting-Community-Inclusion-and-Non-Discrimination/Re-entry-Post-Incarceration (accessed 31 May 2023).

National Commission on COVID-19 and Criminal Justice. (2021). COVID-19 and crime in 2020: A preliminary analysis. www.covid19.counciloncj.org (accessed 22 May 2023).

The National Conference of State Legislatures (NCSL). (2023). Felon Voting Rights. Retrieved from www.ncsl.org/elections-and-campaigns/felon-voting-rights (accessed 26 May 2023).

The National Employment Law Project (NELP). (2021). Ban the Box: Fair Chance Hiring State and Local Guide. Retrieved from www.nelp.org/publication/ban-the-box-fair-chance-hiring-state-and-local-guide/ (accessed 30 May 2023).

National Institute on Drug Abuse. (2020). Substance use and SUDs in LGBTQ* Populations. Retrieved from www.drugabuse.gov/drug-topics/substance-use-suds-in-lgbtq-populations (accessed 1 June 2023).

National Research Council. (2013). *Health and incarceration: A workshop summary*. Washington, DC: The National Academies Press. https://doi.org/10.17226/18372.

Noonan, M. E., Rohloff, H., & Ginder, S. (2013). Sexual Victimization in Prisons and Jails Reported by Inmates, 2011-12. Bureau of Justice Statistics. Washington, DC: U.S. Department of Justice. Retrieved from www.bjs.gov/content/pub/pdf/svpjri1112.pdf.

Pacific Broadcasting Network. (2023a) How many slaves landed in the US? Retrieved from www.pbs.org/wnet/african-americans-many-rivers-to-cross/history/how-many-slaves-landed-in-the-us/ (accessed 31 May 2023).

Pacific Broadcasting Network. (2023b). Incarcerated People Face Barriers to Reentry Post-prison. How One Initiative Aims to Help. Retrieved from www.pbs.org/newshour/nation/incarcerated-people-face-barriers-to-reentry-post-prison-how-one-initiative-aims-to-help. (accessed 31 May 2023).

The Pew Charitable Trusts. (2010). *Collateral costs: Incarceration's effect on economic mobility*. Washington, DC: The Pew Charitable Trusts. Retrieved from www.pewtrusts.org/-/media/legacy/uploadedfiles/pcs_assets/2010/collateralcosts1pdf.pdf.

Pew Research Center (2021). America's Incarceration Rates Falls to Lowest Level Since 1995. www.pewresearch.org/short-reads/2021/08/16/americas-incarceration-rate-lowest-since-1995/ (accessed 31 May 2023).

Physicians for Human Rights. (2021). Praying for Hand Soap and Masks: COVID-19 and Systemic Health Disparities in US Immigration Detention. Retrieved from www.phr.org/our-work/resources/praying-for-hand-soap-and-masks/.

Plata v. Schwarzenegger. (2005). *Findings of fact and conclusions of law re: appointment of receiver*. U. S. District Court for the Northern District of California.

Prison Policy Initiative. (2023). Racial and Ethnic Disparities in the U.S. Criminal Justice System. Retrieved from www.prisonpolicy.org/research/race_and_ethnicity/ (accessed 31 May 2023).

Ranapurwala, S. I., Shanahan, M. E., Alexandrines, A.A., Proescholdbell, S.K., Naumann, R.B., Edwards Jr, D., Marshall, S.W. (2018). Opioid overdose mortality among former North Carolina inmates: 200 -2015. *American Journal of Public Health*, 108(9), 1207–1213. doi: 10.2105/AJPH.2018.304514.

San Francisco Children of Incarcerated Parents Partnership (SFCIPP). (2005). *Children of incarcerated parents: A bill of rights*. San Francisco, CA: SFCIPP. Retrieved from sfonline.barnard.edu/children/SFCIPP_Bill_of_Rights.pdf.

The Sentencing Project. (2021a). Racial Disparities in the United States Criminal Justice System. Retrieved from www.sentencingproject.org/criminal-justice-facts/.

The Sentencing Project. (2021b). Incarcerated Women and Girls. Retrieved from www.sentencingproject.org/publications/incarcerated-women-and-girls/.

Smith, J. P. (2018). The long-term economic impact of criminalization in American childhoods. *Crime & Delinquency*, 64(12), 1568–1587. doi: https://doi.org/10.1177/0011128718787514.

Spaulding, A. C., Kennedy, S. S., Osei, J., Sidibeh, E., Batina, I. V., Chhatwal, J., Akiyama, M.J., Strick, L.B. Estimates of hepatitis C seroprevalence and Viremia in State Prison populations in the United States. *The Journal of Infectious Diseases*. 2023 Sep 13;228(Suppl 3):S160–S167. doi: https://doi.org/10.1093/infdis/jiad227. PMID: 37703336.

Stemen, D. (2017). The Prison Paradox: More Incarceration Will Not Make Us Safer. Evidence brief from Vera Institute. Retrieved from www.vera.org/downloads/publications/for-the-record-prison-paradox_02.pdf (accessed 31 May 2023).

Szalavitz, M. (2009). Prisons: America's Inhospitable Hospitals. Time Magazine. content.time.com/time/health/article/0,8599,1893946,00.html (accessed 31 May 2023).

The 1619 Project. (2023). Educational Materials Collection. https://1619education.org/?gclid=CjwKCAjwg-GjBhBnEiwAMUvNW-Y-lLH_RquSEpaI1CIokvl2u4V93g4Ni_otgnf4GRNJkBdCd22KthoCUUgQAvD_BwE (accessed 1 June 2023).

Torrey, E. F., Kennard, A. D., Eslinger, D., Lamb, R., & Pavle, J. (2010). *More mentally Ill persons are in jails and prisons than hospitals: A survey of the states*. Arlington, VA: Treatment Advocacy Center.

The Transitions Clinic Network. (2023). www.transitionsclinic.org/ (accessed 14 May 2023).

Turner, K. B., Giacopassi, D., & Vandiver, M. (2006). Ignoring the past: coverage of slavery and slave patrols in criminal justice texts. *Journal of Criminal Justice Education*, 17(1), 181–195. doi:10.1080/10511250500335627 (accessed 31 May 2023).

U.S. Census Bureau. (2023). QuickFacts: United States. Retrieved from www.census.gov/quickfacts/fact/table/US/PST045221 (Accessed 31 May 2023).

U.S. Immigration & Customs Enforcement. (2021). Enforcement and Removal Operations Fiscal Year 2021 Report. Retrieved from www.ice.gov/sites/default/files/documents/2022/01/14/ero-fy2021-report.pdf (accessed 27 May 2023).

Vera Institute of Justice. (2023). American History, Race, and Prison. Retrieved from www.vera.org/reimagining-prison-web-report/american-history-race-and-prison (accessed 31 May 2023).

Wang, E. A., Hong, C. S., Shavit, S., Sanders, R., Kessell, E., & Kushel, M. B. (2012). Engaging individuals recently released from prison into primary care: A randomized trial. *American Journal of Public Health*, 102(9), e22–e29. https://doi.org/10.2105/ajph.2012.300894.

Wang, E. A., Lin, H., Aminawung, J. A., Busch, S. H., Gallagher, C., Maurer, K., ... Frisman, L. (2019). Propensity-matched study of enhanced primary care on contact with the criminal justice system among individuals recently released from prison to New Haven. *BMJ Open*, 9(5), e028097. https://doi.org/10.1136/bmjopen-2018-028097.

Wisconsin Poverty Center. (2023). Connections Among Poverty, Incarceration, and Inequality. Retrieved from www.irp.wisc.edu/resource/connections-among-poverty-incarceration-and-inequality/ (accessed 31 May 2023).

World Prison Brief (2021). Incarceration Rates by Country. www.worldpopulationreview.com/country-rankings/incarceration-rates-by-country (accessed 31 May 2023).

Additional Resources

All of Us or None. (2023). https://prisonerswithchildren.org/about-aouon/ (accessed 14 May 2023).

California Coalition for Women Prisoners. (2023). http://womenprisoners.org/ (accessed 14 May 2023).

Campaign for Youth Justice. (2023). http://www.campaignforyouthjustice.org (accessed 14 May 2023).

The Center on Juvenile and Criminal Justice. (2023). http://www.cjcj.org/ (accessed 14 May 2023).

The Council on Crime and Justice. (2023). https://counciloncj.org/ (accessed 14 May 2023).

Critical Resistance. (2023). http://www.criticalresistance.org/ (accessed 14 May 2023).

Detention Watch Network. (2023). http://www.detentionwatchnetwork.org/ (accessed 14 May 2023).

The Drug Policy Alliance. (2023). http://www.drugpolicy.org/homepage.cfm (accessed 14 May 2023).

Families Against Mandatory Minimums. (2023). http://www.famm.org (accessed 14 May 2023).

Human Rights Watch Prison Project. (2023). http://www.hrw.org/ (accessed 14 May 2023).

The Justice Policy Institute. (2023). http://www.justicepolicy.org/ (accessed 14 May 2023).

Legal Services for Prisoners with Children. (2023). https://prisonerswithchildren.org/ (accessed 14 May 2023).

The Real Cost of Prisons Project. (2023). http://realcostofprisons.org/ (accessed 14 May 2023).

The Sentencing Project. (2023). https://www.sentencingproject.org/ (accessed 14 May 2023).

Chronic Conditions Management

Tim Berthold, Mattie Clark, and Lorena Carmona

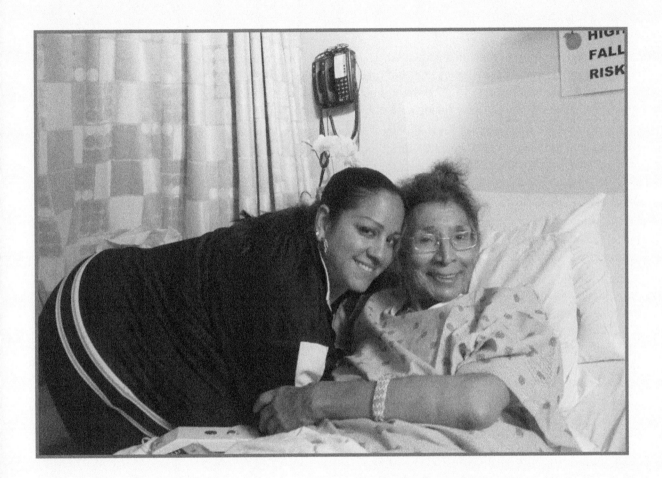

Foundations for Community Health Workers, Third Edition. Edited by Tim Berthold and Darouny Somsanith.
© 2024 John Wiley & Sons, Inc. Published 2024 by John Wiley & Sons, Inc.
Companion website: http://www.wiley.com/go/communityhealthworkers3E

Client Scenario: Rosina Walker

Rosina Walker is 43-year-old. She is raising three children ages one, eight, and nine on her own. After the birth of her youngest son, Mrs. Walker quit her job as a teacher's assistant to care for her children full-time. Childcare was too expensive to cover on her salary.

Since she left her job, Rosina has been dependent on benefits to get by. She receives TANF cash assistance, SNAP benefits to put food on the table, and Section 8 vouchers to help cover the cost of housing. Despite the benefits that Mrs. Walker and her family receive, they never seem to go far enough. Rosina makes sure that her children always have something to eat, even if it means going without food herself for several days each month.

Rosina Walker lives in a small town in a rural area. There is just one grocery store and it is on the far side of town from Rosina's home. There is a bus line that runs close to Rosina's apartment, but it runs infrequently, and it takes more than three hours to go grocery shopping. She leaves her children with a neighbor when she does errands and returns the favor by taking care of her neighbor's children in return.

Rosina was diagnosed with hypertension (high blood pressure) seven years ago. For several years, she was able to manage her blood pressure. However, since her divorce and the birth of her third child, Mrs. Walker has been under increased stress. When she went to the health center three months ago, her blood pressure was too high, measured at 145/105.

Rosina Walker's main priorities are caring for her children. Her two oldest are now in school, but her youngest needs careful monitoring. Rosina's ex-husband lives in another state and is not able to provide much assistance. Rosina is close to her mother, Mrs. Catchings, who lives in a nursing home in the next town over. Her mother is sick with diabetes and arthritis and becoming more disabled.

Each Sunday, Rosina walks her children to church, using a donated stroller for Ben. It is over a mile each way, but the visit is always worth it. Church is the one place where Rosina feels connected and hopeful, and the congregation helps by passing along clothes and toys for her children. Rosina's faith keeps her going, but she has moments of feeling "low" and overwhelmed by parenting on her own and trying to keep the lights on and food on the table. It doesn't leave a lot of time for her to focus on promoting her own health.

If you were the CHW assigned to work with Rosina Walker, how would you answer the following questions?

- *What health risks and challenges does Rosina Walker face?*
- *What factors promote her health and wellness?*
- *How is Rosina doing in terms of the self-management of her hypertension?*
- *What else would you like to know about Rosina in order to best promote her health?*
- *What is your role, as a CHW, in supporting Rosina Walker to self-manage her chronic health conditions and to improve his health and wellness?*
- *What concepts will guide your work with Rosina?*

Introduction

This chapter addresses chronic health conditions (also referred to as chronic illness or chronic disease), the leading cause of illness and death in the United States and globally. CHWs often play an important role in promoting the health of patients living with chronic conditions.

This chapter builds upon information presented elsewhere in the *Foundations* textbook and is best studied after reading Chapters 3, 4, 6–10. We will address how to apply concepts and skills covered in other chapters—including case management and action planning—and the challenge of supporting a patient to manage a chronic disease more effectively.

Please note that this chapter highlights the roles and services provided by CHWs who support patients living with chronic health conditions. This chapter does not present comprehensive information about different chronic diseases such as diabetes, cancer, asthma, lupus, arthritis, and depression. To do so would take up an entire textbook rather than just a chapter. Information about chronic conditions is frequently updated as new research emerges. If you work as part of an interdisciplinary health care team that addresses chronic health conditions, your employer will provide you with information about health conditions as necessary and consistent with your assigned role and scope of practice.

WHAT YOU WILL LEARN

By studying the information in this chapter, you will be able to:

- Identify the most common chronic diseases in the United States, and discuss health inequities in rates of chronic disease among populations
- Apply an ecological model to analyze the causes and consequences of chronic conditions
- Analyze and discuss the limitations of traditional medical models for the treatment of chronic conditions, and the benefits of emerging models that integrate medical and public health approaches
- Discuss team-based approaches to the delivery of primary health care, and the role and scope of practice of CHWs within these teams
- Analyze and explain the concept of patient self-management of chronic conditions
- Discuss the application of person-centered concepts and skills to support patients in learning how to effectively manage their own chronic conditions

C3 Roles and Skills Addressed in Chapter 16

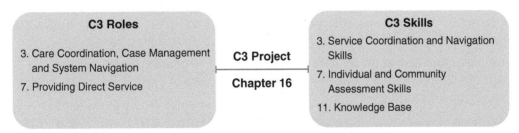

WORDS TO KNOW

Chronic Conditions

Medication Management

Population Health Management

16.1 Defining Chronic Conditions

Chronic conditions are defined as an illness or health condition that lasts for one year or more and requires ongoing health care services or limits daily activities or both (National Center for Chronic Disease Prevention and Health Promotion, 2022a). There are hundreds of chronic conditions. Some of the most common chronic conditions in the United States and worldwide are:

- Cardiovascular diseases including hypertension (high blood pressure), coronary heart disease, and stroke
- Diabetes

- Respiratory diseases including asthma and chronic obstructive pulmonary disease (COPD)
- Cancer
- Depression, post-traumatic stress, schizophrenia, and other mental health conditions
- Substance use, including the current epidemic of opioid use
- Arthritis
- HIV Disease, Hepatitis C, Tuberculosis, and other communicable chronic conditions
- Chronic kidney disease
- Alzheimer's disease, multiple sclerosis, muscular dystrophy, and other progressive and disabling conditions
  - We are still learning about the long-term impacts of COVID-19 infection. Long Covid or Post COVID-19 condition *may become classified as a chronic health condition.* While mild or moderate COVID-19 typically lasts for several weeks, some people experience symptoms such as fatigue, shortness of breath, and cognitive issues that may last for three months or longer (Johns Hopkins Medicine, 2022; World Health Organization, 2021a).

HEALTH DATA

Chronic conditions are the leading cause of illness, hospitalization, and death in the United States. Chronic conditions also contribute to more than 90% of the nation's $4.1 trillion in annual health care costs (National Center for Chronic Disease Prevention and Health Promotion, 2022b).

The CDC estimates that 60% of adults have a chronic health condition and 40% have two or more conditions (National Center for Chronic Disease Prevention and Health Promotion, 2022a). Risks for developing a chronic condition increase with age: approximately 85% of adults ages 65 and older have at least one chronic health condition (National Council on Aging, 2021).

While COVID-19 became a leading cause of death in the United States beginning in 2020, overall, chronic diseases still account for the majority of deaths (Ahmad & Vismara, 2021; Shields et al., 2022). Eight of the top ten leading causes of death in 2021 were chronic diseases including heart disease and cancer (the first and second leading causes of death), stroke, chronic lower respiratory diseases, Alzheimer disease, diabetes, chronic liver disease, and kidney disease (National Center for Health Statistics, 2022).

Globally, chronic conditions accounted for approximately 74% of all deaths (World Health Organization, 2022a). Cardiovascular diseases were the leading cause of death followed by cancers, chronic respiratory diseases, and diabetes (Ibid).

RESEARCH ON CHWS AND CHRONIC CONDITIONS MANAGEMENT

Research demonstrates that CHWs can improve health outcomes for patients living with chronic disease. For example, the Centers for Disease Control and Prevention states that integration of CHWs "as part of cardiovascular disease (CVD) prevention programs can help program participants lower their blood pressure, cholesterol, and blood sugar levels; reduce their CVD risks; be more physically active; and stop smoking. It can also improve patient knowledge and adherence to medication regimens and improve health care services" (Centers for Disease Control and Prevention, 2020).

Integrating CHWs into clinical care teams not only results in improvements to patient health outcomes, it is also cost effective. A review by the Community Preventive Task Force showed that investing in CHWs reduces health care costs (Ibid). A number of studies have shown that hiring CHWs results in a positive return on investment. In other words, CHWs make such positive contributions to promoting health outcomes that they save health organizations money (Christiansen & Morning, 2017; Kangovi, 2020.)

Research on Cardiovascular Disease Risk Reduction and the Role of CHWS: a Study from the Mississippi Delta

Researchers conducted a study in Mississippi to determine the impact of services provided by CHWs to patients at risk for cardiovascular disease. The study was conducted at the G.A. Carmichael Family Health Center, where author Mattie Clark works as a CHW. The study was conducted during the COVID-19 epidemic, so services were provided remotely via telehealth (CHWs were able to see patients in-person in some cases, using personal protective equipment (PPE)). One group of patients received standard clinical care and the other group received enhanced risk management education and monitoring from a team of CHWs.

The group of patients who received enhanced services from CHWs showed a significant increase in knowledge about chronic conditions, including information about blood pressure, diabetes, cholesterol, and strokes (Mayfield-Johnson, 2022). This group of patients also reported significantly higher scores on quality of life measures including energy/vitality, mental health, and social functioning. Study participants reported high satisfaction with CHW education and risk monitoring: 98% reported that they were able to communicate well with CHWs and 97% reported that the CHWs were able to understand their problem.

This study also investigated the use of telehealth care delivery to the same patients, primarily African-Americans living in rural settings. Many patients reported difficulties accessing health care visits due to physical and psychological issues and transportation costs (Mayfield-Johnson, Fastring, Clark, & Crosby, 2022). Most patients agreed with the advantages associated with telehealth utilization and preferred using cell phones to computers to access telehealth care. Researchers identified key challenges with access to technology in rural areas including infrastructure, equipment, and costs. While approximately 93% of the study population had access to cell phone, over a third (36%) had no access to the internet. The study indicated that older African-Americans in the Mississippi delta lacked confidence with some online technologies—such as live chats and social media—and highlighted the need for additional technical support to be provided so that patients can enhance their skills and comfort with these technologies.

For more information about the research study, please see the references at the end of the chapter.

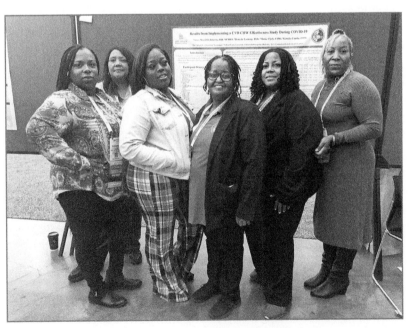

Donishelle Lyons (Mallory Health Center); Kim'eika Crosby (G. A. Carmichael Family Health Center); Brenda Watson (Deltha Health Center); Mattie Clark, Author; (G. A. Carmichael Family Health Center); Linda Newell Johnson (Delta Health Center); Back Row: Willie Mae Horton (Mallory Health Center).

CASE STUDY

Asthma Management Academy Expands Access to Asthma Self-management Education by Community Health Workers

Across the United States over 25 million adults and children have asthma—a chronic disease that affects the airways in the lungs making it difficult to breathe. Asthma costs over $81 billion a year in health care costs—emergency department (ED) visits, hospitalizations, and missed work and school days (Nurmagambe-tov, Kuwahara, & Garbe, 2018). Asthma affects some groups more than others. Black, Latinx, and American Indian/Alaska Native communities carry the largest burden of asthma, experiencing more asthma-related visits, hospitalizations, and deaths than other racial and ethnic groups. Asthma is also especially problematic for children, making it the most common chronic childhood disease.

Community health workers (CHWs) have success in improving asthma outcomes. CHWs delivering asthma interventions, including asthma self-management education (AS-ME) and addressing indoor and outdoor environmental asthma triggers, have demonstrated improved medication adherence and reduced asthma-related ED visits and hospitalizations for people with asthma, and reduced health care dollars spent on asthma (Campbell et al., 2015; Postma, Karr, & Kieckhefer, 2009).

The California Department of Public Health's state asthma program, California Breathing, created the Asthma Management Academy (AsMA) to reduce the burden of asthma in California (California Department of Public Health, 2023). The AsMA teaches evidence-based AS-ME skills to CHWs who work with families with asthma, especially in disproportionately burdened communities. CB believes that CHWs should be trained by other CHWs—those who have experience are best positioned to train others to do the same work. CB partners with several CHW organizations to facilitate the training. These CHW organizations have expertise in delivering asthma programs in high asthma burden communities. The CHW facilitators share their firsthand knowledge of working with families, building trust, and addressing asthma in their communities. CHW facilitators teach participants about the scope of asthma, asthma triggers (e.g., pets, mold, and household cleaning supplies), asthma medications, medication delivery devices, monitoring and assessing asthma control, how to conduct an in-home asthma trigger assessment, and best practices for home visiting.

The AsMA's approach to learning is based on skill building and problem-solving methods. CHWs learn about asthma through short interactive videos, participatory activities, case scenarios, and teach-backs. The teach-back method is a way of checking understanding by asking patients to show or tell you what they learned. As nearly 84% of people with asthma use their medication delivery devices incorrectly, CHWs are encouraged to use the teach-back method with their patients or clients to ensure appropriate medication delivery (Anderson et al., 2019). Collectively, the AsMA has trained over 600 CHWs from 88 organizations that serve people with uncontrolled asthma in high asthma burden communities in California.

All CHWs demonstrated increased asthma knowledge and skills after attending the AsMA. On average, participants scored 97% on asthma knowledge (i.e., scope of asthma, asthma triggers, asthma medications, medication delivery devices, and monitoring and assessing asthma control) and 97% on teaching proper use of spacers and four medication delivery devices. Before the AsMA, CHWs reported having "little" or "no knowledge" of asthma. After the training, most CHWs reporting having "a lot" or "advanced knowledge" in asthma. Most importantly, the AsMA helped to improve health outcomes for people with asthma. CB collected patient-level asthma outcomes from patients with poorly controlled asthma who participated in AS-ME with AsMA-trained CHWs. Eighty percent of patients showed improved asthma control, 70% reported fewer missed work or school days due to asthma, and 83% demonstrated reduced asthma-related ED visits and hospitalizations post AS-ME.

A CHW named Sonya shared her experience after attending the AsMA. Sonya was eager to learn more about asthma. Her son has asthma, and she has friends with asthma. Before attending the AsMA, Sonya felt she

(continues)

(continued)

had a good grasp of what asthma is and how it is managed. She believed her son's asthma was under control despite his symptoms. Sonya enjoyed the participatory virtual AsMA training and working with other CHWs, especially during the teach backs. She shared, "It was the best training I've ever attended." Sonya used the evidence-based tools (e.g., Asthma Control Test and Asthma Action Plan) she learned to advocate for improved asthma management with her son's health care provider. She questioned whether her son's asthma was under control, based on his symptoms, and if he was using the appropriate medications. Sonya credits the AsMA with getting her son's asthma under better control helping her identify asthma early warning signs and advocating for self-management with his health care provider.

To read more about the Asthma Management Academy see the References at the end of the chapter.

16.2 Chronic Conditions and Health Inequities

Chronic conditions are characterized by highly unequal rates of illness, disability, and death between populations nationally and globally, based on factors such as income, ethnicity, immigration status, age, and sex.

Black and Latinx communities in the United States have higher rates of certain chronic conditions than white Americans. For example, while the overall prevalence of hypertension or high blood pressure among all Medicare patients (elders) is 63%, the rates are 60% for white patients, 65% for Latinx patients, and 79% for Black patients (Ochieng, Cubanski, Neuman, Artiga, & Daico, 2021). Data also indicates that rates of diabetes among Medicare beneficiaries are 30% among whites, 45% among Black patients, and 47% among Latinx patients (Ibid).

People of color and low-income individuals are more likely to lack health insurance, resulting in barriers to accessing quality health care. For example, while approximately 7.8% of white Americans were uninsured in 2019, 20% of Latinx and 21.7% of American Indian and Alaska Native communities lacked health insurance (Ndugga & Artiga, 2021).

For more information about health equity, please see Chapter 4. To find out more about inequities in rates of chronic health conditions where you live and work, investigate local city or county data. Your local and state public health departments should post health data and reports on their websites and analyze disparities in health conditions and deaths based on factors that include income, sex, and ethnicity.

16.3 Factors That Cause and Contribute to Chronic Conditions

We use the framework of the ecological model (see Chapter 3) to identify factors that cause and contribute to chronic conditions at the levels of the individual patient, their family, immediate neighborhood or community, and the broader society.

INDIVIDUAL FACTORS

Individual factors that cause or contribute to chronic conditions vary considerably depending upon the disease in question. For example, pathogenic (disease-causing) agents such as bacteria and viruses play a role in certain chronic diseases such as liver and cervical cancer, and HIV Disease. Heredity, or our genetic makeup, also plays a role in the development of many chronic conditions including, for example, cancer, cardiovascular disease, depression, arthritis, diabetes, and disabilities such as muscular dystrophy. The extent to which genetics plays a role depends upon the disease in question. Research highlights the interaction between genetics and our environment in determining the development and progression of many chronic conditions. An individual's age and general state of health, including the health of their immune system, nutritional health, and the presence of infectious or other chronic conditions also influences risks for chronic disease.

Leading national and international health organizations emphasize the role of four (4) key behavioral factors that influence our risks for chronic conditions such as cardiovascular disease and type 2 diabetes:

Levels of physical activity:

- Engaging in physical activity is one of the most effective ways to promote physical and mental health.
- Regular physical activity has been shown to reduce risks for chronic conditions such as cardiovascular disease, diabetes, some cancers, and depression. *Please Note: More detailed information is provided in Chapter 17 on Healthy Eating and Active Living.*

Diet and nutrition:

- The diet of many Americans includes foods and drinks—such as fast and processed foods, sugar, salt, refined carbohydrates, saturated, and trans-fats—that increase risks for cardiovascular disease, cancers and diabetes.
- Eating a healthy diet that features vegetables, fruits, and whole grains can reduce risks for chronic conditions. *Please Note: More detailed information is provided in Chapter 17 on Healthy Eating and Active Living.*

Tobacco use and second-hand smoke:

- Tobacco use—including exposure to second-hand smoke—is considered the most preventable cause of illness and premature death in the United States.
- Tobacco use contributes to cardiovascular disease, cancers, and respiratory conditions.
- The World Health Organization estimates that tobacco kills up to half of its users and accounts for more than 8 million deaths worldwide each year (World Health Organization, 2022b.)

Alcohol consumption:

Excessive alcohol use contributes to chronic conditions including cardiovascular disease, diabetes cancers, and liver cirrhosis.

- *Is there a history of chronic disease in your biological family?*
- *To what extent may your own diet, patterns of exercise, tobacco, and alcohol use influence your health and risks for chronic disease?*

FACTORS RELATED TO FAMILY AND FRIENDS

Our families and friends often play a critical role in promoting our health and well-being. They can also contribute to our risks for illness. For example, family and friends may influence our diet, patterns of alcohol and tobacco use, our level of activity and fitness, and our exposure to stress.

When you work with an individual client to change behaviors, such as their diet, keep the role and influence of the family in mind. For example, the client's family may influence the types of foods that are available in the household. If the rest of the family eats less healthy foods, this will impact, and may limit, the client's ability to eat a healthier diet.

- *To what extent do your family and friends influence your health-related behaviors and risk factors?*
- *In what ways do they support your health and well-being?*

NEIGHBORHOOD AND COMMUNITY FACTORS

The neighborhoods and communities where we live, and work influence our health. This includes the level of access to health-related resources such as quality schools and job training programs, safe drinking water, affordable housing and grocery stores stocked with affordable fresh fruits and vegetables. Exposure to air pollution and mold contributes significantly to chronic respiratory conditions like asthma. Levels of violence in the community, including police and handgun violence, impact levels of stress and risks for chronic conditions (as well as injury and premature death).

Health is also influenced by access to afterschool and childcare services, affordable and quality health care, parks and opportunities for recreation, community-based services, including those provided by nonprofits and faith-based institutions.

- *What health risks are you and your local community exposed to?*

- *What health resources do you have easy access to, and which are lacking?*

What Do YOU? Think

SOCIETAL FACTORS

Social, economic and political factors influence risks for chronic health conditions. Throughout the world, populations with the least access to critical health resources—including healthy food, clean drinking water, affordable housing and health care, safe working conditions at a living wage, and meaningful protection of civil and human rights—are most likely to experience higher rates of illness and premature death from chronic conditions. Access to critical health resources is determined by the interaction of economic and political factors, including actions taken by key policy makers and governments at the local, national and global levels.

The lack of equity is the key driver of health disparities in the United States and globally (Marmot & Bell, 2019). The World Health Organization (WHO) emphasizes the role of social determinants in the causation of chronic disease and describes a vicious cycle of the interaction between poverty, illness, and premature death (World Health Organization, 2022a).

THE ROLE OF STRESS IN THE DEVELOPMENT OF CHRONIC CONDITIONS

Stress operates across all four levels of the ecological model and is a major contributor to chronic conditions (to review basic information about stress, please refer to Chapter 12). This is particularly true for communities exposed to chronic stress arising from factors such as living in poverty, food insecurity and hunger, exposure to violence, institutionalized racism, and other forms of discrimination. Stress raises heart rates and blood pressure and causes our bodies to release hormones such as cortisol. In order to save energy, stress takes energy from the immune system, our bodies' long-term healing system, and uses it for fight, flight, or fat storage. Over time, these biological stress responses increase risks for a range of chronic conditions including diabetes, depression, hypertension, coronary heart disease, and stroke.

Post-Traumatic Stress and Illness

Chapter 18 provides more information about trauma. Post-traumatic stress affects people who survive life's most horrifying events, such as war and armed conflict, torture, sexual assault, incarceration, child abuse, and neglect. Research demonstrates that childhood exposure to trauma increases the risks of developing other chronic conditions including cardiovascular disease, diabetes, depression, and chronic obstructive pulmonary disease (Centers for Disease Control and Prevention, 2021a).

16.4 The Consequences of Chronic Conditions

Chronic health conditions impact the lives of individual patients, their families, as well as the communities and the larger society in which they live.

THE CONSEQUENCES FOR INDIVIDUAL PATIENTS

Consequences for individuals living with chronic conditions depends upon the type and number of conditions they are living with, their age, genetics and family status, their income, and other factors. Common consequences include:

- Fatigue or extreme tiredness
- Challenges with daily living and activities. Due to their symptoms, people with chronic conditions may find it hard to study or work, to live independently and to care for others, including children

- Nausea, bowel, or bladder control problems

- Nerve damage and pain

- Disability such as the loss of mobility, eyesight, or limbs

- Increased levels of stress, anxiety, and depression

- Stigma or negative attitudes from others due to living with certain chronic conditions such as HIV and Hepatitis C disease, addiction, mental illness and diabetes. Stigma also affects people who are perceived as being "overweight," or have engaged in certain behaviors such as drug use

- Shame, isolation and the loss of career, of relationships, of roles within the family and community, of hope, identity, purpose, or faith

- Symptoms often get worse over time and may result in complications, including long-term hospitalization and premature death

  - *Can you think of other consequences for individuals living with chronic conditions?*

THE CONSEQUENCES FOR FAMILIES

The consequences for families may depend upon how many family members have chronic conditions, which family members are ill, the severity of the illness, and the social and economic circumstances of the household. Consequences include emotional distress from witnessing loved ones who are ill or disabled, increased costs for the treatment of chronic conditions and, as a result, fewer funds to invest in other resources such as housing, education, transportation, food, or health care.

When one member of the family falls ill, others typically assume increased caretaking responsibilities. Caretaking roles require time and energy, and sometimes prevent family members from taking on other roles within and outside of the household. Both the family member who is ill, and the caretaker(s) may experience a reduction or loss of employment and income and this, in turn, may result in the loss of other assets such as health insurance or housing.

  - *Can you think of other consequences for families?*

THE CONSEQUENCES OF CHRONIC CONDITIONS AT THE COMMUNITY AND SOCIETAL LEVELS

The consequences at the community and societal levels include increased illness and disability (such as high rates of diabetes, post-traumatic stress or HIV disease), increased costs for treating chronic conditions (chronic conditions account for the majority of all health care costs in the United States), and reduced life expectancy. The funding spent on the treatment of preventable chronic conditions could otherwise have been invested in other key public benefits such as housing, education, or job training.

Chronic conditions also result in a devastating loss of human potential when people die prematurely or are too sick or disabled to fully contribute to the community socially, culturally, politically, or economically. For people living in poverty, health care costs for treating chronic health conditions can exhaust family resources. The World Health Organization estimates that the costs of treating chronic disease drives millions of people into poverty each year (World Health Organization, 2022a).

  - *Can you think of other consequences at the community and societal levels?*

Your Experience with Chronic Conditions

As a CHW, it is important for you to be aware of your own experience with chronic health conditions. Please reflect on the following questions:

- What is your personal experience with chronic conditions? Are you living with a chronic condition? Do members of your family have a chronic condition?
- How do chronic conditions impact your life, and the lives of your family members?
- What types of chronic conditions are most common among the communities that you belong to?
- Do people in your community living with chronic conditions—or risk factors for certain chronic conditions—face stigma and prejudice? If so, which health conditions and risk behaviors are stigmatized?

16.5 Treatment Options

If you work directly with patients who have chronic conditions, you will become familiar with the types of treatments that are available in your workplace and from other local health care and social service providers. Available treatments for chronic conditions depend upon the disease and may include:

- **Changes in health-related behaviors** to reduce risk factors and manage symptoms. These changes typically include:
  - Increasing physical activity levels and fitness
  - Dietary changes such as increased consumption of fruits, vegetables, and whole grains
  - Stopping or reducing tobacco, alcohol, and drug use.
  - Stress management. People can learn techniques to better manage the effects of stress, and limit the harm that stress causes.
- **Medications**: Medications are available that help to reduce the symptoms of certain chronic diseases, and to prevent further progression of the disease. Medications are frequently used to treat chronic conditions such as hypertension, diabetes, HIV disease, cancers, and depression.
- **Physical or occupational therapy:** These treatments help people to regain strength and mobility, and to reduce pain. Physical therapy can help patients to participate more actively in daily activities such as dressing, walking, cooking, or working.
- **Medical interventions:** For example, some patients may receive chemotherapy or radiation to treat cancer. Patients may undergo procedures such as joint replacement surgery to treat conditions such as arthritis, and laser therapy may help others to keep their vision.
- **Mental health therapies:** These include individual, family or group counseling to help people better cope with depression, anxiety and loss, and behavior change.
- **Medical equipment:** For example, an oxygen tank to assist with breathing, or a wheelchair or walker to assist with mobility
- **Access to key resources** such as food, transportation, stable housing, job training, and other services.
- **Physical assistance:** A patient may need someone to help out with daily activities including dressing, cooking, or taking care of a home.
- **Holistic and Integrative therapies** such as acupuncture and other practices.

Please keep in mind that the information provided here about treatment may be different from the guidelines followed in the clinic or hospital you are working for. *The policies and procedures of your employer always take priority in guiding your work with clients. When in doubt about the type of health information to share with clients, always talk with your direct supervisor.*

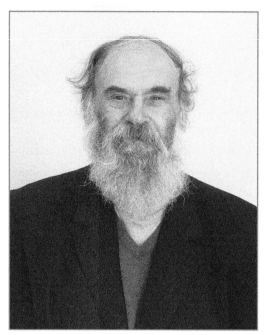

A CHW who supports elderly and disabled patients in a hospital setting.

ACCESS TO TREATMENT

The types of treatments that patients receive depend upon several factors, such as:

- Whether or not the patient has health insurance, the type of insurance they have, the types of treatments covered, and the cost to the patient (such as fees for deductibles and co-payments)

- The health care practice and system providing services to the patient, the level of training and expertise of health care professionals, and the range of services and treatment offered

- Availability of services including mental health services, food, housing and legal assistance, recreational facilities, and programs. Access to services can be particularly difficult for rural and low-income communities, and those lacking reliable and affordable transportation

- Cultural identity and health beliefs, such as a distrust in western approaches to medicine versus other cultural approaches to healing

- **Trust in health care providers**: Trust is in turn influenced by the client's personal history with medical providers, as well as the historical treatment of the client's community by medical providers. Some communities, including immigrants, communities of color, transgender/nonbinary, and formerly incarcerated communities still experience significant discrimination and harm from medical providers.

- Time and competing priorities and responsibilities (such as employment, childcare, or other caretaking responsibilities)

- The stigma associated with the chronic condition and/or risk factors (including issues such as diet, exercise, drug or alcohol use, sexuality, a mental health diagnosis, HIV and Hepatitis C, etc.)

- Depression/mental illness. Having depression or any mental health condition can make it much more difficult for patients to seek or maintain services and available treatments for any health condition

- Health literacy or a person's knowledge about health and their ability to learn new information

- Disability, mobility and the availability and cost of transportation to and from health care services

- The client's experience and perception of the severity of symptoms and the degree to which their illness is interfering with their quality of life. Some patients ignore symptoms and delay accessing care for many reasons including fear, depression, stigma, and denial

- *Can you think of other factors that might influence a client's access to treatment for a chronic condition?*

- *Have any of these factors affected your own access to treatments (or those of your family)?*

Understanding Hypertension or High Blood Pressure

While we are unable to provide detailed information about a wide range of chronic conditions in this brief chapter, we present a basic overview of hypertension to illustrate the type of information that is helpful for CHWs to learn about the most common chronic conditions among the communities they work with.

Definition

Hypertension means having high blood pressure, or the pressure of blood pushing against the walls of our arteries (arteries carry blood from the heart to the rest of the body). Blood pressure is provided in the form of two numbers: systolic pressure, measured while the heart is beating; and diastolic pressure, measured in between heart beats, while the heart is at rest. In general, a healthy blood pressure is less than 120/80. Hypertension is diagnosed when our blood pressure is measured consistently at or over 130/80 (Centers for Disease Control and Prevention, 2022)

Prevalence

Hypertension is one of the most common chronic conditions in the United States. The U.S. Centers for Disease Control and Prevention estimate that *over 116 million Americans, or 47% of adults have high blood pressure* (Ibid). Hypertension is more common among men, people aged 65 and older, and among Black Americans. Approximately 75% of adults with hypertension do not have it under control (Ibid).

Key Causes and Contributing Factors

- Diet, or what we eat and drink. Consuming too much salt, sugar, saturated, and trans fats increases risks for hypertension
- Physical activity. A lack of regular physical activity (including walking) and exercise also increases risks for high blood pressure.
- Stress. Exposure to chronic stress, including post-traumatic stress, increases the risks for hypertension
- Substance use. Tobacco, alcohol and drug use (especially cocaine and methamphetamines).
- Heredity. A family history of hypertension can increase a person's risks.
- Co-existing diseases such as diabetes or kidney disease.

Common Consequences

Over time, high blood pressure can result in damage to and narrowing of the arteries, increasing risks for stroke, heart attack, and death. High blood pressure can also damage the heart, kidneys, brain, and eyes (Centers for Disease Control and Prevention, 2021b).

Symptoms

Hypertension is sometimes called a "silent killer" because people typically do not have noticeable symptoms for many years. For this reason, it is best to have your blood pressure measured regularly by a health care professional. When symptoms do occur, they may include chest pain, irregular heart rhythms, blurred vision, nosebleeds, headaches, and buzzing in the ears. Severe hypertension can also cause nausea, vomiting, fatigue, anxiety, confusion, and muscle tremors (World Health Organization, 2021b).

(continues)

Understanding Hypertension or High Blood Pressure

(continued)

Treatments

Hypertension is typically treated by a combination of medications and changes to diet, exercise, and other behaviors or habits.

- **Medications:** A wide range of medications are used to help control blood pressure. Some clients respond better to certain types of medications, and some may be treated by more than one medication.

- **Tobacco, alcohol and drug use:** Patients are encouraged to stop or reduce their use of tobacco, drug, and alcohol.

- Engaging in regular physical activity can help to control and lower high blood pressure. Patients are encouraged to enhance their participation in daily activity or exercise.

- Patients are encouraged to eat a healthier diet in line with the nutritional guidelines provided in Chapter 17. In general, this means eating more fruits, vegetables, and whole grains, and limiting salt, saturated and trans fats, and sugar.

- Stress reduction and relaxation techniques.

16.6 How to Stay Informed About Chronic Conditions

As a working CHW, you will frequently conduct research to enhance your knowledge of health issues. This is particularly important because research findings, information and practice standards are frequently updated in the fields of health care and public health.

Because there is so much information about health issues, knowing where and how to conduct research on chronic conditions can be challenging. Remember that you have an ethical duty to stay current in your field and to provide accurate information to the client and communities you work with. You must be able to distinguish between reliable and less-reliable sources of information. If you are working directly with people with chronic health conditions, a good place to start is reviewing the information made available by your employer. Talk with your supervisor and colleagues, and study available resources including, for example, practice standards and protocols, journals, reports, and brochures. In general, we recommend that you to rely upon sources from .gov, .edu, or .org websites rather than .com or social media sites.

Become familiar with a range of reputable online sources of health information. These include your local city, county, or state health department as well as leading national sites that feature information including recent research findings and current guidelines for prevention and treatment, such as:

- The US Centers for Disease Control and Prevention http://www.cdc.gov
- National Institutes of Health http://www.nih.gov/
- The National Institute of Mental Health http://www.nimh.hih.gov
- The National Cancer Institute http://www.cancer.gov
- The National Library of Medicine (Medline) http://www.medlineplus.gov

Other recommended sites include national nonprofit professional organizations such as those focused on specific types of chronic health conditions including:

- The American Heart Association www.heart.org
- The American Cancer Society www.cancer.org

- Foundation for Women's Cancer www.wcn.org
- The American Diabetes Association www.diabetes.org

You can also find reliable information at leading educational and health care institutions such as:

- The World Health Organization www.who.org
- The Harvard School of Public Health http://www.hsph.harvard.edu/
- The Mayo Clinic: http://www.Mayoclinic.org

16.7 Emerging Models for Chronic Conditions Management

The delivery of primary health care services in the United States is changing. These changes are perhaps most apparent in clinics or hospitals serving low-income patients living with multiple chronic conditions.

THE LIMITATIONS OF TRADITIONAL MEDICAL MODELS

Traditional medical models are not always effective in managing chronic conditions.

Medicine is concerned with the proximate or most immediate causes of illness in the patient. For example, chronic conditions are generally understood to be caused by physical and biological factors, including genetics and the individual patient's knowledge and behaviors. The medical treatment of chronic conditions generally emphasizes the prescription of available medical treatments, including medications, and changes in individual behavior such as tobacco and alcohol use, diet, and exercise. *This level of focus is vitally important to patients.* Many CHWs work in medical settings, and their work will also focus on engaging individual patients to take medications properly and to change risk-associated behaviors.

However, when health care providers *focus only at the individual level, they fail to consider social determinants that influence a patient's health.* They may fail to diagnose or address issues such as poverty, exposure to racism and other sources of chronic stress, the lack of stable housing, and food insecurity (lack of access to food) that impact a patient's health. Medicine's narrow focus on individual factors sometimes sends a message that the patient is mostly or even completely responsible for their illness. While this may be intended as an empowering message—*"your behaviors contributed to your illness and changing them can make you better"*—it sometimes has the opposite effect, blaming, or shaming patients—*"You wouldn't be so sick if you just followed our directions, took your medications and changed your behaviors!"* This message can have a negative impact on the patient's motivation for change and desire to seek out medical assistance in the future.

At its worse, licensed health care providers and patients end up in a kind of impasse or conflict in which each party grows increasingly frustrated with the other. The physician may be thinking:

> *Why can't the patient understand that if they don't make big changes to their lifestyle now, they are going to end up in the hospital or worse? They nod their heads to say "Yes, doctor," but keep having the same conversation and they aren't doing anything different!*

At the same time, the patient may be thinking:

> *I'd like to see this doctor walk a mile in my shoes! Where is she going to find healthy foods in my neighborhood, and how would she afford them if she did find them? And I'd like to see her go exercise after a day juggling two jobs, a disabled husband and two grandkids! I'm too exhausted to exercise, but that doctor probably thinks I'm lazy.*

16.8 Integrating Medicine and Public Health Models

Increasingly, health care organizations are establishing new models that integrate medicine and public health. These models look beyond a patient's current symptoms and risk behaviors to consider how the broader social environment affects their health. They seek to intervene further "upstream" to prevent the development or progression of illness, to support patients to live healthier lives in a more comprehensive way and, in some instances, to partner with organizations, activists and policy makers to create social change.

To promote better patient outcomes, health care organizations must learn about the social determinants of health. Health care providers can study local data on public health and social issues that impact the health of the communities they serve, such as rates of illness and death—and inequities in these rates among populations—and data on housing, employment, food insecurity, and education (and, again, inequities in rates of access or achievement). Local nonprofit organizations and resident associations understand current health risks and are aware of the key resources that community members most trust. Local media stories often highlight public health and social issues. The more that health care providers understand these issues, they more they will respect the challenges faced by individual patients and their families.

As a working CHW or Promotor de Salud, pay close attention to the environment around you. If you live in the same community in which you work, try to view it with a fresh set of eyes.

- *What do you observe? What types of health and social resources exist?*
- *What types of organizations, programs and services are available?*
- *Which essential resources are missing?*
- *What health risks—including social determinants of health—do you notice?*
- *What types of social change are most necessary for promoting the health of local communities (and particularly for the most vulnerable among them)?*
- *What are the priority concerns of community members?*

As you work with patients and community members, apply the ecological model and person-centered concepts addressed in other chapters of this textbook. When you conduct an assessment to learn about the health status of a new patient, ask open-ended questions and invite them to share more information about their lives, including both the risks that they face and the resources they have. Remember to use a strength-based approach to assess not only the factors that may be contributing to the patient's illness, but also the factors that contribute to their health. By asking about and acknowledging a client's strengths, you are identifying resources that may help to enhance their health. Provide case management and advocacy to support patients in addressing issues that lie beyond the individual level of the ecological model. Health is promoted when you assist clients to access new or improved resources such as stable housing and a regular source of healthy food, or when you support a new patient coming home from prison to re-connect with their family.

People living with chronic conditions often experience social isolation and may benefit from opportunities to connect with others who face similar challenges. By coming together, people can share self-management tips and offer emotional support and motivation for self-care. Connection to others and a sense of belonging are key aspects of emotional, mental, and physical health. There is a strong history of people living with chronic health conditions coming together to provide social support and, as we address below, to take collective social action. Building social support has been essential for people living with mental health conditions, for survivors of trauma, for people struggling with substance use, and for people living with disabilities and chronic conditions such as cancer, HIV disease, and Hepatitis C. We encourage you to learn about the types of social or support groups that exist in the communities where you live and work. Who participates in these groups? What types of health or social issues do they address?

By working to create social change—such as changes to policies that limit or deny access to key resources and rights—we can also change patterns of chronic conditions within our society. For some patients, joining with others to create social change is also a prescription for their wellness. Addressing social issues that we care deeply about, such as issues of equity and justice, not only helps to prevent greater illness and premature death in our communities, it is also good for our own spirits, minds, and bodies. For more information about community organizing and advocacy, see Chapter 23.

Movements for Social Change

Social movements have changed public policies that influence American life and the health of diverse communities. These movements may take many decades to achieve change, and not every effort is successful. Even when victories have been won, new policies may achieve only partial change, may not be enforced or are eroded, and require continued organizing and advocacy. Still, social movements have resulted in meaningful changes. They have changed labor laws related to working hours and conditions, and to the exploitation of children. The civil rights movement resulted in laws to ban discrimination on the basis of sex, ethnicity, and nationality and in areas such as employment, education, and housing. The mental health recovery movement has resulted in changes in the way that people with mental conditions are viewed and treated. Activists changed policies governing research, health care, and benefits for people living with HIV disease and helped lead the movement to find ways to prevent the spread of HIV. Movements across the United States are challenging criminal justice policies that lead to mass incarceration and impose lifelong penalties and barriers for formerly incarcerated people as they try to access employment, housing, education, food stamps, and other key resources.

For the communities that you belong to and work with:

- *Which social movements have created meaningful change for the communities you belong to and work with?*

16.9 Team-based Approaches to Chronic Conditions Management

Primary health care clinics typically rely upon a team-based approach to support the health of patients living with chronic disease. The topic of team-based practice is addressed in greater detail in Chapter 5 of *Foundations*. We will build upon that information here, emphasizing concepts related to chronic conditions management.

The members of a health care team varies across clinical settings. The team always includes the patient (the most important member of the team) and a licensed provider such as a physician or nurse practitioner. Teams may also include key family members (such as parent, guardian, or a partner if they are available and willing), other licensed health care and mental health providers such as a nurse, social worker or psychologist, panel managers (see below), and frontline providers such as medical assistants and CHWs. Some teams may integrate other specialists such as a respiratory therapist or pharmacist.

When CHWs are included as members of the primary care team, they work with clients in a variety of ways and settings. CHWs may meet clients in the clinic and in the community and accompany clients to key medical and social services appointments. CHWs may visit clients in their homes or other setting if clients are homeless, hospitalized, in residential programs, or incarcerated. CHWs may conduct an initial interview or intake with the client, provide health education, and may support the development and implementation of an action plan for the self-management of chronic health conditions. CHWs may facilitate educational or support groups for people diagnosed with chronic disease. For these reasons, CHWs often have more time to build a relationship with the client and to talk in greater depth about the factors that affect their health and welfare. As a result, the CHW is often the critical link between the patient and rest of the clinical team.

Mattie Clark: I work with a large team at the G. A. Carmichael Family Health Center in Canton Mississippi. We are lucky to have nurse practitioners and social workers. We have an internal pharmacy and a dentistry program. We have outreach workers and an HIV program and of course there are other CHWs. So, you are never on your own here.

We have clinical team meetings; it's like our team huddle in the mornings. We get together and one of the nurse practitioners will let everyone know which patients are coming in that day, and what needs they have, and if there are any home visits to do. So, we know if someone has elevated cholesterol or blood glucose or blood pressure. And the nurse will ask us to provide certain types of services, like health education or help with medication adherence or home visits. We CHWs do a lot of the education, talking with patients to see if they understand what hypertension is, or diabetes, and kind of filling in the gaps. We talk with them about basic nutrition, like do they know what kinds of foods they can be eating that are healthier. Home visiting is a key part of this. When I visit the participants in my program, I train them on how to accurately take an accurate blood pressure or blood glucose reading and how to keep a log to track and share the measurements with their health care providers. I bring my laptop with me, and I enter findings into the Mississippi State Department of Health (MSDH) web portal as well as an electronic health record.

Lorena Carmona: I work as part of a large team at Roots Health Center in Oakland California. We have over 50 programs staffed by nurse practitioners, doctors, our behavioral health providers, social workers, medical assistants, and CHWs. We have case conferences twice a month to talk about patients and their progress and what we can do to support them. It is usually the medical director who oversees the program I work for, and our team of 10–12 CHWS. One of the CHWs will present the case of a patient, how they are doing and what they may be struggling with. So, the whole team—the medical director and the CHWs—provides feedback so we can learn together about best ways to support clients with managing chronic health conditions. We talk about how to help with the social determinants of health, like housing and food security resources, or transportation. We learn about referrals both within our agency and to other agencies and programs.

16.10 Population Health Management

Population health management (PHM), sometimes referred to as panel management, is a system for coordinating health care for a group of patients. The primary goal of PHM is to identify patients with the greatest health risks in order to provide timely care and prevent the progression of health conditions. Population health management promotes improved patient health outcomes and reduces health inequities.

Key health information about a clinic or program's group or population of patients is regularly reviewed and analyzed. This data is used to identify "at-risk" patients such as those who have missed one or more clinical appointments, who have not refilled prescribed medications, who have not returned calls or other communications from the clinic, patients with symptoms, or test results that are out of range of "normal" (such as very high or uncontrolled blood pressure readings), or other signs of health risks such as recent hospitalizations or Emergency Department visits. These patients may be at risk for disease progression, disability, and health crises that may include infection, heart attack, and stroke. The goal is to connect with these patients and arrange for the delivery of services that will result in improved health status and/or immediate care such as a clinic appointment or home visit.

Because of their close relationships with patients and the community, CHWs often contribute to PHM. CHWs may reach out to patients by placing calls, sending texts, scheduling telehealth visits or conducting home visits to check in about their health and to ask if they would like to schedule an appointment with a provider.

Population health management has resulted in improved patient care and outcomes (McGough, Chaudhari, El-Attar, & Yung, 2018). Benefits from PHM include (University of Washington, 2018):

- **Better health outcomes:** The ultimate goal of PHM is simple—improving the quality of care while reducing costs.

- **Disease management:** PHM improves the care of those with chronic and costly disease by using IT solutions that track and manage their care.

- **Closing care gaps:** PHM helps to close gaps in care by allowing organizations and physicians to have real-time access to track and address patient needs. Laboratory, billing, electronic health record, and prescription data can easily pinpoint unmet needs and gaps in data or service delivery.

- **Cost savings for providers**: As with all advances in health care management, PHM is a win-win. By leveraging data analytics, PHM improves clinical outcomes while reducing costs.

16.11 Patient Self-Management

The self-management of chronic conditions is rapidly becoming the new standard of care. It is a *person-centered* approach that supports patients to manage their chronic conditions over time, making decisions about the types of treatments and services they want to participate in, and what else they will do to promote their own health.

Self-management is defined as "the ability of the patient to deal with all that a chronic illness entails, including symptoms, treatment, physical and social consequences, and lifestyle changes. With effective self-management, the patient can monitor his or her condition and make whatever cognitive, behavioral, and emotional changes are needed to maintain a satisfactory quality of life" (Multiple Chronic Conditions Resource Center, 2022).

Self-management represents a significant shift in chronic conditions management as well as to the relationship between health care providers and patients. Traditional models of health care view the physician (or other licensed provider) as *the* health expert. In traditional settings, the role of the physician is to share their knowledge and give informed advice to the patient. The role of the patient is to follow the directions of the physician. While this type of relationship may work well for some providers and patients, ultimately, *it ignores the fact that the day-to-day management of chronic disease occurs outside of the clinic or hospital.* If patients don't learn information and skills for the day-to-day management of their illness, including the confidence to make decisions, they may face increased health risks.

Self-management places the patient at the center of a collaborative relationship with their health care team. While it draws on the knowledge and skills that the patient already has, it also builds and enhances knowledge, skills, motivation, and confidence for the day-to-day management of their conditions. This approach fits with the concepts of cultural humility and person-centered practice that will guide your own work, "Sometimes called 'patient empowerment,' this concept holds that patients accept responsibility to manage their own conditions and are encouraged to solve their own problems with information, but not orders, from professionals." (Bodenheimer, Wagner, & Grumbach, 2002)

Self-management education (SME) programs provide structured educational programs for people living with chronic conditions. These programs are designed to help people develop the skills and confidence to cope with symptoms, manage fatigue, handle stress, reduce depression, communicate with doctors, manage medication, eat healthy, and be active (Centers for Disease Control and Prevention, 2018). Some SME groups address a specific chronic health condition. For example, the Centers for Disease Control and Prevention provides information about Self-Management Education programs for specific chronic conditions including Arthritis, Asthma, Cancer, COPD, Depression, Diabetes, Epilepsy, Heart Disease and Lupus (Centers for Disease Control and Prevention, 2019).

Mattie Clark: I am certified in the self-management of diabetes and other health conditions. When a patient is referred to me from the health care provider, I review the patient's electronic health record. If the patient has hypertension, then I'll pull together all my information and resources on hypertension and schedule an appointment. Sometimes, one of the nurse practitioner sits in on the beginning of my appointment with the patient just to introduce me and review the priorities. Then I like to give the patient the floor to tell me what's going on, why they're here, and what they need. They tell me what they know about elevated blood pressure, what they're doing to manage it, and what they are struggling with. I listen with my eyes and my heart and my ears so I can try to see the picture they are painting for me. Many participants struggle with what to eat, and with physical activity and getting enough rest. So, we talk about that, and I always ask them for their ideas first and, if they ask me for recommendations, then I'll offer education or resources. I make sure to address them on their individual level. For example, instead of always having fried food, which is a common thing in Mississippi, we talk about healthier ways to prepare their meals. We just try to have fun with it, coming up different types of styles and recipes. Without fail, I ask about the participant's family, and if they offer them support with their health conditions.

Self-Management commonly includes the following strategies and actions for patients:

- Develop health goals and a realistic action plan to reach those goals
  - Working effectively with their health care team
  - Managing health crises or emergencies
  - Finding and using community resources
- Talk with family, friends, and care-takers about their illness and self-management plan, and asking for help when needed
- Evaluate available treatment options, including medications
  - Taking and using treatments and medications effectively
- Manage symptoms of fatigue, frustration, sleep difficulties, and pain
- Change patterns of behavior such as diet, physical activity, stress management, and the use of tobacco, alcohol, and drugs
- Monitor action plan progress and health symptoms
  - Patients learn to take and keep track of their blood pressure, to monitor blood glucose levels with a home meter, or to keep a record of their level of pain (such as with a scale from 0 to 10).
- Make decisions about when to access health care services
  - *What telse do you consider to be an important part of Self-management?*

What Do YOU Think?

Lorena Carmona: When patients come to the Roots Health Center, we have a kiosk where we take their blood pressure. If I am working with a patient with hypertension, we talk about their blood pressure reading. I'll ask them to tell me what the reading indicates, and what a healthy blood pressure reading should be. This is a chance to find out what they know about hypertension and healthy and unhealthy blood pressure levels. At the same time, I'll ask them if they have a blood pressure monitor at home. If they don't, then I make a note in the electronic health record so that their medical provider can order one for them. I call them when their blood pressure monitor arrives, and I sit with them as they take their blood pressure, and we talk about what it means. If they want some guidance, I will talk with them about how to sit down for a few minutes before taking their blood pressure, how to hold their arm and place the [blood pressure] cuff, and how to record or make a record of their blood pressure. We use the American Heart Association guidelines. Once they feel confident in taking their own blood pressure, this is something that I can check in with them over time, and we can talk about their readings and how they are doing managing their blood pressure.

Please watch the following video interview with David Spero who shares his approach to supporting clients with self-management:

16.12 Chronic Conditions and the CHW Scope of Practice

CHWs are key members of primary health care teams focused on the treatment of chronic conditions. While CHWs can provide a wide range of tasks and direct services, their role is not always well-defined. In some settings, you may find that colleagues don't understand that you can contribute more to the team. In other settings, you may be asked to provide services that lie outside of your prior training and knowledge. As a result, you may need help to clarify the tasks and services you provide.

SELF-MANAGEMENT: FINDING REASONS TO LIVE.

(*Source:* Foundations for Community Health Workers/http://youtu.be/nRChT90HOMM)

The range of services that CHWs perform varies tremendously across clinical sites, based on the specific needs of the clinic or hospital, and the patients they serve. In general, the tasks and services *may* include the following:

- Outreach to local agencies, other clinics, and hospitals to make them aware of the services you provide.
- Outreach to patients (for recruitment, follow-up, and case management).
- Assess the social determinants of health that impact a patient's health, and their needs for better managing their chronic conditions.
- Health education about chronic conditions such as diabetes or hypertension. Many CHWs receive additional training or certification in specific chronic conditions and, in some settings, may provide most of the health education to patients.
- Health education on topics such as dietary and exercise guidelines, smoking cessation, and other health topics.
- Facilitation or co-facilitation of patient education or support groups such as groups for patients newly diagnosed with type 2 diabetes or depression.
- Development of client action plans for the self-management of chronic conditions, including health goals and actions to reach those goals.
- Support for client changes to health-related behaviors, using person-centered counseling.

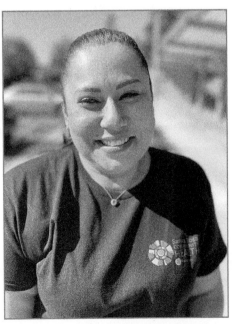

A CHW who supports clients with the self-management of chronic conditions.

- Case management services and providing appropriate referrals to other agencies, programs and services.
- Health system navigation including access to key benefits and services.
- Accompaniment or, at the patients request, attending certain appointments with them. These might include appointments with specialists such as an Oncologist (or cancer specialist), Nutritionist, or with social services agencies in the community (such as a transitional housing agency or residential drug recovery program).
- Medications management to ensure that patients are taking medications as prescribed.
- Measure and document blood pressure; conduct foot exams for patients with diabetes and other health status checks as appropriate.
- Support patients with advocacy. CHWs will encourage and help to prepare patients to advocate for their own health needs with other health and social services providers. When patients are not able to advocate for themselves, they may ask CHWs to advocate for specific health or social needs with other providers or agencies.
- Assistance with population health management
- Home visits to check on patients who are home bound, unable to visit a clinic or health center. As detailed in Chapter 11, home visits can provide additional information about the client's living situation, relationships, access to key resources including food, and their health status.

Ask your employer to clarify your role and scope of practice within the clinical team. *If you are not confident about providing a particular service, tell your supervisor and ask for additional training and guidance.*

Mattie Clark: CHWs provide a variety of services. To be effective in the community, CHWs must meet the core competency skills as a frontline health worker.

Being a part of the community I serve, I recognize the social determinants of health and the lack of resources in my town such as the lack of a hospital, affordable housing, and living in a food desert. CHWs provide health education, case management, home visits and referrals. We assist with medication refills and medications adherence. I teach patients how to check their blood glucose and blood pressure. I talk with them about healthy nutrition. We even run groups! We enter everything we do into the Mississippi State Department of Health (MSDH) web portal as well as the patient's electronic health record, so that the team can see what we're doing, and what questions we document and what referrals we provide. I go out and visit participants in their homes, according to our CHW work protocol. I go out to the rural communities. When I visit with the participants I observe things in the home that other providers don't have an opportunity to see, like if they have food or not. Once a participant was complaining about pain in her feet. She volunteered to show me her feet and they appeared in need of medical attention. But the participant had been hiding what was going on with her feet out of embarrassment. I immediately called and made an appointment for the participant with the podiatrist (foot specialist) and the nurse practitioner to make sure they received medical attention.

Client Scenario: Rosina Walker *(continued)*

CHW: Hello Rosina, it's such a pleasure to meet you. My name is _____ and I'm one of the Community Health Workers here at Southeast Health Center. I'm part of your health care team.

Rosina: Pleased to meet you.

(continues)

Client Scenario: Rosina Walker (*continued*)

CHW: I see here that Mrs. Washington, one of our nurse practitioners, referred you to meet with me about your high blood pressure, is that right?

Rosina: Yes, that's right.

CHW: So, what's going on with your health right now?

Rosina: Well, I just learned that my blood pressure is not doing well, and this gives me a bit of stress.

CHW: Do you know what your blood pressure reading was today?

Rosina: Yes, the nurse took it. She took it twice, actually, and the lowest reading, maybe because I was so nervous, it was 140/95 and I know that's not where it's supposed to be.

CHW: Yes, that's higher than what the goal is for your blood pressure. Do you know what the goal measurement is for your blood pressure.

Rosina: I think it's supposed to be about 120/80 or even lower, right?

CHW: Yes, that's exactly right. Rosina, can I ask how long have you been living with high blood pressure?

Rosina: Let's see, I had it diagnosed after I gave birth to my daughter Louise, so that would be about seven years.

CHW: And how have you done in the past with managing your blood pressure?

Rosina: I did alright at first. I kept my blood pressure pretty well managed. It was mostly in that healthier range we talked about, below 120/80.

CHW: Well, that's impressive. You must have learned a lot about hypertension and how to manage it. Can you tell me what you did to manage your blood pressure so well in the past?

Rosina: I was keeping up with my medications of course, and I was also more active then. I used to work as a teacher's aide at the elementary school and, well, as you can imagine, that kept me busy! I was still married back then, and my husband was at home, and we had more income.

CHW: So, I'm wondering have any of your circumstances changed recently? What do you think is contributing to your higher blood pressure now?

Rosina: A lot has changed. I'm divorced now, and I have a one year old. My husband and I, we tried to reconcile a ways back and I fell pregnant. But he left and I had to quit my job because I couldn't pay for childcare and make ends meet on my salary. So, I went on benefits. And taking care of a toddler, well, I'm older now, and it seems much harder than it was with my first two children.

CHW: So, you're a single parent now, and you're raising three children.

Rosina: Yes. Rosamunde, she's my oldest, then comes Louise and then Ben. The oldest two are in school now, so that's easier. But Ben, he's an active boy and I need to watch him 24/7.

CHW: Can I ask, is your ex-husband helping you and the children out?

Rosina: He does what he can. He takes our oldest girls for a month in the summer and that gives them time with their father, and it gives me a little break. He moved to stay with his brother, in another state. Then he injured his back and is out on disability, so they don't really have much to spare.

(continues)

Client Scenario: Rosina Walker *(continued)*

CHW: So, it sounds like your circumstances have changed a lot since you were first diagnosed with hypertension.

Rosina: It's been a lot of changes that I wasn't expecting. [sighs] I wasn't expecting a divorce, or another child, or to be on assistance for the first time in my life. I'm grateful for the benefits I get but I can barely stretch them out till the end of the month.

CHW: Well, I can't commend you enough for raising three children on your own. Like a lot of single parents, it sounds like you are facing some economic challenges, is that right?

Rosina: It's a struggle to keep the lights on and food on the table. But my kids always have something to eat, even if it means that I go hungry at the end of the month.

CHW: Does that happen every month, running out of food for yourself? [Rosina nods and reaches for a tissue]. Well, Rosina, you're not alone in running out of food by the end of the month. And I'm confident that is something that we can help you with, okay? I know of some good resources. But first, can I ask you a bit about your social support? [Rosina nods]. Do you have support from family or friends? Do you have someone to talk to?

Rosina: Oh, I'm not alone. My mother, she's in a nursing home in _____ [a neighboring town]. She lost her foot to diabetes so she's in a wheelchair and she can't help me out with the children like she used to, but we're very close. I talk with her on the phone two or three times a day if I can't get over to see her.

CHW: Well, I'm so glad to hear that you and your mother are close. There's no substitute for that, is there?

Rosina: No, she's been there for me through the ups and the downs.

CHW: And what about friends or community support?

Rosina: I'm a religious person and I have my church community. I go to the Baptist Church across town and even though it's a long walk with the stroller, I never miss a Sunday service. That's the thing that lifts me up more than anything these days.

CHW: I'm so glad to hear that. Our faith, having a community, that's part of health too.

Rosina: Yes, it certainly is.

16.13 Applying Person Centered Concepts and Skills

The over-arching role of CHWs is to support clients to effectively manage their chronic disease. *This work should be guided by person-centered concepts and skills designed to promote and support the client's independence and autonomy.* These concepts are addressed in detail in Chapters 6–10 of the *Foundations* textbook and include:

Honor a client's right to self-determination: Respect people's right to make their own decisions about their own life, whether you agree with these decisions or not. Strive to let go of your tendencies to control a patient's attitudes, beliefs, behaviors, and choices.

Cultural humility: Work to shift or transfer power away from yourself, providing opportunities for patients or clients to claim greater control and authority for the self-management of their chronic health conditions. Strive to be aware of your own cultural identity, values and assumptions, and to avoid any tendencies to impose these standards as you work with clients. Use person-centered skills to ask clients to share their own cultural values and beliefs.

- For example, in working with Rosina Walker, you don't want to impose cultural standards for a healthy diet. Instead, support Rosina to figure out how to change her diet in a way that fits with and honors her cultural and family traditions.

Ecological models: Our health is shaped and influenced by a broader social, economic, and political context. Learn about the context in which patients live and apply this knowledge as you work together to enhance the patients' health status and autonomy. Consider both the risk factors and resources that may influence a client's health at the level of their family, community, and the broader society.

BIG EYES, BIG EARS, and a small mouth: Don't speak too much. Provide opportunities for patients to share their concerns, priorities, wisdom, and skills. Listen deeply and carefully to what clients tell you. Observe their body language, their behavior, relationships, and surroundings.

Strength-based approach: Never forget to assess a client's strengths such as their knowledge, social support, and accomplishments. Most clients already know something (*and many know a lot*) about their chronic health condition. Ask open-ended questions to draw out the client's knowledge about their health condition and the approaches that have helped them to manage it. Build on the client's strengths as you support them to develop an action plan for the self-management of their chronic condition(s). Remember that the ideas that come from clients are much more likely to be effective in promoting their health than the ideas that come from others.

Harm reduction: Support clients to reduce potential harms to their health. Don't impose an abstinence standard, or expectations that patients will completely stop certain behaviors (such as smoking or eating fast food) or avoid all health risks in the future. Those are not realistic goals for most people, regardless of their health.

- For example, Rosina Walker is struggling to eat healthier foods on a limited budget. By applying a harm reduction model, Rosina may decide to cut back on certain types of food and drinks that pose risks for her high blood pressure, and to gradually increase those that promote her health.

Motivational interviewing (MI): Apply MI skills including the use of OARS. When appropriate, consider using a readiness or motivation scale or ruler to support clients in assessing their readiness for change, their level of motivation, and confidence.

With time and practice, you will become more skilled and confident in using Motivational Interviewing. In working with Rosina Walker, for example, you may

- O = Ask Open-ended questions: *"Rosina, What are some of the skills that you learned from managing your blood pressure in the past that you might be able to apply to your situation now?"*
- A = Provide authentic Affirmations such as: *"You've done a remarkable job raising your family as a single mother on a limited budget—it must take a lot of creativity and determination."*
- R = Use Reflective listening to support Rosina to think about the factors that influence her health, such as the loss of her marriage and her job, her religious faith, and values.
- S = Summarize key information and decisions that Rosina shares with you, such as her goal to manage her high blood pressure, to access resources at the food bank, and attend more services at church.

Person-centered health education: CHWs often provide health education about chronic health conditions and related issues such as stress management, physical activity, and healthy eating. We recommend staying patient-centered as you provide education. Start by asking patients what they already know about their chronic health conditions and other topics such as nutrition. Ask the client if you can share some additional information and be sure to do so a little at a time, rather than in a long lecture. Instead of telling clients what you think they should do—such as take a cooking class at the YMCA or access resources at the food bank—offer this information as a suggestion for them to consider: *"What do you think about the idea of taking a free healthy cooking class at the YMCA?"* When providing health education about topics such as stress, physical activity, and nutrition, keep the client's cultural identity and traditions in mind. Try to share resources and referrals that are based on the client's community and cultural traditions whenever possible. For more information on person-centered health education, please see Chapter 17.

● *What other aspects of person-centered practice will guide your work in chronic conditions management?*

CHW Profile

Joe Calderon (he/him)

Senior CHW, Lead Trainer,

Transitions Clinic Network (TCN)

Providing health care to individuals returning to the community from incarceration

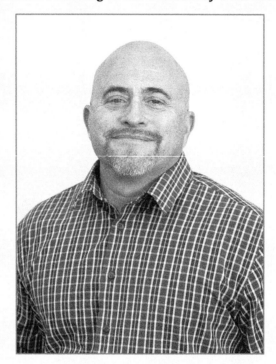

Most good CHWs were CHWS before they knew they were CHWs. My path has been from trauma to medicine to advocacy. When I was in prison, I learned that "for the people and by the people" was not for me or by me. In prison, watching people die, first I felt fear and then anger. I knew that anger wasn't going to get me anywhere, so I asked myself, what part can I play in the solution? And that's what I've been doing since I came home, well before I was a CHW.

It's legal to discriminate against those of us who've made mistakes. Discrimination should never be legal. For the disenfranchised and diverse communities that I serve and love, if we cannot get health equity, then the rest on the table is a façade. Nobody should die of treatable diseases. Health care is reentry.

The Transitions Clinic Network (TCN) includes dozens of primary care clinics across the country and in Puerto Rico. TCN serves a community with a history of incarceration, some of the most stigmatized, with some of the most uphill battles to fight for successful and healthy reentry. I serve returning community members. I use that term specifically because I believe language is important. You can get somebody on board or lose somebody in a word. TCN only hires CHWs who are from the community they serve.

I work with a community historically untrusting of systems to build relationships to keep people in care while they learn to navigate the health system and address their chronic conditions, while on parole, probation, or free. I also teach, consult and train other clinics across the United States on how to successfully integrate a CHW into their medical team.

(continues)

CHW Profile

(continued)

In our clinic in San Francisco, there are always two of us, one person in the office, one in the field. During outreach, we go out and build relationships with transitional homes, probation, parole, emergency rooms, streets, jails, and prisons. I may escort someone to the DMV, Social Security Office, or a medical appointment. I may have coffee with someone having an anxiety attack about family reunification, work, or school.

In the office, I'm making appointments, phone reminders, getting emergency prescription refills, and anything to make it as simple as possible for community members with competing stressors. I'm their advocate. I visit other services we refer to, get to know the people there. Never send anybody someplace you haven't been yourself.

One of my clients, T, was an individual that had a lot going on medically. T had a history of substance abuse and because that history was criminalized, led him to doing half of his life in prison. When he came home he was anxious and he had nobody. I was able to be his ear, with active listening to what his goals were, and aligning them to the goals of TCN. This person who's never had a job, spent a quarter of a century in prison, within 90 days had two jobs and his own apartment in San Francisco, CA. There's people that come in with better circumstances and can't do that. And yet he did that.

What I want a new CHW to know is serve in humility and gratefulness. Motivational interviewing and cultural humility, what I like to call "letting people live in their skin," are two key skill sets to being the best CHW you can be. That puts you in a place to not only be patient-centric, but it puts you in a place to validate anybody in front of you. Validation and active listening keep more people in care.

16.14 Action Planning for Chronic Conditions Management

Chapters 9 and 10 provide guidance on how to work with clients to develop an action plan to promote their health. Your role is to support the patient to develop an action plan that is relevant and realistic. This includes determining one or more achievable health goals for the not-too-distant future (such as within two to six months), and the actions that the patient will take to reach their goals. The actions should be ones that the patient has a good chance of successfully implementing and should include specific details. For example, rather than "exercise regularly," or "Climb Mount Massive," actions might include something like "Walk my dog back and forth to Pine Hill Park. Start walking on Saturdays, and gradually increase to 3 times per week."

Generally, patients have a good idea of what they can do to better manage their chronic condition, but sometimes, they may want support to identify or refine the actions they will take to meet health goals. In these situations, you can provide *suggestions* for the patient to consider, reject, or accept, while keeping in mind that successful behavior change depends upon the extent to which the client can claim ownership of their plan. We always recommend *asking before telling*. In other words, ask clients to share their own ideas or proposals for actions before sharing a suggestion.

We also recommend normalizing the challenge of behavior change. Talk with the patient about how difficult behavior change can be, and the common cycles that people experience, including setbacks or relapse, and re-thinking or revising their plans. Your ability to support a client without judgment, regardless of the challenges they may face as they implement their plan and create positive change, can play a role in their success.

ACTION PLANNING

(*Source:* Foundations for Community Health Workers/http://youtu. be/51J58BJeQak)

Please watch the following video interview about Action Planning:

ESTABLISHING HEALTH GOALS

Developing a health action plan often begins by asking clients to articulate their most important health goals. Health goals will vary among the clients you work with. Keep an open mind about the type of goals that may be most important to clients.

> ## The Patient's Health isn't Always their Top Priority
>
> Sometimes the goals that are most important to clients may not appear to be directly connected to their chronic health condition. Clients may be more concerned about other issues, such as finding employment, permanent housing or access to mental health services for their children. Keep in mind that the action plan belongs to the client and should reflect their authentic priorities and concerns. Remember that by supporting clients to take action to meet any significant goal, you can build trust and rapport, and lay the groundwork for future work to address new goals.

Goals typically represent the client's desire to change or transform some aspect of their health or wellness in order to improve the quality of their life. For clients living with chronic conditions, health goals may include:

- Reducing key health symptoms or indicators
- Slowing the progression of disease
- Sustainable self-management
- Enhancing the ability to engage in daily activities
- Enhancing autonomy or independence
- Improving economic and social circumstances
- Stress reduction
- Promoting mental and/or spiritual health
- Improving medication management
- Family acceptance and support
- Building social connections and a sense of belonging
- Participating in social change/social justice actions or movements

- *What other health goals may people with chronic conditions strive to achieve?*

What Do **YOU?** Think

Lorena Carmona: When I do action planning with members or patients, it is always the patient who comes up with the plan. It has to be the patient's plan, so that it is something they are motivated to do, and something they feel that they can do. I help them to figure out the details and I might provide some guidance or suggestions if they are open to it. Like, if they are taking their blood pressure at home once a day, I might ask what they think about taking it at two different times of the day. They have the power to decide and say yes or no, or to come up with another plan. And if something that they need is missing, like a blood glucose or blood pressure monitor, then that is something I can help them with. I can make sure that they get the equipment. If they have questions about their medications or concerns about it, then I make sure they get an appointment to talk about it with a medical provider. So, I am there to help, but not to lead.

Client Scenario: Rosina Walker (continued)

CHW: Rosina, we ask each patient to develop a personalized plan for managing their chronic health conditions. It includes setting goals that you want to achieve and actions that you will take to meet those goals. Overtime, you can monitor your progress and adjust the plan as needed and, of course, we'll be here to offer support and guidance as you need it. Would you like to start your plan?

Rosina: Yes, I always feel better when I have a plan

CHW: What would you say are your main priorities or goals for promoting your hypertension and your health?

Rosina: Well, I know I'm supposed to be focused on my blood pressure, but honestly, the biggest challenges I have right now are with food and transportation.

CHW: One thing I've learned is that everything is connected to health, Rosina. Not having transportation and food no doubt causes you stress, and we talked about how stress aggravates hypertension, right?

Rosina: Yes, it does.

CHW: So, let's just focus on what your most important priorities are.

Rosina: Well, I don't have a car anymore and the buses don't come as often as they used to. It might take me three to four hours just to go shopping at the SaveMart across town. And I have to arrange for someone to take care of my children now, with my mother in the nursing home. My neighbor Jeannie and I trade off taking care of each other's kids when we need to do errands.

CHW: Are there any family or friends who might be able to help out and give you a ride?

Rosina: My mother used to help us out, but she can't drive anymore. She's in Meadowview, you know, the nursing home over in _____? And, well, I'm not used to asking others for help.

CHW: Why do you think it's hard for you to ask for a helping hand?

Rosina: Well [Rosina sighs] I used to be one that helped others out. As a Teacher's Aide, I knew most of the families in town, and I was a resource for them. I haven't adjusted to being one of the families who needs a hand-up.

CHW: Well, that's how we get by. We help our neighbors who need it when we can, right? [Rosina nods] I can also help out with transportation. There's a company, Reliance Transportation, that we can arrange for anyone on Medicaid. They can't take you everywhere, but they can take you to medical appointments, to the pharmacy, and to pick up groceries. There is no charge for using the transportation service. I can help you set up an account through the clinic and then you need to schedule the rides at least five days in advance.

Rosina: I can do that. I can schedule my trips in advance.

CHW: Great. Where else do you need to go?

Rosina: Well, the other place I go is church. It is a long walk, especially with the stroller. When I was still married, I used to go two or three times a week. I really miss my Wednesday Night Women's Meeting, but I haven't been in . . . Oh, it's been since my pregnancy, so almost two years.

CHW: What would you say to a friend at church if she was in your situation and didn't have transportation?

Rosina: I'd say let's call the Associate Pastor because they want you to be at church and they will arrange a ride!

CHW: So, how is it any different for you? Don't you think your congregation wants to see you at church?

(continues)

Client Scenario: Rosina Walker (continued)

Rosina: [Pauses] I'm sure they do. I know I shouldn't let my pride get in the way.

CHW: So, who will you call?

Rosina: I'll call Reverend Simmons; she's the Associate Pastor.

CHW: Okay then. How does that feel?

Rosina: It's a relief. [Rosina pauses and nods] I've been stuck.

CHW: Well, I'm glad to see you working this out. You're here asking me for help, which I am proud and happy to provide. Your first goal is to improve access to transportation, and we are going to set up an account with Reliance Transportation and you are going to reach out to Reverend Simmons to see if she can arrange a ride to the women's group. Is that right?

Rosina: Yes, that sounds like a plan. [laughs]

CHW: You mentioned that your other priority is food. Can you tell me more about that?

Rosina shares her concern about running out of food each month. The CHW provides information about several organizations that provide families with food assistance including a local Food Pantry that Rosina is familiar with.

Rosina and the CHW write up her Action Plan to include two initial goals, increasing access to healthy and affordable food and increasing access to transportation. The CHW enters the plan into Rosina's electronic health record and prints out a copy of the plan for Rosina to take with her. They schedule a follow-up meeting in a month and agree to add in future goals and actions to Rosina's action plan once she is connected with transportation and food resources.

Please watch the following [▶] that shows a CHW who is working to support a client who has diabetes:

- *What does the CHW do well in supporting the client to develop an Action Plan?*
- *What else could the CHW have done to support this client?*

ACTION PLANNING, DIABETES AND EXERCISE.

(*Source:* Foundations for Community Health Workers/http://youtu. be/XCOQyvhX91A)

USING A MOTIVATION OR CONFIDENCE SCALE

The Motivation Scale (*see Chapter 9*) is a resource to share with clients as they develop or work to implement an Action Plan. The scale from 0 to 10 is a quick and easy way for the client to evaluate their motivation or readiness or confidence in their own plan.

The scale isn't a precise measurement, but it can be useful in assessing a person's readiness for or confidence in moving forward with a certain action. If the client rates their readiness (or confidence or motivation) at a 7 or higher, this is an indication that their Action Plan is relevant or practical, and they have a good chance of moving forward (MacGregor, 2006). If the client rates their readiness or confidence below 7, ask them why, and what might increase it to a 9 or a 10.

- *"Can you tell me why you rated your confidence at a 5?"*
- *"Are there any changes you could make to your plan that could increase your readiness to an 8 or 9?"*

These questions may help the client to refine their plan, address key challenges or doubts, scale back expectations, or add in more detail that will increase the likelihood of their success.

Client Scenario: Rosina Walker *(continued)*

CHW: Rosina, on a scale from 0 to 10, how ready are you to ask Reverend Simmons for a ride to the Women's Group?

Rosina: Oh, that's a 10 for sure; I'm going to call her as soon as I get home.

CHW: Wonderful, and how about scheduling a ride with Reliable Transportation to FoodIsLove, the Food Pantry. On a scale from 0 to 10, how confident are you that you'll give them a call?

Rosina: I'm learning I need to humble myself if I am going to provide for my family. That one's a bit harder, but it's still a 9. The extra groceries are going to make a big difference.

16.15 Medication Management

Many people don't take their medications or don't take them as prescribed. **Medication management**—also known as medication adherence or medication therapy management (MTM)—is the process of working with patients to ensure they take medications as prescribed to achieve their intended impact on their health condition. A wide range of providers—including CHWs—assist patients with medication management to prevent the progression of illness, hospitalizations, and premature death.

MANY PATIENTS DON'T TAKE PRESCRIBED MEDICATIONS

It is estimated that 70% of Americans are on at least one prescription medication and more than 50% take two or more medications. However, an estimated 50% of patients in the United States don't take their medications as prescribed (National Conference of State Legislatures, 2019). About 25% of Americans report not refilling prescriptions, skipping doses, or cutting pills in half due to concerns about the cost of medications (Montero, Kearney, Hamel, & Brodie, 2022). Not taking prescribed medications and not taking them properly can result in poorer health, complications, hospitalizations, and premature death. It is estimated that each year, the lack of adherence to prescribed medications contributes to 25% of hospitalizations in the United States, an estimated 125,000 preventable deaths, and more than $500 billion in avoidable health care costs (Kleinsinger, 2018; Rose, 2022).

Why People Don't Take Their Medication

It is important to try to understand *why* a patient is not taking their medication as prescribed. Some of the reasons may include:

- The clinic or pharmacy made an error, and the medication was never ordered.
- The patient doesn't understand what the medication is for or how to take it.
- The patient can't afford their medication so doesn't refill the prescription regularly, or and may split or skip pills to make them last longer.
- The patient stopped taking the medication due to concerns about side effects.
- The patient is feeling better and assumes they no longer have to take the medication (of course, this could be an indication that the medication is actually working to help control symptoms of the disease and should be continued).

(continues)

Why People Don't Take Their Medication
(continued)

- The patient doesn't believe the medication is effective, so they stop taking it.
- The patient has decided to treat their chronic condition in another way and is not taking the medication. For example, the patient may be going to a different type of health care provider for alternative treatments.
- The patient doesn't want to start a medication that they may have to take for a long time.
- The patient is taking many different medications and it is difficult/confusing to manage. As a consequence, the patient sometimes forgets to take their medication or forgets and takes a double dose of the medication.

CHWS AND MEDICATIONS MANAGEMENT

All levels of health care providers, including physicians, nurses, and pharmacists provide medication management. Increasingly, CHWs also assist patients to manage and take medications as prescribed. A study of CHWs working in four states reported that 79% provide medication management-related services (Jam et al., 2019).

Research has demonstrated that CHWs are effective in providing medication management services. A study of the collaboration between pharmacists and CHWs was shown to improve both medication adherence and patient outcomes among patients with hypertension with or without diabetes (Wheat et al., 2020). A study from Chiapas Mexico showed that CHWs were effective in improving health outcomes and medication adherence among patients with diabetes and hypertension (Newman et al., 2018). The College of Pharmacy at the University of Florida has established a partnership between pharmacists and CHWs to address medication adherence. *"Because CHWs are in a unique position to understand culturally shaped beliefs and health behaviors, they are better able to discover why people are nonadherent to medications compared to pharmacists alone. We propose that many practice barriers faced by pharmacists can be effectively addressed by CHWs."* (University of Florida, 2022).

SUPPORTING PATIENTS WITH MEDICATIONS MANAGEMENT

CHWs can assist with medications management—if assigned to do so by their supervisor and clinical team—by providing patients with education and support in-person and via telehealth. Key tasks for supporting patients with medication management may include:

- Schedule a meeting with the patient and ask them to bring all the medicines they are currently taking (in the bottles, if possible) from all prescribing clinicians (including both those within and outside of your clinical team), and any written prescriptions they may have (even if unfilled).
- Print out a list of medications prescribed by the licensed medical providers from the patient's electronic health record (EHR) to compare with the list and the medications that the patient brings with them. Note any discrepancies or differences between the two lists. For example, the patient may have brought some expired medications that are not currently prescribed or medications prescribed by providers who are not part of the EHR.
- Review each medication with the patient. Check to see that each prescription is current and none of the medications are expired (see how to check the label, below). Ask the patient the following questions about each medication:
  - What do you take this medication for?
  - How do you take this medication?
  - When during the day do you take this medication?
  - When did you last take this medication?
  - Are you taking the medication (and taking it according to the guidelines)? If the patient isn't taking the medication, ask them why not.

- Create a comprehensive list of all current prescribed medications. The patient should have a list and a copy should be entered into their electronic health record. This list can be reviewed and updated when prescriptions change or as needed.

- Ask the patient where they store their medications (note that some medications have specific storage requirements, such as being refrigerated).

- Ask patients how they organize their medications and if they have a system for remembering when to take their medications. Patients may need assistance with organizing their medications in a Medi-Planner (the clinic may provide a Medi-Planner, or it may be covered by their insurance), placing each medication in the designated box for the day of the week when they take it (and/or time of day, as some patients will have AM and PM Medi-kits). Patients may not need or may already have a system in place for remembering to take their medications or may be interested in suggestions such as using a pre-set cell phone alarm or visible notes in places they visit regularly (such as their kitchen or bathroom).

- Ask the patient if they have any questions or concerns about their medications including issues such as cost, dosage, and side effects. Make a note of these questions in the EHR and encourage the patient to discuss these questions directly with their health care provider during their next visit.

- Talk with patients about common concerns such as skipping medications or splitting medications based on concerns about costs or skipping or discontinuing medications because their symptoms or overall health improves. Remind them that any decision about changing their dosage or discontinuing a medication should be discussed with their medical provider to avoid health risks and complications.

- Check to see if the patient fills their prescriptions at more than one pharmacy and, if so, suggest that they inquire if it would be possible to fill all prescriptions at one pharmacy. This way one pharmacist can review all of the medications they take and help with possible drug interactions, dosage, and cost.

- Support the patient to set-up a system to manage refills for prescribed medications. This may be a regular calendar reminder to request a refill or a conversations with their medical provider to ask if it is possible to receive automatic refills of certain medications.

- Follow-up and check in with patients about medication management overtime to ensure that the systems they have set up are still working for them, and any outstanding concerns or questions are referred in a timely fashion to their medical provider or pharmacist.

- As always, document all relevant information in the EHR so that it will be shared with all for all other authorized medical providers.

How to Read the Label on Medications

If you ask patients to bring their medications to an appointment, ask them to do so in the pill bottles they received from the pharmacist. Review the information on the label of the medication bottle with the patient, helping them learn how to read and understand the information provided (Figure 16.1).

The labels include essential information, including:

- The name and strength of the medication
- Instructions for how to take the medication, including how often and when to take it
- Possible side effects and when to see a doctor
- The number of refills before a certain date
- If the medication should be kept out of the reach of children
- The medication's expiration date

(continues)

How to Read the Label on Medications

(continued)

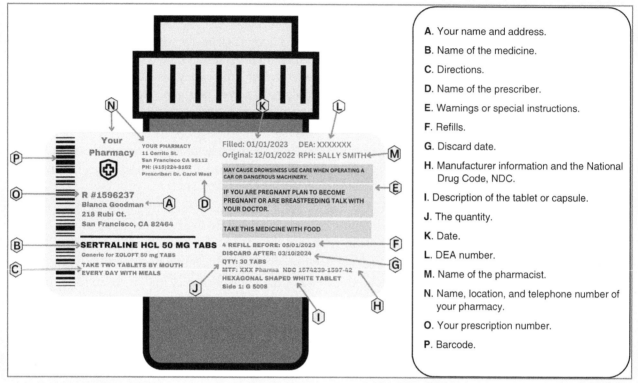

A. Your name and address.

B. Name of the medicine.

C. Directions.

D. Name of the prescriber.

E. Warnings or special instructions.

F. Refills.

G. Discard date.

H. Manufacturer information and the National Drug Code, NDC.

I. Description of the tablet or capsule.

J. The quantity.

K. Date.

L. DEA number.

M. Name of the pharmacist.

N. Name, location, and telephone number of your pharmacy.

O. Your prescription number.

P. Barcode.

Figure 16.1 Medication Label

If the guidelines for prescription labels changes in the future, you can always find updated information by searching online.

Mattie Clark: Medication management always depends on the individual client and what they need. If they are unable to read or understand their medication, I go out to the participant's home, and we go through their medications together to make sure that they understand what each medication is for and how to properly take their medication. Sometimes they can't pronounce the medication or even write it down, and that is okay, but they can still recognize it and tell me what it's for. If they don't have a Medi-Planner then I provide them with one. They put each pill in the little box for that day and tell me what it is for and when they are going to take it. I suggest to some of the participants to put a sticky note on their refrigerator to help remind them to take their medication. If a patient has difficulty remembering, and they have a cell phone, I help them set up a daily alarm to remind them to take their medications. I notice some participants have a lot of different medications, like 10–20 different medications, so I will make a call to our Medications Therapy Management (MTM) Program so the pharmacist can make sure the medications are current and don't negatively interact with one another. If the participant has any questions I can't answer, then I schedule an appointment for them with their health care provider.

Client Scenario: Rosina Walker (continued)

The CHW and Rosina meet via a telehealth visit. The CHW is on her computer with Rosina's electronic health record pulled up on her screen. Rosina is talking with the CHW on her cell phone.

CHW: Thank you for meeting with me to talk about your hypertension medications. Let's start by reviewing which medications you're taking and then we can talk about the dosage and when you take it. Do you have your medications handy?

Rosina: Yes, I have my pills right here [Rosina holds up two bottles of pills for the CHW to see] Let me see. I'm taking two medications now for my blood pressure. The first one is . . .. Well, to tell you the truth, I don't usually remember the names; I kind of go by the green one and the pink one. Okay, the green one, that's Losartan, and I take two 50 mg tablets once a day. I usually take them first thing in the morning when I am getting ready for the day.

CHW: Okay, I'm just going to make a list here so we can compare this with the prescriptions in your electronic health record. [Types on the computer] So, you're taking two 50 mg tablets of Losartan once a day. And what is the other medication, the pink pill?

Rosina: I've got it here, but it is a long name. It's Chlori. . ... No, wait a minute. Why do they make the names so complicated?

CHW: [laughing] Oh, it's hard to remember the names! I like that you've come up with a good system for yourself by remembering the green pill and the pink pill. Can you spell out the name of the pink one for me?

Rosina: Yes, just let me put my glasses on. Okay, its HYDROCHLORO

CHW: Hydrochlorothiazide, is that it?

Rosina: Yes!

CHW: Well, no wonder you couldn't remember the name. It's a real common hypertension medications and all the participants I work with have a hard time pronouncing it. So what dosage are you on?

Rosina: Well, it comes in 25 mg pills, but Mrs. Washington, my nurse practitioner just increased my dose. She wants me to take one and half pills a day instead of just one. So that's a bit complicated because I have to cut some of the pills in half, and they're really small.

CHW: And when do you take the pink pills?

Rosina: Oh, I take them at the same time as the other ones, in the morning. I take two green pills and one and half pink pills.

CHW: And it sounds like you are splitting the pink ones in half yourself?

Rosina: Yes, but it's hard to do it.

CHW: Are the crumbling up on you?

Rosina: Sometimes, but the biggest problem is cutting them even. I do it on my kitchen counter and sometimes I get little bits and pieces.

CHW: I have a suggestion. Talk with your pharmacist and ask them if they can split your pills for you. Sometimes they will split them and make up daily packets for patients. Each packet would have two green pills, the Losartan, and one and half pink pills, the Hydrochlorothiazide. That's what the pharmacist does for me. It makes it much easier to manage.

Rosina: I didn't know they could do that! I will definitely ask them.

CHW: Great, so do you have any questions about your medications or any concerns? Do you remember to take them each day?

(continues)

Client Scenario: Rosina Walker (*continued*)

Rosina: Oh, I do great with that. I have them right out on the counter in my bathroom and taking them is just part of my routine. I take my pills right before I brush my teeth.

CHW: Well, one tip that I share with some of the patients I work with is to write out a little post-it note with the names and dosage of your medication and place them right beside where you take them, like on your bathroom cabinet or vanity. You could write out Green Pill, two a day, Losartan, and so on.

Rosina: Well, I will try that. It's sort of like when we posted the ground rules up in our classroom to remind the students.

CHW: And how are you doing with the new increased dose of the pink pill?

Rosina: I'm doing okay. Now that I have that new blood pressure cuff that you got me, well, I can see that my blood pressure is already a lower. Most of the time, it's in the healthy range, or real close to it.

Please watch the following short videos [▶] feature the work of Juanita Alvarado, a CHW who is supporting a patient with medications management.

Click here to watch the videos

1. Medications Management Part 1: Role Play Demonstration, Foundations

2. Medications Management Part 2: Role Play Demonstration, Foundations

3. Medications Management Part 3: Role Play Demonstration, Foundations

4. Medications Management Part 4: Role Play Demonstration, Foundations

- *What challenges did the patient face in terms of taking his medications?*

- *What did the CHW do well to support the patient with medication management?*

- *What else might you do to support this patient with medication management?*

(*Source:* Foundations for Community Health Workers/http://youtu.be/gleMEwoN72k)

(*Source:* Foundations for Community Health Workers/http://youtu.be/eLRe6wVkLuw)

(*Source:* Foundations for Community Health Workers/http://youtu.be/F2Mndwvfu-c)

(*Source:* Foundations for Community Health Workers/http://youtu.be/SVWbGyEKblk)

16.16 Responding to Ambivalence and Relapse

People living with chronic conditions sometimes feel ambivalent or uncertain about changing behaviors to promote their health. At times, they may resist taking effective action to meet their own health goals. Some patients will relapse or resume older patterns of behavior that increase health risks—such as using tobacco, alcohol, or drugs, or eating a less-healthy diet.

As discussed in Chapter 9, ambivalence, resistance, and relapse are a common part of the behavior change process. Be prepared to respond in a way that honors the autonomy or independence of clients. Your respect may help people to get back on track. As always, let your work be guided by person-centered concepts and skills. For example:

- Listen without judgment to patients' experiences, feelings, and thoughts
- Demonstrate unconditional positive regard.
  - Some clients may worry that their doubts, stalled progress, or relapse will change or harm their working relationship with you and the clinical team. They may fear your disappointment or judgment.
- Use your person-centered skills, including motivational interviewing, to support the client to reflect on what they are thinking and feeling and what they want to do next.
- Roll with Resistance (*see Chapter 9*). Don't try to argue or lecture a client out of their ambivalence or doubts about behavior change. Share open-ended questions and reflections that provide clients with an opportunity to further explore and understand their doubts and concerns. Honor the complex challenge of making and maintaining meaningful changes.
- Support the client's autonomy and decisions. Remember that *this work is about the client's life, their health, their values, beliefs, and decisions.*
- If you find yourself getting stuck, wanting to give advice, or rescue a client, note these impulses and put them aside. Come back to them when you have a chance to reflect on your own or with another (such as a supervisor or other colleague). Strive to understand what was going on for *you* during the session and where the instinct or urge to rescue or direct is coming from. Self-awareness is a critical resource for refining your person-centered approach and ensuring that your own issues don't unduly influence or undermine the health of the client.

Lorena Carmona: It isn't unusual for a client to relapse or stop making progress or to get stuck with their action plan. It happens to all of us. We're not perfect. I never blame the client. I'll ask them what happened between the time they were on track and making progress and when they relapsed. I listen and I ask them what I can I do to help them get back on their feet. I let them know that I'm here to help them be successful.

Please watch the following videos that show a CHW working with a client who wants to better manage her high blood pressure. The client develops a plan to start going to a local Zumba class with her daughter to increase physical activity. However, her plan doesn't go as expected. In the first counter role-play, the CHW struggles to respond effectively. In the role-play demo, the CHW demonstrates a much more person-centered approach to supporting the client.

ACTION PLANNING, REVISING AN ACTION PLAN: COUNTER ROLE PLAY

(*Source*: Foundations for Community Health Workers/http://youtu.be/ g6I5omhDSHU)

- *What got in the way of the client's Action Plan? What factors made it difficult for her to be successful?*
- *What did the CHW do well, and not so well, in these two role plays, and how may the CHW's practice have affected the client?*

- *What else would you want to do or say if you were the CHW working to support the client in this role-play scenario?*

Finally, watch the following video interview about the role plays and the challenge of revising an action plan more generally:

16.17 Follow-up Services

As a CHW providing chronic conditions management, you are likely to work with clients over several months or years. Each additional visit or contact—provided in-person or remotely—is an opportunity to review a client's issues, questions, and plans. Effective follow-up supports clients to learn and apply new knowledge and skills, and to gain confidence in their ability to manage their chronic conditions. Hopefully, these will lead to improved health outcomes. *Remember that the long-term goal is for patients to be able to manage their own chronic conditions and health without frequent assistance from their primary care team.*

Some follow-up services are routine check-ins about the client's current health status and how they are doing with their action plans. Patients whose chronic conditions are not yet well managed—who may still be experiencing uncontrolled high blood pressure or blood glucose levels, for example—are likely to be scheduled for more frequent follow-

ACTION PLANNING, REVISING AN ACTION
PLAN: ROLE PLAY, DEMO

(*Source:* Foundations for Community Health Workers/http://youtu.be/ Clr5pcdz074)

ACTION PLANNING, REVISING AN ACTION
PLAN, FACULTY INTERVIEW

(*Source:* Foundations for Community Health Workers/http://youtu.be/ JUtog9cd29Q)

up appointments. In addition to routine appointments, follow-up visits may be scheduled when:

- A client misses one or more appointments or is no longer in contact with the clinic
- A client is no longer re-filling prescriptions for medications, equipment, or other health resources
- A client reports that their health status is worsening or that they are facing a challenge that will impact their health (such as the loss of housing)
- The clinic learns that a client visited a local emergency department to seek treatment for their chronic condition, such as seeking treatment for an asthma attack, chest pain, or other urgent health symptoms
- A client is discharged from the hospital or another institution (drug treatment facility, the local jail, hospice, etc.)

- *Can you think of other circumstances that might prompt the clinical team to ask a client to schedule a follow-up visit?*

What Do
YOU?
Think

Community Health Workers play a critical role in identifying and reaching out to clients in need of follow-up services. The CHW may contact the patient by phone (or text or e-mail) to see how they are doing. They may schedule a follow-up appointment in the clinic, another setting, or via telehealth technology. When the client cannot be reached in other ways, CHWs may conduct a home visit or seek out the client in other places where they work or live. These locations may include a local shelter, other places where people who are homeless sleep, in residential recovery programs, hospice, hospitals, local jails, and other institutional settings.

In these cases, the goal is to provide the client with an opportunity to re-engage in services or treatment. They may ask for assistance to better control their chronic condition. They may be interested in preventing, if possible, the further progress of their disease. Or they may have other problems to address. Some clients may not want to continue services or treatment, and that must be respected too.

Client Scenario: Rosina Walker (continued)

Rosina comes into the clinic six months after first meeting with the CHW. This is a follow-up visit to check-in on her health action plan.

Rosina: Good morning!

CHW: It's good to see you Rosina; thank you for coming in today. Did you get picked up by Reliance Transportation, like we arranged?

Rosina: Yes, I did, and they'll be picking me up to take me home again at 11. They have been wonderful.

CHW: I'm so glad that it's working. And how is everything going with your family?

Rosina: We're all doing well. You know my daughters just finished school. The youngest graduated from second grade and my eldest finished third grade.

CHW: Congratulations! The time goes by so quickly with our children; it's nice that you're celebrating their achievements along the way. Do you have any photos of your children? [Rosina shows the CHWs photos of her children. They talk about them for a while] And how is your action plan going?

Rosina: My blood pressure is doing much better now. It's down from before, and usually in that desirable range, under 120/80. Getting help with transportation and food, well, that has been a blessing, and it makes me feel much less stressed about managing our family life.

CHW: So, what can I best help you with today? Is there anything you are still struggling with or have questions about?

Rosina: Well, I think my biggest challenge is healthy eating. With the extra help you put me in touch with, the food pantry and all, we're not running out of food at the end of the month. But I want to do better with eating healthier foods and cutting back more on the fried foods and the salt and all that.

CHW: Well, I have a new resource that I'm sharing with patients. [The CHW holds up a book for Rosina to see] It's called the New Soul Food Cookbook and it is all about making healthier versions of our favorite foods. Me and my co-workers have been making the recipes at home and they're easy and fun to make.

Rosina: That sounds good. I've been watching some cooking shows but not many of them are cooking foods like we grew up eating. And you know, I need to cook meals that are good for my hypertension but also foods that my children will eat. And, of course, everything has to be affordable.

CHW: What I really like about this book is that it shares great cultural recipes so you can maintain the same traditions and ingredients we're familiar with. The only thing is that it changes up how the ingredients are prepared, to make them healthier. Instead of adding in a lot of salt, the recipes add in more spices, lots of pepper and garlic and fresh herbs.

Rosina: My biggest challenge is cooking for my children. Getting them to eat vegetables, now that's a struggle!

CHW: One thing I've learned, is instead of taking those vegetables and putting them on the stove, we could take the same vegetables and put them in oven and roast them with just a dap of olive oil, garlic powder, and other herbs. They taste even better because you get a little crunch on them. My grandchildren eat them. And it's so much healthier for your body and your hypertension.

The CHW hands to cookbook to Rosina. She starts flipping through the book. She finds a recipe and talks about it with the CHW.

Rosina: Where can I get a copy of this book?

CHW: Well, we actually just got a bunch of the books. My director ordered them from a grant, and we're able to give out a copy to patients living with chronic health conditions. So, this copy, it's for you.

(continues)

Client Scenario: Rosina Walker *(continued)*

Rosina: Thank you! And this has got me thinking. I know you're busy, but would you ever be able to come out to my church to talk to the women's group about this cookbook? We meet every Wednesday night and a lot of the ladies, well, they have the same struggles—how to eat healthy on a budget and feed their families.

CHW: Well, that would be my pleasure. Let me talk to our nutritionist. I want to see if this is something that she would want to join in on. She's the real expert when it comes to healthy foods. Is there a kitchen at the church?

Rosina: Of course. [she laughs]

CHW: Well, I'll talk with my colleague, but if she can come, and if we can use your kitchen, what about we cook up a healthy meal to share with your group?

Rosina: Yes, I know the group would love cooking a healthy meal together.

CHW: I'll text you and let you know, alright, and then we can set a date.

16.18 Ending Services

Over time, CHWs will begin professional relationships with new clients, while ending services with others. You may work with a client for a week or two, or for months or years, depending upon their interest and needs, and the guidelines of your agency or program.

Ending services may be mutual, meaning that both the client and the provider or agency agree with the decision. Services may also be terminated by the client alone and, in some circumstances, by the clinic/provider alone. Ideally, services come to end because the client's chronic condition is well managed, and they no longer require ongoing and intensive support from a primary care team. But services may end (or be terminated) for many different reasons including:

- The client moves away from the area or passes away
- The client switches to a new medical provider or clinic
- The client may no longer be eligible to receive medical services at your clinic/hospital
- The client is incarcerated
- The client is upset or displeased with some aspect of the services that you and your team have provided and no longer wishes to work with you
- The need for specialized medical care at another clinic, hospital, or hospice

In some situations, you won't have an opportunity to plan for the termination of services or to say goodbye. When you anticipate that services will be ending, you and the patient can manage this process together, along with the rest of the clinical team. For example, consider the case of a long-standing client living with chronic conditions who informs you that she will be moving to another state in three months and will no longer be a patient at your clinic. Suggestions for how to manage the end of the professional relationship with the client include:

- Thank the client for the opportunity to work together
- Ask the client about their plans to seek out another medical provider in their new city and state. If the client is interested, and if you are able, provide referrals for services for their new location
- Ask the client to summarize their key accomplishments so far, including what they have learned that helps them to better manage their health

- Review the client's plan for the self-management of their chronic condition(s) including medications management, behavior change goals, and other actions
  - Check to make sure that the client has sufficient medications with them during their transition (this may depend upon clinic and pharmacy policies)
- Review what the client will do if their health worsens and what signs and symptoms to watch for
- Discuss relapse prevention and what the client plans to do if they relapse to previous behaviors that may place their health at risk
- Affirm the knowledge, skills, and confidence that the client has gained
- Ask the client to share feedback about your own work and the quality of services received by their clinical team

CHALLENGES WITH ENDING SERVICES

Sometimes a client terminates services because they are unhappy, frustrated, or angry about the level or quality of care they received. In these cases, it is important to manage the termination process with generosity, patience, and professionalism. Some patients will cycle in and out of services at the clinic where you work. They may terminate services and re-engage with you six months or two years later. For CHWs, these situations are often awkward, particularly if you live in the same neighborhood or belong to the same community as the client and their family. You may continue to run into the client in community settings, so you want to end this professional relationship as respectfully and peacefully as possible. In these types of situations, our suggestions include:

- Listen without judgment or defensiveness
- Honor and accept the patient's decision
- Stop and reflect on the feedback that the patient provides. What could you and the team have done differently?
- If you can do so authentically, apologize for any mistakes or missed opportunities that you or your colleagues may have made
- Wish the client well.
- If appropriate, keep the door open for their return to service. You might say something like "I know that right now you don't want to continue coming here for services. But, if that ever changes, please don't hesitate to contact me—we will be here for you."
- As above, review current treatment protocols, including medications
  - *What else do you want to do or keep in mind when ending services?*

Chapter Review

After studying the information presented in this chapter, check your knowledge by answering the following questions. Think about how you would explain the concept to a professional colleague or a community member.

1. How would you explain what chronic conditions are?
2. How common are chronic conditions?
3. What are some of the most common chronic conditions?
4. Are the rates of chronic disease the same among all communities? Why or why not?
5. What are some of the causes of chronic conditions (remember to apply the ecological framework!)?
6. What are some of the consequences of chronic conditions—for people living with them, for their families, and for their communities?

7. What are some of the available treatments for chronic conditions?

8. What are some of the key ways that health care practice is changing in terms of chronic condition management?

9. What does "patient self-management" mean, and why is it important?

10. What are some common goals for patient self-management?

11. What are the key roles and tasks of CHWs who work with patients who are living with chronic health conditions?

12. How can CHWs apply person-centered concepts and skills to the task of supporting patients with the self-management of chronic health conditions?

13. What are the three components of medication management and how can they promote a patient's health?

Please review the client scenario about Rosina Walker presented at the beginning of the chapter. If you were the CHW working with Rosina, how would you answer the following questions?

1. What factors may contribute to Rosina's health risks?

2. What factors promote or contribute to Rosina's health and well-being?

3. What would you do or say in working with Rosina Walker to help her to develop an action plan to manage her high blood pressure?

4. How might you use OARS in working with Rosina?
   a. What is an example of an open-ended question that you would ask Rosina, and why would you ask it?
   b. What is an example of an Affirmation that you would share with Rosina, and why?
   c. What is an example of a reflective listening statement that you would share with Rosina, and why?
   d. What would you summarize in working with Rosina, and why?

5. Rosina takes two medications to control her hypertension, but sometimes forgets to take them. How might you help Rosina with medication management?

6. What would you say to Rosina if she relapsed or stopped implementing part of her action plan to manage her hypertension?

7. How will you respond if Rosina tells you that her Action Plan isn't working for her and she wants to change it?

8. Under what circumstances—either positive or negative—might you end your working relationship with Rosina Walker?

References

Ahmad, M. & Vismara, L. (2021). The psychological impact of COVID-19 pandemic on women's mental health during pregnancy: a rapid evidence review. *International Journal of Environmental Research and Public Health*. https://doi: 10.3390/ijerph18137112.

Anderson, W. C., Gondalia, R., Hoch, H., Kaye, L., Szefler, S. J., & Stempel, D. A. (2019). Screening for inhalation technique errors with electronic medication monitors. *The Journal of Allergy and Clinical Immunology: In Practice*, 7(6), 2065–2067.

Bodenheimer, T., Wagner, E. H., & Grumbach, K. (2002). Improving primary care for patients with chronic illness. *Journal of the American Medical Association*, 288(16), 1909–1914. https://doi: 10.1001/jama.288.14.1775.

The California Department of Public Health. (2023). California Breathing. https://www.cdph.ca.gov/Programs/CCDPHP/DEODC/EHIB/CPE/Pages/CaliforniaBreathing.aspx (accessed 8 June 2023).

Campbell, J. D., Brooks, M., Hosokawa, P., Robinson, J., Song, L., & Kreiger, J. (2015). Community health worker home visits for Medicaid-enrolled children with asthma: Effects on asthma outcomes and costs. *American Journal of Public Health*, 105(11), 2366–2372. doi: 10.2105/AJPH.2015.302685.

The Centers for Disease Control and Prevention. (2018). What is Self-Management Education? https://www.cdc.gov/learnmorefeelbetter/sme/index.htm (accessed 6 November 2022).

The Centers for Disease Control and Prevention. (2019). Self-Management Education (SME) Program for Chronic Health Conditions. https://www.cdc.gov/learnmorefeelbetter/programs/index.htm (accessed 6 November 2022).

Centers for Disease Control and Prevention. (2021a). Adverse Childhood Experiences (ACES): Preventing Early Trauma to Improve Adult Health. https://www.cdc.gov/vitalsigns/aces/index.html (accessed 7 November 2022).

Centers for Disease Control and Prevention. (2021b). High Blood Pressure Symptoms and Causes. https://www.cdc.gov/bloodpressure/about.htm#problems (accessed 6 November 2022).

Centers for Disease Control and Prevention. (2022). Facts about Hypertension. https://www.cdc.gov/bloodpressure/facts.htm#:~:text=Nearly%20half%20of%20adults%20in,are%20taking%20medication%20for%20hypertension (accessed 6 November 2022).

Centers for Disease Control and Prevention. Division for Heart Disease and Stroke Prevention. (2020). Integrating Community Health Workers on Clinical Care Teams and in the Community. https://www.cdc.gov/dhdsp/pubs/guides/best-practices/chw.htm (accessed 1 November 2022).

Christiansen, E. & Morning, K. (2017). Community Health Worker Return on Investment Study Final Report. Nevada Department of Health and Human Services. https://dpbh.nv.gov/uploadedFiles/dpbh.nv.gov/content/Programs/CHW/dta/Publications/CHW%20ROI%20Report%209-26-17.pdf (accessed 7 November 2022).

GA Carmichael Family Health Center. (2023). https://gacfhc.com/ (accessed 7 November 2022).

Jam, V. A., McKay, K., & Homes, J. T. (2019). Identifying medication management confidence and gaps in training among community health workers in the United States. *Journal of Community Health*, 44(6), 1180–1184. https://doi: 10.1007/s10900-019-00688-9.

Johns Hopkins Medicine. (2022). Long COVID: Long-Term Effects of COVID-19. https://www.hopkinsmedicine.org/health/conditions-and-diseases/coronavirus/covid-long-haulers-long-term-effects-of-covid19 (accessed 6 November 2022).

Kangovi, S. (2020). Evidence-based community health worker program addresses unmet social needs and generates positive return on investment. *Health Affairs*, 39(2), 207–213. https://doi: 10.1377/hlthaff.2019.00981.

Kleinsinger, F. (2018). The unmet challenge of medication nonadherence. *The Permanente Journal*, 22, 18–033. https://doi: 10.7812/TPP/18-033.

MacGregor, K. Handley, M., Wong, S. Sharifi, C., Gjeltema, K., Schillinger, D., Bodenheimer, T. (2006). Behavior-change action plans in primary care: a feasibility study of clinicians. *Journal of the American Board of Family Medicine*, 19(3), 215–223. www.jabfm.org/content/19/3/215.full.

Marmot, M. &Bell, R. (2019). Social determinants and non-communicable diseases: time for integrated action. *The British Medical Journal*. https://doi.org/10.1136/bmj.1251.

Mayfield-Johnson, S. (2022). Barriers and attitudes toward tele-healthcare delivery with African Americans in the Mississippi dela regions participating in a cardiovascular disease risk reduction education program. *Health Education and Care*. https://doi:10.15761/HEC.1000190.

Mayfield-Johnson, S., Fastring, D., Clark, M., & Crosby, K. (2022). Results from Implementing a CVD CHW Effectiveness Study During COVID-19. A presentation at the American Public Health Association, Boston, Massachusetts (8 November 2022).

McGough, P., Chaudhari, V., El-Attar, S., & Yung, P. (2018). A health system's journey toward better population health through empanelment and panel management. *Healthcare (Basel)*, 6(2), 66. https://doi: 10.3390/healthcare6020066.

Montero, A., Kearney, A., Hamel, L., & Brodie, M. (2022). Americans' Challenges with Health Care Costs. Kaiser Family Foundation. https://www.kff.org/health-costs/issue-brief/americans-challenges-with-health-care-costs/ (accessed 6 November 2022).

Multiple Chronic Conditions Resource Center. (2023). Self-Management in Chronic Conditions. https://www.multiplechronicconditions.org/self-management-guidelines#:~:text=Self%2Dmanagement%20is%20defined%20as,make%20whatever%20cognitive%2C%20behavioral%2C%20and (accessed 23 December 2023).

National Center for Chronic Disease Prevention and Health Promotion (NCCDPHP). (2022a). About Chronic Diseases. Centers for Disease Control and Prevention. www.cdc.gov/chronicdisease/about/index.htm (accessed 6 November 2022).

National Center for Chronic Disease Prevention and Health Promotion (NCCDPHP). (2022b). Health and Economic Costs of Chronic Diseases. Centers for Disease Control and Prevention. https://www.cdc.gov/chronicdisease/about/costs/index.htm (accessed 6 November 2022).

National Center for Health Statistics. (2022). Mortality in the United States, 2021. Centers for Disease Control and Prevention. https://www.cdc.gov/nchs/products/databriefs/db456.htm (accessed 28 December 2022).

National Conference of State Legislatures. (2019). Medication Adherence: Taking Pills as Ordered. https://www.ncsl.org/research/health/medication-adherence-taking-pills-as-ordered.aspx (accessed 6 November 2022).

National Council on Aging. (2021). Chronic Conditions for Older Adults: The Top 10 Most Common Chronic Conditions in Older Adults. https://www.ncoa.org/article/the-top-10-most-common-chronic-conditions-in-older-adults (accessed 7 November 2022).

Ndgugga, N., & Artiga, S. (2021) Disparities in Health and Health Care: 5 Key Questions and Answers. Kaiser Family Foundation. https://www.kff.org/racial-equity-and-health-policy/issue-brief/disparities-in-health-and-health-care-5-key-question-and-answers/ (accessed 6 November 2022).

Newman, P. M., Franke, M. F., Arrieta, J., Carrasco, H., Elliott, P., Flores, H., Friedman, A., Graham, S., Martinez, L., et al. (2018). Community health workers improve disease control and medication adherence among patients with diabetes and/or hypertension in Chiapas, Medico: An observational stepped-wedge study. *BMJ Global Health*, 3(1), e000566. https://doi: 10.1136/bmjgh-2017-000566.

Nurmagambetov, T., Kuwahara, R., & Garbe, P. (2018). The Economic Burden of Asthma in the United States, 2008-2013. *Annals of the American Thoracic Society*, 15(3), 348–356.

Ochieng, N. Cubanski, J., Neuman, T., Artiga, S., & Daico, A. (2021). Racial and Ethnic Health Inequities and Medicare. Kaiser Family Foundation. https://www.kff.org/report-section/racial-and-ethnic-health-inequities-and-medicare-health-status-and-disease-prevalence/ (accessed 6 November 2022).

Postma, J., Karr, C., & Kieckhefer, G. (2009). Community health workers and environmental interventions for children with asthma: A systematic review. *The Journal of Asthma*, 46(6), 564–576. https://doi: 10.1080/02770900902912638. PMID: 19657896.

Rose, J. Z. (2022). Medication Adherence is Not a Zero-Sum Game. American Journal of Managed Care. https://www.ajmc.com/view/contributor-medication-adherence-is-not-a-zero-sum-game (accessed 6 November 2022).

Shields, A. M., Faustini, S. E., Hill H. J., Al-Taei, S., Tanner, C., Ashford, F., Workman, S., Moreira, F., et al. (2022). SARS-CoV-2 vaccine responses in individuals with antibody deficiency: findings from the COV-AD study. *Journal of Clinical Immunology*, 923–934. https://doi: 10.1007/s10875-022-01231-7.

University of Florida, College of Pharmacy. (2022). UF Community Health Worker Medication Therapy Management Services. https://pharmacy.ufl.edu/chwmtms/ (accessed 6 November 2022).

University of Washington Medicine. (2018) Panel Management Lexicon. https://depts.washington.edu/uwmedptn/wp-content/uploads/Panel-Management-Lexicon.pdf (accessed 6 November 2022).

Wheat, L., Roane, T. E., Connelly, A., Zeigler, M., Wallace, J., Kim, J. & Segal, R. (2020). Using a pharmacist-community health worker collaboration to address medication adherence barriers. *Journal of the American Pharmacists Association*, 60(6), https://doi.org/10.1016/j.japh.2020.08.021.

World Health Organization. (2021a). Coronavirus Disease (COVID-19): Post COVID-19 Condition. https://www.who.int/news-room/questions-and-answers/item/coronavirus-disease-(covid-19)-post-covid-19-condition (accessed 6 November 2022).

World Health Organization. (2021b). Hypertension: Key Facts. https://www.who.int/news-room/fact-sheets/detail/hypertension (accessed 6 November 2022).

World Health Organization. (2022a) Noncommunicable Diseases: Key Facts. https://www.who.int/news-room/fact-sheets/detail/noncommunicable-diseases (accessed 6 November 2022).

The World Health Organization. (2022b). Tobacco. https://www.who.int/news-room/fact-sheets/detail/tobacco (accessed 6 November 2022).

Additional Resources

Gaines, F. D & Weaver, R. (2018). *The new soul food cookbook for people with diabetes*, 3rd Edition. American Diabetes Association.

Promoting Healthy Eating and Active Living

Tim Berthold and Jill R. Tregor

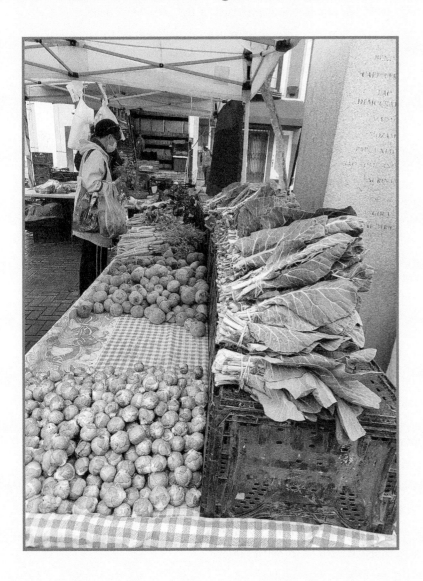

Foundations for Community Health Workers, Third Edition. Edited by Tim Berthold and Darouny Somsanith.
© 2024 John Wiley & Sons, Inc. Published 2024 by John Wiley & Sons, Inc.
Companion website: http://www.wiley.com/go/communityhealthworkers3E

Client Scenario: Janice Sanders

Janice Sanders is a single mother raising a 12-year-old son named Martin. Janice works as a line cook at a busy restaurant on the breakfast and lunch shifts.

Janice has high-blood pressure and suffered a minor heart attack four years ago. Her older sister Vicki died of a heart attack five years ago. Janice quit smoking three years ago after her divorce. "My mother, she died of lung cancer, and she made me promise to quit. I didn't do it before she died, but I kept my promise. I didn't want Martin to grow up watching me smoke like I watched my parents."

Janice has been cooking at the Bluebird Café for nearly five years. It's a popular restaurant focused on comfort foods, led by a female chef. "Restaurant work is long hours, and it gets pretty heated on the line sometimes—stressful, everyone yelling at each other. But at least I'm not smoking with rest of the crew like I used to!"

When you ask Janice what she typically eats, she says: "Because I work so much I usually eat at the Bluebird, you know, burgers and fries. I bring home leftovers for Martin to have for dinner. I must go through four to five Dr. Peppers on a shift to keep me going. I know it's not good for me, but it's my routine."

Janice is self-conscious about her weight. "I hate going to the doctor because they put me on a scale and announce my weight in front of everyone. They tell me that I am obese like it is some big surprise that I am thicc. I've always been big. Everyone in my family is big!"

Janice used to be active in sports; she was the pitcher for her high school's softball team. After she got married, became a mom, and started working full-time, she stopped participating in sports.

Janice is still close with her ex-sister-in-law, Marcie. "She has a daughter about Martin's age—they grew up together." Janice and Marcie try to support each other to get healthier. "She's always telling me to try things like getting off the bus a few stops early and walking the rest of the way to work. But I'm always running late." Marcie took Janice to an aerobics class at the YMCA as her guest. "I couldn't keep up with the class. I felt like everyone was staring at me and wondering what this fat lady was doing in the class. I went out to the parking lot and cried."

"Because I'm working all the time, when I get home, I just want to sit on the couch and watch my programs or, if it's not too late, play video games with Martin. That's our thing."

Janice says, "I probably sound like I'm giving you a lot of excuses, but I don't want another heart attack. So, I just need to figure something that's gonna work for me to get healthier. I don't want to let Martin down."

If you were the Community Health Worker assigned to work with Janice Sanders, how would you answer the following questions?

- What are some of Janice's key internal and external resources?
- What are some of the key health challenges that Janice is facing?
- What barriers or obstacles does Janice face to successfully increasing physical activity and changing her diet?
- How would you address the issues of weight and health in your work with Janice?
- How will you address the topic of healthy eating in your work with Janice?
- How will you address the topic of physical activity in your work with Janice?
- How will you apply person-centered skills in your work with Janice?

Introduction

What we eat and drink and how much physical activity we engage in are key determinants of health. Low levels of physical activity and less healthy diets are highly associated with increased risks for chronic health conditions including heart disease, diabetes, some cancers, as well as increased risks for premature death (for more information, please see Chapter 16).

Many CHWs support clients to increase their level of physical activity and develop and maintain healthier diets.

This chapter addresses the connection between weight and health, and guidelines for promoting the health of people of all sizes, including those who have been labeled as "overweight" or obese. We challenge traditional health care approaches that promote weight loss and introduce the weight-inclusive approach, an emerging model grounded in research evidence and ethics.

This chapter is designed to be used with Chapter 16 on Chronic Conditions Management. It also builds upon and applies concepts and skills presented in other Chapters including Cultural Humility, Person-Centered Counseling, and Case Management.

Your Experience with Healthy Eating and Active Living

The topics presented in this book are relevant for most of us. As you study concepts for supporting the health and well-being of clients, consider how they affect your own life and health status. For example, what challenges and successes have you experienced with maintaining a healthier diet and engaging in physical activity? Have you or your family members ever experienced prejudice or shame related to your body shape and size?

The more that we understand our own experiences and how they shape our lives, the better prepared we are to promote our own health. Self-knowledge also helps us to prevent imposing our own values and beliefs on the clients and communities we work with. This is essential for person-centered practice that truly honors people's identities, knowledge, and values and supports clients to guide and manage their own health.

WHAT YOU WILL LEARN

By studying the information in this chapter, you will be able to:

- Identify key challenges to changing diets and levels of physical activity
- Explain general guidelines for healthier eating and drinking
- Explain general guidelines for physical activity
- Identify key health benefits from healthy eating and physical activity
- Discuss how a focus on health rather than weight is more effective in promoting positive health outcomes
- Apply a seven-step approach to providing health education about healthy eating
- Demonstrate person-centered concepts and skills for supporting clients to establish healthier patterns of eating and activity

C3 Roles and Skills Addressed in Chapter 17

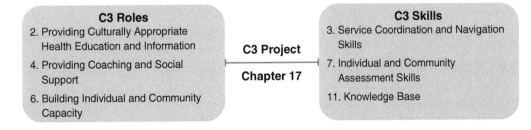

C3 Roles
2. Providing Culturally Appropriate Health Education and Information
4. Providing Coaching and Social Support
6. Building Individual and Community Capacity

C3 Project

Chapter 17

C3 Skills
3. Service Coordination and Navigation Skills
7. Individual and Community Assessment Skills
11. Knowledge Base

WORDS TO KNOW

Body mass index

Food desert

Food insecurity

Food security

Weight cycling

Weight-inclusive

Weight-normative

17.1 What We Eat and Drink

While the foods that we eat in the United States vary considerably based on factors such as culture, income, and geographic region, in general the diet of Americans has become less healthy over time. Today, Americans eat fewer fresh foods—such as fresh fruits and vegetables—than before, and more processed and packaged foods designed to last for months in the grocery store and in our homes, and other foods that are high in salt, sugar, and fats. This pattern of eating is associated with increasing rates of chronic health conditions including cardiovascular disease, diabetes, and cancer.

FOOD POLICY

Changes in the American diet were caused by many factors including the practices of agricultural producers and food manufacturers, and government policies. A few large multi-national corporations now dominate farming and food manufacturing. Their primary interests are market share and profits, and this has resulted in strategies for large-scale production, at low cost, of products that can be easily shipped and stored for many months on the shelves and in the freezers of supermarkets and in our homes.

Corporations have also invested in the development of food products that consumers will literally *crave*. They have applied science to develop food and drink products with just the right balance of salt, sugar, and added fats to keep us coming back for more (Moss, 2021). Visit the middle aisles in almost any supermarket or grocery store in the United States, and you will find thousands of products on the shelves that contain high amounts of sodium or salt, sugar (including high fructose corn syrup and cane sugar), and added fats. Unfortunately, government policies have supported the interests of large agricultural and food corporations at the expense of our health. These practices and policies have contributed to increased rates of chronic conditions across our nation.

Politics Influence U.S. Nutritional Guidelines

Every five years, the U.S. government establishes and promotes dietary guidelines that influence the manufacture, sale, and consumption of foods in our country.

Many public health experts have argued that these policies are not determined by independent scientists with expertise in nutrition and health. Instead, the panels that establish the guidelines are dominated by representatives with close ties to major agricultural and food corporations. The Nutrition Coalition points to the lack of transparency and failure to disclose the financial conflicts and interests of the members of the Advisory Committee (Nutrition Coalition, 2020). The New York Times reported that "half the members of a panel considering changes to the nation's blueprint for healthy eating have ties to the food industry" (Jacobs, 2020). Two-thirds of the of the "Birth-to-24 months" subcommittee members had ties to infant formula or baby food companies (Nutrition Coalition, 2020).

Nutritional guidelines continue to promote the consumption of meat and dairy products which are linked to increased risks for chronic health conditions and climate change. The guidelines "ignore the 60% of the population now diagnosed with one or more diet-related disease" (Ibid). The guidelines have also been criticized for the failure to address and include the diversity of food cultures in America (Giles, 2021).

As a result, the U.S. Dietary Guidelines better represent the interests of large-scale food corporations than evidence-based guidelines for promoting health and wellness.

FOOD SECURITY AND HUNGER

Tens of millions of Americans do not have enough food to eat. The terms **food security** (having enough food to eat) and **food insecurity** (not having enough food to eat) are increasingly used to discuss issues of hunger in America. If you are working with low-income clients, it is likely that some of these clients—and their families—regularly experience times when they don't have enough to eat.

In 2020, more than 38 million Americans were estimated to be food insecure (Food Research & Action Center, 2021). This included 13 million children (No Kid Hungry, 2023), and 5 million people aged 65 and over (Shrider, Kollar, Chen, & Semega, 2021). Approximately 40 million Americans live in **food deserts** or places without access to fresh, affordable, and healthy foods (Rhone, Ver Ploeg, Dicken, Williams, & Breneman, 2017). The COVID-19 pandemic increased the number of people in the United States and worldwide who faced food insecurity: one study found the food insecurity in American households increased from 11% before the pandemic to 14.7% during the pandemic (Parekh et al., 2021).

Global Hunger and Food Insecurity

Globally, it is estimated that approximately 720–811 million people faced hunger in 2020, and more than 146 million children under the age of five suffered from extreme malnutrition (WHO, 2021a,b). To learn more about the global scope and consequences of food security, go to the World Health Organization's website or review the report from 2021 included in Chapter References.

Many American families rely upon school lunch programs to provide at least one hot meal a day for their children. Other families are increasingly relying upon food pantries, the Supplemental Nutrition Assistance Program (SNAP) (formerly known as food stamps and described later on in this chapter), and organizations that provide free meals in the community in order to eat. Food insecurity and hunger can result in chronic under-nutrition that may result in a variety of health problems including, for example, greater risks for low-birth weight, infectious diseases, and premature death (Martins et al., 2011; WHO, 2021b)

If you work with low-income or unhoused clients, you are likely to work with people for whom food insecurity or hunger is their greatest nutritional challenge. Your role may be to help these clients access reliable sources of food—any food—for themselves and their families.

- *Have you or your family ever experienced food insecurity (times when you did not have enough food to eat)?*

- *How may food insecurity or hunger impact a clients' health and well-being?*

- *What local resources are available in your community that provide groceries or meals to people in need?*

Food Equity

Food policies globally and in the United States are not based on principles of equity and leave many people without access to safe, affordable, and healthy foods necessary for good health. The concept and the call for food equity are growing. PolicyLink, a national research and action institute, describes food equity as follows:

An equitable food system is one that creates a new paradigm in which all—including those most vulnerable and those living in low-income neighborhoods and communities of color—can fully participate, prosper, and benefit. It is a system that, from farm to table, from processing to disposal, ensures economic opportunity; high-quality jobs with living wages; safe working conditions; access to healthy, affordable, and culturally appropriate food; and environmental sustainability (PolicyLink, 2022).

- *How could the communities you work with benefit from policies grounded in food equity principles?*

- *Are communities and organizations advocating for food equity in the city, county, or state where you live?*

17.2 Common Barriers to Changing Our Diets

Eating healthy food is essential for overall health. Yet, making lasting changes to our diets can be difficult. As always, we want to encourage you to apply an ecological model to your work. Consider a wide range of factors that make it difficult for people to successfully change what they regularly eat and drink. These factors may include:

FOOD POLICY

As we have highlighted above, the U.S. Government has established policies that better promote the needs of agricultural and food industries rather than public health. Food policies in the United States are not grounded in a concern for equity and are not effective in providing access to quality, affordable, and culturally responsive food for all communities and especially for low-income individuals and families.

TIME AND MONEY

It often takes less time and costs less money to eat the least healthy foods. This includes the food we purchase from fast food restaurants and the processed foods that we buy in grocery stores. Fresh vegetables and fruits are sometimes more difficult to find, depending upon your neighborhood, and more expensive than pre-packaged meals.

LACK OF CONFIDENCE

Some clients doubt their ability to successfully change their diet. Keep in mind that mixed feelings or ambivalence is a natural part of the behavior change process (see Chapter 9), and that many people have tried to change their diet in the past without lasting success. This history of past attempts to change their diet may cause people to doubt their ability to achieve changes in the future.

- *Have you ever lacked confidence that you could change a behavior or another aspect of your life?*

FAMILY AND CULTURE

Food has an important meaning for most families and cultures. People come together to prepare and eat food, and food is often a central focus of family and cultural celebrations. Respect people's food cultures and traditions when working with them to identify healthier choices that will promote their wellness.

PLEASURE

We take pleasure in eating specific types of food. However, some of the foods that we may enjoy the most—such as salty French fries and chips, sugary cookies, or ice cream—can be harmful to our health when eaten too often. Food companies have engineered products with specific ratios of sugar, salt, and fat that consumers crave.

- *What other factors may get in the way of changing what we eat?*

Client Scenario: Janice Sanders *(continued)*

CHW: You mentioned that you quit smoking. That's a major accomplishment. Can you tell me a bit about how you stopped?

Janice: It was really hard. I'd been smoking for over a decade. I tried to stop hundreds of times. I think it was seeing what happened to my mom. Her cancer. She made me promise to stop smoking. And I wanted to do it for Martin too.

CHW: So, your family has been key to your motivation.

Janice: Definitely. The way my mom died—she was in a lot of pain. I don't want to go through that. And I want to do better for Martin.

CHW: Quitting smoking is one of the most difficult health changes to make, and you did it. I'm wondering if there is anything that you learned that could help you to make other changes—like eating healthier—that will protect your health and your family?

Janice: I'm not sure.

CHW: Does anything come to mind? What helped you to quit?

Janice: Every time I was smoking, I thought of my mom and my sister and Martin, and . . . I don't know really, but smoking just wasn't the same. I still sometimes want to smoke. I can smell the tobacco when the guys take their break at work. But I've just . . . I've stayed strong.

CHW: Incredibly strong. I think you may be stronger than you realize Janice.

Janice: Maybe. I remember how scared I was after my divorce. I had to find work and take care of Martin mostly on my own. But I did it. I'm proud of that.

CHW: What does this tell you about yourself?

Janice: I think I'm always hustling so fast, getting Martin to work, going to work, making sure he's keeping up with homework, doing laundry, you know, that I don't realize what I'm managing to do.

CHW: So, when you sit back and reflect on it, what do you think?

Janice: Maybe I *am* stronger than I think. I've managed divorce, losing my sister and my mom, quitting smoking, getting a job, and working my way up. I think I can figure out how to do better in managing my blood pressure.

17.3 Weight and Health

This section addresses the connection between weight and health. It can be a challenging topic for both clients and providers. We will highlight research that questions traditional health care practices that promote dieting and weight loss. We introduce emerging **weight-inclusive models** that honor all body shapes and sizes and focus on health outcomes rather than weight.

People who are judged as being "too" big or heavy face significant prejudice and discriminatory treatment in employment, education, the entertainment industry, housing, and travel (The Association for Size, Diversity and Health, 2022; Sherrell, 2021; Yu, 2022). Children and adults who are judged to be overweight are often harassed and bullied. Prejudice and resulting weight stigma are associated with poorer health outcomes (Lee, Hunger, Tomiyama, 2021). Unfortunately, prejudice and discrimination against people who are perceived as overweight are also common among health care providers.

As a working CHW, we ask you to carefully consider the words you use and the messages that you convey to clients about their body size, shape, and weight. Please don't add to the voices that are already too common in health care and throughout our society that label, judge, and stigmatize people whose bodies are perceived to be bigger or "over" weight. This is a matter of cultural humility and ethics: all of the clients and community members you work with deserve to be fully respected.

A Note on the Language of Size and Weight

Carefully consider the words you use to talk about body weight and size. Our society tends to label people who are perceived to be overweight with a long list of negative and demeaning words. When health care providers echo this prejudice and label patients as fat or obese, they reinforce the stigma of weight and related feelings of shame. While health care providers frequently use the term "obese" as a clinical description, it may be experienced by clients as a judgment and/or an insult.

Speak with the clients and communities you serve without using negative or judgmental language. In most cases, there is no need to assign clients with any label to describe their body shape and size. At the same time, listen carefully to the language that clients may be comfortable using to describe their own bodies. For example, in the Client Scenario presented in this chapter, Janice Sanders uses the word "thicc" to refer to herself ("thicc" is an expression that some people use in place of "thick." It is meant as a complement to someone who is curvy or full-figured). You may wish to let these cues from clients guide you in determining which words to use to talk about weight.

THE TRADITIONAL FOCUS ON WEIGHT-LOSS

Most health care providers are trained to focus on weight as a key indicator of health. One of the first steps taken during a health care visit is for a patient to be weighed and their height recorded. These two indicators (and sometimes the patient's age and sex) are used to calculate **body mass index (BMI)**, which is divided into four categories: under-weight, normal, overweight, and obese (Centers for Disease Control and Prevention, 2022). In health care settings, the BMI is used to identity patients in the higher two categories (overweight and obese) and to counsel them to lose weight. Patients are encouraged to lose weight in a variety of ways including a combination of changes to diet and exercise, participating in dieting programs and, in some cases, surgical procedures.

The focus on weight and dieting in health care is reinforced throughout our society. The dieting industry in the United States generated an estimated $72.6 billion in revenues in 2021 (Marketdata LLC, 2022) by marketing a wide range of products (pills and supplements, books, videos, diet plans, and programs) that promise weight loss. Some products and programs promise rapid weight loss and use dramatic before and after photographs and inspiring testimonials. As a result, many people begin dieting in childhood and continue throughout their adult years, caught in a dangerous pattern of **weight cycling** (or a repeated pattern of dieting and initial weight loss, followed by weight gain, and a new cycle of dieting).

Your Experience

Part of being a CHW is a commitment to self-reflection and cultural humility. As you read this chapter, please take time to reflect and to consider the following questions

- How comfortable are you with your own body shape and size?
- Have you (or members of your family) ever tried to diet to lose weight?
  - What was this process like? What was the outcome?
- Have you (or family members) ever been judged or teased based on your body size?
- Have you ever been told by a health care provider to lose weight?
- To what extent is your own self-esteem (the way that you think and feel about yourself) influenced by perceptions about your body size and shape?

(continues)

Your Experience

(continued)

- What assumptions or beliefs do you have about people based on their body size?
- In what ways may your own experiences, values, and beliefs about weight influence your work with clients in the role of CHW?

THE HEALTH RISKS OF DIETING AND WEIGHT-CYCLING

Dieting to lose weight is not an effective strategy for promoting health. Dieting isn't even effective in promoting sustained weight loss. Research shows that the vast majority of dieters regain the weight they lost, and many gain back more weight than they lost (Ge et al., 2020; Hall & Kahan 2018; Lowe, Doshi, Katterman, & Feig, 2013; Siahpush et al., 2015.).

Because of the combined forces of prejudice and stigma, the promises of the dieting industry, and the prescriptions of medical practitioners, millions of Americans spend many years of their lives caught up in the harmful dynamic of weight-cycling. Many people begin this cycle of dieting to lose weight, gaining it back and dieting again, in childhood. Research links weight-cycling to a wide range of health risks including cardiovascular disease; hypertension; diabetes; cancer; and other chronic conditions, bone fractures, gallstone attacks, and higher risks of mortality or premature death (Brownell & Rodin, 1994; Byun, Bello, Liao, Makarem, & Aggarwal, 2019; Field, Manson, Taylor, Willett, & Colditz, 2004; Rhee et al., 2018; Rzehak et al., 2007.). In addition to the physical health risks, weight-cycling is also harmful to mental health, including lower self-esteem and higher rates of depression (Tylka et al., 2014).

TOWARD A WEIGHT-INCLUSIVE APPROACH TO PROMOTING HEALTH

Research not only demonstrates that traditional approaches of promoting dieting and weight loss are harmful to health, but it also points the way toward strategies and approaches that are effective for promoting health while demonstrating respect for people's bodies and their identities. These new models, including Health at Every Size (HAES), have been classified as weight-inclusive approaches to health.

A **weight-inclusive approach** implies demonstrating respect for people of all body sizes and weight, and is compared to **weight-normative** approaches that identify certain people as having normal weight and others as overweight or obese (or underweight). While weight-normative approaches counsel patients to lose weight, weight-inclusive approaches shift the focus from weight to focus on specific health issues, behaviors, and outcomes.

By taking the focus away from body weight and dieting, weight-inclusive providers are able to support patients in developing their own culturally relevant plans to enhance health and wellness, including self-esteem. These person-centered plans are determined by clients themselves and may include enhancing their level of physical activity by engaging in activities that are practical, enjoyable, and sustainable (discussed at greater length later on in this chapter). Clients may make changes not only to what they eat and drink, but how they think and feel about food (for more information about this, refer to the resources provided at the end of this chapter). Weight-inclusive approaches also support clients to seek out support and build connections with others who are facing similar challenges, including others who are working to accept and love their bodies as they are.

Weight-inclusive approaches are based on research evidence about what works to promote the health of people who have been classified as "overweight" or obese (Hunger et al., 2020). Several studies have investigated the effectiveness of the Health at Every Size approach. People who participated in an intensive HAES approach that included workshops, nutrition counseling, and physical activity resulted in improvements in eating attitudes and practices, improved body image, and psychological health (Ulian et al., 2018). A HAES intervention study showed that women who participated in 14 weekly meetings focused on self-acceptance and healthy lifestyles showed improvements in body and self-esteem, depression, and eating behaviors (Bégin et al., 2019).

A much-cited study published in the Journal of Obesity provides a clear description and justification for the emerging weight-inclusive approach to health (Tylka et al., 2014). This study analyzes existing research evidence to show that weight-normative approaches have failed to promote patient health, and how weight-inclusive approaches, including HAES, offer much greater promise for promoting the health of people who are perceived as overweight. The study questions why health care providers continue to advise dieting and weight loss when they have been shown to be so harmful to both physical and mental health. They remind us that health care providers have an obligation to avoid harming the patients they serve and to promote optimal health.

PRINCIPLES OF THE WEIGHT-INCLUSIVE APPROACH TO HEALTH

The weight-inclusive approach to health is guided by seven key principles presented here (adapted from Tylka et al., 2014):

1. Do no harm.

2. Appreciate that bodies naturally come in a variety of shapes and sizes, and ensure optimal health and well-being is supported for everyone, regardless of their weight.

3. Given that health is multidimensional, maintain a holistic focus.
   a. This principle encourages us to look beyond weight to consider a wide range of other health-related factors and behaviors as we work with clients.

4. Encourage a process focus (rather than end-goals) for day-to-day quality of life.
   a. This principle encourages us to meet clients where they are and help them to engage in realistic steps to improve their life and incorporate into their daily lives.

5. Critically evaluate the evidence for weight loss treatment and incorporate sustainable, empirically supported practices in prevention and treatment efforts
   a. The weight-inclusive approach requires us to think critically about what the research evidence shows us about the effectiveness of advising clients to lose weight. Draw upon existing research evidence about what works to promote the health of clients of all body sizes and shapes.

6. Create healthful, individualized practices and environments that are sustainable (e.g., regular pleasurable exercise, regular intake of foods high in nutrients, adequate sleep and rest, and adequate hydration).

7. Where possible, work to increase health access, autonomy, and social justice for all individuals along the entire weight spectrum. Trust that people move toward greater health when given access to stigma-free health care and opportunities.

This weight-inclusive approach is consistent with the concepts and skills promoted in the *Foundations* textbook including cultural-humility, person-centered practice, motivational interviewing, harm reduction, and support for patient self-management. To read more about weight-inclusive approaches, including Health at Every Size, refer to the list of resources presented at the end of this chapter.

Key Arguments in Favor of the Weight-Inclusive Approach

By shifting the focus of their work from weight to health, CHWs, and other health care providers can

- Uphold CHW ethics and a commitment not to cause harm to clients
- Avoid further stigmatizing or shaming clients based on their body shapes and size
- Apply person-centered concepts and skills to support the autonomy of clients and the development of realistic and sustainable action plans to promote their health and well-being
- Support patients of all sizes to focus on key health goals and indictors such as increasing physical activity and controlling blood pressure and blood glucose levels
- Support patients to significantly improve their physical and mental health
- Develop and maintain professional relationships that enable trust and mutual respect

Please watch the following video role plays that show a CHW talking with a client who has diabetes and has been diagnosed as "obese" by her physician and directed to lose weight. In the counter video, the CHW demonstrates a traditional approach to the issue and also directs the client to diet and lose weight. In the demonstration video, the CHW demonstrates a weight-inclusive approach.

- *What does the CHW do well in supporting the client's health and well-being?*
- *What could the CHW do differently to better support this client's health and well-being?*
- *What else would you do if you were working with this client, and why?*

TALKING ABOUT WEIGHT AND HEALTH, A COUNTER ROLE PLAY
(*Source:* Foundations for Community Health Workers/ http://youtu.be/FLpx7QHjMRY)

TALKING ABOUT WEIGHT AND HEALTH, A DEMONSTRATION ROLE PLAY.
(*Source:* Foundations for Community Health Workers/ http://youtu.be/83EeBQuXOXo)

Talking with Your Clinical Team About Weight and Health

As a CHW, you may work for a health care organization that follows traditional medical models for diagnosing and treating obesity. These traditional approaches may contradict the information we provide here, your own values, and the experience of the clients you work with. *In such a workplace setting, how can you challenge your colleagues to consider different perspectives about weight and wellness?*

If you decide to raise the issue of weight and health, do so with patience and respect for different perspectives. Anticipate that your efforts may be met with defensiveness, and the concept of a weight-inclusive approach may be dismissed by your colleagues. One way to begin is to ask your co-workers or clinical teammates to read and discuss the emerging research that challenges conventional thinking about weight and health. You could ask colleagues to meet together to discuss questions such as

- How does labeling patients as "obese" affect their ability to improve their health?
- Is there evidence to support encouraging patients who have tried dieting many times before—without enduring success—to start another weight-loss diet?
- What approaches are most likely to help patients of all sizes to feel respected and engaged in health care services?
- What type of approach is most likely to support patients to make and sustain meaningful improvements to their health status?

Client Scenario: Janice Sanders (*continued*)

CHW: You don't like how they talk about your weight when you go to the doctor.

Janice: Yes, honestly, it makes me feel like I don't want to go for medical check-ups. I was teased a lot as a kid. My sisters were too. It really got to us, and I think it made us kind of ashamed of our bodies. We were always trying to cover them up.

CHW: How do you think this affects your health today and your management of your high blood pressure?

Janice: Well, it makes me less likely to want to see the doctor because I feel like I'm being talked down to. And it makes it harder for me to want to join an exercise group or something like that.

(continues)

Client Scenario: Janice Sanders *(continued)*

CHW: We still have such a long way to go in terms of treating everyone with respect. I want to let you know that I've been trained not to focus too much on weight in my work with people who have chronic health conditions.

Janice: What do you mean?

CHW: Well, we focus on health rather than weight or size. That means trying to prevent chronic health conditions, like high blood pressure, and helping people who have chronic health conditions to manage them. It means helping every client to figure out how to take medications correctly, to engage in regular physical activity, to eat healthier foods and to practice stress management. These are all actions that can help people better manage high blood pressure and prevent heart attacks and strokes.

Janice: [laughs] So you aren't going to weigh me and tell me that I'm obese?

CHW: Would that help your high blood pressure?

Janice: No, definitely not! [laughs]

CHW: Can you tell me about times when you do feel good or better about your body?

Janice: Oh, wow, it's been a while, I think. [Janice pauses, thinking] When I was playing sports and it didn't matter if you were big; it mattered if you were strong or fast or had good reactions. I played softball and I was a pitcher. It was the one place I felt good about myself in high school.

CHW: What would it be like to feel like that again?

Janice: I don't know. I miss it.

CHW: Are there any times now when you feel more comfortable and confident about your body?

Janice: You know, at work, I don't feel so judged, and a lot of my co-workers are bigger, like me. As a cook you are always multi-tasking and moving, grilling, and frying, plating, running to the walk-in for ingredients. When I am in the zone at work, cooking on the line with my team, I feel good.

CHW: You feel good about your body when you are in the zone at work.

Janice: Yes, I guess I do. I didn't really think about it before.

CHW: That's a great feature of the work that you do. [Janice nods] Would you be interested in considering some other opportunities—outside of work—where you might be able to connect with others and feel good about your body and your health?

Janice: Maybe. It depends.

CHW: What does it depend on?

Janice: Like is it expensive and does it take a lot of time? Do I have to buy an outfit and are they going to judge me if I can't keep up?

CHW: Well, several clients are part of a group that I think meet your criteria. It's called *BigWomenWellness* and they get together a couple of times a month. They go hiking, camping, and swimming. Sometimes they go to a group member's house and cook a healthy meal. I know two women who are members and they've had positive experiences with the group.

Janice: So, you don't have to pay?

(continues)

Client Scenario: Janice Sanders *(continued)*

CHW: No, it's just a group of women who want to support each other to be healthier without any of the types of judgments that you mentioned. The women give each other support and share strategies about how to get good health care without being discriminated against because of their size.

Janice: It sort of sounds like my softball team from high school. We got together all the time. I don't think I would have graduated without them.

CHW: Let me know if you'd like to learn more. I can put you in touch with one of the members and she can tell you more about it.

Janice: Thank you, that sounds good. I think I'll start by talking with one of the group members.

CHW: Okay, here is a card for *BigWomenWellness* and I've written down the name of one of the members, along with her e-mail and phone number.

17.4 Understanding Information about Nutrition

It can be difficult to find reputable and easy-to-understand sources of information about nutrition for several reasons:

- **There are so many sources of information:** The sheer volume of information about nutrition and diet, including scientific, governmental, popular, and commercial sources complicates the task of identifying good sources of information.

- **Distinguishing reputable information:** It can be difficult to determine the most reputable sources of information about nutrition. Agricultural and food corporations and other companies often present misleading information about the nutritional value of their products in order to promote sales. These same corporations have also invested considerable resources to influence government agricultural policies and nutritional guidelines. At times, federal food policy has supported the interests of corporate interests over those of public health.

- **Highly specific scientific information:** Research studies, reports, and guidelines about nutrition often include details that are difficult for most of us to understand. For example, many resources on nutrition and diet include detailed information and calculations about calories, fat grams, glycemic index, vitamins, minerals, and micronutrients.

NUTRITIONAL INFORMATION INFORMED BY RESEARCH

Seek out reputable sources of information from leading health organizations providing nutritional information that is informed by research and presented in a manner that the communities you work with can understand. If you search for information online, prioritize .gov, .edu, and .org sites over .com or commercial sources. While research evidence will continue to refine our understanding of the association between nutrition, chronic disease, and overall health, findings from tens of thousands of reputable studies indicate that diets featuring plant-based foods (vegetables, fruits, beans, and whole grains) are better for our health and life-expectancy than diets that feature red meat, dairy, and refined and processed foods with added sugars and transfats.

Scope of Practice Concerns

As a CHW, you will not be expected to know or share detailed information about nutrition and health. You may provide general information about nutrition, and support clients to develop a healthier diet, often with clear guidelines provided by licensed or certified colleagues. But providing detailed information about nutrition is outside of your scope of practice and should be left to licensed colleagues including physicians and registered dieticians.

If your duties as a CHW include supporting clients to develop healthier diets in order to promote their health, ask your employer to provide you with nutritional guidelines. If you work for a health care organization, it is important for the clinical team to be on the same page in terms of the nutritional information provided to clients.

17.5 Guidelines for Healthy Nutrition

For the purposes of this introductory chapter, we rely on information on healthy eating provided by The Nutrition Source, a website from the Harvard University School of Public Health (Nutrition Source, 2023a). The Nutrition Source provides evidence-based and easy-to-understand information about food, nutrition, and health. It uses a harm-reduction approach. Rather than advising people to stop consuming certain foods and drinks, the Nutrition Source recommends that we reduce consumption of foods and drinks that research shows increase risks for chronic diseases and to eat and drink more of what promotes health.

Please review the **Healthy Eating Plate** presented here (The Nutrition Source, 2023b):

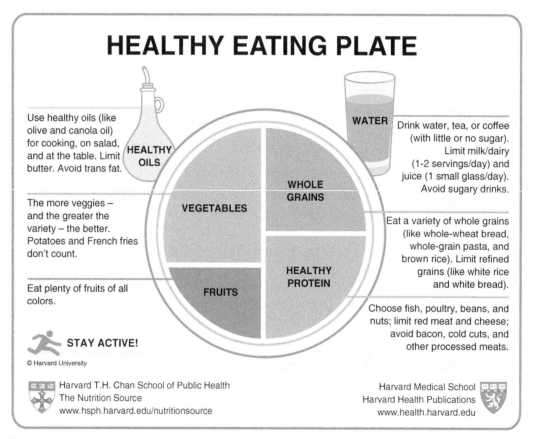

(*Source:* https://cdn1.sph.harvard.edu/wp-content/uploads/sites/30/2012/09/HEPJan2015.jpg.)

KEY GUIDELINES FOR A HEALTHY DIET: THE NUTRITION SOURCE

Make most of your meal vegetables and fruits—½ of your plate: Aim for color and variety, and remember that potatoes don't count as vegetables on the Healthy Eating Plate because of their negative impact on blood sugar.

Go for whole grains—¼ of your plate: Whole and intact grains—whole wheat, barley, wheat berries, quinoa, oats, brown rice, and foods made with them, such as whole wheat pasta—have a milder effect on blood sugar and insulin than white bread, white rice, and other refined grains.

Protein power—¼ of your plate: Fish, poultry, beans, and nuts are all healthy, versatile protein sources—they can be mixed into salads and pair well with vegetables on a plate. Limit red meat and avoid processed meats such as bacon and sausage.

Healthy plant oils—in moderation: Choose healthy vegetable oils like olive, canola, soy, corn, sunflower, peanut, and others, and avoid partially hydrogenated oils, which contain unhealthy trans fats. Remember that low-fat does not mean "healthy."

Drink water, coffee, or tea: Skip sugary drinks, limit milk and dairy products to one to two servings per day, and limit juice to a small glass per day.

(The Nutrition Source, 2023b)

What Did You Eat Yesterday?

Please take a moment to stop and consider *your own diet*. What did you eat and drink for dinner yesterday (or, if you didn't eat dinner, what did you eat for breakfast or lunch)?

- *How typical was the food you ate yesterday in terms of your usual diet?*
- *How healthy—on a scale from 1 to 10—would you rate what you ate yesterday?*
- *What did you eat and drink yesterday that promotes your health?*
- *What did you eat and drink yesterday that may increase your risks for chronic health conditions like high blood pressure and type 2 diabetes?*
- *What one change could you make to the meal to make it healthier?*

Tips for Reading Nutritional Labels

Learning how to read and understand the nutritional labels placed on packaged food products will be helpful to promoting your own health and for guiding your work with clients. The format and content of nutritional labels are updated over time. Current Nutrition Facts Labels, updated in 2020, looks like this (U.S. Food and Drug Administration, 2023a):

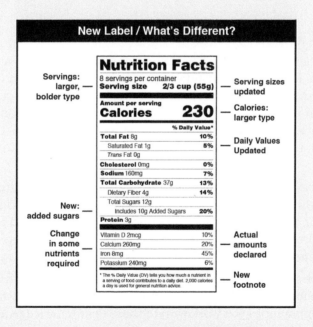

Many of us don't read nutrition labels, but they provide information that can be helpful in making healthier choices about the food products we purchase. Some tips for reading the Nutrition Facts labels include:

- **Serving size:** This provides information on how many servings are in each package of food. Nutritional information is provided per serving size. Note that some packages include many servings.
- **Total calories:** Check the total number of calories per serving size. Compare this to the total number of calories that a person consumes each day (on average, this is about 2000 calories but may vary based on age, sex, height, and physical activity level). If just one serving size of a product has 500 calories, it has 25% of all calories that we are estimated to need in one day.

(continues)

Tips for Reading Nutritional Labels

(continued)

- **Nutrients:** Labels include information about key nutrients in each product.
  - People are encouraged to consume less of certain nutrients including sodium (salt), added sugars, trans fats, and saturated fats.
  - People are encouraged to consume more of certain nutrients including dietary fiber, vitamin D, calcium, iron, and potassium.
- **Percent daily value (%DV):** This estimates the percentage of daily recommended guidelines for each key nutrient that is in a serving size of the food product. In general, a %DV that is less than 5% is considered low and a %DV that is 20% or higher is considered high. When reviewing nutritional labels, look for foods that contain a higher %DV of healthy nutrients such as dietary fiber and lower %DV of the nutrients that are less healthy such as sodium or added sugars.
- Use the Nutritional Facts labels to compare food products that are very similar to help you select the healthiest option.
- Resources to learn more about nutritional labels include the Harvard University Nutrition Source and the U.S. Food and Drug Administration (Nutrition Source, 2023c; USFDA, 2020, 2023b).

CULTURALLY RESPONSIVE HEALTHY EATING

Historically, nutritional policies and programs have imposed culturally specific, and often unhealthy, food guidelines and restrictions on low-income consumers and communities of color. Gradually, government guidelines, policies and programs are beginning to address the fundamental connection between culture and food and to incorporate culturally responsive concepts and goals. Advocates argue that food programs, policies, and guidelines should embrace, respect, and support diverse food cultures in the United States and highlight the unique needs of immigrants and low-income communities to be connected to affordable healthy food from their own cultures.

Local, national, and global organizations are increasingly providing access to nutritional guidelines and recipes that are reflective of a wide variety of cultures and traditions. For example, the Institute for Family Health highlights healthy plates from around the world promoting a wide range of food options that meet and honor cultural food traditions (Institute for Family Health, 2022). The National Institutes of Health includes heart-healthy recipes for African American and Latinx communities (National Institutes of Health, 2022).

Respect the cultural identities and traditions of the communities that you work with as your organization develops guidelines, health education materials, and referrals resources on food and nutrition. Most importantly, ask the clients and communities you work with to share their knowledge, traditions, and ideas for healthy and culturally responsive recipes and meals.

MHP Salud is an organization based in Texas with over 35 years of experience implementing CHW programs to assist Latino communities (MHP Salud, 2022). They provide health education about healthy nutrition and developed a brochure that presents healthy plate options for Latino communities. CHWs cook meals with the community families in local schools, community centers and in people's homes. This type of hands-on approach provides families with the skills and the confidence to plan and prepare healthy meals that are tasty and honor cultural traditions.

- *What food cultures and traditions are common among the communities that you work with?*

- *What local resources are available that support culturally responsive healthy eating?*

What Do
YOU?
Think

FOOD AS MEDICINE

Food as Medicine refers to a range of interventions designed to integrate access to food resources within health care settings. It includes approaches such as co-locating food pantries within health care organizations and providing patients with groceries, cooking supplies, home-delivered meals, medically tailored or therapeutic meals, prescriptions for free or discounted healthy foods, recipes, cooking classes, and more. Food as Medicine programs are still relatively new, but existing research indicates they help patients to access healthy food, to reduce financial hardship, and may result in better self-management of chronic health conditions and fewer hospital admissions (Downer, Berkowitz, Harlan, & Olstad, Mozaffarian, 2020).

The Food as Medicine Coalition is a national network of organizations that provide evidence-based food and nutrition services to people with chronic health conditions. Visit their website to see if there is a member provider in your community (Food is Medicine Coalition, 2022).

The Food as Medicine Collaborative

The Food as Medicine Collaborative (FAMC) is based in San Francisco. It is a coalition of over 20 organizations including the SF Department of Public Health, community clinics, food nonprofits, and businesses. FAMC aims to change health care delivery by integrating food security interventions. Currently serving 11 health clinics, FAMC provides patients with direct access to food in clinic settings, hands-on cooking and nutrition classes, and referrals to local food resources. In 2021, over 3500 patients attended Food Pharmacies in 11 clinics and received more than 15,000 bags of healthy food. Ninety-two percent of these patients reported adopting healthier eating habits.

(Food as Medicine Collaborative, 2022)

Food, Sustainability, and Environmental Health

Shifting to a more plant-based diet is better for human health and the environment.

Growing plants for direct human consumption is much more efficient than raising livestock (such as cattle, sheep and pork) for meat and dairy products. Significantly more resources—land, water, grain to feed to the livestock, fuel, fertilizer, pesticides, and other resources—are required to produce meat and dairy products than to grow grains or vegetables. More than half of the world's habitable land is used for agriculture and approximately 77% of these lands are used for raising livestock (Ritchie, 2019).

> If half of the crops used to feed livestock were instead used for human consumption, "we could feed all the starving populations around the world and solve the problem of world hunger." (Dopelt, Radon, & Davidovitch, 2019)

Livestock production is also highly destructive to the environment (Lynch, Johnston, & Wharton, 2018). The livestock industry contributes to global warming and is estimated to produce between 14.5 and 18% of the worlds' greenhouse gas emissions and 35–40% of methane emissions (Dopelt, Radon, & Davidovitch, 2019; Gustin, 2019). Animal waste pollutes groundwater, rivers, and oceans. The increasing demand for meat and dairy products creates pressure for more pastureland resulting in clearing forests to grow corn and soy for livestock, decreasing the earth's biodiversity and its ability to absorb carbon dioxide from the atmosphere (Ritchie, 2021)

Shifting away from livestock production to cultivating crops for direct human consumption would not only promote food security and improved health outcomes, it would also protect the environment and help to slow climate change.

To learn more about this topic, please see the Additional Resources provided at the end of this chapter.

17.6 Practical Guidelines for Healthier Eating

As you work with people to change their diets, we recommend the following strategies. Support clients to develop food plans that are:

AFFORDABLE

Any healthy eating plan must be affordable for the people you work with. Keep the client's budget in mind. Unfortunately, some of the healthiest foods—like fresh fruits and vegetables—are sometimes more expensive than unhealthier options, especially processed and packaged foods.

ACCESSIBLE

Not every neighborhood has affordable sources of healthy food. Many rural areas and lower-income neighborhoods are "food deserts" or places where it is difficult to find fresh vegetables, fruits, and other healthier foods. People may have to travel some distance to find an affordable grocery store, and time and transportation are significant barriers.

SNAP Benefits

Previously known as Food Stamps, the Supplemental Nutrition Assistance Program or SNAP is the largest food and nutritional support program in the United States.

SNAP recipients receive an Electronic Benefit Transfer (EBT) card that can be used to buy groceries at authorized food stores. Benefit amounts are automatically loaded onto the card each month. Eligibility for SNAP benefits depends upon income and strict asset tests. In 2022, household income must be at or below 130% of the federal poverty line (FPL) or, for example, $28,550 a year for a family of three. In 2021, 41 million Americans received SNAP benefits and the average SNAP benefit per household member per day in 2022 is estimated at $5.34 (Hall & Nchako, 2022).

While SNAP helps millions of Americans to purchase food, advocates argue that the income and asset eligibility guidelines are too strict, and the level or amount of the benefits too low (Carlson, Llobrera, & Keith-Jennings, 2021). Research indicates that the level of SNAP benefits aren't enough for recipients to afford healthy foods (Mulik & Haynes-Maslow, 2017). Larger SNAP benefits would increase food security, promote child health, and reduce child poverty (Carlson, Llobrera, & Keith-Jennings, 2021).

REALISTIC

- Don't set a client up for disappointment by encouraging them to make dramatic changes to their diet overnight. If a client eats at fast food restaurants four times a week, it isn't a realistic for them to stop eating fast food. Keep harm reduction in mind. Encourage the client to begin by gradually reducing the number of times they eat at fast food restaurants, or to change what they order at fast food restaurants.

- It can be helpful to steer clients away from viewing any food as purely "good" or "bad" or for cutting some foods out of their diet forever. Apply harm reduction concepts (Chapter 9) to the challenge of health eating. Every food may be enjoyed in moderation or on occasion.

Please watch the following video [▶] Role Play of a CHW working with a client who is interested in changing her diet to improve their health:

CLIENT-CENTERED COUNSELING AND NUTRITION, ROLE-PLAY, DEMO.

(*Source:* Foundations for Community Health Workers/ http://youtu.be/ 73-ebSBGQU0)

- *What did the CHW do well in terms of supporting this client to make changes to her diet?*
- *Which client-centered concepts and skills did the CHW use?*
- *What would you do differently if you were the CHW who is working with this client?*

WITH THE FAMILY IN MIND

- For many clients, attempts to change their diet may be influenced or limited by their family. Changing a diet may conflict with family cultures and traditions. This is especially true if other members of the family do most of the grocery shopping and cooking.
- Ideally, family members will support the client and make at least some adjustments to what the entire household eats and drinks. However, it is unlikely that all family members will be persuaded to adopt similar changes to their own diets. The client may have to make changes on their own, and to find ways to manage the challenge of having less healthy food and drink in their home.

ENJOYABLE

- Most people enjoy food. Unfortunately, some of the foods that we enjoy the most are the least healthy. We have become conditioned by food manufacturers to crave certain foods high in sugar, salt, and fat.
- A healthier diet may be less pleasurable, especially at first. Acknowledge this. Support clients to talk about it and listen patiently.
- Support clients to find healthier foods and drinks that they enjoy. What is their favorite healthier meal? What is a healthier meal that their whole family enjoys?

NONJUDGMENTAL

Judgment—and the shame it causes—isn't helpful to changing behaviors or for our health in general. Clients are often sensitive to the judgments that health care providers and other professionals make about their behaviors and their health status. When clients feel judged, they may distance themselves from providers and the health information those providers share.

Francis Julian Montgomery: For people without a kitchen or cooking facilities, it can be difficult to manage diabetes, high cholesterol, or other things related to diet because they cannot really cook for themselves. Because a lot of my clients eat at fast food restaurants, I bring menus from those places, and we go over the choices and things like sodium, carbohydrates, and sugar content of different items. We look for the healthiest items. That way I don't end up in the unwanted position of reprimanding a person due to the choices they make based on their income. They can go to an inexpensive fast-food restaurant and still make healthier choices. Also, some congregant meal sites [places that provide free meals such as soup kitchens] are healthier than others. By learning to think about how healthy different foods are, my clients have the tools to navigate those meals.

CHW

COMMUNITY GARDENS

Urban and community gardens provide improved access to affordable and healthy foods for local community members, schools, and other organizations. They use public, donated, or private lands and teach community members how to grow, tend, harvest, and prepare crops for healthy meals. Participating in community gardening is also associated with improved nutrition and health outcomes (Garcia, Ribeiro, Germani, & Bógus, 2018; Gregis, Ghisalberti, Sciascia, Sottile, & Peano, 2021). One research study found that participants in an urban home gardening program experienced improved food access, increased consumption of fresh produce, reduced consumption of fast food, and more home cooking (Palar et al., 2019).

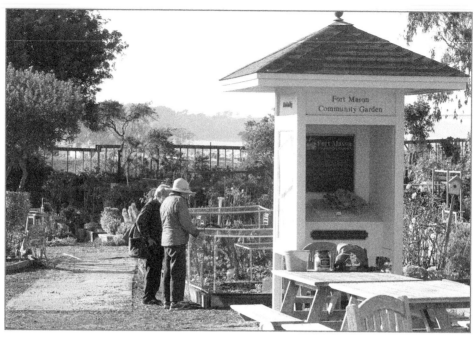

Many communities have started Community Gardens to increase access to healthy food.

- *Are there any urban or community gardens in the communities where you live or work?*

17.7 Approaches to Providing Health Education About Nutrition

CHWs provide information about a variety of health topics to the clients and communities they work with. *How you provide health information matters.* Consider the following the Seven-Step Guideline for sharing health information about nutrition with clients:

1. **Determine what the client already knows**: We recommend that you begin by asking people to share what they already know about nutrition (or any health topic when you are providing health education). Most clients know something (and many know a lot) about the topics that impact their health. Many people have experience trying to change their diet and have learned a lot along the way.

   Start by asking the client what they understand about the foods and drinks that are best for their health, and those that are associated with increased risks for chronic health conditions. Let the client's level of knowledge set the agenda for providing any additional health information.

2. **Determine the client's interest in learning more**: Before you share any new information about nutrition, ask the client if they are interested in learning more. If the client isn't interested, change the topic and move on. Respecting a client's wishes and priorities is essential to providing person-centered services and maintaining a strong positive connection or rapport.

3. **Share general information:** Nutritional information and guidelines are often highly detailed and difficult to comprehend. Remember that you are not a certified nutritionist; your role is to provide more general information about healthy nutrition, and to link your clients to additional resources such as access to nutritional counseling, affordable food (including, as necessary, food pantries and hot meal programs), and other resources.

   We propose the *Healthy Eating Plate* (discussed in Section 17.5) as a good place to start with general health information. Information is presented in a simple graphic and incorporates a harm reduction approach that presents both the types of food and drinks that increase health risks, and those that promote good health.

   A reasonable goal for clients is to be able to summarize:

   - Foods and drinks that promote health and well-being
   - Foods and drinks that increase health risks, such as risks for chronic health conditions

4. **Keep culture—and cultural humility—in mind:** When clients plan to change their diet, their decisions are often influenced by their own cultural values and practices. When people are able to eat healthy foods that are also part of their food culture(s), they are more likely to enjoy and maintain these food habits.

5. **Provide more detailed information or referrals:** In some situations, you will be asked to provide detailed nutritional information to clients about how to maintain a healthier diet given their day-to-day realities, including their budget, culture, and health status. Note that nutritional guidelines may change depending on the type of chronic condition that the client is living with. For example, there are special dietary guidelines for the self-management of diabetes or for patients undergoing radiation or chemotherapy. As always, follow the guidance of your supervisor or your clinician; ask for nutritional guidelines approved by your employer. If you have not been trained and authorized by your organization to provide this information yourself, make a referral to a trained colleague or local program.

6. **Keep the information practical and specific to the client's life circumstances:** A key role of CHWs is to support clients in translating information about healthy nutrition into specific and practical guidelines for their daily lives. Don't overwhelm clients with too much information all at once. Let them control the pace of your conversation and how much information you provide. Rather than talking about more general or abstract issues such as "what is healthy nutrition?" or "What food does your family usually eat?"—our suggestion is to keep the discussion highly focused on their specific life circumstances. For example, try asking the client:

- *What did you eat for lunch today?*
- *What did you eat for dinner last night?*

These questions are more likely to generate very detailed information about the client's diet. Follow-up questions might include:

- *How could you change the meal (what you ate last night) to make it healthier? Can you think of one or two changes you could make?*

There are many ways to make a meal healthier, such as:

- Not eating or drinking a particular item (e.g., drinking soda)
- Eating less of a particular item (a smaller order of fries)
- Eating or drinking more of an item (such as more vegetables)
- Substituting one food or drink for another (such as substituting water or tea for soda)

Another practical approach is to support clients in developing a plan for how to shop for and prepare a healthy meal for their family. This meal should be affordable and something that the client and their family are likely to find appealing. The plan could include:

- Where the client will shop
- A budget
- A shopping list
- Accompanying a client to shop for healthier foods together
- A menu for the meal
- Recipes. Note that the recipes should be easy to follow and probably shouldn't include too many steps or ingredients or require too much time to prepare. We recommend sharing recipes that take less than 30 minutes to prepare.

7. **Follow-up with the client:** Follow-up with the client during the next few weeks or during a next appointment. Ask them about their experience. Have they tried to implement any changes? What was their experience like? Do they have any outstanding questions or needs for additional resources or referrals? Stay person-centered, open to feedback and the possibility that clients may want to revise their health plan. Provide affirmations for their hard work and accomplishments. With experience, you will learn what types of information and resources are most relevant to clients.

CHW: What do you want to work on in terms of managing your blood pressure?

Janice: Well, I know I could eat better. I mean, I'm a cook, so I do know about food; I just don't really eat healthy foods.

CHW: You mentioned that you eat a lot of meals at the Café where you work.

Janice: Yes, I usually eat lunch at the Bluebird and sometimes I bring leftovers home for dinner.

CHW: Would you like to start talking about the foods you eat at work, or at home?

Janice: Let's start with what we eat at home.

CHW: What did you have for dinner last night?

Janice: Oh, I'm so busted! [laughs] We had frozen pizza and frozen French fries.

CHW: Well, that's a pretty typical meal for a lot of us, right?

Janice: Yeah, but I can do better.

CHW: Okay let's focus on what you already eat at home that is healthier. Do you have a favorite healthier meal that you make at home?

Janice: Probably the tacos we make. They're pretty simple. We add in a lot of veggies. My neighbor down the street makes homemade corn tortillas. Sometimes I get a rotisserie chicken and we also make some amazing fish tacos. They don't take long but are crispy and they taste great. In the summer, we grill up some chicken and the veggies. And salsa. That's pretty healthy, right?

CHW: That sounds great.

Janice: Yeah, and Martin loves making them and eating them. He's starting to help out more and more with the prep.

CHW: How often do make the tacos?

Janice: It's been a couple of weeks, maybe longer.

CHW: What would help you to make the tacos, or another healthy alternative, more frequently?

Janice: Well, I think I could manage doing this pretty much every weekend. And I can ask Marcie to help—we're usually at each other's houses. During the week is the hardest. I cook all day at work and when I come home the last thing I want to do is cook some more.

CHW: So, maybe you want a super easy meal to prep for dinner on the days that you work.

Janice: Yes. I think that's why I've gotten into a rut with frozen meals.

CHW: Okay. Could I share a suggestion or two?

Janice: Sure, that would be great.

CHW: Okay, for now, maybe you could focus on cooking healthier meals on the weekends and checking in with Marcie about it. Maybe next time we meet, or whenever you're ready, we could brainstorm ideas for healthier meals during the week that are also easy and quick. Maybe even some different frozen options. How does that sound?

Janice: That's sounds good.

CHW: The thing with making big changes like this, especially to what we eat, is that slow and steady wins the race. If you can have one success that will help set you up for another. I'm here to help, but it needs to be at your pace and ideas that truly work for you and Martin.

Janice: Thanks, I appreciate it. And I'll talk with Marcie and Martin about this and see what ideas they may have for better meals during the week.

Depending upon the guidelines of your agency, other options for supporting clients to improve their regular diet may include:

- Keep some packaged food or soups at your office. Together with clients, examine the labels and recommended portion sizes of the foods in order to enhance understanding of the levels of key ingredients and components such as sugar and transfats.
- Visit the client's home (if they invite you) to talk about the foods that they have on hand and how they may impact their health (and the health of their family).
- Share quick, culturally relevant, affordable, and healthy recipes, videos, and websites.
- Join the client on a trip to their local grocery store or supermarket to talk about healthy and not-as-healthy food choices.

Finally, become an expert in local resources—other agencies, programs, and services—that may be of interest to the clients you work with. Conduct your own research in the community to identify possible referrals to resources such as:

- The Supplemental Nutrition Assistance Program or SNAP (if clients meet the eligibility guidelines)
- Educational and support groups related to healthy nutrition
- Food as Medicine programs
- Food pantries
- Hot meal programs
- Urban and community garden projects
- Programs that teach people how to prepare healthy and culturally relevant meals for their families

Please watch the following three-part video series that show a CHW providing nutritional information to a client who wants to better manage his high blood pressure.

1. HYPERTENSION AND HEALTHY EATING, PART 1:
(*Source:* Foundations for Community Health Workers/ http://youtu.be/ aGuViTC42G4)

2. HYPERTENSION AND HEALTHY EATING, PART 2:
(*Source:* Foundations for Community Health Workers/ http://youtu.be/271pMgUluNg)

2. HYPERTENSION AND HEALTHY EATING, PART 3:
(*Source:* Foundations for Community Health Workers/ http://youtu.be/ gVlV_8iM_HA)

- *What did the CHW do well in terms of supporting the client to better understand guidelines for healthy nutrition?*
- *What else would you do as a CHW to enhance this client's understanding of healthy nutrition?*

17.8 Physical Activity

Physical activity is vital for overall health and the management of most chronic health conditions. Physical activity is defined as *anything* that gets the body moving. For clients who are struggling with health conditions or body image, enhanced physical activity can offer a sense of control and self-mastery.

Activity or Exercise?

You may note that we use the words *physical activity* or *activity* more than *exercise* in this book. We do this because, for many people, exercise implies strenuous physical actions that are beyond their capacity (such as jogging). When some patients hear the word exercise they may translate that into *"something that other people do."* Increasingly, public health and health care organizations are using the words *activity* or *physical activity* because these words include a full spectrum of actions such as walking, playing, gardening, stretching, dancing, and riding a bicycle. Physical activities include anything that gets the body moving (even if you are doing the activity while sitting down).

THE HEALTH BENEFITS OF PHYSICAL ACTIVITY

Extensive research has documented the clear health benefits of physical activity. More recent research indicates that any amount of physical activity has some health benefits, and that physical activity also has immediate health benefits including reducing blood pressure and anxiety and improved sleep quality (U.S. Department of Health and Human Services, 2018).

Long-term health benefits of physical activity are highlighted in the second edition of *Physical Activity Guidelines for Americans* (Ibid) and include:

- improved cardiovascular health
- improved bone health
- reduced risks for depression and dementia
- prevention of eight types of cancer
- reduced risks of mortality and stroke
- reduced risk of fall and injuries from falls for older adults
- improved overall physical functioning and quality of life

17.9 Guidelines for Healthy Activity

Guidelines for healthy activity levels are available from leading health organizations such as the World Health Organization, the U.S. Department of Health and Human Services, and the American Heart Association. There are specific guidelines for children and youth, active adults, seniors, people who are pregnant, and people living with illness or disability. These guidelines are regularly reviewed and updated to reflect new research evidence.

The U.S. Department of Health and Human Services revised physical activity guidelines in 2018. The guidelines emphasize that any level of physical activity is better than none. They encourage us to sit less and move more throughout each day. People who have been inactive for a long time, who are living with a disability or pain should re-engage with low levels of physical activity and build up their level of intensity or duration slowly (if possible).

The recommendations (USHHS, 2018) for healthy physical activity for adults ages 18–64 are:

Two and half hours a week (150 minutes total) of moderate-intensity aerobic activity (such as brisk walking, yard work, and bicycling).

The health benefits from physical activity can be enhanced by:

- Engaging in more vigorous activities such as bicycling, hiking, exercise classes, swimming, playing basketball, or dancing (the list of activities is detailed in the full Guidelines).
- Adding in muscle-strengthening activities (working with weights, push-ups, carrying heavy loads) that involve all muscle groups at least twice a week.

The types of physical activities that people engage in are numerous and depend upon factors like our age, health-status, flexibility, disability, and cultural identities. The most important message is to move our bodies as much as possible throughout the day and to find types of activities that we enjoy and can engage in regularly.

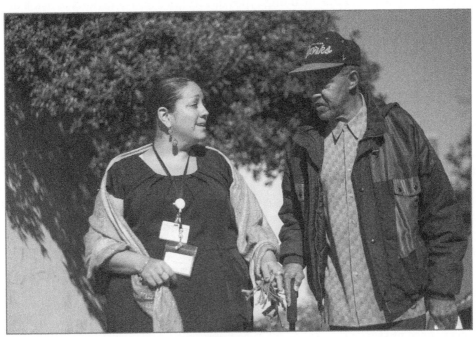

[Some CHWs schedule walking meetings with clients]

WALKING AND ROLLING

Walking is perhaps the most common form of physical activity. It has the advantage of being readily available to most people and does not require any special equipment, training, or fees. Research evidence has shown that walking is highly effective in promoting short- and long-term health outcomes.

Keep in mind that not everyone lives in a neighborhood where it is safe to walk and that access to safety and green spaces is a health equity issue. As a CHW, you want to support clients in identifying safe options for walking or other forms of physical activity. Brainstorm together and respect their knowledge, goals, and limitations.

The National Center on Health, Physical Activity and Disability (NCHPAD) has launched a campaign—"How I Walk"—to challenge the way that we think about walking and physical activity, and to encourage more inclusive perspectives. (NCHPAD, 2022). The campaign reminds us that there are many ways to walk including with wheelchairs, walkers, and other resources.

ELDERS, DISABILITIES AND PHYSICAL ACTIVITY

Engaging in physical activities helps to prevent injuries and disabilities as we age, as well as to promote independent living (National Institutes on Aging, 2020). Yet engaging in physical activity can be more challenging as we age or if we are living with a disability. Unfortunately, many programs and resources don't take this into account. If you are working with elders or people with disabilities, be sure to consult with your colleagues and seek expert advice about safe physical activity guidelines and resources.

Encourage people to start with realistic physical activity goals and to build slowly from there. Walking to the mailbox may be an initial goal that, over time, could lead to walking around the block or to a local park and back. Research emphasizes the importance of self-efficacy for sustained physical activity (Blom et al., 2021). In other words, when people feel confident, comfortable, and in-control of their physical activity levels and choices, they are more likely to be successful.

There are local and national agencies and programs that focus on serving seniors and people living with disabilities. Seek out local and online resources to share with the clients and communities you work with. For example, senior centers almost always provide physical activities designed to be accessible for elders, including activities designed to be done sitting down or standing with the support of a walker. The National Institute on Aging provides guidelines for older adults including types of activities and questions to ask a doctor before beginning new activities (National Institutes on Aging, 2020). Look for the information provided under Additional Resources at the end of this chapter.

A Realistic and Holistic Approach to Movement: The Body Positive

The Body Positive highlights the importance of exercise being joyful and authentic, rather than motivated by a desire to lose weight (The Body Positive, 2013):

> When exercise becomes intuitive [natural] and is more than just a means of burning calories, we find that people exercise more frequently and put an end to their stop and start (yo-yo) exercise patterns. The goal of exercising intuitively is to do it for the purposes of pleasure and release of physical and mental stress, as well as for fitness.

When clients are new to exercise, or unsure of where to begin, consider asking the following questions:

1. **What type of movement will make me feel great in my body today?**

2. **Are there any obstacles in my life that make it difficult for me to exercise regularly? Is so, what can I do to remove these obstacles?**

17.10 Supporting Clients to Increase Activity Levels

As you work with clients who want to increase their physical activity, please keep the following concepts in mind:

INJURY PREVENTION

Ask clients to consult with a health care provider about plans to increase activity levels and to clarify any possible risks or limitations. Physicians or other providers, including physical therapists, may provide guidelines designed to prevent injury and further harm to existing limitations or disabilities. This is particularly important if the client is recovering from an injury or serious health condition (such as treatments for cancer), has a disability, or has not been active in a long time.

GRADUAL OR INCREMENTAL CHANGE

Increasing physical activity should be done incrementally or in small steps. Some clients want to start out with intensive activities such as an aerobics class, jogging, or long hikes. However, they may not be ready to succeed with such an ambitious plan, and their lack of success may become a significant obstacle for implementing more realistic actions in the future.

Talk with clients about the feasibility of their action plan. Support them to develop a plan for increased physical activity they can have immediate success with (such as within the first day or week), and to build gradually from there, never taking on more than they can manage at the time. An action plan to increase walking is a good starting place for many clients. Some clients may start out walking a relatively short distance and at a relatively slow pace. Over time, they may gradually increase the distance they walk and/or the pace of their walking. Remember that any level of physical activity is better than none, and that, within reason, more activity is always better for our health.

When clients are developing plans for increased activity, consider using a Motivation or Confidence Scale (see Chapter 9). Ask the client how confident or ready they are, on a scale from 0 to 10, to implement their plan. When clients rate their confidence or readiness at a 7 or above, they are more likely to have success.

Please watch the following video interview with David Spero, RN, a nurse, and chronic conditions management coach. In the video, David talks about his work to support a client to start walking. She, and her physician, doubted her ability to increase her physical activity.

THE VALUE OF TAKING SMALL STEPS.
(*Source:* Foundations for Community Health Workers/ http://youtu. be/4ILopSTH7lk)

- *What health issues and barriers did David's client face?*
- *What approach did David take to support the client in increasing her level of physical activity?*
- *What did you learn from this video that you may wish to apply to your work as a CHW?*

REALISTIC AND AFFORDABLE

Support clients to establish physical activity plans that are easy for them to implement and maintain over time. For example, talk with clients about the types of activities they can do close to where they live and work, or even on their way to and from home or work. What activities can they engage in for 10 minutes or more several times a week? What activities can they do without additional expense, such as the costs of equipment or membership fees?

> **Francis Julian Montgomery:** My overall goal when I am working with a client who has expressed an interest in increasing their physical activity, is to help them to do it in small, obtainable increments. The client will set their goal, and I will ask them questions to help them figure out the rest—what they are willing to do, what their capacity is, and what may be too much for them to take on. Then I help them put this into an Action Plan with specific steps and activities and all the other details.

NONJUDGMENTAL

Some people don't feel positive about their bodies and may feel embarrassed, frustrated, or ashamed about engaging in physical activity. They may have been teased or discriminated against in the past based on their perceived body size or shape, and these experiences and the emotions they generate can pose significant barriers to physical activity in the present. Demonstrate cultural humility and don't impose similar judgments about body shape or size, fitness, or physical abilities. Strive to be aware of any prejudices that you may have. If you have internalized common negative perspectives and assumptions about weight, seek out opportunities to learn more about these topics and to enhance your cultural humility.

ACCESSIBLE

For many clients, maintaining ongoing physical activity requires that the activity be easily accessible to them. However, many people live in areas where participating in physical activity is limited by factors such as the weather, safety concerns, or the lack of sidewalks or green spaces. Support clients to brainstorm ideas for where and how they can engage in physical activities as safely and efficiently as possible. For example, what activities can they do at home?

ENJOYABLE

People are more successful participating in regular physical activity when they enjoy it. If the activities are uncomfortable, painful, or boring, they are more difficult to maintain. Keep the focus on pleasurable movement and activities, and not on unattainable fitness goals. An action plan that includes dancing, or walking a child to school, may make more sense for a client than daily visits to a gym. As you think about how to talk with clients about physical activities, keep the weight-inclusive approach in mind. Dr. Michael Loewy, suggests

> *No one is too big to move around as much as feels good. I found that motivational interviewing techniques that meet a person where they are now and assesses their motivation to change, with no judgment, worked great.* (The Association for Size Diversity and Health, 2013)

Consider asking people what kind of movement or activities they enjoyed in the past. Those memories can often provide insight about how to move forward, in the present, to be more active.

WITH OTHERS, OR ON THEIR OWN?

Some people prefer to engage in physical activity on their own. Others find that engaging in physical activity with a friend or a group can provide motivation, companionship and safety. Honor the client's preferences and, if they enjoy being active with others, support them to identify opportunities to do this. This may include taking a daily walk with a friend or family member or joining a local (and free) neighborhood or community walking, bicycling, or tai chi group.

COMMUNITY RESOURCES

Ask the clients you work with if they know about local parks and other green spaces, organizations, or programs that support people to engage in physical activity. Conduct research to identify local resources. There may be free or low-cost programs offered in the community by nonprofit or faith-based organizations, or local health departments and community colleges. Programs may include walking or swim clubs, Tai Chi classes, or even water aerobics. There may be programs or services for people who share a specific identity such as activities for women, people with disabilities, or chronic conditions such as arthritis, cancer, or chronic pain. Increasingly, there is also a wide variety of online programs that support people with physical activity, and many of these are free. You may search online with a client for programs or activities that appeal to them or provide some suggestions.

Client Scenario: Janice Sanders (continued)

CHW: Janice, can you tell me a bit more about your experience with physical activity or exercise?

Janice: Well, I used to love it. When I was young, I played a lot of sports and hung out with my brothers. But lately, I've kind of . . . [Janice stops and considers]

CHW: [listens patiently]

Janice: I've tried. My sister-in-law Marcie, she encourages me to do more exercise. I went to some kind of a workout class with her at the Y, but I just felt big and out of shape. I couldn't keep up and I felt embarrassed. I didn't go back.

CHW: I've felt that way too. Can I ask about what was going on for you?

Janice: I just felt like people were staring at the fat lady and . . . I don't know. I used to get teased a lot as a kid.

CHW: About your body?

Janice: Yeah

CHW: What if we could think about ways to increase your physical activity that you were more comfortable with?

Janice: What do you mean?

CHW: Well, for any plan to work, it needs to be realistic for you.

(continues)

Janice: I didn't mean to sound so negative.

CHW: You don't sound negative to me. You sound realistic. You work long hard physical hours and don't have a lot of energy left over. You already get a workout at work.

Janice: I do, don't I?

CHW: Remember that anything that gets our body moving counts as physical activity. So being on your feet all day, doing physical work like cooking, that *is* physical activity.

Janice: Oh, good. I thought you were going to tell me to go back to the class at the Y! [laughs]

CHW: Is there anything else that you might want to try or that you've done before on your days off? Maybe something with Martin? What does he like to do?

Janice: Well, his first love is video games, but he's been asking me to throw a baseball around with him lately. I used to play softball.

CHW: Have you had a chance to do it yet?

Janice: A couple of times. Now that the days are longer, we can even throw a ball around after dinner.

CHW: What was it like for you, playing catch with Martin?

Janice: It was fun. We laughed a lot, but he's also improved after just a few times and . . . I think that makes him proud, and that makes me happy.

CHW: Okay, so it sounds like you are already adding in some new activities, and you're enjoying them.

Janice: Well, yes, I guess so. But, I mean, does that count as physical activity?

CHW: It does. Remember the guideline; anything that involves moving your body.

Janice: Okay, I'm still getting used to thinking this way.

CHW: Is there anything else that you might want to try?

Janice: [thinks] We went biking, Marcie and me and our kids. We rented some bikes out at Big Lake.

CHW: What was it like?

Janice: It felt really . . . free. We had a good time.

CHW: Is that something you might want to do again?

Janice: Definitely. Martin has a bike and he's asked me to go riding with him. Let me talk to Marcie. I'm sure we can come up with something.

CHW: Wonderful. And remember that physical activity doesn't have to happen all at once or be done for a long time. Every time you do something, it counts. So, a bike ride or a walk can involve stops along the way.

Janice: Well, that's good because we definitely stop a lot!

CHW: When we started talking about physical activity, it seemed like you felt a bit. . . [CHW pauses]

Janice: Depressed.

CHW: How do you feel about it now?

Janice: This is not how I thought it would go. I thought you'd be trying to get me into some spandex and to go back to the Y. [laughs] So I feel relieved and . . . I think I feel more positive about the whole thing. If I start just adding some things on the weekend, things that I can do with my family, that feels more like fun.

CHW: I look forward to hearing how it goes, Janice.

Please watch the following video that shows CHW supporting a client to enhance his level of physical activity and to improve his diet.

- *What did the CHW do well in terms of supporting the client to make changes to his diet and level of physical activity?*
- *What else would you do (or do differently) if you were the CHW working with this client?*

ACTION PLANNING AND EXERCISE: (*Source:* Foundations for Community Health Workers/http://youtu.be/ x9kt4EusdwA)

CHW Profile

Fadumo Jama, she/her

Community Health Worker

Somali Family Service, San Diego

Refugee and Immigrant Communities

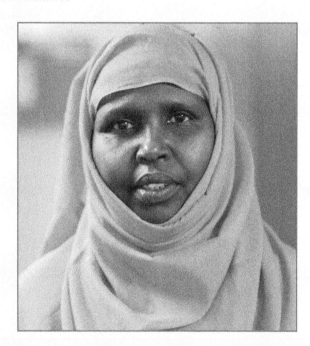

I am a refugee myself. I know what it feels like to come to a new country, being discounted and not speaking the language. When I came to the United States from Somalia, I started from the ground up. I went to school, learned English and started working while raising seven children. My motivation to work as a CHW is to give back to the community. I've been working as a CHW with Somali Family Service of San Diego (SFS) for 12 years.

SFS has been addressing the critical needs of refugees, immigrants, and underserved communities living in San Diego County for the last 22 years with programs that include Health and Wellness, Youth, Microenterprise, and Workforce Development Program. Our clients speak more than 75 languages. Our doors are open for everyone who needs assistance—we never turn anyone away. Refugees face a lot of challenges including the barrier of language, transportation, housing, and becoming citizens.

(continues)

CHW Profile

(continued)

The people in my community call me Google because I find information for them and connect them with resources. I take them to the welfare office and advocate for them. I help them get benefits like CalFresh (Food Stamps), Supplemental Security Income (SSI), and In-Home Supportive Services (IHSS). I enroll them in English as a Second Language (ESL) classes and help them apply for citizenship.

For our program for seniors, I teach them how to use gas stoves, how to use phones to call their families, and how to dial 911. I take them to doctor, fill out applications for benefits, and provide health education. I got training from the county and facilitated a six-week health education workshop called Healthy Living that included important health issues for seniors like depression and mental health.

I love my job as it enables me to make a positive impact in people's lives. I want to share the story of a woman who came into my office. I helped her get a doctor's appointment and join an ESL class. One morning she asked to talk with me. I made her some coffee. She told me her daughter was abusing her and she doesn't feel safe in her home. She had Section 8 housing, so I wrote a letter to Section 8, and her daughter had to move out. Nobody should suffer that kind of abuse. I helped her get in-home support services. Yesterday she drove her home after her eye surgery. She is doing well now: she is able to live independently. I feel so good for being able to help her.

Being a CHW has changed my life. In my culture, you don't to go to the doctor unless you are very sick. It's a shame to have cancer or a mental health issue—people hide it. I worked with a group of women, who believed that mammogram machine gives you cancer. So, I made an appointment for all of us at clinic and told them that I will be the first one to get a mammogram. After I went first, the others felt comfortable. At one of our workshops, a woman spoke out to share that she is a cancer survivor because it was caught early.

I would tell new CHWs that one of the most important things is cultural humility and awareness. That is why CHWs are mostly hired from inside the community. For refugee communities, what is seen as normal in America is not normal for them. People don't trust you if you don't respect their culture. They don't open up and share their problems with you. And if you tell a client you are going to do something, Do It. If you don't, they are going to stop trusting you.

Chapter Review

Review the chapter, including the Client Scenario about Janice Sanders. Based on what you have studied and learned so far, do your best to answer the following questions:

Food and Health

- How does our diet (what we eat and drink) influence our health?
- What are general guidelines for a healthier diet?
  - What can people eat and drink less of to promote their health?
  - What can people eat and drink more of to promote their health?
- What types of factors get in the way or make it difficult for people to eat a healthier diet?

- How do culture and family influence what people eat and drink?
- What challenges does Janice Sanders face in terms of healthy eating?
- Identify three ways that Janice might be able to change her diet to improve her health (what changes could she make to what she eats and drinks)?
- What guidelines will you keep in mind as you work to support clients to change what they eat and drink?

Weight and Health

- How effective is dieting in terms of sustained weight loss and improvements to health?
- How does repeated dieting or weight-cycling impact people's health?
- What are the key principles of a weight-inclusive approach to health promotion?
- How do issues of weight and body image affect Janice Sanders?
- What messages would you want to share with Janice Sanders about weight and health?

Physical Activity and Health

- How does physical activity improve health?
- What types of physical activities are beneficial to health?
- What challenges or barriers does Janice Sanders face in terms of physical activity?
- What strategies might you use in working with a client to increase their level of physical activity?
- How might you apply person-centered concepts and skills to working with Janice or another client to increase levels of physical activity?

References

The Association for Size Diversity and Health. (2013). HAES Matters: Exercise and HAES Model (Part 2). [Blog]. http://healthateverysizeblog.org/2013/01/15/haes-matters-exercise-and-the-haes-model-part-2/ (accessed 9 November 2022).

The Association for Size, Diversity and Health. (2022). Health at Every Size (HAES) Principles. https://asdah. org/health-at-every-size-haes-approach/ (accessed 9 November 2022).

Bégin, C., Carbonneau, E., Gagnon-Girouard, M-P., Mongeau, L., Paquette, M-C., Turcott, M., & Provencher, V. (2019). Eating-related and psychological outcomes of health at every size intervention in health and social services centers across the province of Québec. *American Journal of Health Promotion*, 33(2), 248–258. https://doi:10.1177/0890117118786326.

Blom, V., Drake, E., Kallings, L. V., Ekblom, M. M., & Nooijen, C. F. J. (2021). The effects on self-efficacy, motivation and perceived barriers of an intervention targeting physical activity and sedentary behaviours in office workers: A cluster randomized control trial. *BMC Public Health*, 21, 1048. https://doi.org/10.1186/s12889-021-11083-2.

The Body Positive. (2013). Practice Intuitive Self-care. https://thebodypositive.org/model.html (accessed 9 November 2022).

Brownell, K. D., & Rodin, J. (1994). The dieting maelstrom. Is it possible and advisable to lose weight? *American Psychologist*, 49(9), 781–791. https://DOI: 10.1037//0003-066x.49.9.781.

Byun, S. S, Bello, N. A, Liao, M., Makarem, N., & Aggarwal, B. (2019). Associations of weight cycling with cardiovascular health using American Heart Association's Life's Simple 7 in a diverse sample of women. *Preventive Medicine Reports*, 2(16), 100991. https://doi: 10.1016/j.pmedr.2019.100991.

Carlson, S. Llobrera, J., & Keith-Jennings, B. (2021). More Adequate SNAP Benefits Would Help Millions of Participants Better Afford Food. Center on Budget and Policy Priorities. https://www.cbpp.org/research/food-assistance/more-adequate-snap-benefits-would-help-millions-of-participants-better (accessed 9 November 2022).

Centers for Disease Control and Prevention. (2022). Body Mass Index (BMI). https://www.cdc.gov/healthyweight/assessing/bmi/index.html (accessed 9 November 2022).

Dopelt, K., Radon, P., & Davidovitch, N. (2019). Environmental effects of the livestock industry: The relationship between knowledge, attitudes, and behavior among students in Israel. *International Journal of Environmental Research and Public Health*, 16(8), 1359. https://doi: 10.3390/ijerph16081359.

Downer, S., Berkowitz, S. A., Harlan, T. S., Olstad, D. L., & Mozaffarian, D. (2020). Food is medicine: Actions to integrate food and nutrition into healthcare. *BMJ*, 369, m2482. https://doi:10.1136/bmj.m2482.

Field, A. E., Manson, J. E., Taylor, C. B., Willett, W. C., & Colditz, G. A. (2004). Association of weight change, weight control practices, and weight cycling among women in the Nurses' Health Study II. *International Journal of Obesity and Related Metabolic Disorders*, 28(9), 1134–1142. https://DOI: 10.1038/sj.ijo.0802728.

Food as Medicine Coalition. (2022). http://www.fimcoalition.org/ (accessed 9 November 2022).

Food as Medicine Collaborative. (2022). https://www.foodasmedicinecollaborative.org/ (accessed 9 November 2022).

Food Research & Action Center. (2021). Hunger Quick Facts for 2020. https://frac.org/hunger-poverty-america (accessed 9 November 2022).

Garcia, M., Ribeiro, S., Germani, A., & Bógus, C. (2018). The impact of urban gardens on adequate and healthy food: A systematic review. *Public Health Nutrition*, 21(2), 416–425. https://doi:10.1017/S1368980017002944.

Ge, L., Sadeghirad, B., Ball, G. et al. (2020). Comparison of dietary macronutrient patterns of 14 popular named dietary programmes for weight and cardiovascular risk factor reduction in adults: Systematic review and network meta-analysis of randomised trials. *The BMJ*, 369, m696. https://DOI: 10.1136/bmj.m696.

Giles, C. (2021). Food Guidelines Change but Fail to Take Cultures Into Account. Kaiser Health News. https://khn.org/news/article/food-guidelines-change-but-fail-to-take-cultures-into-account/ (accessed 9 November 2022).

Gregis, A., Ghisalberti, C., Sciascia, S., Sottile, F., & Peano, C. (2021). Community garden initiatives addressing health and well-being outcomes: A systematic review of infodemiology aspects, outcomes, and target populations. *International Journal of Environmental Research and Public Health*, 18(4), 1943. https://doi.org/10.3390/ijerph18041943.

Gustin, G. (2019). As Beef Comes Under Fire for Climate Impacts, the Industry Fights Back. Inside Climate News. https://insideclimatenews.org/news/21102019/climate-change-meat-beef-dairy-methane-emissions-california/#:~:text=Emissions%20from%20livestock%20account%20for,for%20grazing%20and%20feed%20crops. (accessed 9 November 2022).

Hall, K. D., & Kahan, S. (2018). Maintenance of lost weight and long-term management of obesity. *Medical Clinics of North America*, 102(1), 183–197. https://doi: 10.1016/j.mcna.2017.08.012.

Hall, L. & Nchako, C. (2022). A Closer Look at Who Benefits from SNAP: State-by-State Fact Sheets. Center on Budget and Policy Priorities. https://www.cbpp.org/research/food-assistance/a-closer-look-at-who-benefits-from-snap-state-by-state-fact-sheets#Alabama (accessed 9 November 2022).

Hunger, J. M., Smith, J. P., & Tomiyama, A. J. (2020). An evidence-based rationale for adopting weight-inclusive health policy. Social issues and policy. *Social Issues and Policy Review*, 14(1). https://spssi.onlinelibrary.wiley.com/doi/abs/10.1111/sipr.12062 (accessed 9 November 2022).

Institute for Family Health. (2022). Healthy Plates Around the World. https://institute.org/health-care/services/diabetes-care/healthyplates/ (accessed 9 November 2022).

Jacobs, A. (2020). Scientific Panel on New Dietary Guidelines Draws Criticism from Health Advocates. *New York Times*. https://www.nytimes.com/2020/06/17/health/diet-nutrition-guidelines.html (accessed 9 November 2022).

Lee, K. M., Hunger, J. M., Tomiyama, A. J. (2021). Weight stigma and health behaviors: Evidence from the Eating in America Study. *International Journal of Obesity.* https://www.ncbi.nlm.nih.gov/pmc/articles/PMC8236399/ (accessed 9 November 2022).

Lowe, M. R., Doshi, S. D., Katterman, S. N., Feig, E. H. (2013). Dieting and restrained eating as prospective predictors of weight gain. *Frontiers in Psychology*, 4, 577. https://doi: 10.3389/fpsyg.2013.00577.

Lynch, H., Johnston, C., & Wharton, C. (2018). Plant-based diets: Considerations for environmental impact, protein quality, and exercise performance. *Nutrients*, 10(12), 1841. https://doi.org/10.3390/nu10121841.

Marketdata LLC. (2022). The U.S. Weight Loss Market: 2022 Status Report & Forecast. https://www.marketresearch.com/Marketdata-Enterprises-Inc-v416/Weight-Loss-Status-Forecast-30974038/?progid=91794 (accessed 9 November 2022).

Martins, V. J., Toledo Florêncio, T. M., Grillo, L. P., do Carmo P, Franco, M., Sawaya, A. L. (2011). Long-lasting effects of undernutrition. *International Journal of Environmental Research and Public Health*, 8(6), 1817–1846. https://doi.org/10.3390/ijerph8061817.

MHP Salud. (2022). Adding Better Nutrition to Cultural Dishes Doesn't Have to Be a Challenge (CHWs Know How). https://mhpsalud.org/adding-better-nutrition-to-cultural-dishes-doesnt-have-to-be-a-challenge-chws-know-how/ (accessed 9 November 2022).

Moss, M. (2021). *Hooked: Food, free will, and how the food giants exploit our addictions.* New York: Random House.

Mulik, K. & Haynes-Maslow, L. (2017). The Affordability of MyPlate: An analysis of SNAP benefits and the actual cost of eating according to the dietary guidelines. *Journal of Nutrition Education and Behavior*, 49(8), 623. https://doi: 10.1016/j.jneb.2017.06.005.

National Center on Health, Physical Activity and Disability (NCHPAD). (2022). How I Walk: A Campaign to Rebrand the Word Walking. https://www.nchpad.org/howiwalk/ (accessed 9 November 2022).

National Institute on Aging. (2020). Maintaining Mobility and Preventing Disability are Key to Living Independently as We Age. https://www.nia.nih.gov/news/maintaining-mobility-and-preventing-disability-are-key-living-independently-we-age (accessed 9 November 2022).

National Institutes of Health. (2022). Delicious Recipes for Heart Healthy Eating. National Heart, Lung and Blood Institute. https://www.nhlbi.nih.gov/health/healthdisp/recipes.htm (accessed 9 November 2022).

No Kid Hungry. (2023). How Many Kids in the United States Live with Hunger? https://www.nokidhungry.org/blog/how-many-kids-united-states-live-hunger (accessed 23 December 2023).

Nutrition Coalition. (2020). 2020-2025 Dietary Guidelines Not Applicable for Majority of Americans; Not Scoped for 60% of U.S. With at Least One Diet-Related Chronic Disease. https://www.nutritioncoalition.us/news/2020-2025-dietary-guidelines-final-release (accessed 9 November 2022).

The Nutrition Source. (2023a). Harvard University School of Public Health. https://www.hsph.harvard.edu/nutritionsource/ (accessed 27 May 2023).

The Nutrition Source. (2023b). The Healthy Eating Plate. https://www.hsph.harvard.edu/nutritionsource/healthy-eating-plate/ Harvard University School of Public Health (accessed 27 May 2023).

The Nutrition Source. (2023c). *Understanding food labels.* Harvard University School of Public Health. https://www.hsph.harvard.edu/nutritionsource/food-label-guide/ (accessed 27 May 2023).

Palar, K., Lemus Hufstedler, E., Hernandez, K., Chang, A., Ferguson, L., Lozano, R., & Weiser, S. D. (2019). Nutrition and health improvements after participation in an urban home garden program. *Journal of Nutrition Education and Behavior*, 51(9), 1037–1046. https://doi.org/10.1016/j.jneb.2019.06.028.

Parekh, N., Ali, S. H., O'Connor, J., Tozan, Y., Jones, A. M., Capasso, A., Foreman, J., & DiClemente, R. J. (2021). Food insecurity among households with children during the COVID-19 pandemic: Results from a study among social media users across the United States. *Nutrition Journal*, 20, 73. https://doi.org/10.1186/s12937-021-00732-2.

PolicyLink. (2022). Equitable Food Systems Resource Guide. https://www.policylink.org/food-systems/equitable-food-systems-resource-guide (accessed 9 November 2022).

Rhee, E., Cho, J., Kwon, H., Park, S.E., Park C., Oh, K., Park, S., & Lee, W. (2018). Increased risk of diabetes development in individuals with weight cycling over 4 years: The Kangbuk Samsung Health Study. *Diabetes Research and Clinical Practice*, 139, 230–238. https://doi.org/10.1016/j.diabres.2018.03.018.

Rhone, A., Ver Ploeg, M., Dicken, C., Williams, R., & Breneman, V. (2017). Low-Income and Low-Supermarket-Access Census Tracts, 2010-2015. U.S. Department of Agriculture, Economic Research Service. https://www.ers.usda.gov/webdocs/publications/82101/eib-165.pdf?v=0 (accessed 9 November 2022).

Ritchie, H. (2019). Half the World's Habitable Land is Used for Agriculture. Our World in Data. https://ourworldindata.org/global-land-for-agriculture (accessed 9 November 2022).

Ritchie, H. (2021). Cutting Down Forests: What Are the Drivers of Deforestation? Our World in Data. https://ourworldindata.org/what-are-drivers-deforestation (accessed 9 November 2022).

Rzehak, P., Meisinger, C., Woelke, G., Brasche, S. Strube, G., & Heinrich, J. (2007). Weight change, weight cycling and mortality in the ERFORT Male Cohort Study. *European Journal of Epidemiology*, 22, 665–673. https://DOI: 10.1007/s10654-007-9167-5.

Sherrell, Z. (2021). What is Weight Discrimination? Medical News Today. https://www.medicalnewstoday.com/articles/obesity-discrimination-in-healthcare#summary (accessed 9 November 2022).

Shrider, E., Kollar, M., Chen, F., & Semega, J. (2021). *Income and poverty in the United States: 2020*. Census Bureau: Current Population Reports. U.S. https://www.census.gov/library/publications/2021/demo/p60-273.html (accessed 9 November 2022).

Siahpush, M., Tibbits, M., Shaikh, R. A., Singh, G. K., Sikora Kessler, A., & Huang, T. T. (2015). Dieting increases the likelihood of subsequent obesity and BMI gain: Results from a prospective study of an Australian national sample. *International Journal of Behavioral Medicine*, 22(5), 662–671. https://doi:10.1007/s12529-015-9463-5. PMID: 25608460.

Tylka, T. L., Annunziato, R. A., Burgard, D., Danielsdottir, S., Shuman, E., & Davis, C. (2014). The weight-inclusive versus weight-normative approach to health: Evaluating the evidence for prioritizing well-being over weight loss. *Journal of Obesity*, 1. https://doi:10.1155/2014/983495.

Ulian, M. D., Pinto A. J., de Morais Sato, P., Benatti, F. B, Lopes de Campos-Ferraz, P. Coelho, D., Roble, O. J., et al. (2018). Effects of a new intervention based on the Health at Every Size approach for the management of obesity: The "Health and Wellness in Obesity" study. *PLoS One*, 13(7), e0198401. https://doi: 10.1371/journal.pone.0198401.

U.S. Department of Health and Human Services. (2018). Physical Activity Guidelines for Americans, 2nd Edition. https://health.gov/our-work/nutrition-physical-activity/physical-activity-guidelines/current-guidelines (accessed 27 May 2023).

U.S. Food & Drug Administration. (2020). Quick Tips for Reading the Nutrition Facts Label. https://www.fda.gov/media/131162/download (accessed 27 May 2023).

U.S. Food & Drug Administration. (2023a). Changes to the Nutrition Facts Label. https://www.fda.gov/food/food-labeling-nutrition/changes-nutrition-facts-label (accessed 27 December 2023).

U.S. Food & Drug Administration. (2023b). How to Understand and Use the Nutrition Facts Label. https://www.fda.gov/food/new-nutrition-facts-label/how-understand-and-use-nutrition-facts-label (accessed 9 November 2022).

World Health Organization. (2021a). Malnutrition. https://www.who.int/news-room/fact-sheets/detail/malnutrition (accessed 9 November 2022).

World Health Organization. (2021b). The State of Food Security and Nutrition in the World, 2021: Transforming Food Systems for Food Security, Improved Nutrition and Affordable Healthy Diets for All. https://www.who.int/publications/m/item/the-state-of-food-security-and-nutrition-in-the-world-2021 (accessed 9 November 2022).

Yu, A. (2022). *The unspoken weight-discrimination problem at work.* Equality Matters: British Broadcasting Corporation (BBC). https://www.bbc.com/worklife/article/20220411-the-unspoken-weight-discrimination-problem-at-work (accessed 9 November 2022).

Additional Resources

Brown, S. (2019). How Livestock Farming Affects the Environment. DownToEarth. https://www.downtoearth.org.in/factsheet/how-livestock-farming-affects-the-environment-64218 (accessed 9 November 2022).

California Mobility. 21 Chair Exercises for Seniors: A Comprehensive Visual Guide. https://californiamobility.com/21-chair-exercises-for-seniors-visual-guide/ (accessed 9 November 2022).

Centers for Disease Control and Prevention. (2022). Making Physical Activity a Part of an Older Adult's Life. https://www.cdc.gov/physicalactivity/basics/adding-pa/activities-olderadults.htm (accessed 9 November 2022).

Food and Agriculture Organization of the United Nations (FAO). https://www.fao.org/home/en (accessed 9 November 2022).

Food and Agriculture Organization of the United Nations. (2022). Tackling Climate Change Through Livestock: Key Facts and Findings. https://www.fao.org/news/story/en/item/197623/icode/ (accessed 9 November 2022).

Food Research & Action Center. https://frac.org/ (accessed 9 November 2022).

Grossi, G., Goglio, P., Vitali, A., & Williams, A. G. (2019). Livestock and climate change: Impact of livestock on climate and mitigation strategies. *Animal Frontiers*, 9(1), https://doi.org/10.1093/af/vfy034.

Lindberg, S. (2020). Chair Exercises for Seniors. Healthline. https://www.healthline.com/health/chair-exercises-for-seniors (accessed 9 November 2022).

National Center on Health, Physical Activity and Disability (NCHPAD). https://www.nchpad.org/ (accessed 9 November 2022).

National Institute on Aging. (2020). How Older Adults Can Get Started with Exercise. https://www.nia.nih.gov/health/how-older-adults-can-get-started-exercise (accessed 9 November 2022).

Partnership for a Healthier America. Food Equity. https://www.ahealthieramerica.org/articles/food-equity-868 (accessed 9 November 2022).

Robinson, L. Segal, J. (2022). How to Exercise with Limited Mobility. HelpGuide. https://www.helpguide.org/articles/healthy-living/chair-exercises-and-limited-mobility-fitness.htm (accessed 9 November 2022).

Science Direct. Nutrition Policy. https://www.sciencedirect.com/topics/food-science/nutrition-policy (accessed 9 November 2022).

Supporting Survivors of Trauma

18

Tim Berthold

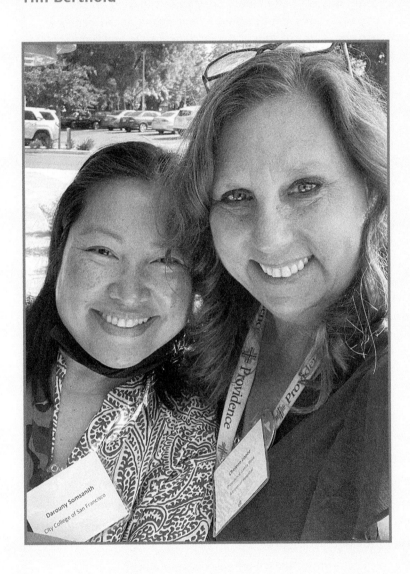

Foundations for Community Health Workers, Third Edition. Edited by Tim Berthold and Darouny Somsanith.
© 2024 John Wiley & Sons, Inc. Published 2024 by John Wiley & Sons, Inc.
Companion website: http://www.wiley.com/go/communityhealthworkers3E

Client Scenario: Tony Hernandez

You are a CHW at a neighborhood health center. You have worked with Tony Hernandez and his father in the past, helping to manage Tony's asthma. Because his asthma has been well-controlled for some time, you haven't seen Tony in several years.

Tony Hernandez is now 20 years old. He calls the clinic and asks for an appointment with you.

Tony tells you that two months ago, his friend Leroy was shot and killed. They were standing on the street a few houses down from Tony's house. Tony says, *"One minute we were hanging out, then I went to my dad's house to go to the bathroom. I heard the 'pop pop' sound of guns. If you live where I live, you know that sound. When I came out, people were screaming and there was all this blood and . . . Leroy was dying. He looked at me."*

Tony tells you he isn't sure what to do. His father is so busy working that they hardly see each other. *"My dad, he told me to just put it behind me and like, stand strong and get on with my studies. He's so focused on me being the first one in the family to graduate college. But I can't stop thinking about what happened to Leroy, and I just. . . I need to figure this out. It's like this war is happening around me and I don't know what to do."*

Tony has been too scared to stay at home. He's staying with an ex-girlfriend's family across town. *"They're cool, but I can't stay there forever."*

Tony hasn't been sleeping much and is having bad dreams. *"I went to the funeral, but I just didn't know what to say to Leroy's family. I just kept thinking about Leroy dying and that maybe if I hadn't gone into the house, I could have said something, and he'd still be alive. I can't stop replaying it over and over in my mind and thinking that I should have done something."*

Tony is taking classes at a local community college. He is doing well in his Psychology class. *"The professor, he's okay. The stuff he teaches is like . . . it's just more real life than my other subjects. But I haven't gone to my other classes. I don't know what to do because if I drop out, they'll cancel my financial aid and my dad will freak out. I don't want to fail, but I don't really care about anything right now because this is the third person killed in my neighborhood this year, and my second friend who died from bullets."*

If you were a CHW and Tony Hernandez was your client, how might you answer the following questions?

- How might Tony's exposure to trauma affect his health and his life?
- When Tony first tells you about his trauma experience, how will you respond? What will you say?
- How can you support Tony in his recovery from trauma? What concepts and skills will guide your work?
- What is the proper role and scope of practice for a CHW who is working with a survivor of trauma? When and how will you provide a referral to another provider?
- What resources exist for survivors of trauma in the communities where you live and work?
- How are you (and other helping professionals) affected by working closely with survivors of trauma?
- What can you do to practice self-care and enhance your resilience for working with survivors of trauma?

Introduction

Because trauma is so common—over half of Americans have been exposed to one or more traumatic events—Community Health Workers are likely to work with survivors of trauma.

Social support—or the lack of it—is one of the most important factors that influences how a person responds after experiencing trauma. CHWs are an important part of providing support and linking vulnerable individuals and communities to additional sources of help.

The goal for this chapter is to better prepare you for the moment when a client tells you about their trauma experience or asks for help in addressing their traumatic stress. How you respond in these moments can have a significant impact on the client and their healing or recovery.

While CHWs and other nonlicensed helping professionals frequently assist survivors of trauma, this work raises questions about scope of practice (SOP) (defined in Chapter 5). It is clearly outside of a CHW's SOP to provide therapy, and it is clearly within a CHW's SOP to apply person-centered skills to listen with compassion to a client's story and provide a relevant referral. Between these two ends of the spectrum, however, are situations that raise questions about the role and SOP of CHWs. We address questions of SOP more fully in Section 18.6.

WHAT YOU WILL LEARN

By studying the information in this chapter, you will be able to:

- Define trauma and post-traumatic stress
- Discuss how common exposure to trauma is
- Identify common responses to trauma (symptoms and effects)
- Discuss a variety of strategies for healing from trauma
- Analyze the CHW scope of practice when working with survivors of trauma and when and how to provide referrals
- Explain and demonstrate key skills for working with survivors of trauma
- Discuss secondary trauma and resilience and strategies for self-care

C3 Roles and Skills Addressed in Chapter 18

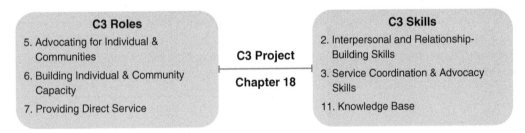

C3 Roles

5. Advocating for Individual & Communities
6. Building Individual & Community Capacity
7. Providing Direct Service

C3 Project

Chapter 18

C3 Skills

2. Interpersonal and Relationship-Building Skills
3. Service Coordination & Advocacy Skills
11. Knowledge Base

WORDS TO KNOW

Historical Trauma

Secondary Trauma

Secondary Resilience

Somatic

Trauma-informed Care

Preparing to Address the Topic of Trauma

Trauma can be a difficult topic to address. To prepare CHWs for their work with survivors of trauma, we talk openly and explicitly about traumatic events such as rape and war, and how they affect us. We do this with the intention of better preparing you to work effectively with clients when they tell you about a trauma experience.

(continues)

Preparing to Address the Topic of Trauma

(continued)

Whenever we teach about trauma, regardless of the audience, we assume that some of the participants are survivors. We assume that others know someone close to them—a family member or a friend—who is a survivor of trauma. We assume that some of you who are reading this chapter are also survivors of trauma. Please know that you are not alone.

Do your best to stay present as you read this chapter, just as you must do when listening to a survivor.

At the same time, don't forget to take care of yourself along the way. Pay attention to thoughts and feelings that may arise. Draw upon the skills and techniques that you have already learned. When something happens that stirs up strong emotions, what do you do to stay grounded and present? This may include deep breathing, taking a short break, or drawing upon spiritual or religious practices. Over the course of this training, you will be supported to enhance your knowledge and skills related to self-care (see Chapter 12).

If you are a survivor of trauma, we hope that the information provided in this chapter supports your health and healing. It is also possible that studying this material, and working directly with clients who are survivors, may re-stimulate memories of your own trauma stories and trauma responses. Your challenge is to develop skills for putting your own story aside when you are working with clients, so that you don't unintentionally impose your own assumptions, beliefs, or values. Clients require you to be fully present to focus on their needs. After your work is done, it can be helpful to revisit your personal memories or stories of trauma, as part of your own path for healing or recovery. You may find time to address your experiences during meetings with a clinical supervisor or on your time, by yourself or with the help of family, community, or professionals.

While the topic of trauma can be difficult to study, it also brings tremendous hope. The efforts of people who have faced and survived terrible experiences are inspiring. Witnessing the healing of survivors will bring you face to face with extraordinary people and the opportunity to enhance your own resilience to face the difficult moments that inevitably arise in everyone's life.

Faith Fabiani: Most of us get into this line of work because we or someone we are close to have been impacted by trauma. Even with the best intentions, it's imperative that you work on your own trauma first or inadvertently you may create more harm. No matter how similar your story is, it's important to remember we all experience trauma differently. It's not about you. As harsh as this sounds, it is a principle to live by when working with other survivors.

- *What are your thoughts and feelings about working with clients and communities who have experienced trauma?*

- *How can you practice self-care as you study this chapter and prepare to work with clients who are survivors of trauma?*

CHW Profile

Faith Laterza Fabiani, She/Her

Training Associate, West Coast Children's Clinic

Commercial Sexual Exploitation of Children Department

Training Providers working with At-Risk and System-Involved Foster Youth

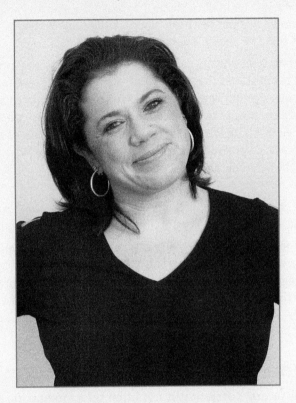

I was motivated to become a CHW based on my lived experience. I am a survivor of sexual and physical trauma, homelessness, and incarceration. The resources presented to me at the time were better in theory than reality. After seeing so many other people struggling around me, I wanted to provide realistic solutions for my community.

I work for Westcoast Children's Clinic (WCC), a large nonprofit that provides direct mental health services for at-risk youth, research and evaluation, training, and advocacy. We have contracts to provide trainings throughout the United States for anyone who works with at-risk youth including professionals working in areas such as foster care, juvenile justice, probation, and parole.

I work in the training department that addresses commercial sexual exploitation of children. I facilitate 16-hour trainings about how trauma affects our youth. The trainings encourage providers to view youth from a different perspective, not just a trauma-informed lens but also a health equity lens. Some providers look only at the individual behaviors or choices of youth who end up in the juvenile justice or foster care systems. We help them to develop a broader perspective about the social determinants that influence the health of youth WHO have experienced trauma.

(continues)

CHW Profile

(continued)

I used to provide direct services and I worked with client who had fallen through the cracks in the systems. She was released from juvenile hall to no one. She was out on the streets with an ankle bracelet, and the court expected her to check in with five different providers each day while she was homeless, trying to survive and to charge her ankle bracelet. She had an impossible task because the system was set up to fail her. I accompanied her to court, and she would just put her head down on the table while the adults were talking about her—not to her—using terms that she couldn't understand.

As a trainer, I always think of that client and my community. I bring their stories into trainings because I want providers to really think about the obstacles that youth face that they might take for granted. Like, what is it like to be dope dependent and unhoused and trying to get across town for a mandated appointment when you don't have money for the bus? The clients they work with are more than a diagnosis or a case number. They need to get to know the person, not their labels. In the trainings we do a lot of case studies and small group discussions, and we ask providers how they would work with a client. How will they listen? What will they say? How will they build rapport? And it's beautiful when they are honest about how hard their work is, and I can see that they are learning to approach their work differently with transparency, creativity, and more respect for the youth.

I have never forgotten where I came from. I appreciate how far I've come, but I'm constantly considering what solutions I can bring that best serve the community. This is my main purpose, my main drive.

Don't forget why you started doing this work in the first place, and don't lose yourself trying to please other people. Any education you have is just a bonus, but you still need to be able to connect with your community and be authentic. It took me a long time to find a job that I love where they allow me to be my authentic self. It may take you while to find the right job too, but just keep trucking until you find it.

18.1 Defining Trauma and Post-traumatic Stress

Trauma is a term that is used in several different ways. It often refers to horrific events, such as child abuse and neglect, domestic violence, war, torture, and incarceration. It can also refer to physical injuries—broken bones or burns that are treated in a "trauma unit" in a hospital. In this chapter, we are most concerned with a third meaning of trauma—the thoughts, feelings, and behaviors we experience as a response to traumatic events, whether or not those events resulted in physical injuries.

According to the American Psychological Association:

> *Trauma is an emotional response to a terrible event like an accident, rape, or natural disaster. Immediately after the event, shock, and denial are typical. Longer-term reactions include unpredictable emotions, flashbacks, strained relationships, and even physical symptoms like headaches or nausea. While these feelings are normal, some people have difficulty moving on with their lives. (American Psychological Association, 2023)*

Trauma affects us in many ways—physically, emotionally, spiritually, communally. Trauma experiences are typically characterized by:

- Bodily harm or the threat of bodily harm
- Loss of control
- Threat or fear of annihilation (death—one's own or that of a loved one—or even of a group one belongs to, such as in the case of genocide)
- Intense fear or horror
- Helplessness
- Rupture or loss of meaningful social relationships

Even if a person affected by a traumatic event does not experience overwhelming fear or helplessness during the event, the severity of the event itself can generate a post-traumatic stress reaction.

Responses to traumatic events vary considerably. In the immediate aftermath of a traumatic event, most people experience a trauma response, along with normal grieving or other reactions. For some people, that response will diminish or disappear over time, especially if they receive meaningful social support and the traumatic event is not ongoing or chronic. Other people experience symptoms of trauma that may endure for months, years, or even decades. Trauma can affect every part of a person's life—their health, welfare, work, and relationships, as well as their sense of emotional well-being.

Keep in mind that how people experience, respond to, and are affected by events is often highly subjective or individual. In other words, people who experience the same event can be affected in quite different ways. After an earthquake, for example, one person might bounce back quickly from the initial fright and begin rebuilding with optimism, while another person may not be able to stop thinking about the disaster, and as a result, feel a persistent sense of danger and instability months after the earthquake.

IDENTIFYING TRAUMATIC EVENTS

A *partial* list of events that may be classified as traumatic includes:

- Child abuse and neglect
- Sexual assault
- The death of a loved one, especially if it is sudden, unexpected, or violent
- High levels of neighborhood violence, including shootings, killings, and threats
- Domestic violence, including physical, verbal, and emotional abuse
- Incarceration
- Sudden unexplained separation from a loved one
- State-sponsored violence including, for example, police brutality/assault, terrorism, armed conflict, or war
- Racism and other types of prejudice and discrimination
- Torture
- Natural disasters such as earthquakes, tsunamis, and hurricanes
- Accidents such as fires and car crashes

- *What types of trauma are most common in the communities where you live and work?*

What Do
YOU?
Think

HOW COMMON IS EXPOSURE TO TRAUMA?

Unfortunately, exposure to traumatic events is very common, and much more common than many people think. Judith Herman, a physician and the author, writes:

> *"It was once believed that such events were uncommon. In 1980, when post-traumatic stress disorder was first included in the diagnostic manual, the American Psychiatric Association described traumatic events as" outside the range of usual human experience. "Sadly, this definition has proved to be inaccurate. Rape, battery, and other forms of sexual and domestic violence are so common a part of women's lives that they can hardly be described as outside the range of ordinary experience. And in the view of the number of people killed in war over the past century, military trauma, too, must be considered a common part of the human experience; only the fortunate find it unusual" (Herman, 1997, p. 33).*

It is challenging to research and document how often people are exposed to trauma. In general, rape, child abuse, and other acts of violence are under-reported due to factors that include fear of retaliation or alienation (loss of family or friends), distrust of the police and/or criminal justice system, shame, self-blame, and stigma. Nations often have a compelling self-interest to distort the reporting of traumatic events such as war-related injuries and deaths.

The National Center for Post-Traumatic Stress Disorder or PTSD estimates that approximately 60% of men and 50% of women in the United States experience one or more traumatic event over the course of their lifetime (The National Center for PTSD, 2023c). Some studies estimate exposure to traumatic events is even higher. The National Council for Behavioral Health estimates that 70% of adults—or approximately 223 million people—in the United States have experienced some type of trauma (NCBH, 2023). They estimate that 90% of clients seeking public behavioral health or mental health services have experienced trauma (Ibid).

Exposure to traumatic events is extremely common among U.S. combat veterans. These events include being shot at, seeing dead bodies, receiving rocket or mortar fire, and knowing someone who was seriously injured or killed is highly common. It is estimated that 95% of army veterans in the Iraq war saw dead bodies and 93% experienced being shot at (National Center for PTSD, 2023a). A study of veterans of the Iran-Iraq war estimated that 27.8% had experienced PTSD (Barzoki et al., 2021). An analysis of multiple studies of civilian communities exposed to war and armed conflict indicates that over 23% experienced PTSD (Lim et al., 2022).

Exposure to trauma and resulting traumatic stress is also common among children and youth. The national Substance Abuse and Mental Health Services Administration estimated that "more than two thirds of children reported at least 1 traumatic event by age 16" (SAMHSA, 2022). Each year, approximately 14% of children experience child abuse or neglect (Ibid) and Child Protection Services receives approximately 3 million reports of abuse (National Center for PTSD, 2023b). Approximately 3–10 million children witness family violence each year (Ibid) and 33% of youth who are exposed to community violence experience post-traumatic stress disorder (National Council for Behavioral Health, 2023). The National Council for Behavior Health states, "Nearly all children who witness a parental homicide or sexual assault will develop Post Traumatic Stress Disorder. Similarly, 90% of sexually abused children, 77% of children exposed to a school shooting and 35% of urban youth exposed to community violence develop PTSD" (Ibid).

Studies show that people in prison experience high rates of trauma and that 30–60% of men in prison have post-traumatic stress disorder (Widra, 2020). The prevalence of PTSD among incarcerated women was estimated at 53% by a study commissioned by the Urban Institute (Ervin, Jagannath, & Zweig, 2020).

Francis Julian Montgomery: Most of the clients I work with are managing multiple traumatic experiences, including being homeless in this city [San Francisco]. It's important for me to remember that trauma is invisible most of the time. A lot of people still have a misguided belief that only veterans or women who have experienced sexual assault have trauma, but the people I work with have survived all kinds of trauma.

Trauma is common throughout the world. The World Mental Health survey was conducted by the World Health Organization in 24 countries and including data from over 68,000 people. This survey estimated that 70% of people experienced traumatic events (Benjet et al., 2016; Kessler et al., 2017). Each year, millions of people across the world are displaced and forced to move from their homes due to armed conflict, war, and related threats. The World Health Organization estimated that over 270 million people were displaced in 2019 by war, and PTSD and other mental health conditions were found to be common among these populations (WHO, 2021).

Exposure to traumatic events is not equally experienced by all populations. Some communities experience higher rates of exposure to trauma including veterans and people with a history of incarceration, LGBTQIA+ people, immigrants and refugees, communities of color, and people living in poverty. The presence or absence of resources to overcome, escape or transform the sources of trauma, and to support healing from their impacts has a significant effect on whether the symptoms of traumatic stress become chronic or not.

The Legacy of Historical Trauma

Historical or intergenerational trauma refers to the way that post-traumatic stress can be passed down across generations within communities that have faced extreme trauma such as slavery and genocide. Exposure to chronic trauma can shape coping mechanisms, parenting practices, and life expectations in lasting ways—especially when institutionalized discrimination continues, in new forms, into the present day. Dr. Joy Degruy Leary coined the term "post-traumatic slave syndrome" to describe "a condition that exists as a consequence of the multigenerational oppression of Africans and their descendants resulting from centuries of chattel slavery . . . This was then followed by institutionalized racism which continues to perpetuate injury" (DeGruy, 2023).

Historical trauma affects many communities across the world that have experienced trauma on a mass and enduring scale (American Psychiatric Association, 2021; Franco, 2021; Stanford, 2023; Stress & Trauma Evaluation and Psychological Services, 2022.).

THE LANGUAGE WE USE TO TALK ABOUT TRAUMA

There are many ways of conceptualizing trauma. There is a difference, for example, between the medical language used to diagnose trauma among survivors and the language that most people use to communicate about trauma and its consequences. Our goal is to use words and concepts that are accessible to the clients and communities you work with as a CHW.

Questions about the Term "PTSD"

Not everyone is comfortable with the term post-traumatic stress disorder (PTSD). Some survivors of traumatic events don't want to label their reactions as a "disorder" (and point out that the events they survived, rather than their reactions to these events, are where the "disorder" lies). Others live in situations of ongoing danger where the P in PTSD might stand for "persistent" instead of "post." As we discuss later in this chapter, some have argued that PTSD is a culturally specific concept that should not be applied universally to all communities. Some people describe their response to trauma in terms that are culturally or personally meaningful to them—they may not relate to the clinical language of post-traumatic stress at all.

18.2 Post-Traumatic Stress Disorder (PTSD)

While trauma has always been a part of our history, it hasn't always been acknowledged. Post-traumatic stress disorder was formally defined as a health condition in 1982 when it was included in the Diagnostic and Statistical Manual (DSM) of the American Psychiatric Association. The DSM is the basis for diagnosis and treatment of all mental health conditions in the United States and informs mental health practice globally as well (keep in mind that only a licensed medical or mental health care professional is qualified to provide a diagnosis).

Since 1982, research has resulted in revised diagnostic criteria for PTSD. Today, when licensed medical and mental health professionals assess and diagnose people with PTSD, they follow the clinical criteria from the Fifth Edition of the DSM (DSM-5) published in 2013 and the Text Revision of the Fifth Edition of the DSM (DSM-5-TR) published in 2022 (American Psychiatric Association, 2023). There are several different diagnostic categories for PTSD including, for example, one for children six years old and younger, and one for complex PTSD. For the purposes of this chapter, we will review the most commonly used diagnostic criteria for people ages seven and older. If you are interested in reading more about PTSD and its various subcategories for diagnosis, please see the references and resources included at the end of this chapter.

PTSD is diagnosed in people ages seven and older if they have been exposed to one or more traumatic events characterized by death or death threats; bodily harm or threats of bodily harm; sexual assault or threats of sexual assault. This includes people who were directly exposed to a traumatic event, such as an assault, and those who directly witnessed the trauma.

To be diagnosed with PTSD, the survivor must show symptoms in each of four different categories, and the symptoms must last for at least one month. The four categories or symptom clusters from the DSM-5-TR are: (1) intrusion symptoms [such as persistent trauma-related thoughts or dreams]; (2) avoidance [avoiding thoughts, feelings, people, places, and situations that are associated with the trauma], (3) negative alterations in cognition [thoughts] or mood [including the inability to remember key aspects of the trauma, persistent negative emotions or beliefs, and the inability to experience positive emotions, etc.], and (4) alterations in arousal and reactivity [including hypervigilance, an exaggerated startle response, problems with concentration and sleep disturbances, irritable or aggressive behavior or self-destructive behaviors].

18.3 A Common Language for Trauma Responses

Rather than trying to use the language of the DSM-5, we will use more accessible language in this chapter to talk about how trauma affects our lives. We begin by discussing how individuals may respond to trauma, using six broad categories of trauma responses. Please keep in mind that these are not comprehensive lists of all possible trauma responses and that some responses may belong in more than one category.

Exposure to trauma can have profound and lasting impacts on survivors. *Yet, how people respond to trauma is often unique. There is no formula to predict how an individual will respond to or be affected by a certain type of trauma.* Two individuals exposed to the same traumatic event may respond in very different ways. Survivors may experience some, most, all, or none of the most common responses to trauma described below. Trauma symptoms or responses may last a few months or many years and can range in terms of severity and the degree to which they harm the survivor and interfere with day-to-day life.

PHYSICAL RESPONSES

Physical responses to trauma may include:

- Anxiety, agitation, and startle responses (strong physical responses to stimuli such as sounds, sights, smells, sudden movements, being approached from behind, etc.),
- Hypervigilance, or constantly scanning the environment for possible risks or threats.
- Increased heart and respiratory rates and blood pressure, and the release of stress hormones such as cortisol and adrenaline. These biological responses prepare the body for "fight or flight" in the face of danger. When stress responses are repeated over time, such as when someone is exposed to ongoing trauma (child abuse or neglect, domestic violence, war, or torture), these same biological responses are associated with an increased risk for chronic health conditions such as heart disease.
- Changes to patterns of sleep and dreaming including difficulty sleeping, sleeping a lot, and having dreams related to trauma experiences.
  - Chronic and recurring nightmares about some element of the trauma story accompanied by strong emotions such as fear or dread.
- Chronic health conditions including heart disease, diabetes, and cancer
- Chronic pain such as headaches, stomach pain, or nausea.
  - This pain can be extreme. For some survivors, for example, it may feel as if they have had a headache that lasts for years.
- Injuries such as bruises, broken bones, burns, disabilities, and loss of sight.
  - Chronic disability such as the complete or partial loss of sight, balance, movement, speech, or paralysis.
- Pregnancy (such as the unintended pregnancy resulting from a sexual assault) and sexually transmitted infections (STIs) including HIV disease.

EMOTIONAL RESPONSES

Common emotional responses and feelings *may* include:

- Numbing or the inability to feel
- Irritability, anger, or rage

- Fear or terror
- Sadness or despair
- Self-blame and guilt (including survivor's guilt)
- Humiliation and shame
- Feeling detached

- *Can you think of other common emotional responses to trauma?*

Please note that because trauma encompasses the most extreme events that people can experience, it can provoke extreme emotions such as rage rather than anger, terror rather than fear, or despair rather than sadness. These extreme emotions can be overwhelming and difficult to manage. They may inspire survivors to seek relief, escape, or regulation, such as through the use of alcohol and drugs.

It is important to understand that some survivors are numb or devoid of feeling. This is a highly common response. It can be very confusing, however, for family, friends, and helping professionals.

Trauma and Numbness

Tim Berthold: I worked for a rape crisis center. I was sometimes called out to the local county hospital to provide accompaniment and support to a survivor of a recent sexual assault (the survivor was always asked if they wanted someone from the rape crisis center to accompany them, and if they would accept the male counselor on call, or if they would prefer a female counselor). The survivors were highly diverse and experienced a wide range of trauma responses. Numbness was common.

While I had been trained to accept numbness as one of many common responses to trauma, other helping professionals, including nurses, physicians, and the police, were sometimes confused when survivors didn't display strong emotions. They didn't understand and, in some instances, it made them doubt the survivor's experience and story. These helping professionals held assumptions about how survivors should respond, and numbness in the face of extreme violence was difficult for them to comprehend or believe. The lesson for me was about honoring the unique responses of individual survivors and the importance of pushing aside assumptions about other people's experiences.

Survivor's Guilt

Survivor's guilt can affect those who witness or survive a traumatic event in which others were harmed or killed. Survivors are left with a feeling of guilt that they survived or escaped harm or were not as deeply affected as others. Consider, for example, someone who survives a car crash in which other passengers were killed or a soldier who witnesses the death of a fellow combatant. Consider this chapter's Client Scenario and the experience of Tony Hernandez.

Tim Berthold: I volunteered briefly in Guatemala with children from Mayan communities who had been orphaned during the war. One of the boys I worked with witnessed the destruction of his village and carried with him the burden of survivor's guilt. He had been sent to the river to gather water by his mother. He was there when the helicopters arrived. He rushed back to his village and hid in some bushes as soldiers descended to torture and kill his family and neighbors. He watched as the soldiers cut the fetus from his pregnant mother before slitting her throat.

This young boy was haunted by survivor's guilt. He blamed himself for the death of his family. He told me: "If I hadn't been at the river, I would have heard the helicopters early and warned everyone to run and hide." In his mind, "If my mother had gone to fetch water, I would have been killed, and she would still be alive."

BEHAVIORAL RESPONSES

Common behavioral responses to trauma *may* include:

- Isolation and avoidance (of others, including friends and family, of work or school, or public spaces or particular types of places),
- Alcohol and drug use
  - The use of alcohol and drugs is common among survivors. One theory is that alcohol and drugs are used to alter, numb, or forget feelings or thoughts arising from the trauma. Early childhood trauma is seen by some researchers as the root cause of substance use, abuse, and addiction (International Society for Traumatic Stress Studies, 2023).
- Changes in sexual feelings, relationships, and behaviors
  - Including difficulty feeling safety, connection, or pleasure; avoidance of sexual experiences; or increased sexual activity.
- Changes in appearance (such as the way that someone dresses or presents themselves)
- Changes in diet (eating more or less, and disordered patterns of eating such as binging or anorexia)
- Frequent arguments or conflicts
- Acting out through hurting others emotionally or physically, including through retaliation
- Hurting oneself, including self-injury and suicide
- Risk-taking behaviors, such as driving too fast or engaging in unsafe sexual practices
- Re-enactment or returning to situations or locations, including dangerous situations, that are similar to the original traumatic experience

- *How else may trauma impact the behavior of survivors?*

THE IMPACT ON RELATIONSHIPS

Trauma can touch upon all aspects of life, from performance at school and work, to relationships with family and friends. Survivors may find it difficult to trust others or to tolerate intimacy and may push others away, including loved ones. They may stop going to work or school or stop performing well in these environments. They may find it difficult to feel comfortable or safe in sexual relationships, to believe that they can love others or are deserving of love themselves. Survivors may feel betrayed by family or friends (or the church or school) and act out in anger or simply disengage or abandon these relationships altogether.

In contrast, some survivors develop deeper relationships or connections with others. Some find a sense of refuge or safety at school or at work, a realm where they can exercise greater control. Some become closer to their family or friends or develop new friendships among others who have survived similar events or share common values.

COGNITIVE RESPONSES

Trauma can influence what people think about as well as how their mind functions. It can also affect the way that people think about themselves, and the future. Common trauma responses include:

- Recurring thoughts or memories about the trauma
  - Such thoughts are sometimes triggered by specific factors such as physical environments, social dynamics, objects, physical sensations, sounds, or smells.
- Lack of an ability to remember the trauma or key aspects of the trauma
  - Dissociation is characterized by a disconnection between what's happening and one's awareness of what's happening. During a traumatic event, a person may disconnect from their thoughts and feelings, or later may seal off the memory of those events, as if they didn't happen. The continued dissociation, after the trauma has ended, can make it difficult for survivors to reclaim or integrate memories,

thoughts, and feelings related to the trauma experience. They may continue to experience dissociative responses in daily life when memories, flashbacks, sights, or smells re-stimulate some aspect of the original trauma experiences. Survivors may "zone out" or shut down or in some way retreat from the memory of what happened in the past or what is happening in the present.

- Anxiety about safety and future exposure to trauma
- Thoughts of death (including more passive death thoughts or wishes, and active plans for suicide)
  - Thoughts about death are common among survivors. These may resemble a passive desire to die or be killed in an accident. These thoughts are often related to a desire for current symptoms and suffering to end. Having death thoughts is different than being suicidal—which is defined as having a specific plan and an intention to kill oneself.
- Thoughts or fantasies of revenge
- Self-blame, shame, worthlessness
- Self-hatred
- Confusion and doubt
- Questioning why such horrible things happen, and why they happened to me, or my family. *Why did it happen to me? Why did I survive? Why did I survive when others did not?*

While we tend to focus on the negative impacts of trauma, survivors can also be affected in more positive ways. For example, survivors may, with time, gain self-confidence and self-esteem. They may identify as a strong person, as a survivor, as someone with wisdom and skills to guide their life or to share with others. They may actively seek ways to help others and strengthen community ties. They may become a CHW or another type of helping professional.

Traumatic Memories

Trauma can affect memory. It may cause intrusive or recurring and unwanted memories of traumatic events, including flashbacks. It causes some survivors to avoid thinking about or recalling the original trauma events. For others, trauma may distort or result in the repression or inability to remember part or all of the trauma experience (Government of Canada, 2023; National Institute for the Clinical Application of Behavioral Medicine, 2023).

Most people have difficulty remembering, in a precise or detailed way, all of life's major or minor events (*Can you remember every difficult or wonderful thing that happened in your life?*). Because of the nature of trauma and of dissociation, some survivors are unable to recall what happened to them or to remember it in a clear, chronological and complete way.

Yet it can be difficult for others—such as family, friends, police, judges, and providers without specialized training—to understand how survivors can forget key aspects of the traumatic events. They may think, *"If something so horrible happened to me, I'd certainly remember it!"*

As a CHW, your job is to accept that trauma can alter, suppress, or banish memories. Keep this in mind as you work with clients who may be trying to avoid memories, experiencing flashbacks, or struggling to remember and reconstruct what happened to them.

THOUGHTS ABOUT ONE'S SELF

Trauma can influence the way that survivors perceive or think about themselves. Some survivors develop a more negative self-image that may stem from a sense of self-blame. They may doubt their own value or worth, or see themselves as damaged, poisoned, or poisonous. They may view themselves as limited or incapable of loving or being loved. They may experience self-hatred.

Survivors may also develop a renewed sense of their own self-worth, courage, wisdom, capability, or resilience. By witnessing their own healing and their connection with others, they may develop a deeper sense of their own strengths and values.

CONCEPTS OF THE FUTURE

Research shows that trauma can influence the way that survivors think about the future in the following types of ways:

- Loss of a sense of meaning in life
- A belief that the future will never be different from the present, that trauma symptoms will always persist and at an elevated level
- A sense of doom
- Difficulty in imagining the future or setting any future goals
- An expectation of dying early and through violence

Or, in contrast, survivors may also experience:

- Acceptance of human fallibility or vulnerability
- A deeper commitment to creating a meaningful life
- A focus on the next generation (children or grandchildren) as a way to envision the future

The Kidnapping in Chowchilla, California

In 1976, a school bus with 26 elementary school students was stopped by armed men; the children were held captive underground for 16 hours in a buried van. They were eventually able to escape by digging and climbing their way out. Everyone was rescued; nonetheless, the experience caused trauma responses among the survivors that continued for decades.

Among other things, the children's view of the future was strikingly bleak. One boy explained that he didn't plan to have children because "in case of an emergency there will only be time for me." An 11-year-old survivor, interviewed several years after the kidnapping, expected to die at age twelve, saying "Somebody will come along and shoot me." The children lived with a fear of the future and an expectation that bad things were more likely to happen than not. (Terr, 1990, p. 164)

SPIRITUAL, RELIGIOUS OR PHILOSOPHICAL RESPONSES

Trauma may affect a survivor's spiritual, religious, or philosophical values and beliefs. Not everyone is religious or identifies as being spiritual, but they may hold values and ideas that provide a sense of meaning for life. This may include, for example, a commitment to family, compassion, generosity, or social justice.

Some survivors may lose their faith or sense of meaning. They may question god, creator or religion. They may feel betrayed or abandoned. They may stop praying or going to the temple, mosque, or church. They may feel that life has no purpose or meaning.

Toni Hunt Hines: My sister used to go to church regularly, but after my son was killed, it shook her faith. She is angry with God. She can't go back. She and I, we only go to church for funerals.

Others may find that their sense of faith or meaning deepens or is strengthened. They may feel closer to god or the creator. They may establish closer relationships with their mosque, temple, church, or other religious or faith-based community. They find a renewed sense of purpose or meaning in the world. They may dedicate their life to educating or helping others. They may join together with others who are advocating for change or social justice.

● *How else can trauma affect our sense of meaning, faith, or religion?*

The Long-Term Impacts of Childhood Trauma

Exposure to trauma can result in long-term harm to health. Some of the best evidence of the long-term health consequences of exposure to trauma comes from the Adverse Childhood Experiences (ACE) Study. ACE is a large-scale research study about the long-term health impacts of childhood exposures to "adverse" experiences such as child abuse and neglect, including childhood sexual abuse. The study demonstrated that exposure to childhood abuse is common and results in significant, widespread, and long-lasting impacts to physical and mental health, increasing rates of post-traumatic stress, chronic illness, and premature death (Centers for Disease Control and Prevention, 2021).

Sixty-one percent (61%) of adults from 25 states reported at least one type of adverse childhood experience before the age of 18 and nearly 1 in 6 reported four or more ACEs (Centers for Disease Control and Prevention, 2022). Exposure to childhood abuse is linked to comprehensive health risks including chronic disease such as cancer, diabetes, heart disease, and suicide along with persistent challenges with issues such as learning, employment, and relationships (Ibid). People exposed to adverse childhood experiences are 7 times more likely to consider themselves alcoholic, 10 times more likely to have injected street drugs, and 12 times more likely to have attempted suicide (Trauma-Informed Care Implementation Resource Center, 2023).

To learn more about the ACE study, please see the references and resources provided at the end of this chapter.

OTHER TRAUMA RESPONSES

When we train CHWs, we always leave space for them to identify trauma responses that may not fall into the categories provided above. It is important for you to leave the question of trauma response open as you work with clients. The longer you work directly with survivors of trauma, the more you will learn about how trauma can shape and impact human lives.

● *What other categories or examples of trauma responses would you add to this list?*

Faith Fabiani: Trauma responses can look widely different from person to person, and they can show up in ways the individual may have never considered was connected to their trauma. When experiencing complex trauma, where each day brings new experiences and the individual is in survival mode, there is little time to process and heal resulting in the individual remaining in fight or flight mode. Familiarize yourself with different types of trauma responses. With survivors, validate that the stress responses they're experiencing are natural and common consequences of trauma.

Trauma Responses at the Community Level

This chapter focuses on the work that CHWs do with individual survivors of trauma. It is important to acknowledge that trauma also impacts communities as a whole. Communities that experience violence such as state-sponsored violence or armed conflict or natural disasters such as hurricanes, floods, or famine also experience trauma responses. These collective trauma responses may include damage to social connections within a community. Trauma often separates families and community members through displacement such as in the wake of armed conflict or natural disasters. Trauma can also result in distrust within communities, conflict, blame, and alienation.

Collective trauma can result in fear and insecurity within the community, especially when the nature of the trauma is ongoing. It can cause people to avoid each other, to limit or stop communicating with others, and sometimes results in increased interpersonal violence.

At the same time, trauma can also result in closer connections among community members when they turn to each other for comfort and survival, and when they take action to try to prevent or respond to traumatic events and dynamics.

For more information about the impact of collective trauma at the community level, see the Additional Resources at the end of the chapter.

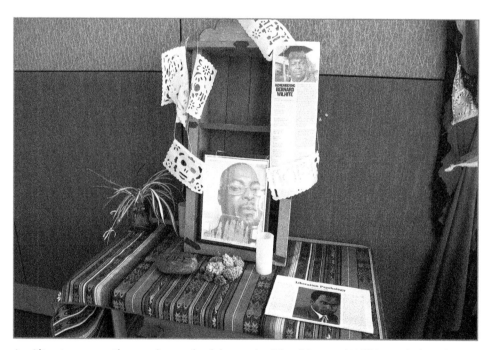

An Altar to mourn the passing and celebrate the life of Bernard Wilhite, a beloved CHW and graduate of City College of San Francisco.

18.4 How Culture and Status Influence Trauma

One of the most common mistakes that helping professionals make is to assume that others share their own understanding and beliefs about trauma and recovery. Research has shown that the way that people respond to traumatic experiences, and the way that they define and seek healing from trauma, are influenced by culture, identity, and status (Chentsova-Dutton & Maercker, 2019; Health Care Toolbox, 2023; Mollica, 2009).

Some research has led to questions about cultural bias in the definition and diagnostic standards for PTSD in the American Psychiatric Association's (APA) DMS-5. In some cultures, certain symptoms associated with PTSD may not appear at all, while others appear but are named and understood in culturally specific ways. Programs that pay attention to cultural traditions and support a variety of approaches to healing are more likely to resonate with clients and communities.

Refugees and asylum seekers living in the United States are also likely to have experienced multiple and severe traumatic experiences in settings with very few resources for basic survival, let alone psychological support. Their symptoms are compounded by being displaced from their country of origin and their support networks and, for some, by long stays in a refugee camp or a detention center while waiting to immigrate or receive legal status. Adjusting to life in a new country and culture also adds to their stress. CHWs should be aware of these multiple sources of stress in the lives of refugees and asylum seekers and may find similar stresses in the lives of immigrant clients in general.

> **Toni Hunt Hines:** Working with Latino families, especially if they are undocumented, there is such a fear of fighting back (after something traumatic has happened.) They are afraid that someone will be deported if they make a complaint or do anything. It's hanging over the family's head.

Status, privilege, bias, and discrimination affect all aspects of our lives and health including exposure to and recovery from trauma. In the United States, people of color, immigrants, members of the LGBTQIA+ community, people with disabilities, and others are at greater risk of experiencing traumatic events and of encountering biased responses from the agencies charged with providing support. Among veterans of the Vietnam War, for example, ethnic minority veterans were more likely to be exposed to war zone stressors than whites. Institutionalized forms of racism both in the Armed Services and in U.S. society as a whole added to the stressors that veterans of color experienced, prior to deployment, during their time in the war zone, and after the war (Loo, 2014). It's important for a CHW to understand this larger context. As CHWs often come from a similar background as their clients, the client may feel more comfortable talking with the CHW about the role that discrimination, exclusion, or bias has played in their experience of trauma.

USING PERSON-CENTERED CONCEPTS AND SKILLS

Perhaps the most significant concern is the risk of imposing culturally biased ideas and standards onto the clients and communities you work with, unintentionally causing injury or harm.

- Let person-centered concepts and skills, including cultural humility (Chapter 7), guide your work with all clients.
- Don't assume that you know about the experiences, beliefs, values, and emotions of others.
- Don't make assumptions about how clients identify with their culture or cultures—instead, support them to explore their own choices around identity and how that impacts their well-being, especially when historical trauma is present.
- Stay curious and ask open-ended questions to learn from the only true experts in the room—the clients and community members you work with.
- Don't tell people what to do or think or believe; use your "Big Eyes and Big Ears" to provide clients with an opportunity to share their own stories and wisdom.
- Let people determine their own route to healing (or not healing), at their own pace.
- Keep learning about trauma and about the history and culture of the communities you work with. Learn about the resources within these communities that can provide culturally relevant guidance and support to survivors.
- Remember that you are not responsible for rescuing, "fixing" or healing the client. You are there as a support for the client, to help the client mobilize internal and external resources to overcome the challenges they face.

- Discuss with the client (and with your co-workers, if you work as part of a team) how cultural identities and norms may conflict with the practices of your agency. For example, mixed-gender or mixed-generation support groups may feel inappropriate to some clients.

18.5 Healing from Trauma

Many survivors, especially those who have recently experienced trauma, question whether or not it's possible to heal or recover. Healing may seem daunting, remote, or impossible in the moment.

It is possible to heal from trauma. But healing may be quite different than what the survivor initially hoped for. And healing is not universal; for some survivors, the effects of trauma continue to dominate significant aspects of their lives.

Finding the right language to talk about healing from trauma is challenging. While some people talk about "recovery" from trauma, others find this language confusing, especially when they compare it to the process of recovery from drug or alcohol abuse. In the mental health field, "recovery" is used to refer "a process of change through which individuals improve their health and wellness, live self-directed lives, and strive to reach their full potential" (Substance Abuse and Mental Health Services Administration [SAMHSA], 2014a). Another term that many people favor is "healing from trauma." Something we like about this language is that it implies a process ("I am healing") rather than a destination or outcome ("I am now healed").

- *What are your beliefs about healing or recovering from trauma?*

- *What language do you use to talk about this concept?*

GOALS FOR HEALING

Trauma survivors have a broad and diverse understanding of what healing means to them. Some may hope to be restored to the person they were before they were harmed. They may wish to be restored to an earlier and/or more innocent state of being; this is a common wish among survivors of childhood abuse. However, it isn't possible to travel back in time or erase the trauma or its impacts. The trauma happened, and trauma changes us. Accepting this can be difficult and often takes time, patience, and courage.

Some survivors have specific goals for reducing or eliminating trauma responses or symptoms. These may include being able to sleep without being disturbed by night terrors, to return to work or school, to build close and trusting relationships with family and friends, to enjoy a satisfying romantic and sexual life, to be more present or comfortable with their children, or to feel joy in more aspects of their life. For trauma survivors who have acquired a disability or a physical change in their body as a result of the traumatic experience—for example, the loss of a leg or an eye—their goals may include adapting to their injury, learning to use assistive devices, and increasing their sense of independence.

Depending upon your role and scope of practice, it can be helpful to explore the survivor's goals for their health and recovery, just as you would explore a client's goals for the self-management of diabetes or depression. For example, you may ask them, "What are some of your goals and priorities?" or "What do you hope to change or accomplish?" And, just as you would in supporting any client to establish an Action Plan, assist them to establish realistic steps to take to meet goals or milestones over time. Keep in mind that gradual and incremental change is likely to be more successful than attempts to create dramatic change quickly.

MULTIPLE PATHS FOR HEALING FROM TRAUMA

Healing from trauma takes many forms. *Deciding which path to follow is a highly individual matter* and may be influenced by factors such as the survivor's current symptoms, their cultural and family traditions, housing and financial situation, spiritual and political beliefs, and knowing other survivors who have experienced meaningful healing or recovery.

Faith Fabiani: Since we all experience trauma differently, the same goes for the healing process. There is no wrong or right way, no timeline or expected end date. It can be a lifelong journey, but the bottom line is it can get better, and things can change! I am a walking, talking, breathing example of this. Think outside of the box and be creative. Take chances. Consider your clients' barriers and resources and let them guide you in supporting the client to create a case plan that is customized to their needs. There is no one-size-fits-all.

Consider the ecological model and reframe the way you provide services by identifying resources and barriers on each level. For instance, maybe under community, you list that a client has a bus stop directly in front of their house, but as a barrier, you note that client's neighborhood is heavily influenced by gang activity and crime. You could use that information to better develop a time and place at which to meet your client. Maybe it's at school where they feel safe or maybe you arrange a Zoom chat so that your client doesn't have to ride the bus into the evening hours. A case plan or safety plan is only useful if your client will really utilize it; otherwise, it's about just as useful as the piece of paper it's written on.

There are many different strategies, approaches, treatments, and resources for healing from trauma. New resources are developed through research and practice. We provide an overview of commonly used resources for healing from trauma below. Please continue to talk with clients and colleagues and to do your own online research to identify emerging approaches and resources. The National Center for PTSD includes resources to support people in making an informed choice about treatment and healing options (National Center for PTSD, 2023d).

Many trauma survivors choose to combine several different paths to support their healing. Just because a client is not interested in a specific path to healing at one point in time does not mean they won't be open to that path at a later time. Develop a list of referrals related to these various paths or options, including those that have a specific focus on trauma recovery, as well as some (for example, a free yoga class) that could be supportive of healing more generally.

Survivors may want to engage in one or more, or none, of the following pathways for healing:

Counseling or Therapy

There are many different types of therapy provided by licensed mental health professionals. Therapy often seeks to create a safe environment for clients to talk about and reflect upon key aspects of their trauma story, gaining new insights, knowledge, and skills. Counseling goals vary among survivors but commonly include reducing trauma responses/symptoms that are interfering with their current quality of life. Therapy may be offered as individual sessions, family sessions, or group sessions. While most counselors or therapists have *some* knowledge of trauma, there are benefits to working with a counselor or therapist who has specialized training and experience in the field of trauma.

No one approach works for *all* people. A client might need to meet with more than one counselor before selecting the best one to work with.

Cognitive-behavioral therapy is commonly used approaches with survivors of trauma. Cognitive-behavioral therapy usually consists of a series of sessions (over weeks or months) designed to assist the client in understanding how their thought patterns and behaviors may affect them, and to learn tools to change ingrained thought patterns or behaviors that may be harmful. It often helps survivors to better understand their physical and emotional responses to trauma, to manage stress, explore their trauma story (see below), distinguish between current and past experiences, and develop new coping skills.

Seeking Safety is a model for supporting adult survivors of trauma who also experience substance use (Najavits, 2002). Most addiction treatment models do not address trauma explicitly. The seeking safety model is used for both individuals and groups.

Exposure therapy is another approach used with trauma survivors and with veterans in particular. Survivors gradually expose themselves to images and other stimuli (situations, sounds, etc.) that are similar to key aspects of their trauma experience, with the goal of reducing anxiety and other post-traumatic symptoms. Exposure therapy using video games that simulate combat experiences has been used with military veterans. Exposure starts slowly and progresses over time *at the client's pace.*

Eye movement desensitization and reprocessing (EMDR) is another form of therapy that has been used to support survivors of trauma. EMDR is conducted by a trained professional and asks survivors to talk about their trauma experiences while engaging in certain types of physical actions such as rapidly moving the eyes from side to side or tapping alternating sides of the body. The theory behind EMDR is that this process allows the client to store the memory of the trauma in a different way than it was stored previously. The result for some survivors is a meaningful reduction in post-traumatic stress symptoms.

New types of counseling or psychotherapy approaches continue to emerge including Cognitive Processing Therapy, Present-Centered Therapy, Written Exposure Therapy, and others. Please see the resources posted at the end of the Chapter for more information.

Social or Support Groups

Survivors often benefit from meeting with others who have experienced similar traumatic experiences and symptoms. This can be particularly beneficial because trauma can be stigmatized and isolating. The rape crisis movement was built upon the idea that survivors benefit from meeting and forging connections with others, breaking silence, shame, stigma, and isolation. Peer support and understanding can open up possibilities of healing and recovery for many groups, such as survivors of intimate partner violence, veterans, parents grieving the death of a child, survivors of natural disasters or state-sponsored violence, and others. Some groups are facilitated by mental health professionals, while others are peer-led.

- *What type of social or support groups exist in your local communities?*

What Do
YOU?
Think

Educational Groups

An educational workshop, or series of workshops, about trauma often includes aspects of emotional or psychological awareness, skills, and support. These groups or workshops are sometimes called psycho-educational. They may be designed and offered specifically for people living with the effects of trauma or other types of psychological distress (such as depression, anxiety, or compulsive behaviors).

Another approach is to weave information about trauma into a more general educational group or workshop. As trauma, violence, and loss are a common part of life, there is a great likelihood that any group includes people for whom trauma is a concern. In addition, such groups may reach people who would not seek out a workshop on violence and trauma, but who would be open to a workshop on family life or wellness.

Medications

Some survivors choose to take medications that may reduce and relieve anxiety, depression, or other trauma symptoms. Clients should talk with a medical or mental health provider and carefully consider different treatment options. Clients taking medications should also meet regularly with a medical provider in order to assess the effectiveness of the medications they are taking, to monitor side effects and to revise dosages or change medications as necessary.

Acupuncture or Other Forms of Complementary Medicine

Some survivors find that acupuncture can be helpful in managing the physical and emotional effects of trauma. Acupuncture is a practice of Chinese medicine that uses needles to stimulate specific channels of energy in the body. Other survivors choose to consult with naturopaths or other practitioners of complementary and alternative medicine. As with selecting a medical doctor or therapist, it is helpful to work with reputable practitioners who have training and experience in trauma.

Somatic Therapies

Biomedical researchers have found that the effects of trauma are stored in the body and can change or re-wire our neurobiology. Some survivors seek out **somatic** therapies that engage the body in ways that promote healing. Somatic therapy may include physical movements designed to help the client recognize and work with bodily sensations that arise in the present moment, as a result of the past traumatic experience or memory. Somatic therapies sometimes may use dance, theater or yoga to engage the mind and body, to revisit memories in a new way or to create new pathways for relaxation and expression.

Healing Arts

The creative and performing arts support the healing of many survivors. Music, dance, drumming, poetry, drawing/painting, theater, drama therapy, and other art forms can provide survivors an opportunity to express aspects of their trauma experience that may be more difficult to tell in conventional settings. Approaching healing through the arts is also an opportunity to incorporate cultural practices or traditions that resonate with survivors.

Social and Political Action

Some people approach healing by taking action to advocate for social change and social justice. Especially when people have been exposed to trauma at a community level, such as survivors of state-sponsored violence and armed conflicts, they may find healing in taking collective action. Survivors of war, rape, police violence, domestic violence, and incarceration have formed organizations and movements to create social and political change. Some survivors, in fact, are not comfortable with the concept of "healing" or "recovery," as it implies an internal or individual process; they identify their journey toward wholeness with the collective pursuit of truth, justice, and peace.

Spiritual and Religious Practices

Spiritual or religious beliefs and practices, including spiritual or faith-based counseling, prayer, and meditation, are beneficial to many survivors. They may increase a survivor's sense of safety and connection to others and offer hope and purpose. Healing work in a faith community can draw upon the power of tradition and ritual to help address the hard questions that inevitably arise. Survivors may create meaningful connections with others through participating in a faith community or other spiritually oriented groups.

Mindfulness

Mindfulness cultivates awareness and being present in the moment with our thoughts, feelings, physical sensations, and environment. While the practice of mindfulness arose out of religious meditation practices, it is now widely practiced in both religious and secular or nonreligious ways to support those living with mental and physical health conditions. Mindfulness practices include breathing exercises and meditation, yoga, chanting, and prayer. Mindfulness supports survivors to notice and accept thoughts and feelings related to their trauma and healing stories. For many, it helps to create a state of awareness and clam, reducing stress symptoms. For more information about mindfulness, see the resources provided in Chapter 12.

Support from Family and Friends

The support of family and friends is often critical to a person's success and well-being. Many of us naturally turn to family and friends first to talk about intimate and difficult issues, and how those loved ones respond—whether they are supportive or not—can have a significant impact on survivors.

- *What are some other strategies or resources for healing from trauma?*

TELLING THE TRAUMA STORY

For many survivors, telling stories about their trauma experience(s) is a key aspect of healing. *There are many different ways to tell these stories.* Stories may be told in whole or in part, chronologically or in an out-of-time sequence. They may be told literally or metaphorically, in words or images, through art, theater, dance, or other methods. Stories may be kept private or shared with a witness such as a friend or family member, a group of other survivors, a CHW, physician, or social worker.

Regardless of whom the story is shared with and how, the most important audience for the story is the survivor themselves. By telling their trauma stories, survivors can better understand their experiences including what happened, how they responded in the moment, how they have been affected since, how they live with trauma today, as well as their story of survival and healing. In this sense, the story itself can serve as a critical resource for healing.

Please keep in mind that not every survivor will choose to tell their story, or to tell it to you. Not every survivor remembers their story. Consider, for example, children who were harmed at a very young age, or survivors who were sexually assaulted after losing consciousness, or survivors for whom memory has been banished and cannot be recalled.

For some survivors, telling their trauma story is an overwhelming or terrifying prospect. Many people spend years trying to escape or run away from the story of what they survived. And for others, they may begin to talk about their trauma experience and find that it is too difficult to continue. This is one reason why we never want to nudge or pressure a survivor to tell their story. Only the survivor can decide if, when, and how they want to tell their story.

My Trauma Story: Anonymous

Over time, I came to think of my trauma story like a book. At first, I buried it in the garage. I didn't want to look at it, much less read it. It felt like, if I looked at it, I might burst into flames. But, at the same time, it was like a book that you can't throw away or, if you did, you would keep finding that it had been returned to your home.

My healing has been a slow and gradual path of learning to pick up that book—the story of what was done to me. I started by reading just a few words or pages at a time. Sometimes I waited months or years before I could read any further. What I noticed, over time, is that the more I read the book, the less afraid of it I became.

Gradually, I stopped thinking of my story as this shameful secret that could destroy me, but as something that hadn't destroyed me, as something that I had been strong enough to survive. Eventually, the book disappeared. It isn't a book anymore—some object outside of myself that I can pick up or hide away—it is simply another part of me. Not the most important part. Not the part that defines me or controls me. And not just a negative part anymore. Now, when I think about the trauma, I don't just see all the horrible things that happened; I see my own strength, the part of me that survived and is becoming a person capable of love and joy. Now I think of the future more than the past.

Telling a trauma story can also be a political act. A public reckoning with traumatic acts, especially when those acts were carried out by the government or with the government's acquiescence, can contribute to healing, especially if the survivors of those traumatic acts are treated with dignity and respect throughout the process.

18.6 The CHW Scope of Practice

Scope of practice is a concern for CHWs who provide direct services to survivors of trauma (SOP was defined in Chapter 5). It provides a framework for CHWs regarding the types of tasks and services that they are qualified to provide and those that should be provided by other types of helping professionals.

The most serious concern is that CHWs might exceed their SOP when working with a survivor. It is important to emphasize that CHWs cannot provide therapy and should not continue to work independently with a client who discloses severe trauma symptoms such as behaviors of self-harm or suicidal ideation (thoughts and a plan to kill themselves).

CHWs have an ethical duty to stay within their SOP and to "do no harm" to the clients and communities they serve. The risks or potential harms of working beyond your SOP include:

- **Harms to the client**: This may include complicating, delaying, or harming a client's recovery or healing from trauma. It may also cause clients to feel less secure reaching out for professional support in the future.
- **Damaged relationships between clients/community and the CHW**: By exceeding your SOP, you may damage professional relationships and any trust that you have built up with a client or the community.
- **Harm to the CHW**: By exceeding your SOP, you could risk disciplinary action, re-assignment, reduced SOP, or loss of employment. Your professional reputation as a CHW may also be damaged.
- **Harm to the agency you work for**: This could include a diminished or damaged reputation among clients and the community and possibly among other service providers and funders.

A secondary concern, at the other end of the SOP spectrum, is that CHWs will hold themselves back from providing the services they are qualified to offer to survivors of trauma. The topic of trauma has become so "medicalized" that people who are not licensed providers are sometimes cautioned from addressing it. Medical and mental health professionals may forget that trauma is a common part of life and that survivors and witnesses need a variety of opportunities to talk about it and receive support. Finding ways to talk openly about trauma is key for healing and building resilience. If we caution all unlicensed providers from ever addressing trauma with the clients and communities they work with, we may unintentionally reinforce the shame and isolation that is so common among survivors. We may also give the impression that survivors of trauma should just put the trauma behind them and not talk about it, or that trauma should only be discussed by licensed professionals.

FACTORS THAT INFLUENCE THE CHW SCOPE OF PRACTICE

Unfortunately, there is no simple formula or hard and fast rule to tell CHWs what they can and cannot say or do in every circumstance. The SOP of CHWs regarding trauma varies depending upon factors such as:

- Prior training, skills, and comfort level.
  - Some CHWs have not received specialized training related to trauma, while others, for example, have been trained and certified as a Sexual Assault Counselor or Violence Prevention Specialist.
- The type of program you work for. Some CHWs work for agencies and programs that primarily address trauma (such as a domestic violence shelter) and may provide direct services to clients. Other CHWs work in settings where they rarely if ever address trauma directly with clients.
- The employer's policies and protocols. Some agencies have adopted trauma-informed policies (more information is provided later on in the chapter) that provide additional training and clear guidance for considering and addressing trauma as a routine part of service delivery.
- The quality of the supervision you receive. If you work with communities in which trauma is common, you should receive ongoing supervision from a qualified professional who can support you in providing quality services to clients, staying within your SOP. Supervision also provides support for identifying and managing signs of secondary trauma and risks for burnout.
- The severity of the client's trauma response, risk behaviors, and level of distress.
  - In general, CHWs work with survivors who have already made some progress toward establishing safety (see below) and are coping day-to-day with trauma responses. Clients who have recently experienced trauma (or recently started to face a past trauma) and who are experiencing greater distress in terms of emotional, behavioral, or cognitive responses should be referred to work with licensed colleagues and trauma-focused programs.
- The availability of quality services for survivors in the community.
  - When quality services are accessible to all clients, CHWs and the agencies they work for can develop collaborative relationships and provide referrals to other providers and programs.

We encourage you, and the program or agency you work for, to carefully define the limits of your SOP for working with survivors of trauma. In what circumstances, and to what extent, are you authorized to address trauma? How and when should you consult with other colleagues, including licensed professionals? What types of referrals sources are you encouraged to share with clients (including those within and outside of the agency you work for)? What professional opportunities exist for you to enhance your knowledge and skills?

- *To what extent do you address the topic of trauma with the clients and communities you work with?*

- *How well is your scope of practice defined by your employer or supervisor?*

- *Do you receive ongoing professional development and supervision related to trauma?*

Some CHWs Specialize in Addressing Trauma

Throughout the world, some CHWs work very closely with survivors of trauma. They may work with individuals, groups, or at the community level. For example, many rape crisis centers and domestic violence shelters train volunteers and hire nonlicensed staff who provide a wide range of direct services. These CHWs and other unlicensed providers may accompany sexual assault survivors during forensic medical exams at local hospitals, and during criminal or civil court proceedings. They may provide individual peer counseling, by phone and in person, and co-facilitate support groups with the supervision from a licensed professional. Throughout the world, in situations of armed conflict and civil war, in refugee camps and detention centers, licensed mental health therapists are rare. Often CHWs and other peer or unlicensed providers take the lead in providing support to their community (Kok, 2021. Werner et al., 2022).

WITHIN THE SCOPE OF PRACTICE OF ALL CHWS

We believe that every CHW who has been well-trained in person-centered concepts and skills can provide the following types of services to survivors of trauma:

- Listening with patience and respect, and with Big Eyes, Big Ears, and small mouth as discussed in Chapters 6 and 9. Sometimes what survivors most need is an opportunity to talk about what they are going through. In this way, CHWs bear witness to the client's stories.

- Validating and normalizing the experience of surviving trauma. Survivors often feel isolated and alone and may believe that their experience is unusual or shameful. By acknowledging that trauma is all too common, CHWs can help to reduce the stigma that some client's face, as well as their sense of being alone.

- Reinforcing the message that help is available and that healing from trauma is possible.

- Providing linkages and referrals to local services. CHWs can support clients to connect with available quality services, including services provided by licensed mental health providers, physicians, and local programs specializing in supporting survivors of violence (including rape crisis centers, domestic violence shelters, reentry programs, and programs serving Veterans).

- Accompanying clients as they access new medical, mental health, legal, or other services. Sometimes, at the request of the client, a CHW will go with a client during a first meeting with a local organization such as a rape crisis center or mental health agency.

- Supporting clients to re-establish safety by focusing first on immediate physical and emotional safety, and not rushing to tell the details of their trauma story until they feel ready to do so. CHWs can help clients consider when and how they wish to address their trauma and their healing, and with whom.

- Providing a strength-based approach that highlights the survivor's key strengths and resources for health, coping, and healing.

- Assess a client's risk for suicide and provide an immediate report and/or referral, as necessary.

- Keeping the focus, to the extent possible, on the present, and what the client can do now to cope, seek safety, and find a way forward in their recovery.

Faith Fabiani: While we don't diagnose clients, or prescribe medicine, our role as CHWs is essential. You don't need a degree to hold space for someone who is suffering. Truly hearing your client's needs, prioritizing their wants and holding space for their pain is a unique skill set. Never minimize the power you have and your ability to make a difference.

Inez Love: I'm the first line of support. In this work, you do some counseling, but it's not the same as therapy. I would advocate and link youth to services to receive therapy, help them navigate the system. I would let them know that I can offer them what I know from my experience and my classes, and let them know that if they want more, I would recommend therapy.

OUTSIDE THE CHW SCOPE OF PRACTICE

The following types of services lie outside of the CHW SOP, and should be provided by other professionals with the relevant training and skills:

- Working independently (or on your own) with a trauma survivor without seeking consultation and/or supervision from a well-trained colleague.
- Guiding the client regarding actions or decisions that they should make in order to promote their healing. Recommending treatments or medications or paths to healing or recovery.
- Addressing issues or challenges for which you have no training and skills.
- Crossing the line from peer counseling into therapy. Examples may include extensive exploration of the client's past, in-depth discussion about the details of the trauma experience, or providing interpretation of the meaning of a client's story.
- Continuing to work with a client who discloses or demonstrates acute symptoms of trauma-related distress. If clients are highly distressed (anxious, scared, angry, etc.) and unable to maintain a calmer state, they should be referred to a qualified professional. If you aren't sure where to refer a client, refer them to a trusted colleague who can, in turn, provide an appropriate referral to a specific provider, program, or agency.
- Continuing to work with clients who indicate that they are acting out in ways that pose risks to their health (or risks to others), such as a client who has suicidal thoughts or is engaged in cutting (cutting their bodies with a razor, knife or other sharp object) or other risk behaviors.

SIGNS THAT YOU MAY BE EXCEEDING YOUR SCOPE OF PRACTICE

As we have discussed before, some of the lines between the types of services that lie within and outside of your SOP may be a bit fuzzy or unclear. And sometimes, despite your best intentions, you may find yourself in a situation in which you are exceeding or at risk of exceeding your SOP. A conversation with a client may change into one in which you feel in over your head.

Signs that you may be exceeding your SOP include:

- The client may be highly distressed and unable to contain their thoughts and strong emotions (such as fear or terror, despair or rage).
- The client may begin to talk about issues properly addressed by well-trained professionals such as:
  - Suicide
  - Self-destructive behaviors such as putting themselves at risk for further exposure to trauma
  - Signs of another mental health issue or confusing state (thoughts or behaviors that are highly confusing to you and/or the client)
  - Acting out in ways that hurt others or planning to harm others

- ○ Inability to stay or return to the present, or to shift to a safer and more neutral topic (away from their trauma story). The client may seem "stuck" in the past, in their trauma story and memories.
- You feel overwhelmed, unprepared, uncertain about what to do or say, and worried that you could cause harm to the client.
- The client is asking or pressuring you to exceed your SOP by asking for a diagnosis, treatment recommendations, or to talk explicitly and in-depth about trauma experiences that they have not addressed before.

Talk with your supervisor and licensed colleagues to learn more about other possible signs that you could be working beyond your SOP.

WHAT TO DO WHEN YOU ARE RISK OF EXCEEDING YOUR SCOPE OF PRACTICE

When in doubt about whether or not you are at risk of exceeding your SOP:

- **Clarify your scope of practice**: Sometimes, it is helpful to clearly state your own limitations as a provider. For example, you may wish to explain that you been trained to support clients with many issues, but that when it comes to trauma experiences, your role is to help clients to connect with a professional who has further training and expertise, so that they can benefit from the best possible support. In general, clients will appreciate your compassion and honesty, and your desire for them to receive quality services.
- **Focus on the present**: Try to support the client to shift their focus and talk with you about the present and, if necessary, a different topic. Sometimes shifting physically can be helpful in shifting the client's immediate focus. For example, you may try standing up, sitting in a different location, moving to a different office or, if possible, taking a walk with the client.
- **Demonstrate respect and kindness**: No matter what you are feeling or thinking, or what the client says or does, continue to demonstrate respect and kindness. Often, this has value in itself in terms of supporting the client's welfare and recovery from trauma.
- **Pause, stop, or take a break**.
- **Comment on the process** (see Chapter 9): Speak up to draw the client's attention to the current problem or challenge that is happening in the moment between you. Sometimes naming what is happening—such as the client's immediate distress or your own concern about SOP—can help to interrupt a dynamic that could do harm to the client. It can also be helpful to shift the conversation to the present.
- **Encourage the client to consider a referral**: Describe local options for therapy, counseling, or other services.
- **Seek consultation**: Sometimes a qualified colleague may be just a few rooms or a phone call away. If necessary, step out of the room for a moment to consult with or ask for the immediate support of a well-trained colleague. With the client's permission, you may be able to bring a qualified colleague into the room or meeting to address the issues that are beyond your SOP.
- **End the session**: While it may be uncomfortable, sometimes you may need to interrupt the client, such as when a client is talking about issues that you aren't qualified to address. The risk of causing harm to the client by continuing the conversation may be greater than any risks from ending the session in a clear, kind, and firm manner. When your other attempts to interrupt conversations that stray beyond your SOP fail, consider ending the session. You might explain that you have an ethical duty to find a qualified professional to help the client with their current concerns.

Anonymous: I worked as a CHW in a busy primary care clinic. One time, a client told me that she had recently been raped. She broke down sobbing. I reached for tissues and just sat with her. I wasn't sure what to do. I told her how sorry I was to know that she had been raped, and she just started to cry even harder. I didn't want to run out of the room right then, but when she was able to catch her breath and talk a bit, I told her that I wanted to bring in a colleague who had training around trauma, and would she agree to meet with someone? She agreed, so I left and returned with a social worker. We sat together and it was really amazing to watch how the social worker was able to talk with the client. I was just so relieved, and I knew that I had done the right thing because of how the client responded. She thanked us both and made an appointment to talk again with social worker later that same week.

18.7 Guidelines for Working with Survivors

In some ways, working with a client to support their recovery from trauma is similar to working with a client to support their self-management of depression or diabetes. As a CHW, you have a limited SOP and work in collaboration with other health care and social services providers. With all clients, you are in a facilitative role, and you apply skills such as Motivational Interviewing to support clients to identify challenges and strengths, to establish goals and actions to meet those goals. You support clients to identify and gain access to culturally relevant agencies, programs, services, and providers.

What may distinguish your work around issues of trauma are your own feelings and beliefs about the issue, heightened concerns about SOP, and the need to consult more regularly with your supervisor and other colleagues. With more experience working with survivors of trauma, we trust you will find that your knowledge and skills are relevant and meaningful to promoting the health and healing of clients.

TO DO AND NOT TO DO

As part of the training at City College of San Francisco, we ask CHWs to brainstorm a list of things TO DO or say when working with a survivor of trauma and a second list of things that they DON'T want to do or say. The lists are meant to fit with and build upon concepts of person-centered practice. Here is a sample list:

Not to Do

- **Judge the client's experience or trauma responses**.

- **Blame the client** for not responding to trauma in a different way (*Why didn't they fight back? Why didn't they tell someone right away? Why didn't they call the police?*).

- **Take away or undermine autonomy and control** such as by directing or telling the client what they should do or think or feel. Helping professionals may do this unintentionally. Keep in mind that a central feature of trauma experiences is a loss of control and that supporting the client to reclaim control is a key part of their recovery.

- **Interrogate the client** about their experience by asking too many questions and inquiring about details of the trauma story.

- **Make physical contact** with the client. Some people are conditioned to comfort others through touch (such as a touch on the arm or shoulder, or a hug). But unwanted touch may also be part of the trauma experience. Instead of touch, use words, and your person-centered skills to demonstrate and share your unconditional positive regard for the client.

- **Try to "rescue" a client**: Rescuing may take the form of telling the client what they "need" to do or making decisions for the clients, and sometime threatens to violate ethical standards. This often happens when working with youth and others who are particularly vulnerable to harm. The desire to rescue is understandable—it comes from a desire to help. But it can also get in the way of person-centered practice. Slow down and let the client guide their own recovery and determine how you may best support them. Reach out for consultation, supervision, and assistance from your colleagues.

- **Pressure a survivor to report** a sexual assault or other crime, or to expect justice from the criminal or civil justice system. This is a decision that only the survivor can make. There is no way to predict how the police may respond, whether or not a District Attorney will decide to prosecute a case, how the courts will treat the survivor, much less the ultimate outcome of a court case. Decisions about reporting, filing for a protective order, or participating in a criminal trial are difficult to make, and should be carefully considered by the survivor.

- **Let your own experiences and assumptions dominate**: Be aware of how your own experiences—including experiences with trauma—may influence your work with clients. For example, helping professionals may guide discussions to address topics or questions that are based on their own experience and needs, rather than on the expressed desire or interest of the client. Try to notice any tendencies for your own issues to influence how you work with a client. Put these aside in the moment and return to tend to them later, on your own time (and not during the client's appointment).

- **Tell a client** *"I know how you feel."* You don't! You may know how *you felt*, or can imagine how *you might feel*, but this is very different from knowing how a client feels. Even if you experienced a similar trauma, remember that how people respond to trauma is unique and subjective. Telling a client how they feel may engender feelings of anger and undermine rather than build trust and rapport.

- **Focus on a particular aspect of a trauma event or story**: Helping professionals sometimes ask about a particular part of the client's experience. For example, with a survivor of sexual assault, providers may inquire about the sexual aspects of the story. This is an unintentional way of taking control away from and may feel like a type of manipulation. Follow the lead of the client regarding what they do and don't want to discuss with you.

- **Promise more than you can do**: Promises create expectations, and when you fail to deliver or follow through, you are likely to undermine trust and rapport with the client.

  - *What else would you NOT want to do when working with a survivor of trauma?*

To DO

- **Be aware of your own tendencies for denial**: We sometimes doubt trauma stories because we don't want to believe that such horrific things truly happen, or we don't want to consider that they could also happen to us or our loved ones. If it is difficult for you to stay present and to focus on the client's story, this may be a sign that you require additional training about trauma (and/or time for your own healing).

- **Listen**: Listening is sometimes more difficult than it seems. It can be difficult to do well, especially if what the client has to tell you is disturbing or horrifying, or similar to something that you or a loved one has experienced. Breathe and lean in to the client's story. Don't worry about what you will say next. *Know that the act of listening and trying to hear what a survivor is telling you can, in itself, support their healing.*

Listening can be Hard To Do

Tim Berthold: The first day I was training to become a certified sexual assault counselor, I was asked to participate in a role-play. Because we were being trained to do phone counseling on a rape crisis hotline, we did our role plays seated back to back (so that we couldn't see each other). My role was to play the counselor, and my fellow volunteer was given a role-play script about a client who had recently been assaulted.

As the role-play began, I kind of blanked out. The story of the caller was so similar to something that had happened to one of my family members. I interrupted the caller to ask questions that were really about my family member's experience ("Is he still in the house?" "Can you get out of the house?" "Did you call 911?").

It was a bit embarrassing, but a great training lesson. I learned how my own issues can get in the way and keep me from focusing and truly hearing the experience of a client. This topic became an area of focus for me and for the training group that I was a part of: How can we push aside our own concerns in the moment in order to be present and listen to the story of another?

- **Learn to be comfortable with silence**: Let the client take the time they need to reflect, to feel, and to consider what they want to say.

- **Use your OARS and other motivational interviewing skills** (see Chapter 9): Ask open-ended questions and demonstrate reflective listening to provide clients with the opportunity to reflect upon and express their experience, feelings, and values (*while keeping your scope of practice in mind*). Provide authentic affirmations, sparingly, to support clients to recognize their own strengths and accomplishments. Summarize key messages shared by the client and any plans or agreements that you make.

- **Let the client guide the pace, focus, and manner of telling their story**: Be gentle in inquiring about the client's experience and responses. Let them guide the discussion and determine what they wish you talk about, when, and how.

- **Encourage clients to consider working with licensed professionals** who have advanced training in trauma and recovery. Explain the limits of your SOP and why it is important for survivors of trauma to work closely with a trained professional who has expertise in this topic.

- If you make a mistake (and all service providers make mistakes), **apologize**. Let the client know that you are sorry if you did or said something that was unintentionally hurtful. This may be particularly important for a survivor who was harmed by another person, perhaps someone they knew or loved who has not acknowledged or taken responsibility for what they did. Providing a sincere apology often helps to restore and enhance the professional connection or rapport between CHWs and clients.

- There may be times to share specific messages with a client, such as:

  - **It's not your fault:** Many survivors, including survivors of childhood abuse and neglect, and survivors and witnesses of domestic violence, believe that they are at fault. Many were told that they caused the trauma. Depending upon the circumstances and the survivor, it may be helpful for them to hear that you don't believe it is their fault. They may need to hear this more than once. Hearing it from others may help them to internalize this message.

  - **I'm here to support you:** Some survivors have been told not to talk about the trauma events or to put it behind them. They may feel embarrassed or ashamed, and they may worry that you will be harmed if you hear what they survived or that you may reject them. It may be helpful for you to let the client know that you are grateful that they disclosed their story to you and that you want to do your very best to support their healing and recovery.

- **Practice self-care**: Whether you are a survivor or not, working with survivors can be stressful, and it can lead to secondary trauma (discussed below). Enhance your skills for self-care and put them into practice each day. Reach out to others—including family, friends, colleagues, and professionals—as needed, for support. If you are a survivor, watch for signs that your own trauma responses are returning or increasing, and continue to do your own healing.

Faith Fabiani: Prepare for the worst, hope for the best, and throw expectations out the door. Healing from trauma is not linear, there are a lot of ups and downs and sometimes your clients might walk out the door and never come back. Your job is to plant a seed, even if it means not seeing the moment the seed grows. Transparency with everything you do is the first step in providing quality care to diverse populations; we give them the information with the understanding that the choices they make from there are out of our control and regardless of the path they choose, we hold them in positive regard. It also means understanding how the same systems we may work for have historically wronged the communities they were meant to serve. We can't move forward, rebuild, and gain trust without understanding and addressing the impact of the past.

THE MOMENT WHEN A CLIENT FIRST TELLS YOU ABOUT TRAUMA

Not all clients will share their trauma experiences with you, but some will. Consider the moment when a client tells you that they are a survivor of trauma.

- *What may be at stake for the client?*
- *What concerns may they have?*
- *What hopes may they have?*
- *What are your primary goals in this moment?*
- *Are you grounded and prepared to assist the client?*
- *How do you want to respond?*
- *How will you stay within your scope of practice?*

Some clients are accustomed to talking about their trauma experiences. They may have talked about their trauma many times, to many people, and made significant progress in their healing. Others may never have shared their story with anyone before. Or they may have told someone who did not respond in a supportive or helpful manner.

Keep in mind that some survivors may feel nervous about telling you—or anyone—about their trauma experience and may be fearful of how you may react (Will you believe them? Will you blame them? Will you view them or treat them differently?). Others may be terrified of confronting their own experiences in a new way, by voicing them out loud in the presence of a witness.

How people respond when survivors share a history of trauma can have a significant impact on their healing and welfare. Consider the example of a survivor who tells a family member about their trauma, and their family member doesn't believe them, or blames them in some way, or responds in way that enhances their embarrassment or shame. In contrast, if survivors are met with patience, kindness, and respect when they share their stories, this can support them in taking action toward healing or recovery.

Suggestions for how to respond when a client first tells you they are a survivor include to:

- Remain calm and patient
- Thank them for sharing part of their story with you
- Express or demonstrate your compassion and concern for the welfare of the client
- Assess physical and emotional safety (addressed in greater detail later in this chapter)
- Follow the lead of the client. If they indicate that they don't want to talk further, or talk about a particular question or topic, accept this decision.

CASE STUDY — Tony Hernandez (continued)

CHW: It's good to see you, Tony. How have you been? How's your asthma?

Tony: Okay. Well, I mean . . . my asthma's okay. I'm here for something else.

CHW: How can I help you?

Tony: Well, you know the neighborhood where we live, right?

CHW: Of course. I grew up just a few blocks away.

Tony: Did you hear about the shooting on 4th street?

CHW: Yes, I did. There have been a lot of shootings this year.

Tony. It was my friend. It was Leroy. (Tony starts to cry and puts his arm over his face)

CHW: I'm so sorry, Tony.

Tony: (cries)

CHW: (Listens and waits patiently) I'm glad you came in to today Tony. I'm here to support you.

Tony: I don't know what to do (he looks up at the CHW). There've been other shootings in our neighborhood and two guys I knew in High school were killed. But . . . (Tony looks down and pulls the cuffs of his shirt over his hands).

CHW: I'm here, Tony. You can tell me whatever you want to.

Tony: I don't know even know how to begin.

CHW: There isn't a right or wrong way to begin.

Tony: I was hanging out with Leroy on the street, like we always do. He was showing me a video. I went back in the house and then I heard this 'pop pop' sound, you know? I knew it was a gun. When I ran back out

CASE STUDY   Tony Hernandez *(continued)*

Leroy was lying on the sidewalk, and everyone had scattered. He was bleeding real bad. I called 911, but he died right there before they came. He was looking at me.

CHW: Oh Tony, how horrible.

Tony: I don't know what to do.

CHW: Have you been able to talk with others about this? Have you been getting support?

Tony: I don't know. My dad. You know how he can be. He just keeps telling me I need to put it behind me . . . He's worried about it affecting my studies.

CHW: What do you want?

Tony: I want help. I can't handle this on my own. I need to talk about Leroy.

CHW: How does it feel to be talking about it today?

Tony: It feels right. (pauses) But it's hard too. I keep thinking, what if I'd seen something and I could have warned him and told him to come inside with me? What if I'd done something? I just keep replaying it in mind over and over.

CHW: I think what you're experiencing—feeling guilty or blaming yourself for not being able to prevent Leroy's death, replaying it over and over in your mind—that's common for people who experience a trauma like witnessing the death of a friend.

Tony: It is?

CHW: (nods) Too many people have lost loved ones to guns. Some of them—like you—were right there when it happened. And they also struggled to understand what to do.

Tony: What do they do?

CHW: People respond to and heal from trauma in their own ways. That's important. We work with a lot of survivors of trauma right here at the clinic.

Tony: How do you help them?

CHW: Well, I have some training on trauma, and I'm here to support you like always, but I'd like you to consider meeting with one of the social workers here. They have more training and more skills than I do to help you with what you're going through. Trauma can take a deep toll on our physical and mental health. Counseling—with the right person—can help you to process your experience and how it's affecting you and help you to decide what steps you want to take to for your own healing.

Tony: I don't know.

CHW: What are your concerns?

Tony and the CHW continue to talk.

Topics that you *may* wish to explore with a new client (always with their consent and in a manner that is consistent with your SOP within the agency where you work) include:

- Are they open to seeking support and services from a qualified professional?
- What skills and resources do they have that can help them to cope with or heal from trauma?
- How can you best support them? What are their key priorities?
- What is it like to be talking about the trauma now, in this moment?

HOW TO PROVIDE A REFERRAL

How you provide a referral is sometimes just as important as the quality of the referral. Referrals should be offered in a way that encourages the client to consider the value of the resource, while supporting their autonomy and maintaining a positive professional connection (for more information about providing referrals, see Chapter 10 on Case Management).

Sometimes, when a CHW provides a referral to another provider—such as a social worker or psychologist with expertise in the field of trauma—a client may feel as if you are saying, *"Now that you have told me _____ [about the trauma], I can't work with you anymore. Talk with someone else. I don't want to listen to these horrible things."* It can feed into a survivor's shame or embarrassment about their trauma story and, unintentionally, harm rapport and erode trust. It may also make the survivor more reluctant to disclose their trauma story to another.

We encourage you to take extra time when providing a referral related to the topic of trauma, especially if you haven't worked with the client for very long. Explain why you are providing the referral and how it may benefit the client. You may want to explain that you have a more limited SOP and, when it comes to the topics of trauma and counseling, you have an obligation to refer clients to opportunities to work with highly trained professionals. Finally, to the extent that you are able and willing to continue to play a role in supporting the client's health, reinforce your interest in doing so.

CASE STUDY | **Tony Hernandez** *(continued)*

CHW: Tony, my job is to support clients to get healthier, and this means connecting you with opportunities to work with professionals who have the most training and skills for working with survivors of trauma. I have some knowledge and experience, but I'm not qualified to serve as your primary support in healing from trauma.

Are you open to considering referrals to some counselors and local programs that work with survivors? If you decide to work with one of these counselors, I could also continue to meet with you when you come to the health center. What are your thoughts about this?

Tony: I guess so; I mean that makes sense to me. Could you continue to meet with me at least until I find someone that . . . . Someone I feel good about?

CHW: Yes, I'd like that, Tony.

Tony: (nods and looks up)

CHW: I'll do my best to help you find a qualified counselor, someone who you feel good about working with. I have a couple of people in mind who have a lot of experience supporting survivors of trauma. Do you have any thoughts about the type of counselor you would like to meet with?

Tony: I guess I'd want to work with someone from our community, you know? Someone I can talk to in Spanish and English, like I do with you. Are there any guy counselors?

CHW: Yes, one of my colleagues here, Mr. González, is a social worker and I've heard great things about him from other clients. He speaks Spanish and English.

Tony: Okay. I'll meet with him, with Mr. González. But I've never gone to a counselor before. I mean, what is supposed to happen there?

CHW: Well, let's talk a little more about that . . . .

Identifying Local Services for Survivors of Trauma

Work with your colleagues to research and develop a list of the best local services for survivors of trauma. Identify agencies and providers that offer services in the community. What type of services do they provide? What level of training have they received? Are there any eligibility requirements for clients? What is the cost of services, and what type of health insurance do they accept (Do they accept Medicaid)? What languages do the providers speak?

ESTABLISHING SAFETY

Establishing safety is often the first step toward healing and restoring a sense of control that trauma has taken away. Safety is an inclusive concept that includes both physical and emotional safety. It may begin with gaining greater control and comfort with physical sensations and dynamics such as sleeping and eating and coping with responses and behaviors that put the survivor at risk. The next stage may focus on the survivor's living environment and establishing safe and stable housing and income. After these first stages of safety have been achieved, survivors are better prepared to address their trauma story more directly, and to focus on remembrance, integration, and mourning (Mendelsohn et al., 2011).

Not every client is ready to talk about their trauma experiences or to engage in more active forms of treatment, such as counseling. Doing so may result in increased stress, heightened symptoms (or responses), and risks. You don't want to inadvertently cause harm to a client. So, just as you would with many other clients, start by talking about more basic issues of safety and survival.

If the client demonstrates great anxiety, stress, fear, or concern:

- Don't continue to engage in dialogue about their trauma story
- Provide a referral to a licensed colleague or community-based provider
- Consult with your supervisor and/or clinical team

To learn more about supporting clients to establish safety, please see the Additional Resources listed at the end of the chapter. Please note that safety is also established by assessing for the risk of suicide as described later in this chapter.

CASE STUDY   Tony Hernandez (continued)

It may take time for Tony to build a foundation of safety because of the nature of the trauma he experienced and the fact that it occurred at his home. He is feeling overwhelmed, experiencing anxiety and nightmares, and has moved away from his neighborhood.

As a CHW, you can talk with Tony about issues of safety and stability. You can explain that it is often important for survivors to address basic issues of physical safety and stability before they begin to talk about their trauma experiences. First steps for Tony may include finding a place to stay away from his own neighborhood, and engaging in daily activities that help to reduce stress. Tony may also want to consider whether or not he is ready to start talking with others—including the social worker—about Leroy's death. It is important for Tony to be in control of what he focuses on next and the steps he takes to promote his own health and to heal from trauma.

FACILITATING THE END OF A MEETING WITH A CLIENT

Related to the topic of establishing safety is the question of how to end a meeting or conversation about trauma. You don't want to suddenly end an appointment in the middle of an important or challenging discussion, or when the client is feeling highly emotional or distressed. As discussed in Chapter 10, you are responsible for time management and helping clients to anticipate the end of an appointment or meeting.

You may need to gently interrupt a conversation to support a client to prepare for the end of a meeting (*"I'm sorry to interrupt, but we only have about 10 minutes left, and I want to make sure that we make time for . . . ."*). This is an opportunity to schedule a follow-up appointment and to support the client to transition from the meeting to the rest of their day. For example, you might ask them what they will do after the appointment. If they are facing challenges or having a difficult day, ask them to consider what they can do to take care of themselves. Will they take a walk, talk to a friend, prepare a healthy meal, or read a book? This is an opportunity to help clients to enhance their stress management and self-care skills, and to put them into practice when they are most needed.

ACTION PLANNING

The concepts that guide you in supporting people to establish an action plan for managing diabetes or depression are the same for working with a survivor of trauma (see Chapters 10 and 16 for more information about Action Planning). Assist the client in establishing clear goals for their healing. With survivors of trauma, it may be helpful for them to articulate their long-term goal and then to select a more near-term goal, something that they may be able to achieve in the next three to six months. Next, ask them to identify a series of steps or actions that they are ready to take to help them reach their goals.

Ask clients to anticipate challenges they may face in implementing their plan and how it may feel to achieve or not to achieve their goals. Identifying and discussing challenges can help to normalize the complex process of recovering from trauma, which seldom happens in a clear and straightforward path.

CASE STUDY   Tony Hernandez *(continued)*

Tony has started working with Mr. González, a social worker at the Central City Clinic. All parties agreed that the CHW will help Tony to develop his Action Plan.

CHW: Tony, I'm happy to learn that you feel good about the connection you're building with Mr. González.

Tony: Yeah, I'm glad you recommended him. I'm also glad that you and I can keep working together because I've known you for so long.

CHW: I'm happy to be working with you too. You're doing counseling with Mr. Gonzalez and talking about your healing. We've agreed that I can help you come up with an Action Plan, right? (Tony nods) Do you remember the Action Plan that you developed for managing your Asthma?

Tony: Yeah, I still use it. It's why I haven't had to go to the Emergency Room in a long time.

CHW: That's great. You can use the same sort of approach to develop an action plan for your recovery from trauma. You can start by laying out some goals and then identifying some actions to meet your goals. How does that sound?

Tony: Okay. I think that will be helpful. I've kind of been . . . almost reacting to what happened rather than thinking about the future.

CHW: What goals do you have for your recovery?

Tony: (wipes his eyes)

CHW: What are you feeling just now?

Tony: I think I'm feeling guilty that I get to move on and have a life and Leroy's dead. It feels weird to leave him behind. I thought we'd always be connected.

CHW: You're feeling guilty about leaving him behind.

Tony: Yeah. I mean, I know I'll always remember him. It's still hard to remember that he's gone. . . .

CASE STUDY   Tony Hernandez *(continued)*

CHW: It takes time to process the loss of someone close to us.

Tony: Yeah. But I know he'd want me to move forward. Me and Mr. Gonzalez talked about it. Leroy was a big supporter of me going to college.

CHW: So what do you want now. What are your goals?

Tony: I want to finish college and get my degree, but it may take me longer than what my Dad wants. And I want to be able to go back to my Dad's house without . . . (Tony shakes his head). I haven't been able to go back since it happened. I think I also want to do something to help stop all these killings. It's got to stop.

CHW: These are three great goals. Let's take them one by one. Which one do you want to start with today?

Tony: Well, I guess with the easiest one. Not that any of them are easy (laughs). But I should come up with a plan for college.

CHW: Okay, let's start there. How should we write down what your goal is for college?

Tony: (thinking) I want to keep making progress toward getting my A.A. degree and transferring to State.

CHW: (writing) Okay. I like how you phrased that goal. So what actions do you want to take that will help you keep making progress toward your degree?

As you continue to work with the client, check their progress in implementing their action plan. Continue to normalize the challenge of recovery. Be open to the client's need or desire to question or change their plan. And remember to roll with resistance rather than digging in to lecture or try to persuade the client to stick to any aspect of their plan (see Chapter 9). Be sure to notice and reflect back on the client's accomplishments—big or small—as they move forward. Remember that survivors may have a harder time noticing or taking credit for these accomplishments and, a growing awareness of their strengths will help them to gain confidence and a greater sense of self-determination.

How Trauma may Influence Action Planning and Behavior Change

Anyone attempting to change health-related behaviors may experience ambivalence and self-doubt. These challenges may be even more pronounced for survivors of trauma. Survivors may fluctuate back and forth between different emotions and states of readiness, and their efforts to achieve change may be complicated by trauma responses such as fear, anxiety, numbness, guilt, shame, and isolation. Remain patient, and keep in mind that neither behavior change or healing from trauma typically happens in a linear way—from Step 1 to Step 2, and so on. As discussed in Chapters 6 and 9, the process of behavior change often includes ambivalence, doubts, relapse to prior patterns of behavior, and the need to revisit and revise Action Plans.

ANTICIPATING CONSEQUENCES

It can be helpful to ask clients to consider the possible consequences of their plans and decisions. It may be particularly important to do so when you work with a survivor of trauma who is contemplating decisions that may have a significant impact on their health and relationships, such as:

- Whether to disclose or tell someone else about their trauma experience
- Whether to report an assault or other type of harm to a third party such as an employer or the police

- Whether to provide testimony in a criminal or civil court case
- Whether to "confront" someone who harmed them, such as a parent who neglected or abused them
- Whether to make a significant life change such as ending or beginning a relationship or job or moving to a new city or state

Sometimes trauma survivors rush into big decisions related to their recovery. They may be influenced by friends or families or assumptions about what they "should do." As a CHW, your role isn't to tell a client what to do, but to support them to carefully consider key decisions, possible consequences, and the impact on their recovery and health (and to provide referrals as necessary).

18.8 Conducting a Suicide Assessment

Many CHWs are trained to assess a client's potential risk for suicide and, when necessary, to consult immediately with a licensed colleague and/or make a report to a third party such as an emergency response team. We provide guidelines for assessing a client's risk for suicide in this section. However, once you are working in the field, please ask your supervisor for additional training, and carefully review your agency's policies and protocols for screening and reporting the risk of suicide.

THE RISK OF SUICIDE

Suicide is not as rare as many people think. It was the twelfth leading cause of death in the United States in 2020. It was the second leading cause of death among people ages 10–14 and 25–34 and the third leading cause of death among people ages 15–24 (National Institutes of Health, 2022). Thoughts about suicide are also much more common than most people think: in 2020, 4.9% of adults thought of suicide and 11.3% of young adults ages 18–25 (Ibid).

WARNING SIGNS

Some people who commit suicide do so without ever talking about it. While it can be difficult to determine if someone is suicidal, research has identified several common warning signs that may indicate an increased risk for attempting suicide. The national Substance Abuse and Mental Health Administration (SAMHSA, 2023) provides the following information about warning signs of suicide:

- Talking about wanting to die or kill oneself
- Looking for a way to kill oneself
- Talking about being a burden to others
- Increasing the use of alcohol or drugs
- Acting anxious or agitated; behaving recklessly
- Sleeping too little or too much
- Withdrawing or feeling isolated
- Showing rage or talking about seeking revenge
- Displaying extreme mood swings

The risk of suicide is greater if the behavior is new, or has increased, and if it seems related to a painful event, loss, or change.

CONDUCTING A SUICIDE ASSESSMENT

When helping professionals suspect that a client may be at risk for suicide, they conduct an immediate risk assessment and take appropriate action.

Keep in mind that thoughts of death are common among survivors of trauma. Trauma, after all, is characterized by a threat of death or annihilation, so thoughts and dreams (or nightmares) about death are fairly common. The challenge is to distinguish between these common passive thoughts of death and an intention to kill oneself. Suicidality is not having a dream that you die or wishing or fantasizing about death. Suicidality is defined as having a desire and a specific plan to kill yourself, including the means or method (such as guns, poison, pills, or a plan to drown, etc.).

The Substance Abuse and Mental Health Services Administration emphasizes that *"Everyone has a role in preventing suicide."* They provide the following guidelines for what to do if you think someone is considering suicide (SAMHSA, 2023):

- **Call or text 988** to reach the 988 Suicide and Crisis Lifeline to talk to a caring professional.
- **Ask them** if they are thinking about killing themselves. This will not put the idea into their head or make it more likely that they will attempt suicide.
- **Listen without judging** and show you care.
- **Stay with the person** or make sure the person is in a private, secure place with another caring person until you can get further help.
- **Remove any objects** that could be used in a suicide attempt.

The key to screening a client for the risk of suicide is to speak directly and in plain language. Ask them if they have any plans to kill themselves or commit suicide (don't use vague language like "Are you planning to hurt yourself?"). You may also explain why you are asking these questions, emphasizing your concern for the client's safety and welfare. If a client tells you that they plan to kill themselves, ask them how and when they plan to kill themselves. The risk for suicide is higher if the client has a specific plan in mind.

CASE STUDY   Tony Hernandez *(continued)*

CHW: Tony, we have a protocol that requires us to ask about suicide whenever we work with someone who has experienced trauma. Can you tell me if you've had any thoughts of killing yourself?

Tony: Well, I have dreams and thoughts . . . . Sometimes I think about what would have happened if Leroy had gone in the house instead of me. Like, why did it have to be him, you know? It could've been me.

CHW: Those dreams and thoughts are really common for people who survive trauma.

Tony: They are?

CHW: Yes. Have you had thoughts of killing yourself?

Tony: No, nothing like that.

CHW: Have you ever tried to kill yourself before?

Tony: No. I mean, I've been depressed . . . Thinking about my mom and after my break-up. But I've never thought about killing myself.

CHW: The reason we ask is to try to protect your safety. Other providers may also ask you about your risks for suicide, so I want you to be prepared and to try to understand why we bring up this topic.

Tony: I understand.

CHW: If you did start to feel suicidal, is there someone who you think you would talk to about this?

Tony: I don't know. I guess what I can say is that If I started to feel that way I'd try to tell someone. But I'm here because I want to move forward with my life.

If a client tells you they intend to kill themselves, you have a legal and ethical duty to report it immediately. **Contact your supervisor—or any available licensed colleague or supervisor—right away.** For example, if you are in the office, clinic, or hospital, ask for a supervisor to join you and the client. When the supervisor arrives, let them take the lead in assessing the client and determining what further actions may be necessary. If a licensed colleague is not available, call the designated number for the local Crisis Response Team. Some cities and counties designate EMT/Paramedics or other emergency response providers to respond to reports of a suicidal person and others use the police. Make sure to review your employer's policies and know what agency and number to call to report that a client is suicidal.

Wait with the client until the crisis response team arrives. If the crisis response team finds an immediate threat of suicide, they will transport the client to a local hospital for further assessment. The client may be held in a hospital unit for several days (typically up to 72 hours) and closely monitored to prevent harm.

Sometimes a client who reports that they are suicidal will ask or plead with you not to call a supervisor or 911. They may be highly emotional and possibly very angry with you. Keep in mind that—regardless of what the client wants in this situation—if they have disclosed that they are suicidal, you have a legal and ethical duty to make a report right away. Your duty to protect a client from potential harm outweighs any other ethical duties such as the duty to protect their privacy.

Remember to document the incident as soon as possible. Write down the date, time, and location of your interaction with the client, what they reported to you, the actions that you took, and the names of any other professionals or agencies involved.

> **Juanita Alvarado:** I worked with a client who had recently been released from prison and he was utilizing all of the CHW services. He had a lot of mental health issues and was receiving medication from the primary care doctor here at Transitions. He tested dirty [a test indicated that he was using drugs] and was denied pain medications. He was very upset and was determined to jump in front of the T train. I stood by him, calmed him down, and just listened to him; I didn't care how long it was going to take. Just really listening to him, talking positive to him and what he had to look forward to instead of focusing on the pain meds and how he could get back on them. I tried to reassure him that not everyone was going to look at him like a liar and gave him a lot of positive reinforcement. After two hours, he was able to calm down. I got him something to eat and I took him to Bayview Mental Health, where a mental health provider evaluated him further. He didn't kill himself and I felt like I did what I could to prevent that.

18.9 Trauma-informed Care

Trauma-informed care is a widely used model for supporting the health and healing of survivors of trauma. It is commonly referenced in the fields of public health, health care, mental health, substance use, child development, education, and other disciplines. It encourages agencies, programs, and professionals to incorporate trauma knowledge and skills into their policies and the services they provide to clients and communities.

The U.S. Substance Abuse and Mental Health Services Administration (SAMHSA) developed a framework for a trauma-informed approach (also called trauma-informed care) that can be adapted and applied to any agency serving the public (SAMHSA, 2014b). **Trauma-informed care** includes:

- Understanding the prevalence of trauma and the impact on health and behavior
- Recognizing the effects of trauma on health and behavior
- Training leadership, providers, and staff on responding to clients or patients with best practices in trauma-informed care
- Integrating knowledge about trauma into policies, procedures, practices, and treatment planning
- Avoiding re-traumatization by approaching survivors of trauma with nonjudgmental support

SAMHSA further defines six guiding principles for a trauma-informed approach (Centers for Disease Control and Prevention, 2020; Trauma-Informed Care Implementation Resource Center, 2023; Menschner and Maul, 2016).):

- Safety including the physical and psychological safety of clients and staff
- Trustworthiness and transparency. Policies and decisions should be shared openly with clients.
- *Peer support including people—like CHWs—with shared experiences as part of the direct services team.*

- Collaboration and mutuality including a commitment to naming and working to resolve conflicts and to shift power and share decision-making.
- Empowerment, voice, and choice. The strengths of clients and staff should be recognized, validated, and developed.
- Cultural and historical issues including a recognition historical trauma and discrimination and the goal of promoting health equity.

These principles are intended to guide all aspects of an agency's operations including how clients are viewed and treated, how services are delivered and how staff are trained and supervised. It requires a commitment from the highest levels of the organization; policies and procedures that support recovery and avoid re-traumatizing clients; budgets for appropriate services including peer support; ongoing training and workforce development; and the engagement and involvement of trauma survivors and family members in designing and improving programs.

For CHWs and other direct service providers, trauma-informed practice means:

- Being well-trained to understanding what trauma is, how common it is, and how survivors are affected (trauma responses)
- Understanding how trauma exposure can influence current health, mental health, and addiction risks and status
- Paying attention to signs that a client may have a trauma history
- Learning to talk comfortably with clients and to assess for trauma symptoms/responses
- The application of harm reduction principles to avoid unintentional harm to survivors who disclose a history of trauma
- Practicing person-centered skills—including cultural humility and a strength-based approach—that promote client autonomy and their unique paths for healing
- Providing referrals to appropriate community-based resources including resources for mental health and legal services.

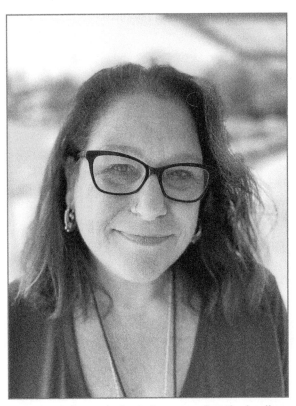

CHWs can play a vital role in supporting the healing of survivors of trauma.

While the trauma-informed care model is widely promoted within the United States, some people have critiqued how well it fully encompasses diverse experiences of trauma and the extent to which it is fully implemented (Hunger, 2018). Others have called for new models such as healing-centered engagement (Ginwright, 2018). Ginwright argues for an approach that promotes a more holistic view of healing from trauma, including civic action and collective healing rather than emphasizing individual experiences. Healing-centered engagement is strength-based and supports people's autonomy or independence in setting aspirations or goals, taking action, and creating meaning of their own experiences. It emphasizes the importance of people's cultures, identities and relationships (Holdsworth & Ash, 2023).

Over the course of your career as a CHW, new concepts, language, and approaches to working with survivors of trauma will continue to emerge. The more you learn about trauma responses and recovery, and the more confidence you gain in listening to your client's stories, the better prepared you will be to support clients in their healing. For more information about trauma-informed practice, see the resources provided at the end of this chapter.

18.10 Secondary Trauma, Secondary Resilience

Licensed and unlicensed helping professionals, including CHWs, who work closely with survivors of trauma are at risk for developing signs of secondary trauma. However, they also benefit from secondary resilience.

SECONDARY TRAUMA

CHWs can be profoundly affected by their work with survivors of trauma. Over time, through witnessing the trauma stories of clients or community members, you may begin to develop **secondary trauma** or signs and symptoms of traumatic stress. These symptoms may include intrusive thoughts related to trauma stories, nightmares, and difficulty concentrating. Common emotional responses include sadness or despair, numbness, fear, anger, guilt, or shame. You may also experience irritability, fatigue, avoidance, isolation, and nightmares. Your perceptions of situations may become distorted, seeing threats where there are none, or the opposite reaction, becoming insensitive to violence or danger.

In other words, even if the helping professional themselves is not a survivor of trauma, they may develop trauma responses/symptoms through their exposure to the stories of the survivors they work with.

> **Christina**: Working with victims of sexual exploitation and trafficking, I saw directly how important it was for the organization to have safeguards and support for the staff. When that wasn't in place—not enough supervision, unclear boundaries and protocols, unreasonable workload—it made me feel overwhelmed and isolated. I was essentially the duck appearing to be calm on the surface but, underneath, desperately paddling to stay afloat. I was definitely experiencing secondary trauma, such as a sense of hopelessness and despair in the world, intrusive thoughts, and inability to be intimate with my partner. I found myself hiding away from the world, smoking marijuana, and playing video games. What helped me most was the support and understanding from my friends and taking a step back from my work to focus on my education and self-care.

Of course, some helping professionals are also survivors of trauma and working with clients can re-stimulate or intensify their own stories and responses.

If you work closely with survivors of trauma, it is important to know that you may be at risk for developing secondary trauma, and to adapt a regular practice of self-care (addressed later on in this chapter).

SECONDARY RESILIENCE

Helping professionals who work closely with survivors of trauma may also be positively affected by the extraordinary strength and resilience of clients who have faced and survived horrific trauma (**secondary resilience**).

Working closely with survivors provides an opportunity to witness their creativity, courage, generosity, and resilience. Over time, CHWs and other helping professionals may begin to internalize and benefit from these positive qualities. In this way, working with survivors can be tremendously hopeful and inspiring.

In the Presence of Perseverance

Janey Skinner: Whenever I think something is too hard or too inconvenient for me—that I just can't make it to another meeting, rally, or fundraiser—I think of Simon, a subsistence farmer in Guatemala who was active in a human rights organization I knew well. Simon always made it to the protests in the capital. He didn't miss one—he came to march, or to speak, or just to be counted among the many rallying for human rights and against the state-sponsored repression that was all too common then. To do so, Simon had to get up at three in the morning, walk four hours to the road, then take a bus another four hours to the capital. The busses were crowded—he often made the whole trip standing in the aisle. But what touched me most was his quiet seven-year-old son, always stuck to his father's side. He too had walked those four hours to the road, every time, and ridden the bus standing in the aisle. I think of Simon and his son, and all my excuses for not showing up just fade away. Their persistence seemed to spring from unshakable beliefs and the strength they found in taking action with others. I'm grateful if even a little bit of their resilience rubbed off on me.

While it's impossible to control how you are affected by working with survivors, we believe that focusing on the client's resilience can enhance your own. Take time to apply a strength-based analysis and to identify and consider aspects of a survivor's recovery that you find courageous, creative, or inspirational.

- *In what ways do survivors of trauma teach or inspire you?*

What Do
YOU?
Think

18.11 Self-care

The work of CHWs can be both highly rewarding and highly stressful. The success and longevity of your career will be significantly enhanced by your ability to regularly practice skills for stress management and self-care. Self-care is even more important if you work closely with survivors of trauma because of the risks of secondary trauma.

Please review Chapter 12 on Stress and Health. Take a few minutes to reflect on your own history of practicing self-care:

- *What time in your day (today or yesterday) provided a moment of calm, relaxation, or relief from stress?*
- *How do you care for yourself at the end of a difficult working day?*
- *What types of activities best help you to release and reduce the impacts of stress?*

If your self-care practices aren't providing enough relief from stress, research and identify new practices that might work for you. If you need help, reach out and talk with someone who may be more accomplished in their self-care practice. This may be a co-worker or supervisor, your own physician or therapist, or someone else in your local community. Some self-care practices that may be relevant to you include:

- Ongoing counseling, therapy or other healing practices
- Mindfulness, meditation, prayer, and other stress-reduction techniques
- Taking time to reflect on your accomplishments and skills. Provide yourself with the same type of Affirmations that you offer to the clients you work with
- Regular self-assessment for developing signs of secondary trauma
- Regular supervision in which you talk about how working with trauma survivors is affecting you

- Movement, yoga, stretching, exercise, or other physical activity to reduce anxiety and manage stress
- Prayer or other spiritual or religious practices
- Seeking support from your own external resources such as family, friends, or community-based programs and organizations

Faith Fabiani: Besides practicing strategic self-care, which means identifying where your stress symptoms are showing up (mentally, emotionally, cognitively, etc.) and using a self-care strategy that addresses that specific category, you need to have your own line of support.

You need people you can call to either talk to about your day or perhaps the opposite; maybe it's folks you can go out with and have some fun with. Whatever works for you, but you cannot do this alone.

One of my favorite quotes regarding this subject is by Rachel Naomi Remen, "The expectation that we can be immersed in suffering and loss daily and not be touched by it is as unrealistic as expecting to be able to walk through water without getting wet" (Remen, 2023). You will be affected. That's not in question; it's about making sure you're supported when it happens.

Work to develop and refine your own realistic action plan for self-care. *Start today.* Take five minutes to write down one or two ways that you can better manage stress. Then take the time—as soon as you can—to put one of these ideas into action. Remember that self-care doesn't need to be complicated, expensive, or time consuming. A good option for many people may be some form of mindfulness practice (again, see Chapter 12) such as five of deep breathing. It can be as simple as:

Breathe in through your nose as you count to four, hold your breath for four counts, and breath out through your mouth for six counts. Repeat. Do it two or three more times.

- *How do you feel now?*
- *Do you notice a difference?*

Swimming Laps at the End of the Day: Anonymous

I worked at a rape crisis center. I talked with survivors and their family members in person and over the phone. Sometimes I accompanied survivors undergoing forensic exams at the local county hospital in the aftermath of a rape. This work was deeply meaningful. I had amazing co-workers, and the agency provided regular supervision with a therapist to help me talk about how the work affected me, and to identify challenges along the way.

Still, it was sometimes difficult for me to separate work and my personal life. I brought the stories and the emotions home with me. I had nightmares that included details that clients told me about their own experiences. And I had nightmares about not being able to help my clients.

On my way home from work, I noticed a pool. I started to swim laps after work. I swam until I was exhausted and, as I swam, I imagined the stories that clients told me, their fear and sorrow, melting into the water. When I stepped out of the pool, I imagined leaving the stories, and their emotions, behind in the water, a safe and protected place.

This routine helped me to create a better transition back to my personal life. I started to sleep better. And this, in turn, gave me more energy for my work.

18.12 Ongoing Professional Development

We encourage you to participate in opportunities to enhance your knowledge and skills for working with survivors of trauma. Workshops and trainings are available online and local organizations may also offer training and, in some cases, certification. Many organizations offer free training in exchange for a volunteer commitment of a certain number of hours each week or month for a specified number of months. Options may include:

- Suicide prevention and crisis intervention agencies and hotlines
- Rape crisis centers
- Domestic violence shelters and hotlines
- Hospitals and departments of public health/health services
- Local colleges and universities. For example, City College of San Francisco offers several courses designed to prepare frontline providers to work in preventing violence and providing services to survivors of trauma.

Chapter Review

To review the key concepts and skills addressed in this chapter, take time to reflect upon the following questions.

1. **Test your general knowledge about trauma by answering the following questions:**
   - How would you define and explain trauma if you were making a presentation to a local community group?
   - What kinds of events or situations are likely to cause traumatic stress?
   - How does trauma impact survivors? What are some common responses to trauma?
   - What are some possible pathways or strategies for healing from trauma?
   - How does culture, status, and identity impact trauma responses and healing?
   - What are some local resources, such as agencies, programs, or providers who offer services to survivors of trauma?
   - If you currently work as a CHW, how does trauma show up in your work? What do you currently do to support clients and communities affected by trauma, and what new ideas did you get from the chapter that might enhance your practice?

2. **Consider how you will work with a client who decides to tell you about a trauma experience.**
   - As a CHW, what is your scope of practice when working with survivors of trauma? If you currently work as a CHW, what policies or programs at your organization might be important when working with a trauma survivor?
   - Why are issues of autonomy and control particularly important to someone who has experienced trauma?
   - How might you use person-centered counseling in your work with this person?
   - What is something that you would not want to say to this client? What is something you probably would want to say?
   - How will you assess the client's possible risk for suicide?
   - What fears or concerns come up for you when you imagine working with a client who wants to talk about a trauma experience? Where can you go to get advice, support, or information to help you address those concerns?

3. **Review the Client Scenario about Tony Hernandez presented throughout this chapter (including each of the conversations between Tony and the CHW).** What person-centered skills does the CHW demonstrate? For example, can you identify examples of when the CHW:
   - Demonstrates a strength-based approach
   - Supports the client's autonomy and self-determination

- Asks open-ended questions
- Provides an affirmation
- Demonstrates reflective listening
- Assesses Tony's risks for suicide
- Provides Tony with a referral to a licensed provider
- Supports Tony to develop an action plan

4. **Professional Development and Self-care**
   - What are secondary trauma and secondary resilience? How may they affect you, personally and at work? Have you experienced either one?
   - What self-care practices do you regularly practice to manage your stress and prevent burnout? What additional self-care practices would you like to try?
   - What is your professional development plan for learning more about trauma? What aspects of trauma do you most want to explore? Which skills for working with survivors do you most want to enhance? Where or how can you access resources to build your knowledge and skills?
   - Identify one professional development opportunity that you can engage with in the six months that will enhance your knowledge and skills for working with survivors of trauma.

References

The American Psychiatric Association. (2021). How Historical Trauma Impacts Native Americans Today. https://www.psychiatry.org/News-room/APA-Blogs/How-Historical-Trauma-Impacts-Native-Americans (accessed 20 April 2023).

The American Psychiatric Association. (2023). Diagnostic and Statistical Manual of Disorders (DSM-5-TR). https://www.psychiatry.org/psychiatrists/practice/dsm (accessed 25 January 2023).

American Psychological Association. (2023). Trauma. https://www.apa.org/topics/trauma#:~:text=Trauma%20is%20an%20emotional%20response,symptoms%20like%20headaches%20or%20nausea. (accessed 22 April 2023).

Barzoki, H. S, Ebrahimi, M., Khoshdel, A., Noorbala, A. A., Rahnejat, A. M., & Avarzamani, L. (2021). *Studying the prevalence of PTSD in veterans*. Combatants and Freed Soldiers of Iran-Iraq War: A Systematic and Meta-analysis Review. Psychology, Health & Medicine. https://doi.org/10.1080/13548506.2021.1981408.

Benjet C. B. E, Karam, E. G., Kessler, R. C., McLaughlin, K. A., Ruscio, A. M., Shahly, V., Stein, D. J., et al. (2016). The epidemiology of traumatic event exposure worldwide: results from the World Mental Health Survey Consortium. *Psychological Medicine*. https://doi: 10.1017/S0033291715001981.

The Centers for Disease Control and Prevention. (2020). Infographic: 6 Building Principles to a Trauma-Informed Approach. https://www.cdc.gov/orr/infographics/6_principles_trauma_info.htm (accessed 21 April 2023).

The Centers for Disease Control and Prevention. (2021). Adverse Childhood Experiences (ACEs). Vital Signs. https://www.cdc.gov/vitalsigns/aces/index.html. (accessed 21 April 2023).

The Centers for Disease Control and Prevention. (2022). Fast Facts: Preventing Adverse Childhood Experiences. https://www.cdc.gov/violenceprevention/aces/fastfact.html (accessed 21 April 2023).

Chentsova-Dutton, Y. & Maercker, A. (2019). *Cultural scripts of traumatic stress: Outline*. Illustrations and Research Opportunities: Frontiers in Psychology. https://doi.org/10.3389/fpsyg.2019.02528.

Degruy, J. (2023). Post Traumatic Slave Syndrome. https://www.joydegruy.com/ (accessed 20 April 2023).

Ervin, S., Jagannath, J., & Zweig, J. M. (2020). Addressing Trauma and Victimization in Women's Prisons: Trauma-Informed Victim Services and Programs for Incarcerated Women. The Urban Institute. https://www.urban.org/sites/default/files/publication/103017/addressing-trauma-and-victimization-in-womens-prisons.pdf (accessed 26 January 2023).

Franco, F. (2021). Understanding Intergenerational Trauma: An Introduction for Clinicians. Good Therapy. https://www.goodtherapy.org/blog/Understanding_Intergenerational_Trauma (accessed 21 April 2023).

Ginwright, S. (2018). The Future of Healing: Shifting from Trauma Informed Care to Healing Centered Engagement. https://ginwright.medium.com/the-future-of-healing-shifting-from-trauma-informed-care-to-healing-centered-engagement-634f557ce69c Ginwrigt.medium.com (accessed 23 April 2023).

Government of Canada. (2023). The Impact of Trauma on Adult Sexual Assault Victims. https://www.justice.gc.ca/eng/rp-pr/jr/trauma/p4.html (accessed 24 April 2023).

Health Care Toolbox. (2023). What is Culturally-Sensitive Trauma-Informed Care? https://www.healthcare-toolbox.org/culturally-sensitive-trauma-informed-care (accessed 21 April 2023).

Herman, J. L. (1997). *Trauma and recovery: The aftermath of violence—from domestic abuse to political terror.* New York, NY: Basic Books.

Holdsworth, S. Ash, M. (2023). RECOVER. https://www.urbanwellnessedmonton.com/stories/from-trauma-informed-to-healing-centered (accessed 23 April 2023).

Hunger, N. (2018). Trauma Outside the Box: How "Trauma-Informed" Trend Falls Short. Mad in America. https://www.madinamerica.com/2018/11/trauma-informed-trend-falls-short/ (accessed 23 April 2023).

International Society for Traumatic Stress Studies. (2023). Traumatic Stress and Substance Abuse Problems. https://istss.org/ISTSS_Main/media/Documents/ISTSS_TraumaStressandSubstanceAbuseProb_English_FNL.pdf (accessed 22 April 2023).

Kessler, R. C., Aguilar-Gaxiola, S., Alonso, J, Benjet, C., Bromet, E. J., Cardoso, G., Degenhardt, L, et al. (2017). Trauma and PTSD in the WHO World Mental Health Surveys European Journal of Psychotraumatology. https://doi: 10.1080/20008198.2017.1353383 (accessed 21 April 2023).

Kok, M. (2021). *The role of CHWs in fragile and conflict-affected settings.* CHW Central: KIT Royal Tropical Institute. https://chwcentral.org/twg_article/the-role-of-chws-in-fragile-and-conflict-affected-settings/.

Lim, I. C. Z. Y., Tam, W. W. S., Chudzicka-Czupala, A., McIntyre, R. S., Teopiz, K. M. Ho, R. C., & Ho, C. S. (2022). Prevalence of depression, anxiety and post-traumatic stress in war-and conflict-afflicted areas: a meta-analysis. *Frontiers in Psychiatry.* https:// doi: 10.3389/fpsyt.2022.978703.

Loo, C. M. (2014). PTSD Among Ethnic Minority Veterans. National Center for PTSD, U.S. Department of Veterans Affairs. http://www.ptsd.va.gov/professional/treatment/cultural/ptsd-minority-vets.asp (accessed 22 April 2023).

Mendelsohn, M., Herman, J. L., Schatzow, E., Coco, M., Kallivayalil, D., & Levitan, J. (2011). *The trauma recovery group: A guide for practitioners.* New York, NY: Guilford Press.

Menschner, C. & Maul, A. (2016). Key Ingredients for Successful Trauma-Informed Care Implementation. Center for Health Care Strategies. https://www.samhsa.gov/sites/default/files/programs_campaigns/childrens_mental_health/atc-whitepaper-040616.pdf (accessed 24 April 2023).

Mollica, R. F. (2009). *Healing invisible wounds: Paths to healing and recovery in a violent world.* Nashville, TN: Vanderbilt University Press.

Najavits. (2002). *Seeking safety: A treatment manual for PTSD and substance use.* New York: The Guilford Press.

The National Center for PTSD. (2023a). Combat Exposure. U.S. Department of Veterans Affairs. https://www.ptsd.va.gov/understand/types/combat_exposure.asp (accessed 26 January 2023).

The National Center for PTSD. (2023b). How Common is PTSD in Children? U.S. Department of Veterans Affairs. https://www.ptsd.va.gov/understand/common/common_children_teens.asp (accessed 26 January 2023).

The National Center for PTSD. (2023c). How Common is PTSD in Adults? U.S. Department of Veterans Affairs. https://www.ptsd.va.gov/understand/common/common_adults.asp (accessed 26 January 2023).

The National Center for PTSD. (2023d). Choosing a Treatment. https://www.ptsd.va.gov/understand_tx/choose_tx.asp (accessed 26 January 2023).

The National Council for Behavioral Health. (2023). How to Manage Trauma. National Council for Mental Wellbeing. https://www.thenationalcouncil.org/wp-content/uploads/2022/08/Trauma-infographic.pdf (accessed 26 January 2023).

National Institute for the Clinical Application of Behavioral Medicine. (2023). Infographic: How Trauma Impacts Four Different Types of Memory. https://www.naadac.org/assets/2416/2019NWRC_Michael_Bricker_Handout4.pdf (accessed 24 April 2023).

National Institutes of Health. (2022). Suicide. https://www.nimh.nih.gov/health/statistics/suicide (accessed 20 April 2023).

Remen, N. R. (2023). Leaning In. Supportive Care. https://supportivecarecoalition.org/cultivating-professional-resilience/2018/7/10/leaning-in (accessed 19 June 2023).

Stanford Medicine. (2023). Historical Trauma. https://geriatrics.stanford.edu/ethnomed/alaskan/introduction/history.html (accessed 20 April 2023).

Stress & Trauma Evaluation and Psychological Services. (2022). What is Intergenerational or Historical Trauma? https://traumaprofessionals.com/what-is-intergenerational-or-historical-trauma/ (accessed 20 April 2023).

Substance Abuse and Mental Health Services Administration (SAMHSA). (2014a). Recovery and Recovery Support. http://www.samhsa.gov/recovery (accessed 24 April 2023).

Substance Abuse and Mental Health Services Administration. (2014b). SAMHSA's Concept of Trauma and Guidance for a Trauma-Informed Approach. https://store.samhsa.gov/sites/default/files/d7/priv/sma14-4884.pdf (accessed 23 April 2023).

Substance Abuse and Mental Health Services Administration. (2022). Understanding Child Trauma. U.S. Department of Health & Human Services. https://www.samhsa.gov/child-trauma/understanding-child-trauma (accessed 26 January 2023).

Substance Abuse & Mental Health Services Administration. (2023). Preventing Suicide. https://www.samhsa.gov/suicide#:~:text=Everyone%20has%20a%20role%20to,painful%20for%20family%20and%20friends. (accessed 20 April 2023).

Terr, L. (1990). *Too scared to cry: Psychic trauma in childhood.* New York, NY: Basic Books.

Werner, K., Kak, M. Herbst, C. H., & Lin, T. K. (2022). The role of community health worker-based care in post-conflict settings: a systematic review. *Health Policy and Planning.* https://doi.org/10.1093/heapol/czac072.

Widra, E. (2020). No Escape: The trauma of Witnessing Violence in Prison. Prison Policy Initiative. https://www.prisonpolicy.org/blog/2020/12/02/witnessing-prison-violence/#:~:text=Even%20before%20entering%20a%20prison,of%20the%20general%20male%20population. (accessed 26 January 2023).

The World Health Organization. (2021). Mental health and forced displacement. https://www.who.int/news-room/fact-sheets/detail/mental-health-and-forced-displacement (accessed 26 January 2023).

Additional Resources

The Columbia Lighthouse Project. (2023). The Columbia Suicide Severity Rating Scale (C-SSRS). https://cssrs.columbia.edu/the-columbia-scale-c-ssrs/about-the-scale/ (accessed 20 April 2023).

Beristain, C. M. (2010). *Manual sobre la perspectiva psicosocial en la investigación de los derechos humanos.* Bilbao, Spain: Hegoa.

de Jong, K. (2011). Psychosocial and Mental Health Interventions in Areas of Mass Violence: A Community-based Approach (2nd ed.). Retrieved from http://www.msf.org/sites/msf.org/files/old-cms/source/mentalhealth/guidelines/MSF_mentalhealthguidelines.pdf.

Dillman, S. M. (2010). Phases of Trauma Healing: Part 1, Establishing Safety. Good Therapy. https://www.goodtherapy.org/blog/phases-of-trauma-healing-part-i-establishing-safety/ (accessed 21 April 2023).

Malchiodi, C. A. (2020). *Trauma and expressive arts therapy*. New York. The Guildford Press.

Manion, L. (2020). What Safety Means as a Trauma Survivor. National Alliance on Mental Illness. https://www.nami.org/Blogs/NAMI-Blog/September-2020/What-Safety-Means-as-a-Trauma-Survivor (accessed 21 April 2023).

National Center for PTSD. (2023). PTSD and DSM-5. U.S. Department of Veterans Affairs. https://www.ptsd.va.gov/professional/treat/essentials/dsm5_ptsd.asp (accessed 20 April 2023).

Saul, J. (2014). *Collective trauma, collective healing: Promoting community resilience in the aftermath of disaster*. New York, NY: Routledge.

Stevenson, K. M. & Rall, J. (2007). Transforming the trauma of torture, flight and resettlement. In M. Bussey & J.B. Wise (Eds.), *Trauma transformed: An empowerment response* (pp. 236–258). New York, NY: Columbia University Press.

Substance Abuse and Mental Health Services Administration. (2023). Suicide Assessment Five-step Evaluation and Triage (AFE-T) cards. https://store.samhsa.gov/product/SAFE-T-Pocket-Card-Suicide-Assessment-Five-Step-Evaluation-and-Triage-for-Clinicians/sma09-4432 (accessed 20 April 2023).

Trauma-Informed Care Implementation Resource Center. (2023). What is Trauma-Informed Care? https://www.traumainformedcare.chcs.org/what-is-trauma-informed-care/ (accessed 21 April 2023).

WORKING WITH GROUPS AND COMMUNITIES

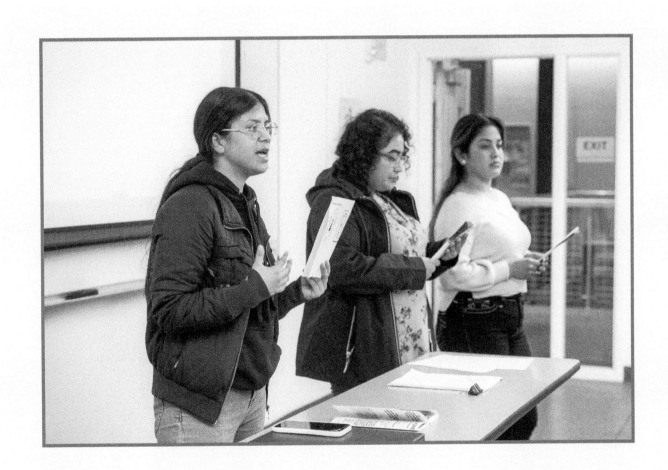

Community Health Outreach

Thelma Gamboa-Maldonado

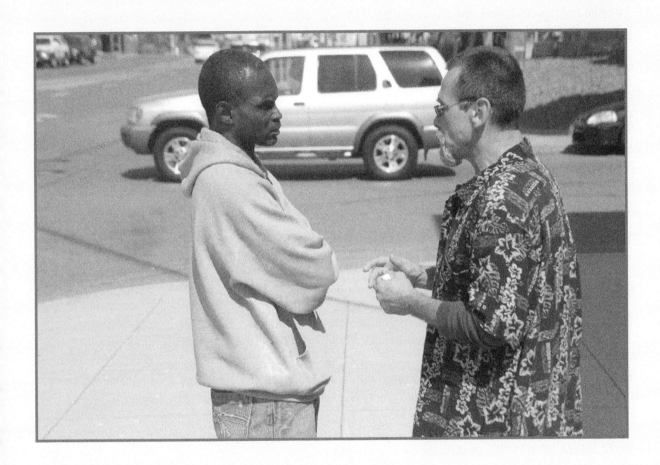

Foundations for Community Health Workers, Third Edition. Edited by Tim Berthold and Darouny Somsanith.
© 2024 John Wiley & Sons, Inc. Published 2024 by John Wiley & Sons, Inc.
Companion website: http://www.wiley.com/go/communityhealthworkers3E

CHW Scenario

Imagine that it is the height of the COVID-19 pandemic (or that another highly infectious airborne virus has emerged), and an effective vaccine has been developed.

The number of infections, hospitalizations, and deaths are still rising in your community and around the world. There is much uncertainty, fear, and conflicting information about the vaccines.

You have been hired as a CHW by a local health department that is concerned about the increasing rates of COVID-19 in an immigrant community of the county.

Your job is to conduct outreach to the immigrant community, to provide them with information about the disease, address vaccine hesitancy, and to support them in preventing new infections and in accessing local clinics for screening and vaccination.

How would you begin your outreach work?

- What do you want to know before you start to conduct outreach? What types of information will you gather?
- How will you build relationships with the community to be served? How will you gather community input into the design of your outreach efforts?
- What types of outreach methods will you use?
- How will you document the outreach services you provide?
- How would you know if your outreach program was successful?

Introduction

This chapter is an introduction to community health outreach. Outreach links vulnerable communities to programs and services designed to promote their health. Most CHWs participate in some level of outreach during their career.

We hope that by the end of the chapter, you feel more prepared to answer the questions posed above and to bring your own experience, personality, and creativity to the task of conducting health outreach.

WHAT YOU WILL LEARN

By studying the information in this chapter, you will be able to:

- Define community health outreach
- Discuss the types of communities served and the health issues addressed through outreach
- Identify and provide examples of different outreach levels and methods
- Describe and apply strategies for approaching people you do not know
- Identify key safety concerns and strategies for outreach workers
- Document outreach services accurately and explain the importance of doing so

C3 Roles and Skills Addressed in Chapter 19

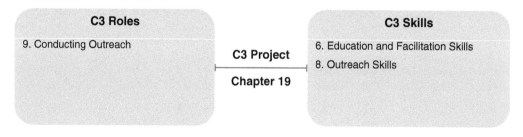

C3 Roles	C3 Project	C3 Skills
9. Conducting Outreach	Chapter 19	6. Education and Facilitation Skills 8. Outreach Skills

WORDS TO KNOW

Cost-effectiveness

Key Opinion Leaders

Priority Population

Reach

Social Marketing

Venue

19.1 Defining Community Health Outreach

Community health outreach is the process of identifying and establishing positive relationship with communities to engage them in services or to assist with the development of community-specific health programs. Outreach provides health-related services to vulnerable communities. Typically, the community to be served is selected due to higher rates of health conditions or challenges such as cancer, cardiovascular disease or other chronic health conditions, an infectious disease, substance use, or challenges such as food insecurity or being unhoused. Community health outreach is a temporary initiative that engages the community to collaborate in undertaking a purposeful health intervention to reach the population at health risk (Shin, Kim, & Kang, 2020).

Additional goals for health outreach may include to:

- Increase awareness about a particular health issue (such as breast cancer)
- Promote health knowledge and changes in health behaviors (such as regular breast self-exams and mammogram screenings)
- Recruit participants for research (such as research on the effectiveness of specific breast cancer treatment options)
- Establish links to and partnerships between existing communities and existing health programs (such as between a local church and a women's health clinic)
- Increase community participation in the design, implementation, and evaluation of health programs and policies (such as development of new outreach programs to assist women of color in gaining access to breast cancer screening and treatment services)
- Mobilize community members to participate in community organizing and advocacy efforts (such as expanded access to health care)

- *Can you think of other goals for conducting health outreach?*

19.2 Qualities of Successful Community Health Outreach Workers

Health outreach programs are often designed to work with communities who have experienced discrimination and who may face significant prejudice from the larger society, such as people with a history of incarceration, drug use, homelessness, or mental health conditions. It is sometimes difficult for an outsider to gain entry to the identified community and to build the trust required to provide effective services. For these reasons, public health programs typically recruit outreach workers from the communities to be served, with an emphasis on hiring culturally and linguistically competent CHWs.

At the height of the COVID-19 pandemic, CHWs were well-positioned to reach communities that were hardest hit and at high risk for COVID-19 exposure, infection, and illness. CHWs were key in providing culturally appropriate health education about disease prevention and promoting testing and vaccination to stop the spread of the disease (National Association of CHWs, 2023; Salve et al., 2023). At the risk of contracting COVID-19 themselves or spreading it to their loved ones, CHWs played a pivotal role during the pandemic by bridging gaps between health care systems and communities. CHWs served as trusted sources of information, disseminating accurate and up-to-date knowledge about COVID-19 transmission, prevention measures, and vaccination. They conducted community outreach programs, distributed educational materials, and organized awareness campaigns to ensure that individuals had access to reliable information and understood the importance of following public health guidelines. They helped address the unique challenges faced by marginalized communities during the pandemic, including language barriers and cultural considerations.

Of course, not all outreach workers come from the communities to be served. Regardless of whether or not they are already familiar with the community, successful CHWs tend to share the personal qualities outlined in Chapter 1, including self-awareness, open-mindedness, and interpersonal warmth. In addition, because all CHWs spend so much of their time building new relationships in the community, it is helpful to be:

- A "people person" who is good at talking with strangers as well as acquaintances
- Easy-going and approachable
- *Extremely* patient
- Viewed as trustworthy by others, someone people feel comfortable talking to about personal issues
- Capable of earning the respect of all members of the community (and, sometimes even more important, someone who will not alienate particular subgroups within the community)
- Flexible and able to adapt to a variety of different working conditions
- Creative and willing to "think outside the box" to engage people
- Attentive to the needs of communities and individual contacts
- Highly organized in maintaining outreach information, resources, and materials

- *What other qualities do you think may be especially important for outreach workers?*

One of the biggest mistakes that new outreach workers make is to imitate the style and personality of more experienced CHWs. However, the clients and communities you work with have a sixth sense for anything that is false or fake. Be your authentic self: if you pretend to be something or someone you are not, you will alienate the community and make it harder for them to trust you.

There are as many styles of outreach as there are outreach workers. There is room for all personality types in this profession. Be patient with yourself: with time and experience, you will develop your own unique approach to conducting outreach. Whether you are quiet, energetic, calm, or outgoing, your personality can inform and guide your work as a CHW.

CHW Profile

Francis Julian Montgomery (they/them)

Street Wellness Specialist

Heluna Health

San Francisco Fire Department Street Wellness Response Team

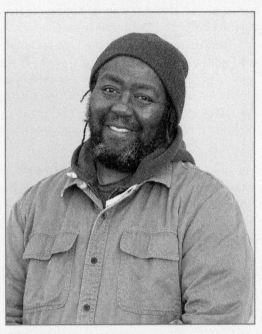

I know where the pain points are and how to connect to people in my communities to appropriate services. What motivated me to become a CHW was the lack of native San Franciscans, African American, and gender nonconforming folks providing direct services in our own communities. I had a strong desire to represent the communities that I participate in, and a desire to help people that look like me.

I am a Street Wellness Specialist working with Community Paramedics as part of the San Francisco Fire Department's Street Wellness Response Team. The goal of the collaboration is to be a team, answering calls, participating in joint field operations anywhere in the city where there are encampments or clusters of unhoused people in tents, or folks in the community, maybe on the sidewalk, experiencing some sort of concerns.

It's a gentle dance, you know. The community paramedics outreach to folks, introduce themselves and complete a wellness check, and if the person is interested in services, I will engage them. I inquire what their priorities are, medical, mental health, treatment, shelter, food, benefits, and other issues they bring up. I complete the consent, enroll, and assess them then link them up with a district outreach specialist, so I don't carry a caseload. We go where we get the call and we're always moving.

Becoming a CHW, learning the structure, the ethics, how to engage folks and have them lead the work has influenced me greatly. I rely heavily on motivational interviewing, continuously honing my skills to prioritize the client's voice, their needs, their readiness, and their priorities. It has always been a privilege to partner with folks who are experiencing some of the most difficult circumstances in their life.

(continues)

CHW Profile
(continued)

In a previous role, I worked with a client in their early thirties, living in their car. Their chronic condition at that time was poorly maintained, and they often ended up in the emergency department through not understanding their medications and the importance of taking them on a regular basis. For the first several weeks, I just spent time building trust, and we got to know each other. What they wanted first was to be safe, a place to get their mail and also work on getting a medical provider. I helped them get into a safe place where they could park their car and there were support services on site - a bathroom, showers, laundry, a microwave. I helped them find a new medical provider, who helped them understand the difference between an intended and unintended side effect of the medication, which improved their health and their trust in health care. And 22 months along in our relationship, they'd applied for and located permanent housing. It sounds bucolic, but it was a lot of hard work. Some folks feel like they're just following someone else's plan rather than their own plan, and it doesn't work for them. This person's success was all due to their trust and hard work. They followed the process, and they stuck to it; that's great.

What I'd say to new CHWs is this: be prepared to listen without preparing a response. You know how sometimes we're talking and we're already thinking about the solution? Be prepared to listen without preparing a response. Be in the moment. After you introduce yourself and share why you are reaching out to them, ask the most open-ended question that will have the greatest profound foundation for the work. How can I help? When people allow you to be a part of their crises or their situations, they already have a sense and an idea about what they need. So ask it. Just put it out there. How can I help?

19.3 Communities to Be Served Through Outreach

The **priority populations** served by outreach efforts are defined by a variety of factors, including epidemiologic and other public health data that document a clear risk for a specific disease or health condition. The communities are also defined by geographical boundaries that may be nationwide, statewide, or within the boundaries of a particular county, city, school district, ZIP code, or neighborhood. Other factors include age, ethnicity, nationality, immigration status, housing status, primary language, income, sexual orientation, gender, gender identity, behaviors (such as the use of injection drugs), and affiliations (such as the members of a particular labor union or religious organization).

Most communities served by outreach lack access to essential health resources and face significant barriers to health, such as poverty, lack of legal status, a history of discrimination, lack of access to educational programs or primary care services, geographic isolation, or homelessness.

Lee Jackson: I do HIV outreach where it's needed most, like in areas where there's a lot of drugs and sex work. If a lot of people are injecting drugs, and people are trading sex for drugs or money, and they don't always use condoms, there's gonna be a high rate of STDs (sexually transmitted diseases), especially HIV.

19.4 Health Issues Addressed by Outreach

Outreach programs address a wide range of health issues including:

- Infectious diseases such as tuberculosis, HIV, malaria, syphilis, hepatitis, COVID-19, and the need for immunizations, contact tracing, and treatment.

- Chronic diseases such as cancer, diabetes, asthma, hypertension, and heart disease

- Drug, alcohol, and tobacco use

- Mental health issues such as depression, posttraumatic stress, schizophrenia, and bipolar disorder

- Accidents and injuries including automobile and pedestrian injuries

- Violence, including domestic violence, police violence, and gun violence

- Environmental and occupational health issues, including exposure to toxins and infectious agents where people live and work

- Access to key health and social services including income, housing, utilities, food, transportation, alcohol and drug treatment, employment, legal services, and primary health care

- Enrollment in free and low-cost health insurance programs including Medicaid and linking community members to new and existing services

- Enrollment in research studies

- Community planning efforts related to local health concerns

- Organizing and advocacy efforts related to health issues

- School-based interventions for children and/or parents.

- Emergency preparedness and response, climate change, and community resilience

- Farm worker health and rights

- Immigrant and employee rights (such as for day laborers)

- *Can you think of other health-related issues to address through outreach?*

What Do
YOU?
Think

The San Francisco Homeless Outreach Team

Cities and counties across the United States are developing new models for responding to public and behavioral health crises. Many of these models incorporate CHWs in prominent roles.

Through the San Francisco Department of Homelessness and Supportive Housing (HSH), the San Francisco Homeless Outreach Team (SFHOT) works to engage and stabilize the most vulnerable individuals by voluntarily placing them into shelter and housing or connecting with other available resources. To make these placements, SFHOT works seven days a week to provide outreach and case management to people experiencing homelessness living on the streets of San Francisco. Services are provided by small, skilled teams with expertise in the complex issues that are barriers to stability for this population. For individuals who are not ready to accept the services HSH has to offer, SFHOT continues to outreach and build motivation to ensure services are available when they are needed.

SFHOT works collaboratively with the Department of Public Health's Street Medicine, San Francisco Fire Departments Community Paramedics, and other teams to address medical and behavioral health needs, using an individualized approach that includes wrap-around services and promotes harm reduction and stability-based recovery.

(continues)

The San Francisco Homeless Outreach Team
(continued)

The Street Wellness Response Team consists of community paramedics and EMTs from the San Francisco Fire Department (SFFD) and Homeless Outreach Team members from the Department of Homelessness and Supportive Housing (HSH). They are dispatched to focus on well-being checks and situations that require immediate attention, but do not meet the threshold of an acute behavioral health crisis. This includes situations such as someone with obvious wounds, people who are lying down or sleeping, or someone inappropriately clothed for the weather.

Francis Julian Montgomery is a CHW with the Street Crisis Response Team. Francis highlights his work and the value of CHWs in crisis response work:

> *It's so important for community health workers to be incorporated in these types of street interventions because CHWs are on the frontlines already. We see people who are unhoused and not accessing services. CHWs know the local providers for health care, shelter and housing assistance, substance use, and mental health services. We have the ability to engage people in a conversation about their priorities and immediate needs.*

> *The SF HOT Team has vans that are equipped to transport more than one person, so we can take people directly to services that they want or need. We'll take them to the hospital Emergency Department if that is necessary, or to a health clinic or a shelter or a drop-in center for people who are not doing too well as a result of using substances like fentanyl.*

> *Last month, winter storms started in San Francisco. We came across a community member who we know well. He was unhoused and, in the past, he was not interested in anything we offered. I said, "You know it's really cold and wet out. There are these safe sleep sites where you can go during the day. Nobody's required to stay. There is no check-in or check-out. It's warm and they have blankets and coffee. They have a bathroom, too. It's up to you." And the person said, "Yeah, I'll check it out." They had been telling us "No, no, no," so it was a win that they were willing to accept some assistance. We were worried about what could have happened to him if he'd stayed outside.*

> *We don't take it personally if someone doesn't want to talk with us or if they tell us "No," but it is a success when they start to engage with us and to access services on their own terms."*

For more information about the San Francisco Homeless Outreach Team, please go to https://hsh.sfgov.org/services/the-homelessness-response-system/outreach/homeless-outreach-team/. To learn more about the Street Crisis Response Team go to https://sf.gov/street-crisis-response-team

19.5 Outreach Levels

Outreach programs can operate on the level of the individual, group, institution, or population.

- **Individual level**: CHWs talk one-on-one with individuals, using person-centered practice. The CHW responds to the individual's questions and concerns, and provides health information, counseling, and referrals, as appropriate. CHWs may also provide testing or screening services such as blood pressure screenings.

- **Group level**: CHWs speak with a group from the priority population, such as clients at a homeless shelter, a youth group at a local church, or mothers at a local Supplemental Nutrition Clinic for Women, Infants, and Children (WIC). The CHW provides health education and referrals and addresses the group's questions and concerns.

- **Institutional or community level**: CHWs work with representatives of a specific institution to reach their membership including, for example, schools, labor unions, employment sites, churches, mosques, or temples.

- **Population or society level**: Outreach efforts sometimes focus on a particular population within a city, county, state, or nation. This may include campaigns to reach elders, families with uninsured children, pregnant women, or smokers. Because these populations are large, the outreach methods usually include the use of media such as television, radio, print media, and social media, such as Facebook, Instagram, and TikTok, to promote particular actions such as enrolling in health insurance programs, getting the COVID-19 vaccine, testing for HIV antibodies when pregnant, or the importance of engaging in regular physical activity.

19.6 Common Outreach Methods

CHWs use a wide variety of outreach methods depending on the characteristics of the priority population and their preferred means of communication, the nature of the health issue to be addressed, and the type of health outcomes the program aims to promote.

STREET AND NEIGHBORHOOD OUTREACH

Street outreach requires spending time in a neighborhood with the goal of talking with members of a specific community, such as unhoused or unsheltered youth. CHWs approach clients to start a conversation. While the outreach workers will have specific goals, such as promoting the services of safety net health clinics, the community often has different priorities. In order to build trust and ongoing relationships, CHWs need to listen first to the concerns and questions of community members.

CHWs usually carry outreach materials with them. These may include brochures, lists of referrals, first aid kits, socks and gloves, health resources such as condoms and lubricant, and other incentives such as hygiene kits (including soap, toothpaste and toothbrushes, and so on) for people who are trying to survive on the streets.

Olivia Ortiz: I've worked with people experiencing homelessness in various capacities for 20+ years. When conducting street outreach, it is important for me to approach people's space in the same way I would if I were in someone's home. I am in someone's home. I wait to be invited or asked to enter. I don't touch their positions, move things around, or sit down unless invited to. I begin by making small talk, pleasantries. If I notice we have something in common, like being dog parents, we talk about our commonalities. I carry my supplies like paperwork, vouchers, socks, Band-Aids, etc., in a bag over my shoulder. I would never approach someone with a clipboard in hand or assume that they want socks or toiletries. When working with people experiencing homelessness, it is easy to feel that you are working in a state of emergency, in many ways, you are. As a CHW conducting street outreach it is important for me to conduct myself in a way that allows me to connect with people, not the emergency.

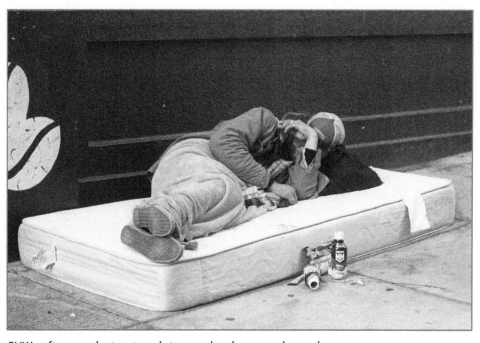

CHWs often conduct outreach to people who are unhoused.

VENUE-BASED OUTREACH

In the public health field, the term *venue-based outreach* refers to outreach strategies that target particular places (a **venue** is a place) where the priority population spends significant time. Venues may include schools, homeless encampments, public housing units, marketplaces and cafes, public transportation stations, barber shops and salons, job sites, day laborer centers, bars and clubs, sports events, parks, and churches, mosques, temples, and other places of worship.

- *Can you think of other venues or places to conduct outreach?*

> **Phuong An Doan Billings:** *At Asian Health Services, we go out and try to connect the underserved populations to our clinic because one of the most important challenges for some communities is getting access to health care. The newcomers (or new immigrants) might be eligible for Healthy Families (health insurance for low-income families) or Medicare, but they don't know about these programs, and they are scared that they will have to pay, or their sponsors will have to pay, so they just stay home. That's why we need the outreach workers to be from the community. We go to English as Second Language (ESL) classes and nail salons and other places where the community is. For the Korean community, we go to small stores, like dry cleaning stores, markets, or churches. To reach the Vietnamese, we also go to the churches. And to temples, pagodas. We go to senior centers too.*

Black and African American beauty salons and barber shops have a long history of serving as venues for health outreach and engagement efforts. These health outreach efforts address a wide variety of health issues including cardiovascular disease, cancer, and type 2 diabetes (Palmer et al., 2021).

Historically, these businesses are places where community members gather and talk about important issues in their lives. Salons and barber shops often have a relaxed atmosphere that fosters social connection and dialogue. Hair stylists are trusted by their clients and therefore serve as a confidante and reliable source of information. This trust is in stark contrast to the mistrust of the medical system and research community common among African Americans. Because of this trust/mistrust, lack of access to quality health care, and culturally appropriate health interventions, Black women are less likely to have a primary care provider. However, it is more common for them to have a regular hair stylist illustrating the significance of routine hair care service.

Beauty salon and barber shop-based interventions have been successful in providing health screenings—such as blood pressure readings—health information and referrals to local services. In one neighborhood, health organizations partnered with a barbershop to screen more than 700 people for high blood pressure in one day (Thomas, 2022). Black beauty salons and barber shops have also been key resources for providing their communities with access to COVID-190 information and vaccinations (Ibid).

RECRUITMENT OF VOLUNTEER PEER EDUCATORS

Sometimes the best way to connect with a particularly hard-to-reach community is to recruit volunteer peer educators. CHWs identify **key opinion leaders** (people whom the community respects and looks to for guidance), build relationships, and ask the leaders to participate in the outreach effort on a volunteer basis. These volunteers may receive formal training in a workshop or informal training via conversations with CHWs. Depending on the nature of the outreach program, volunteers may pass out information or other health resources, provide basic education, and make referrals to local services. Volunteers can assist in an outreach program to reach more members of the priority population. While recruiting volunteers from the community can expand the reach of an outreach program, it is also time consuming and requires thoughtful recruitment, training, and supervision of volunteers. Sometimes these volunteer positions can become paid positions. Agencies may be able to award stipends to volunteers or hire them on a part-time or full-time basis.

Check with your agency to see if there is funding to support the contribution of volunteer peer educators. It is important to recruit diverse and multigenerational members for the outreach team. One way to increase reach is to create a core team of educators and then recruit a web of peer educators.

● *Who are some of the key opinion leaders in the communities where you live and work?*

What Do
YOU?
Think

Working with Key Opinion Leaders

In Oakland, California, the Asian Health Center has organized Patient Leadership Councils to assist in reaching new immigrants. Phuong An Doan Billings: We do outreach to recruit people to be part of the Patient Leadership Council. We try to recruit people from each community that we serve—people who we think have potential, and we train them. We train them in leadership skills and basic knowledge about the clinic and health issues that are big in the community, and they go out and do more outreach to spread the word about the clinic. They talk to their neighbors: "Hey I just came back from Asian Health Services today, and there is something so good about this place." They share this news, answer questions, and encourage people to get health care if they need it. And they advise us about how we can do a better job serving their community.

INSTITUTIONAL OUTREACH

Many communities belong to or are represented by institutions that they trust and respect. Outreach programs can establish partnerships with these institutions to reach a specific community more efficiently. These institutions may include schools, churches, labor unions, clinics or health plans, or artistic, professional, political, or community membership groups.

INTERNET AND MOBILE WEB OUTREACH

As access to the internet, computers, smartphones, and other electronic technology continues to expand, CHWs have developed outreach strategies to take advantage of technology. Electronic and technology-based outreach can take many forms, such as:

● Add a web page to your agency's existing website (or create a new website) that focuses on your program and key information that you want the audience to discover. Include culturally appropriate graphics, photographs and other visual features to hold the interest of the audience. Share updates about what has been happening with your program, events that you've held, volunteer opportunities, social marketing campaigns, and so on.

● Create a social networking community page or group that people can view, join, participate in, and receive updates from. Use Facebook, Pinterest, Twitter, LinkedIn, Instagram, TikTok, Discord, or any current and popular social media.

● Create an electronic mailing list that can serve as an internet forum. People can join the list on their own, or you can add them to it, so they can communicate by e-mail. Examples include Yahoo Groups, Google Groups, and so on.

● Develop a list of community members who are able and willing to be contacted by e-mail, text, or mobile app such as WhatsApp. Send out group e-mails and texts with news of interest, information, event announcements, and your outreach schedule so that they can visit your site (this is different from an electronic mailing list because *you* are the only one who sends information out and participants can respond only to *you* and not to the entire list).

● Add your program to the Links section of related websites, resource listings, and so forth. Make sure the word gets out about the services you're providing and how to reach you.

- Use video-conferencing, such as Zoom or Google Meet, to connect a community of people at the same time, providing information and facilitating dialogue and support.

- Host a web seminar (webinar) when you want to reach a large number of people at a planned and scheduled time.

- Consider adding scannable graphics (such QR codes) to existing printed materials to provide a direct link to online information.

- *Can you think of other technology that you could use to conduct outreach?*

Benefits to using the internet to conduct outreach include:

1. **Privacy:** Much of your information can be provided on your website without the consumer being asked to provide any personal information.

2. **Cost-effectiveness**: You can reach many people via the internet at little cost. You may be able to add a page to your agency's existing website, or you may be able to create a free web page or other internet resource.

3. **Reach**: Your internet presence can be accessed by almost anyone at any time in any country all around the world.

Limitations to using the internet or mobile web to conduct outreach include:

1. **Access:** Many people still do not have access to a computer, smartphone, or other mobile device because of the cost of equipment and internet or data access.

2. **Cultural appropriateness:** For web-based outreach to be successful, the technology used, and the information presented should be aligned with the cultural identities and values of the priority populations. Many communities may not want to engage with you via the internet and may prefer in-person opportunities for education, counseling, and relationship building.

3. Client concerns about the privacy of their communication and information online.

Priority populations with whom internet and mobile outreach can be particularly effective include:

- Youth and young adults
- Participants in social media sites
- People using the web to make romantic or sexual connections with others

- *Can you think of a way that you could use the internet or mobile web to provide outreach to your community?*

- *Do you belong to any social media groups that address community health or social concerns?*

SOCIAL MARKETING

Social marketing applies the same methods that private businesses use to sell products (such as soft drinks or cell phones) to promote specific health outcomes. Social marketing campaigns may seek to promote immunizations or screening for breast cancer, or to prevent smoking or domestic violence. Social marketing techniques include the use of social media, posters, billboards, comics, and brochures as well as public service announcements on television, radio, the internet, or cell phones. To be successful, social marketing campaigns need to analyze and understand their "target market" (the community), select a medium (such as radio or social media) that is popular with the target market, and develop a persuasive and culturally relevant message. CHWs sometimes participate in the development of social marketing campaigns, and they often work in concert with social marketing to reach specific audiences.

SOCIAL MEDIA

Social media sites—such as Facebook, Instagram, Twitter, and others mentioned above—have been used to promote a wide range of public health issues, health behaviors, resources, and organizations. For example, social media has been used to address nutrition and healthy eating, cancer screening, physical activity, vaccine promotion, mental health, and other health issues (Mendoza-Herrera et al., 2020; Plackett et al., 2020; Stellefson, Paige, Chaney, & Chaney, 2020; Wadham, Green, Debattista, Somerset, Sav, 2018)

Social media has also been used to spread misinformation about a wide variety of health issues often resulting in confusion, mistrust, or fear. These messages sometimes undermine or damage the efforts of public and private organizations to effectively promote community health.

An example of a multifaceted social media marketing campaign is El Sol Neighborhood Educational Center's NEW COVID-19 CHW Toolkit. It includes a wide variety of outreach resources including cartoons, comic strips, an activity book, posters, video testimonials, and songs that can be played on the radio to tackle vaccine hesitancy in vulnerable communities (El Sol Neighborhood Educational Center, 2022).

Alexander Fajardo, Executive Director of El Sol Neighborhood Education Center (El Sol): The COVID-19 pandemic challenged us beyond our imagination, but these trying times were the catalyst for creativity, connection, and survival. As a result of the COVID-19 pandemic, El Sol quickly transitioned from in-person outreach to electronic/virtual outreach within a matter of weeks. While we anxiously awaited the time when we would be able to do more person-to-person contact/outreach, El Sol was resilient. Our team launched us into a modern, virtual form of engagement while also utilizing our traditional methods of popular education. Our social media outreach has evolved as we adapted to transmit messages of prevention, recovery, hope, and community resilience through the arts: music, poetry, dance, drama, games, and graphic arts.

What Do YOU Think?

- *Have you recently viewed or listened to a social marketing campaign?*
- *Where did you encounter the campaign (social media, TV, radio, the internet, a poster, billboard, or pamphlet)?*
- *What health outcome did the campaign attempt to promote?*
- *Are you a member of the "target" audience?*
- *What do you think of the social marketing message? Is it effective for you?*

19.7 Planning Health Outreach

Careful planning and preparation will enhance the quality of community health outreach. At the end of this chapter, we ask you to develop a preliminary health outreach plan for a community that you are already familiar with. Remember, a plan is not static: it should change as you analyze your work and learn from the community you are serving.

Outreach workers are often hired to work for a health outreach program that has already been designed, hopefully with extensive planning. In these circumstances, the priority population has already been determined, along with the health issue to be addressed, goals and objectives, and outreach methods. In other circumstances, CHWs will play an important role in developing the core elements of a health outreach plan.

DEFINE THE COMMUNITY TO BE SERVED BY OUTREACH

To learn about the community you will be working with and its health status, review available literature and reports, including reports generated by state and local health departments. Seek out available epidemiological data that will provide you with an understanding of the prevalence of the health condition you are addressing. How many people are affected by the health issue? Which parts of the community are at the greatest risk?

Read local papers and internet sources (web pages, online newsletters, newsfeeds, etc.) to find out what is currently happening in the community.

The most important research you will do is with the community. Take your time getting to know members of the community—including key opinion leaders—and talking with them about the work you plan to do. It is particularly important to learn what the community is thinking about the health issues you plan to address (Is it a priority for them?) and any past attempts to address these issues in the community (Were these efforts welcomed by the community? Were they successful?). You also want to understand what the community thinks about the agency that you work for (Does it have a good reputation? Were mistakes made in the past that require accountability and time to build trust and collaboration?). Identifying past successes and mistakes can help you avoid making errors and assist you in building positive relationships.

- **Visit local agencies and/or agency websites** to find out about the services they provide. For example, learn about health clinics, counseling programs, educational institutions, food pantries and soup kitchens, and shelters. Some benefits of visiting local agencies in-person include relationship building, fostering coalitions, and maintaining contacts for future referrals.

   - *Be sure you research an agency before your first visit so that you can maximize your time while you are at the site. Be prepared!*

- **Identify potential outreach methods and sites**: What type of outreach strategies do community members and local agencies recommend? What types of media and social media are most popular in the community? What types of venues might be most successful for conducting in-person outreach? These may include parks, schools, bars, churches, hair and nail salons and barber shops, homeless encampments, syringe exchanges, drug treatment programs, or soup kitchens, depending on the population you wish to reach.

- **Gather community input for outreach messages and materials**: Ask local community members to help you to develop or to review outreach and media messages to help ensure that the language and images will be effective in reaching the intended audience.

Ramona Benson: I do street outreach and we have a flyer that talks about our services at the Black Infant Health Program. I also go out and visit local businesses and organizations like nail and beauty salons and churches. I tell them who I am and if they have time, I tell them about our program. I ask if I can post my flyer or if they may want to pass it out. I always get some ladies who come to our program saying that they saw the flyer in their church or at a nail shop, so I know that it works to get the word out about our services.

IDENTIFY THE HEALTH ISSUE AND THE HEALTH OUTCOMES YOU WILL PROMOTE

Most outreach programs are funded to address one or more specific health issues such as breast cancer, hepatitis C, depression, or gun violence. Remember that the issues you are paid to focus on may not always be the greatest priority for the community you work with (we will address this later on in greater detail).

Your outreach efforts will be most effective if you are clear about the health outcomes you are trying to achieve. Is your goal to prevent further hepatitis C infections among injection drug users? Is it to promote testing for hepatitis C? To link people living with hepatitis C to treatment resources? All of the above?

By defining your goals, and researching the health issue and the community, you can develop outreach strategies that are more likely to promote your desired outcomes. If some of your strategies aren't effective, you will be better prepared to adapt or develop new ones because you have a clear sense of what you want to accomplish.

ORGANIZE THE OUTREACH TEAM

Take time to talk with your supervisor and colleagues in order to determine:

- The number of people you will need on the outreach team (Are you going solo, or will you have a partner or two?)

- The key messages you wish to communicate to the community

- The materials you should bring to the site (written materials or pamphlets, business cards, safer health supplies, promotional materials, hygiene products, resource listings or directories, and so on)

- Always ask someone else to carefully proofread your flyer, webpage, or information because they many times can see errors or mistakes in language, spelling, etc.

- The referrals that you will provide

- The forms you will use to document your contacts with people and the services that you provide

- How will you dress when conducting outreach? Will you wear casual clothing, professional attire, or an outreach shirt that identifies you as an outreach worker with your agency? While this may seem like a trivial issue, how you dress often sends a message to the community. For more information about dress codes and code-switching, please refer to Chapter 14.

- If you are providing outreach online or via social media, who will monitor responses and other postings, and how often? How often will you respond to the messages of others in order to build dialogue and relationships?

19.8 Conducting Health Outreach

This section discusses how to build relationships in the community, approach new clients, handle rejection, work as part of a team, manage outreach materials, and enhance your safety. While this section emphasizes outreach conducted in-person in the community, the key concepts can also be adapted and applied to conducting outreach via technology (such as social media).

BUILDING RELATIONSHIPS IN THE COMMUNITY

When you are conducting health outreach, the community will closely observe what you do and say, how you treat people, and if you remain true to your word. You will need to be patient, giving the community time to get to know and accept you. While this is particularly challenging for CHWs who work in communities that they are not a part of, even when you come from the community you are serving, it may take time for your work to be understood and accepted.

When you are initiating a new health outreach project, begin by developing relationships with the community. Here are some suggestions for how to do this:

- If you come from or are already familiar with the community, *contact people you already know*. Tell them about your new role as a CHW and the agency you are working for. Let them know what services you plan to provide and how you think these will benefit the community. Ask for their assistance and advice about how to get your message and services out to the community, and to make introductions to key opinion leaders. Ask them if they would like to help or volunteer.

- **Identify key opinion leaders in the community**: Don't assume that you already know who they are. Key opinion leaders are not always those with formal authority (such as elected leaders). They are the people in every community whom others listen to, respect, and turn to for advice. If, for example, your job is to conduct outreach to homeless and runaway youths, observe and ask whom they turn to for guidance and support. Introduce yourself, explain the work you will be doing, and ask for their assistance in building relationships in the community. Take time getting to know these opinion leaders, and when the moment is right, ask them for their guidance regarding your outreach work: ask for their advice regarding how, when, and where to conduct health outreach in the community. Remember that relationships require constant nurturing: keep returning to visit key opinion leaders and to continue this dialogue. Keep a confidential list of these key contacts and where to find them.

  - If you are conducting outreach via social media, you will also identify and build relationships with key opinion leaders, learning from the information they provide and the suggestions they may make.

- *Network with the community* at local events and meetings and let people know what services you offer. Bring business cards and be prepared to quickly introduce yourself and explain your role as a CHW. You will need to repeat this information many times before people begin to understand who you are and what you will be doing.

- *Identify community agencies* that share common goals. Introduce yourself, explain what you will be doing, and explore options for strategic partnership and collaboration. For example, you may refer clients to their agency. Other agencies, in turn, may invite you to conduct outreach to community groups that they work with.

- *Organize a community forum* to introduce yourself and your program. Invite as many people as you can. Make sure that you advertise the forum well. You can print flyers to announce the forum and carry these with you so that you can hand them out at every opportunity.

- **Encourage community involvement**: Let people know that their guidance and suggestions are welcome. Let them know how they might be able to volunteer or become more involved with your program and your outreach work. Invite them to visit your agency to find out more about your services.

- **Listen and observe**: Your first priority should be to get to know people. Remember the diagram of the client-centered CHW with big ears and big eyes: you shouldn't be doing most of the talking. Create an actual or virtual space for community members to share information, concerns, and opinions with you. Ask them what they know about the health problem you will be addressing, the key resources in the community, and whom they think you should be talking with.

- **Be patient**: Don't push your agenda. Your top priority should be to listen.

- **Keep your promises**: If you say that you will show up at a certain location at a certain time—or post new information on a specific date—follow through with these expectations. Unfortunately, the communities you serve are likely to recall a long list of broken promises from health and social service providers—don't add to this list!

- *What else have you learned about how to build effective relationships in the community?*

HOW TO APPROACH NEW OUTREACH CONTACTS

When you are conducting in-person outreach and approaching someone for the first time, do what comes naturally—introduce yourself. At most outreach locations, you will be able to make a full introduction. Speak clearly and with a friendly, welcoming tone. Let the person know your name, which agency you represent, and why you are at the outreach location.

> *Hi, I'm Janet from the Center City Health Center. I work with a breast cancer prevention project and I'm out here tonight to let people know about the services we provide.*

Depending on the circumstances, you may or may not have a chance to share more information. Be ready to continue a conversation and to share information about health issues and your services. At the same time, be ready to back off if you need to—don't be too pushy. Be respectful of people's time and interests: at the moment, they may not have time to speak with you. If the person appears to be in a hurry, or if the outreach site is in a difficult setting, keep your message simple and brief, while taking the opportunity to distribute outreach materials if appropriate.

- *Have you ever been approached by an outreach worker?*

- *How do want to be approached by an outreach worker?*

  - *How do you <u>not</u> want to be approached?*

> **Chelene Lopez:** When working with Farmworkers and Day Laborers, you have to gain their trust first before they access the services. Because many of them do not have legal status, they can be wary of government agencies. When I introduce myself, I always let them know that I'm there to assist them and I'm not affiliated with a government agency. Additionally, you may have to work with the ranch owners or employer groups to provide services for the employees. You must gain their trust too. If they believe that you are going to organize the employees, they will normally not allow you access to the employees. I have learned ways to provide information to the employees about their rights and how to organize without the employer knowing.

Every outreach setting really is unique. Because of this, it is important for you to learn as much as possible about the setting and the community before your first visit. If you are providing outreach in a new setting, you may feel nervous. If the location becomes a site for regular outreach, you will adapt and tailor your approach with time, gaining confidence. You will begin to recognize some of the community members and develop ongoing conversations and relationships. If you are preparing to conduct outreach online or through social media, take time to visit and explore the site and the technology before you begin. Pay attention to what people are talking about.

Depending on the outreach site and the target population, you may develop creative ways to gain access and acceptance into the community you are attempting to reach. For example, you may want to expand your outreach focus to *address more generalized needs* of the community. If you are providing outreach to migrant farm workers, brainstorm and network with people at the site to find out what they need. Do they need food, clothing, or school supplies for their children? You may be able to provide some things that are really needed at this location, even if these items have not been explicitly stated as part of your outreach services and goals. By meeting some of the basic needs of the priority community, you will accomplish several goals at once. Not only will you provide important resources, but you will also build relationships with members of the community so that you can work with them more closely each time you visit their camp.

Training Outreach Workers at City College of San Francisco

At City College of San Francisco, we offered a course on conducting health outreach. During the first month, students are divided up into teams of two, provided with a backpack with HIV prevention materials, and given 10 minutes to go out on campus, introduce themselves to someone they don't already know and initiate a conversation related to HIV issues. When students are preparing to conduct outreach for the first time, they often feel nervous, embarrassed, shy, or worried about whether or not they will be able to initiate a conversation with anyone.

Once the students return to the classroom, they analyze their experience and the factors that made it easier or harder to connect with potential clients.

As a final assignment, the students design and manage a three-hour campus outreach event that reaches hundreds of students. With repetition, the students gain confidence and skills in conducting health outreach. They learn to relax, have fun, and focus on their successes rather than their disappointments.

Break the ice with humor, games, or fun interactive exercises. At City College of San Francisco, outreach workers have used a variety of participatory activities such as the Spinning Wheel Game and a Talking Wall. The Spinning Wheel Game is a large colorful wheel that CHWs set up in a prominent location.

Outreach workers invite people to spin the wheel, which lands on a number matched to a question about a health issue (such as sexual health, diabetes or nutrition). As other people gather around to see what is happening, the CHWs facilitate discussions about related topics such as "What types of food and drink are best for preventing chronic conditions like high blood pressure?" or "Name two locations on campus where you can buy fresh whole fruits and vegetables." Players are provided with prizes whether they win or lose.

The Talking Wall is simply a big piece of paper—we have used paper as large as 10 feet high by 15 feet wide—with a series of questions or quotes, and colorful pens also and markers available so that people can add their own comments and questions, building a dialogue through their posts. Typically, the wall focuses discussion on particular topics or themes, such as "What factors contribute to risks for diabetes in our communities?" As the wall fills up with anonymous comments and opinions, CHWs stand by to talk with participants, pass out health materials, and make referrals.

Hold an event in the community you are trying to reach. Work with your outreach team and volunteers to come up with something that will be fun. Make sure that the event allows members of the target population to participate in a way that will energize them so that they will want to get involved.

Community Health Workers/Promotoras de Salud from El Sol Neighborhood Education Center recruited community members in Cathedral City, California to host a series of fun and engaging community multi-generational events including a cultural potluck, cooking classes, teatime, Zumba sessions, a bike parade, community theater, and movie nights. During these events, they shared messages on our individual and collective roles to prevent domestic and sexual violence. The CHWs invited community members to be part of domestic and sexual violence prevention seminars, trainings, and advocacy efforts.

HANDLING REJECTION

When you conduct health outreach, most people will respect your role and your contributions. But not everyone will be interested in what you have to offer, be welcoming, or polite. Expect and prepare to handle *a lot* of rejection as an outreach worker.

- *Have you ever encountered a pushy outreach worker or sales representative who didn't take no for an answer?*

- *Have you ever been followed down the street by someone who wanted to give you a flyer, ask you to sign a petition, or sell you something?*

- *What do you think of these outreach strategies?*

Many people don't like to be approached by strangers. If you continue to bother a prospective outreach contact after they have clearly indicated, by their words or actions, that they are not interested in speaking with you, you risk making a strong and lasting negative impression that could hurt future efforts to conduct outreach in the community. If potential outreach contacts try to ignore you or avoid you, *don't pursue them.* If they let you know that they aren't interested (by shaking their head or saying something like "I don't have time" or "I'm not interested"), accept this and move on immediately. Remember that you may return to the same locations again and again, and therefore to encounter the same people in the future: leave a positive first impression. At a future visit to this location, you may very well have a chance to interact with the person who could not speak with you today.

Some people will be rude or disrespectful. Try not to take it personally. Even if a prospective contact is angry or says something vulgar or disrespectful to you (this *will* happen!), don't retaliate in kind. When you get a chance, debrief these encounters with a colleague, supervisor, friend, or family member. Vent your feelings in a safe place, and never with the clients and communities you work with. One angry outburst or nasty comment to a prospective client may quickly become news in the community and seriously damage your reputation.

With time, you will find that your skills as an outreach worker become more developed and fine-tuned. Encountering rejection and indifference will aid you in learning to tailor your outreach messages and interactions to reach more people in more effective ways.

> **Rosaicela Estrada:** The community, in general, continues to lose interest in COVID information and incentives. In addition, many people are not interested in receiving our free COVID test kits because their children receive them at school. So, it's hard to use them as incentives during our outreach. Since the President announced the termination of the national COVID-19 emergency, many community members believe that COVID no longer exists, and they are not interested in listening to us. Families no longer open their doors to our CHWs. We have to remain patient.

RECOGNIZE AND ACKNOWLEDGE YOUR LIMITATIONS AND MISTAKES

As a CHW, you will be confronted with questions that you don't know how to answer and situations that you are not sure how to handle. Don't be afraid to acknowledge the limits of your knowledge and skills to clients or coworkers. Choose your own words and say something along the lines of: *"I don't know"* or *"I'm not certain about that"* or *"I don't want to tell you anything that may not be true. Let me research this question when I get back to the office, and next time I see you, I'll let you know what I have learned."* Trust us: You will need these words often!

Many of the clients you work with have experienced prejudice, discrimination, isolation, or loss. These experiences often influence their interactions with helping professionals, and they may be watching, waiting, and expecting you to be yet another person who lets them down in some way. Inevitably, despite your best efforts and intentions, you will disappoint some potential outreach contacts and clients. For example, you might arrive late for an appointment, run out of food vouchers, forget an important detail that a client told you about their life, misinterpret a statement that a client makes, make an incorrect assumption, or say or write something that triggers previous bad experiences for a client. These are natural, common, and inevitable mistakes that we all make at some point in our careers.

As a result of these types of mistakes, some clients will stop working with you and may avoid you and your agency in the future. Others may show their disappointment or anger and say something about your action. We encourage you to view these moments as an opportunity to repair and perhaps deepen the working relationship. A sincere apology often has remarkable power to defuse and transform anger and conflict. It shows that you are a fallible human being who makes mistakes, not someone who thinks that you are better than your client. An apology communicates your commitment, your desire to be supportive, and your intention to treat your clients with the respect they deserve. In many cases, it will actually result in renewed trust in the working relationship and open up dialogue that will assist you to get to know your clients in a deeper way.

What words do you use when you apologize or otherwise take responsibility for doing something you wish you hadn't done? Don't apologize simply because someone suggested it to you as a professional technique: whatever you say, *it has to be authentic.*

Please see Chapter 13 for more information about the Power of Apology.

YOUR REPUTATION AS AN OUTREACH WORKER

As you conduct health outreach, you will get to know the community. People will begin to recognize you and associate you with your work and your agency. Your reputation, both on and off the clock, will follow you wherever you go in the community, and will become one of your most important professional resources. When we asked senior CHWs how they have built and maintained positive reputations in the communities they serve, they shared ideas for what to do—and what not to do:

GUIDELINES FOR BUILDING A POSITIVE REPUTATION

DON'T	DO
DON'T break confidentiality in any way. This is the quickest way to end your career.	Let the client know that your discussions are confidential (and don't forget to explain the limits of confidentiality and the types of information that you may need to report—see Chapter 5). Maintain confidential client information including notes, discussions, disclosure forms, etc.
DONT ever act like you are better than anyone else; talk down to them or criticize anyone behind their back.	Treat everyone with equal dignity and respect.
DON'T pretend to be something or someone you're not. The community will always see through your act, and you will lose their respect.	Be clear about your role as a CHW and acknowledge your own strengths and limitations. Act and speak in a way that is authentic to who you are.
DON'T make things up. If you don't know about a particular topic or how to answer a question, just explain this to the community.	Be honest and do your best to get the information needed by your client and follow up as appropriate. You can say, "I'm not sure about that, but I will do research and get back to you."

(continues)

(continued)

DON'T	DO
DON'T spend all of your time speaking with *one* outreach contact. Other people may want to speak with you, and they may feel ignored if you don't give them a chance to interact with you.	Spend your outreach time wisely and reach as many members of a community as possible without compromising the quality of your interactions.
DON'T discriminate against any part of the community you are serving. As an outreach worker, your duty is to provide services and information to *everyone* you interact with—not just the ones you are more comfortable speaking to or the ones you would *rather* approach. Review your own reporting data to make sure that you aren't leaving anyone out—for example, are you serving women as well as men, Latinos as well as African Americans?	Be mindful of ALL people around you, and be sure not to ignore, miss, or leave anyone out!
DON'T pick sides when the community you are working with is in conflict.	Stay neutral, to the extent possible, and work to maintain positive relationships with all sectors of the community.
DONT rush through engagements with people who want to speak with you.	Take the time to listen to and be kind to everyone you interact with. When you have to cut a conversation short, do so as politely as possible.
DONT make promises you can't keep. It can damage your reputation if clients feel that you do not keep your word or care enough to follow through with promises.	Know your limitations and your scope of practice. Refer clients or contacts to other professionals or relevant programs and services.
DON'T flirt or have inappropriate conversations. This may be perceived as sexually charged, inappropriate, unprofessional, or unwanted.	Be friendly and professional but also mindful when a conversation is moving in a direction that it should not. Interrupt conversations that cross a line. Steer them back to an appropriate topic or find a polite way to end the conversation.
DONT use language that is unfamiliar to the community (such as *epidemiology*): everything you want to say can be communicated using language that is accessible to your audience.	Use language that is accessible to the community. Be mindful of the words and terms that you and your colleagues use among outreach contacts. Stop to clarify any confusion or misinformation.
DON'T ignore a mistake you may have made. Don't argue or try to prove that you are "right."	Apologize if you mess up or make a mistake. Owning your mistake is critical to building and strengthening your relationship with clients.
DON'T push your own agenda on clients.	Listen to the immediate needs and priorities of contacts and clients. If you are talking about prostate cancer and the client is telling you he is hungry, listen to him and see if there is anything you can do to help him out. Maybe there is a soup kitchen or food pantry nearby. If you assist clients with their priorities, then they will be ready to listen to yours.
DON'T forget or violate your code of ethics! For example, do not sleep with clients, do drugs with them, or give them money.	Maintain ethical and legal boundaries that support your work as a CHW.

SAFETY ISSUES

Some members of the community may view outreach workers with suspicion or fear and treat you as an outsider or intruder. This is one of many reasons why it is essential to get to know the community you will be working in, and to build respectful relationships with key opinion leaders.

Depending on the type of outreach you are providing, safety issues and concerns may include:

- Losing sight of your outreach partner
- Injuring yourself in dark or dimly lit areas
- Witnessing arguments, threats, or violence (such as incidents of domestic violence)
- Encountering an angry, aggressive, or threatening person
- Experiencing harassment, including sexual harassment
- Witnessing illegal or underground activities such as selling or using drugs
- Unintentional involvement in police actions
- Theft and assault

- *Can you think of additional safety concerns?*

Your job as a CHW is to provide services to the most vulnerable and at-risk communities, such as people who are unhoused. Society often stigmatizes these communities, and others fear them and assume they are dangerous. *Sometimes your own prejudices may influence your assessment of safety issues. Try to be aware of the tendency for this to happen and guard against discriminating against clients or communities that have already been harmed in this way. Remember that safety issues are present in any work setting and with clients of all backgrounds.*

Chapter 11 discusses safety issues in relation to home visiting and presents safety tips that apply to conducting health outreach as well. Review the safety discussion in that chapter. Here, we present additional tips and issues that are specific to doing outreach.

If you are conducting in-person outreach in the community, work with a partner or outreach team. Keep your teammates within view at all times and check in with each other regularly. Develop a system to "signal" one another if you need some assistance, whether it be a hand signal or a code phrase ("Hey, Marcos, did you check in with **Dr. Strong?**") and come together immediately after the signal is given. Keep cell phones with you if possible and keep them turned on with the sounds/notifications on for receiving text messages in case a colleague tries to reach you this way. Always allow for quick communication with other team members if you or someone else should run into a difficult situation. Listen to your instincts, which will develop over time, and pay attention to them when you feel particularly ill at ease, anxious, or unsafe.

If you find yourself in the midst of a conflict, try to deescalate the situation using conflict resolution skills (Chapter 13). If necessary, ask your team members for assistance. Here is where a code phrase or hand signal can come in handy ("Dr. Strong"). If the situation is too intense, however, shout out for assistance. If no other team members respond and the situation is dangerous and immediate, ask for assistance from anyone who is nearby and might be able to assist you. If you don't see any hope for calming the situation, leave. File an incident report with your organization and document the contact information of witnesses in case you will need to file for workers comp or legal action. Only call the police if it is absolutely required. Most situations will not require such a drastic measure. You want to avoid bringing the police into a community that has a history of tensions with law enforcement. You could find yourself losing the trust and respect of this community.

Rosaicela Estrada: CHWs have experienced challenges when conducting outdoor outreach. Specifically, CHW's feel hesitant to leave their tables to talk to community members due to fear of having items stolen from their tabling stations. Outreach materials (including 200 COVID tests, table, and wagon) were stolen from the truck bed of one of our CHWs while she went inside a building to use the restroom. Due to this fear, CHWs prefer to work in pairs. Working as a team is the best way to serve the community.

TIPS FOR SUCCESSFUL TEAMWORK

We strongly encourage CHWs to work with a partner or as a part of an outreach team for several reasons:

- It is safer to work in a team.
- You can reach a larger number of clients.
- You can provide more than one service at the same time. For example, some CHWs can conduct general outreach in a club, and others may provide confidential risk-reduction counseling or screening services in a more private area.
- The more diverse the outreach team, the more choice you offer potential clients about who to talk with.

Successful teamwork often comes down to good communication. When conducting health outreach with a partner or team, here are a few tips for working together:

- Meet with your team to clarify your goals, objectives, expectations, and the policies and protocols that will guide your work.
- Make time to review and discuss your outreach plan, including locations, outreach materials, and referrals you will provide.
- Develop a system for responding to safety concerns, including a code that will alert you and your partners to potential danger.
- Ask for and listen to the ideas and opinions of your teammates.
- Accept and respect the different experiences, cultural perspectives, and opinions of your partners.
- Assert your opinions clearly, calmly, and respectfully.
- Be ready and willing to compromise.
- Learn to provide and accept feedback calmly and respectfully (see Chapter 14).
- Make time to debrief your work together after every shift. Share your successes and your challenges. Acknowledge the positive contributions of teammates and outcomes of your collaborative efforts. Make plans to improve aspects of your teamwork that didn't go as well as you had hoped.

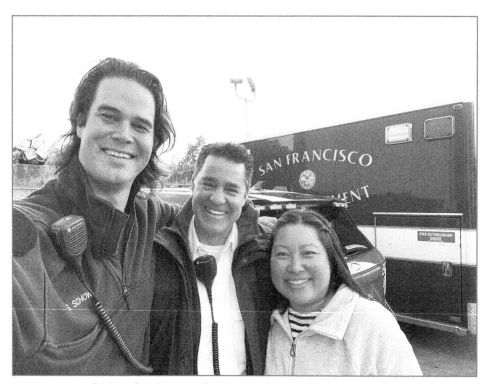

Emergency Medical Technicians conduct outreach in San Francisco.

DEVELOPING AND MANAGING OUTREACH MATERIALS

CHWs use a variety of outreach materials in the course of their work such as printed brochures, pamphlets, flyers, posters, health promotion comics or books, and referral cards. They may include promotional materials such as key chains, pens, cups, toys, tote bags, and so on that have your agency logo and contact information printed on them. Some outreach workers bring food, clothing, hygiene materials (toothpaste, toothbrushes, soap, and so on), or other items that are needed by members of the priority community.

Outreach materials may also be digital, such as messages, graphics, videos, and other resources posted online and shared via social media. Depending on your agency and your program, you will find that some materials work better than others with your priority audience. You will want to develop a tailored mix of outreach materials that you can take to different venues or distribute in other ways. The messages should mirror the health program's goals and objectives.

You should plan your collection of outreach materials carefully, based on the demographics and needs of the priority population. Trial and error will guide you as you determine what has and hasn't worked in prior visits to that site or to similar sites. Most importantly, ask the community you are serving what they think about the materials you are using. They can help tailor your outreach for optimal success.

Your agency may also be able to provide incentives for community members that will support your outreach efforts. These could be gift certificates, food vouchers, or stipends in exchange for community member participation in events, services, or research.

Making the Most of Outreach Materials

A CHW conducting outreach to the homeless always made a point of carrying clean socks in his backpack. Many of his clients slept on the streets and in parks and lacked clean, warm clothes, and they truly appreciated a pair of clean socks. By providing clean socks, he was able to start off a new relationship by offering something valuable to a client. This was often useful in creating an opportunity to start other conversations. For example, if a client pointed to the backpack and asked, "What else do you have in there?" the CHW was able to talk about the full range of services that he could provide.

Keep your outreach materials well organized. Be sure that they are up-to-date and undamaged. Giving a client outdated or damaged goods is a sure way to damage their trust in you.

CHWs often participate in the development of new outreach materials such as flyers, brochures, or resource guides. When developing any outreach materials, or using those produced by other sources, be sure to pay close attention to the content and the messages being provided. Gather members of the priority population and ask for their input and opinions on the materials you are considering developing or distributing. Coordinate focus groups (see Chapters 19 and 23) to ask the community what they think about the materials. Test the visuals, graphics, and language with a multi-cultural and multi-generational audience. Collaborate with other agencies who serve the priority population to see what they think. If you are purchasing or otherwise acquiring materials produced by another source, make sure that the message is culturally appropriate for your priority population(s). Make sure you examine the materials, reading every page of the brochures, reviewing websites thoroughly, watching every minute of the videos, testing out the equipment and promotional materials, and so on. The last thing you want to do is discover that you have been handing out materials that are offensive or inaccurate. Offensive materials are worse than none at all.

Leticia Olvera Arechar: The pamphlets, brochures, posters, and the t-shirts we wear when we do outreach and tabling at multiple community health and resource fairs were co-created with community members. Their input was central to designing our logo and slogan.

19.9 Documenting Health Outreach Services

One of the most important tasks of outreach work is the documentation of the services you provide. The health program's goals, objectives, and work plan should guide the development of the forms you will use to document your work.

Documentation of community health outreach services has become increasingly important for a variety of reasons:

- Documentation can show what you've accomplished and if you have met program goals and objectives.
- It provides data that can be used to find additional funding to continue or expand the program.
- It reveals the history of the program and builds a timeline of program development.
- The information gathered can assist your agency and others in developing plans to better promote the health of the community in the future.
- It enables you to be accountable to funders including, in the case of public funding, the general public (taxpayers).
- Documentation makes it possible to evaluate your program. Data are gathered in order to:
- Determine who you have and have not reached, and highlight opportunities to reach underserved segments of the community
- Analyze the strategies and resources, including technology, that have been most and least effective in reaching the priority community and promoting desired outcomes
- Better understand the clients and communities served
- Refine and improve the quality of services provided
- Guard against discriminatory practices, such as the exclusion of certain groups from programs and services
- Advocate for the continuation and expansion of necessary services
- Provide evidence that can assist others in developing similar programs and services

- *Can you think of other reasons why documentation is so important?*

What Do
YOU?
Think

Lidia Benitez: I became a CHW because I wanted to work with people and provide them services for their well-being and prosperity. As a new CHW, I did not understand why I had to complete so many forms. Now as a CHW team lead, I understand the importance of correctly and thoroughly completing the forms in order to meet the funder's goals, objectives, and requirements. Now I make sure my team takes pride in completing the outreach logs and other forms correctly. Quality documentation increases our chances for continued funding, which sustains our employment and provides much-needed resources to our communities.

Depending on the agency you work for, you may be asked to provide a weekly, monthly, quarterly, or annual report. You may have a supervisor who completes some of these reports for the program. Whatever the requirements are, it is a good idea to keep track of every outreach session you complete. Use the outreach tracking forms your agency provides or talk with your supervisor about creating such a form (increasingly these are digital forms that permit you to enter data on a computer, tablet, smartphone, or other digital device). Your agency will maintain some form of database or a calculating or totaling system to keep track of the numbers and demographics of outreach contacts. This is especially helpful if you provide outreach many times throughout the month or to many different contacts. You will also need a simplified method of totaling the number of contacts and other services you provide to prepare accurate, detailed reports and to determine if you are reaching program goals.

For the documentation to be useful, data about the outreach services you provide are likely to include the following types of information:

- The date and time when the outreach was provided.
- Outreach location(s) including physical places and addresses as well as online "locations."
- The names of the outreach worker(s).
- A count or estimate of the number of people you reached and their demographic profile:

  Often you will be asked to record demographic information about the identities of the people you serve, such as their sex, ethnicity, age, substance use, sexual orientation, homeless or marginally housed, or health status. You won't always be able to gather this information. Sometimes, you will be asked to make an educated guess about the identities of those to whom you conduct outreach, but be careful not to jump into stereotypes or assumptions. Ask for guidance about how to do this from experienced CHWs and your supervisor.

- Key services provided, if any (such as blood pressure screening or health education).
- The number and type of supplies, materials, brochures, and so on that you distributed.
- Key referrals provided.
- Any outstanding problems or challenges encountered (such as conflicts or complaints).
- Other information that is required for your specific program.

We don't recommend that you fill out outreach reports as you talk with clients, as it is likely to distract you from focusing on your interaction with them and may harm your relationship (this type of documentation is different from what you will do when you provide case management or other person-centered services). However, don't wait too long before you document the services that you provide. Take time during each day to stop and document your work: you won't be able to remember the details later on.

19.10 Ethics and Health Outreach

Because of the independent nature of their work, outreach workers frequently face ethical challenges, including:

- Requests for food, money, vouchers, or transportation
- Offers of gifts, sex, or drugs
- Witnessing violence, including incidents of domestic violence
- Maintaining confidentiality when working in public places
- Developing personal relationships with clients, including romantic relationships

We strongly encourage you to anticipate and prepare to respond to common ethical challenges. Review the section on ethics in Chapter 5. Talk with more experienced CHWs to learn how they handle these situations and consult with your supervisor. Be ready to clearly explain your policies to clients—what you can and cannot do, and in some instances, why. For example, be prepared to explain the following to clients:

- Why you cannot give or loan them money
- Why you cannot accept gifts
- Why you cannot develop personal relationships with them, including romantic or sexual relationships
- Why you need to preserve confidentiality, and the exceptions to this policy (specific types of harm to the client or harm to others)
- That you don't know the answer to a relevant question, but will do your best to find out

To be successful in your career as a CHW, you will need to develop strong interpersonal boundaries that protect both you and your clients (again, please refer to Chapter 5). Be prepared to set and maintain your limits and to stand behind them. You will often have to say "no" to clients or otherwise communicate that you cannot provide a service or type of assistance they have asked for. Some clients won't accept the boundaries you attempt to establish and may continue to push for what they want.

Try not to let yourself get placed in a defensive position or to spend too much time repeating your ethical obligations and professional policies to clients. Find ways to refocus the conversation on the client's issues and on the services that you *can* offer. For example, you could say: *"I'm sorry, as we discussed before I can't give you money, but I can walk with you to the food kitchen which opens soon. Do you know the staff there?"*

Make sure to always maintain your professionalism: handling these challenges with grace and compassion often results in renewed trust and the opportunity to do more substantive work with a client. If you are unable to change the focus of the conversation or the client becomes increasingly assertive or aggressive, remember that you can always walk away from the encounter. If you need to do this, however, don't do it in anger. Explain yourself clearly, calmly, and politely.

Sometimes CHWs complain that clients are trying to "manipulate" them. We encourage you to reframe the way you think about this. It may be helpful to remember that for some clients, what you perceive as manipulation is how they learned to get the resources they need in order to survive. For some clients, these strategies may be connected to drug or alcohol use. Try not to take a client's behavior personally; it isn't about you. Practice the words you will use to end an encounter with a client when you feel the need to walk away. How will you explain this in ways that assert your own professional boundaries and preserve their dignity?

Chelene Lopez: When working with the unhoused and day laborers, we got many requests to drive clients to appointments or to go pick up medicines for them. This is strictly prohibited by our organization, so our department requested our supervisor to help us figure out how to help our patients without breaking our policy. The solution was to provide free bus passes for those patients who could take the bus. Additionally, we have arranged for Uber or Lift to take patients to appointments. Also, we have worked with a few pharmacies to deliver medicines to patients, which helps so we don't have to go pick up medicines.

19.11 Supervision and Support

While we hope you have the opportunity to work with a knowledgeable and supportive supervisor, the truth is that not all supervisors have the skills necessary to provide effective guidance and support to CHWs. Despite this, you have a professional responsibility to do your best to develop and sustain a positive working relationship with your supervisor. A positive relationship with your supervisor is essential for doing effective work, preventing stress and burnout, and maximizing your job satisfaction and opportunities for advancement. Ask for regular meetings with your supervisor and take the opportunity to inform them about your accomplishments as well as the challenges that you face in the field. If necessary, discuss how outreach strategies can be changed and provide some possible solutions. Remember to turn in documentation of your work in a timely fashion.

When you face an immediate challenge and do not have a supervisor (or another coworker) nearby to consult, rely on what you have learned about ethics, safety, and representing your agency. You will not always know how best to respond to problems that arise in the field. Sometimes, it is better to remove yourself from a situation as soon as possible rather than to try to respond or resolve it in the moment. When this occurs, document what happened and report to your supervisor as soon as possible. For more information about supervision, see Chapter 14.

Outreach workers sometimes feel isolated and wish for more professional support. Other outreach workers will best understand the nature of the challenges that you face and are best equipped to provide meaningful support in terms of how to handle the stresses of the job and to enhance the quality of services that you provide. Try to identify someone you trust to talk with about the challenges you face on the job. Our recommendation is to seek out a mentor who has years of experience conducting health outreach. This senior CHW may work at your same agency or with another organization. In many parts of the country and around the world, CHWs have formed local support groups that provide them with an opportunity to meet regularly with peers. These groups function both as a source of support and of ongoing professional development.

Chapter Review

To review the CHW competencies covered in this chapter, we would like you to develop a health outreach plan for a community that you belong to or know well. Please do your best to answer the following questions based on what you already know about your community and the information presented in this chapter.

1. Select a community that you know well. Define the community to be served (demographics, location, and so on). Be as specific as possible.
2. Define the health issue to be addressed by the outreach program.
3. What is the objective of your outreach program (what do you want to accomplish as a result of the outreach services provided)?
4. Who are the key opinion leaders in the community? How will you identify others? What are three questions that you would like to ask these key opinion leaders?
5. Identify actual or virtual (online) places (such as social media sites) where you can reach and contact community members.
6. List three institutions that are respected by the community that you can work with.
7. What outreach level might you use to conduct your outreach?
8. Which types of outreach methods would you select?
9. What types of outreach messages or materials will you share with the community?
10. What types of information will you gather to document the outreach services you provide? How might this information be used to improve the quality of your program?

References

El Sol Neighborhood Educational Center. (2022). Covid-19 Resources. https://www.elsolnec.org/blog/2020/09/04/covid-19-response/ (accessed 26 February 2023).

Mendoza-Herrera, K., Valero-Morales, I., Ocampo-Granados, M. E., Reyes-Morales, H., Arce-Amaré, F., & Barquera, S. (2020). An Overview of Social Media Use in the Field of Public Health Nutrition: Benefits, Scope, Limitations, and a Latin American Experience. Preventing Chronic Disease. http://dx.doi.org/10.5888/pcd17.200047external icon (accessed 25 February 2023).

National Association of Community Health Workers. (2023). NACHW COVID-19 Resources, Publication and Webinars. https://nachw.org/covid-19-resources/ (accessed 26 February 2023).

Palmer, K. N. B., Rivers, P. S., & Melton, F. L., McClelland, D. J., Hatcher, J., Marrero, D. G., Thomson, C. A., Garcia, D. (2021). Health promotion interventions for African Americans delivered in U.S. barbershops and hair salons- a systematic review. *BMC Public Health*, 21, 1553. https://doi.org/10.1186/s12889-021-11584-0.

Plackett, R., Kaushal, A., Kassianos, A. P., Cross, A., Lewins, D., Sheringham, J., Waller, J., & von Wagner, C. (2020). Use of social media to promote cancer screening and early diagnosis: Scoping review. *Journal of Medical Internet Research*, doi: https://doi.org/10.2196/21582PMID: 33164907PMCID: 7683249.

Salve, S., Raven. J., Das, P., Srinivasan, S., Khaled, A., Hayee, M., Olisenekwu, G., & Gooding, K. (2023). Community health workers and Covid-19: Cross-country evidence on their roles, experiences, challenges and adaptive strategies. *PLOS Global Public Health*, 3(1): e0001447. https://doi.org/10.1371/journal.pgph.0001447.

Shin, H. Y., Kim, K. Y., & Kang, P. (2020). Concept analysis of community health outreach. *BMC Health Services Research*, 20(1), 417. https://doi.org/10.1186/s12913-020-05266-7.

Stellefson, M., Paige, S. R., Chaney, B. H., & Chaney, J. D. (2020). Evolving role of social media in health promotion: updated responsibilities for health education specialists. *International Journal of Environmental Research and Public Health*, doi: 10.3390/ijerph17041153. PMID: 32059561; PMCID: PMC7068576.

Thomas, S. B. (2022). Leveraging Barbers' & Stylists' Trust to Promote Health Equity & Healthier Communities. Physician's Weekly. https://www.physiciansweekly.com/the-covid-19-pandemics-silver-lining-leveraging-the-expertise-of-barbers-stylists-to-promote-health-equity-create-healthier-communities/ (accessed 19 December 2023).

Wadham, E., Green, C., Debattista, J., Somerset, S., Sav, A. (2018). New digital media interventions for sexual health promotion among young people: a systematic review. *Sexual Health*, https://doi.org/10.1071/SH18127.

Additional Resources

Choi, K., Romero, R., Guha, P., Sixx, G., Rosen, A.D., Frederes, A., Beltran, J., Alvarado, J. et al. (2022). Community health worker perspectives on engaging unhoused peer ambassadors for COVID-19 vaccine outreach in homeless encampments and shelters. *Journal of General Internal Medicine* 37, 2026–2032. https://doi.org/10.1007/s11606-022-07563-9.

deBeaumont. (2019). Social Media in Public Health: A Vital Component of Community Engagement. https://debeaumont.org/news/2019/social-media-in-public-health-a-vital-component-of-community-engagement/ (accessed 12 May 2023).

El Sol Neighborhood Educational Center. (2023a). El Sol Neighborhood Education Center Instagram. https://www.instagram.com/elsolnec/?hl=en (accessed 12 May 2023).

El Sol Neighborhood Educational Center. (2023b). El Sol NEC YouTube. https://www.youtube.com/c/ElSolNEC/videos?app=desktop (accessed 12 May 2023).

Hannah Payne, H., Arredondo, V., West, J. H., Neiger, B., Hall, C. (2015). Use and acceptance of social media among community health workers. *Journal of Community Medicine Health Education*, 5, 354. doi: 10.4172/2161-0711.1000354.

National Healthcare for the Homeless Council CHW Voices Podcasts. https://soundcloud.com/user-459520516/sets/chw-voices (accessed 12 May 2023).

Stellefson, M., Paige, S. R., Chaney, B. H., & Chaney, J. D., (2020). Evolving role of social media in health promotion: updated responsibilities for health education specialists. *International Journal of Environmental Research and Public Health*, 17(4), 1153. https://doi.org/10.3390/ijerph17041153.

Facilitating Trainings

Jill R. Tregor and Joe Calderon

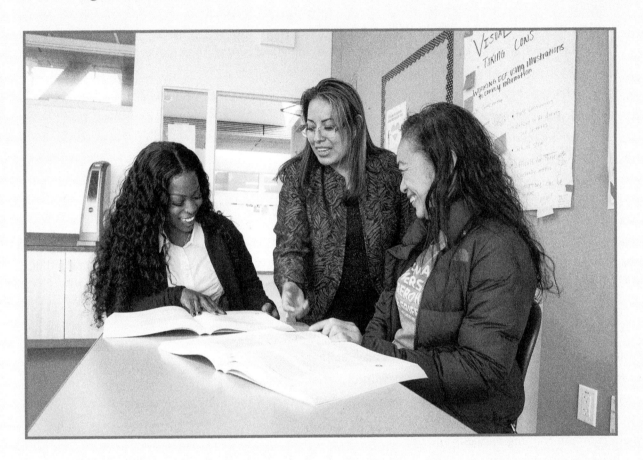

Foundations for Community Health Workers, Third Edition. Edited by Tim Berthold and Darouny Somsanith.
© 2024 John Wiley & Sons, Inc. Published 2024 by John Wiley & Sons, Inc.
Companion website: http://www.wiley.com/go/communityhealthworkers3E

CHW Scenario

You are a Community Health Worker at a nonprofit agency that provides behavioral health services. Your supervisor has asked you to develop and facilitate a 90-minute training on the topic of cultural humility for a regional meeting of CHWs. This group is interested in enhancing understanding and skills for working with clients of all cultural identities and backgrounds.

You have a strong understanding of cultural humility and do your best to apply it in your work with clients and community members. However, you feel a bit nervous about facilitating a training on this topic.

Please consider how you would answer the following questions:

- What else do you want to know about the proposed training and how will you gather this information?
- How will you plan and prepare for the training?
- What training objectives or learning outcomes could be appropriate for this training?
- How will you engage the training participants?
- What training methods will you use?
- How will you know if the training is successful?

Introduction

This chapter introduces knowledge and skills for facilitating a training or educational presentation. For the purposes of this chapter, we will use the word "training" for any type of class, presentation, or workshop that CHWs facilitate.

WHAT YOU WILL LEARN

By studying the information in this chapter, you will be able to:

- Identify different types of trainings that CHWs may facilitate
- Discuss some of the ways that people learn new information and skills
- Describe and apply approaches to training commonly used by CHWs, including popular education, participatory learning, and problem-based learning
- Explain common training methods and tips
- Identify and respond to common challenges that facilitators may face
- Develop a training plan, including learning outcomes
- Develop a simple evaluation of a training

C3 Roles and Skills Addressed in Chapter 20

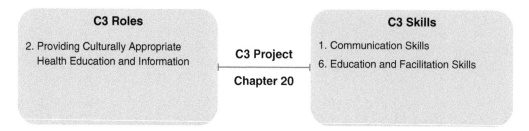

C3 Roles

2. Providing Culturally Appropriate Health Education and Information

C3 Project

Chapter 20

C3 Skills

1. Communication Skills
6. Education and Facilitation Skills

WORDS TO KNOW

Auditory Learners

Conscientization

Kinesthetic Learners

Learning Outcomes

Popular Education

Participatory Learning

Problem-based Learning

Visual Learners

20.1 An Overview of Training

As a CHW, you may be asked to facilitate or co-facilitate all or part of a training. These trainings vary in many ways.

AUDIENCE OR PARTICIPANTS

CHWs facilitate trainings for a wide variety of audiences including youth, parents, co-workers, clients, members of a faith community or other group, people diagnosed with chronic illness, and professionals such as teachers, CHWs, or other health care and social services providers, police, and the staff and volunteers of community-based organizations.

- *Can you think of other groups who might participate in trainings?*

LOCATIONS

Trainings take place in a wide variety of locations, such as:

- Clinics, hospitals, and local health departments
- Community-based organizations
- Housing sites, including public housing and homeless shelters
- Churches, mosques, temples, and other religious or faith-based organizations
- Juvenile hall, jails, or prisons
- Work sites
- Schools and colleges
- After-school programs
- Recreational sites
- Cultural and arts organizations
- Online, using online learning platforms and videoconferencing applications such as Zoom

- *Where do trainings take place in your community? What are some of the locations where you have participated in trainings?*

FOCUS OR MAIN TOPIC

CHWs facilitate trainings that address a wide range of public health topics, such as:

- Stress management
- Chronic health conditions such as diabetes, high blood pressure, substance use, depression, and cancer
- Infectious diseases such as hepatitis, tuberculosis, HIV and COVID-19
- Reproductive health topics, including family planning and pregnancy
- Violence, including domestic violence
- Healthy relationships, including parenting
- Environmental or occupational health
- Civil rights and human rights
- Skills such as outreach, case management, motivational interviewing, or cultural humility

- *Can you think of other topics that you might address in a training?*

> **Joe Calderon:** I am the National Trainer for the Transitions Clinic Network, a group of 48 clinics across the country and in Puerto Rico that provide primary health care to individuals returning home from incarceration. I facilitate trainings primarily for CHWs who are part of the national clinic network and for several groups of CHWs in California. Some of the CHWs are just starting out and some are seasoned. Because the participants are working all over the country, I mostly facilitate trainings online. I train on a wide range of topics such as how to support patients who are coming home from prison, self-care, motivational interviewing, systems navigation, suicide assessment, medication-assisted treatment (or MAT), and working with survivors of trauma.

PURPOSE OR GOAL

The primary purpose or goal of trainings may include:

- To share and learn new health-related information
- To promote changes in health-related behaviors
- To promote self-management of chronic conditions
- To share and learn new skills such as stress management, risk reduction, health outreach, or advocacy skills
- To build leadership skills, capacity, and autonomy
- To promote teamwork and community building
- To support a community planning or organizing process

  - *Can you think of other goals for trainings?*

What Do **YOU?** Think

> **Francis Julian Montgomery:** It's vital for people like myself—African American and middle-aged—to have a chance to learn about chronic conditions. Many trainings leave out people, such as people of color or gender minorities, by not including language and information that is geared for them. I want to make sure that a person like me can get the information they need.

DURATION

Trainings may last anywhere from thirty minutes to eight hours or more and may even take place over many days or weeks.

NUMBER OF FACILITATORS

Sometimes you will facilitate trainings on your own, and sometimes with a co-facilitator or as part of a training team. When you are starting out, it is helpful to observe other facilitators and to facilitate trainings as a part of a team. This provides opportunities to learn new skills and approaches from trusted colleagues, and to give and receive critical feedback. In our experience, having a co-trainer is generally the best option for effective trainings as it allows for sharing the challenges of group management, makes it easier to facilitate more complex learning activities and to address more challenging topics, and allows facilitators to work as a team to adjust the training plan as needed.

PREPARATION

Facilitating trainings can be intimidating, especially if you feel uncomfortable speaking in front of groups. Most people who lead trainings start out feeling nervous and unsure about what to do. Even those of us who have been facilitating trainings for many years may still feel nervous before a training session. The good thing about feeling a bit nervous is that it provides energy and motivation to do your best.

By the end of this chapter, our hope is that you will have the building blocks to develop engaging and effective trainings and will feel more confident as a facilitator.

20.2 Understanding How People Learn

TYPES OF LEARNERS

Many people think of the process of learning as one in which an "expert" talks about what they know, and the "learners" simply listen. The learners are assumed to have understood what they heard, even though there may be no steps in place to evaluate whether or not they did. Perhaps you experienced (or still experience) school that way: the teacher lectures or gives an assignment, and then you, the student, are assumed to have understood. In reality, people learn in many different ways, including:

- **Visual learners:** Who need to see the material they are learning. They might prefer films, photographs, drawings, or observation. For example, if you are a visual learner, you will probably benefit from being able to watch others as they facilitate trainings.

- **Kinesthetic or tactile learners:** Who need to interact with the material they are learning, to move around, touch, or practice doing what it is they are trying to learn. This type of learner may want to practice how to facilitate a training by doing part of one with an experienced co-facilitator.

- **Auditory learners:** Who learn by listening. This learner might enjoy a lecture, a film, or a small or large group discussion. To learn how to facilitate a training, this type of learner may want to listen to a detailed lecture or presentation about training skills.

Of course, there are other types of learners as well. Both of this chapter's authors find that we are most likely to learn if given the opportunity to interact with the trainer/educator *and* the material. For us, having the opportunity to ask questions, have discussions, and to understand how the ideas being presented can be applied to our own lives and work provides the best opportunity for learning.

While some people may be *primarily* one type of learner, all of us learn in more than one way. In any training, you will be working with a diverse group that learns in a variety of ways. If you rely on just one teaching method, you will limit the effectiveness of your trainings. A two-hour training that consists of the facilitators lecturing, reading PowerPoint slides aloud, or even just talking (without a lot of listening) is not likely to engage most learners.

ADULT LEARNING THEORY

While you may facilitate trainings for participants of all ages, many CHWs principally work with adult learners. Adult learning theory—a loose collection of ideas about how adults learn—has several things in common with popular education (described below). Both acknowledge that adults learn best when they are invited to share and build upon what they know. Both emphasize active learning through simulations, games, case studies, and role plays that engage the body, mind, and emotions. Key principles of adult learning include:

Relevance: Trainings should be relevant to the social environments and day-to-day experiences of participants.

Respect: The most effective trainings will acknowledge and build upon participants prior experience, knowledge, interests, and skills. Effective adult learning also establishes group norms that encourage mutual respect and support.

Immediacy: Adults are more likely to commit to learning when the goals and objectives are realistic and important to them. Training content should be something that participants can apply to their daily lives or work.

Application: Adults appreciate direct concrete experiences in which to apply the knowledge and concepts they are learning. Applied training activities—such as case studies and role plays—should be reflective of the real lives, circumstances, and challenges experiences by participants.

Safety and challenge: Adult learners tend to resist activities when they feel judged or shamed. Trainers must create a safe environment for discussion, discovery, and practice. Training content should be sequenced appropriately and sufficiently complex to engage adult learners.

Feedback: Adult learners often wish to receive timely feedback on what they are doing. Constructive feedback from peers and trainers increases the impact and value of training.

WHAT IS YOUR EXPERIENCE AS A LEARNER?

Think about a training session or class that *was not effective* in facilitating your learning:

- What made it difficult for you to become actively engaged in learning?
- Did the trainer or teacher talk too much?
- Did the training value your own experience and knowledge?
- Did the training or class invite your participation?
- What could the trainer or teacher have done to improve the class?

Now think about a training or class that *was effective* in facilitating your learning:

- How did you know that this training or class was effective for you?
- What did the trainer or teacher do to make you feel comfortable?
- What kind of activities most engaged you?
- What styles of teaching worked best for you?

An Early Experience as a Trainer: Jill Tregor

My first paid job in the community was with an organization that worked to prevent and respond to hate-motivated violence (when people are threatened or attacked due to their real or perceived ethnicity, religion, immigration status, sexual orientation, gender, or gender-identity). We often received requests for presentations about hate violence from schools and other organizations. Occasionally, I had time to learn something in advance about the group I would present to, but more often I showed up to the training without knowing much about the participants because I really didn't understand how important it was to do so. I thought my material should be what guided the format for the training, not the audience, and not even what I hoped would be the outcome(s) for the training.

Because I knew a lot about my topic, I wanted to just *tell* people about hate violence. But quite often the people in the trainings already knew a lot about the topic, because their communities had been the targets of hate-motivated violence themselves. I didn't think about how boring it might be for them if I just stood up at the front of the room and talked for thirty minutes or more, although I knew I did not like to be a participant in trainings like this. Because I didn't always have a training plan, or the training plan I had was overly simplistic, it was also possible (or likely) that I would end a training without covering topics or concerns that the participants were most eager to learn about.

Eventually, I realized that I needed help and looked for opportunities to become a better trainer. I talked with my co-workers. I read books, went to workshops, and participated in trainings for trainers. I observed what experienced trainers did. I finally learned to prepare for *every* training I do and to tailor each training to fit the needs of the group I am working with. Now my first step is to make sure I know who my participants are and what it is they want to know or learn about. While doing that research, I can ensure that I am actually capable of meeting the goals identified for the training, or if I need to ask for help from others.

20.3 Approaches to Teaching and Training

There are many approaches to facilitating trainings. For the purposes of this chapter, we will emphasize three approaches that are commonly used in the field of public health to actively engage training participants in learning and teaching: popular education, participatory learning, and problem-based learning.

POPULAR EDUCATION

Paulo Freire is considered one of the world's most important thinkers about education. He is widely known in the field of public health as a key theorist and practitioner of "popular education." Freire lived and worked in Brazil, where it was illegal to vote unless one was literate (able to read and write), leaving many people without a voice in elections. Freire worked to address the problem of illiteracy, teaching sugarcane workers how to read in just forty-five days. He initiated a national literacy campaign, which ended when the Brazilian government was overthrown.

Freire recognized that unless a learner's own experiences were recognized and valued, truly significant learning could not occur. Education that starts *where people are* has the potential to transform lives. Freire's approach suggested that education that supported people in identifying and analyzing important problems in their lives, and in better understanding how those problems are connected to larger social issues and dynamics, could lead them to develop and implement actions to change and improve their circumstances.

Freire called this process **conscientization,** or the development of a critical consciousness about social and political realities. He also strongly believed that the true purpose of education should be liberation and the promotion of social justice.

> Freire wrote: *One cannot expect positive results from an educational or political action program which fails to respect the particular view of the world held by the people. Such a program constitutes cultural invasion, good intentions notwithstanding* (Freire, 1970, pp. 68).

When Freire taught farmworkers how to read, the workers also talked about and analyzed their personal experiences with poverty and injustice. They came to realize that these were not individual problems, but larger problems created by social inequities and oppression. Freire believed the final step of the popular education process comes when the development of critical consciousness leads to *praxis*—when the participants use their knowledge to take collective action to promote social justice and the welfare of their community.

Have you ever taken a class in which the teacher lectured the entire time? Freire called this "banking"—a traditional teaching method that treats learners as though they are containers into which information is poured, with the expectation that the learner will be able to repeat back the information exactly as it was told to them. As a learner, it is easy to become so accustomed to this approach that we may have difficulty adjusting if we are invited to more actively participate in our education. In contrast to this approach, Freire encouraged teachers or trainers to recognize, value, and call forth the experience, the knowledge, and the wisdom of students or participants. Though it can be comfortable to be taught via the banking method instead of being an engaged participant, there is research to show that learners actually retain much more of what was intended if they are given opportunities to apply the information/learning as soon as possible.

Popular education supports learners in "speaking their own word," rather than repeating back the language, analysis, and ideas of trainers, or anyone else. To learn more about popular education, review the resources provided at the end of this chapter, including the Paulo Freire Institute.

PARTICIPATORY LEARNING

When CHWs engage people in all aspects of the learning experience, when they presume that a learner is also a teacher, the process of **participatory learning** has begun. Other ways to describe participatory learning are interactive or active learning. As with popular education, participatory learning views the learner as more than a recipient of information. This approach identifies what participants want to learn, how they would like to learn new information, and engages them in all learning activities. You might say that the learners identify not only what their problems are, but the solutions to these problems as well. This approach to learning eliminates the idea of there being one expert: we are all experts when it comes to figuring out the solutions to our own questions and challenges.

PROBLEM-BASED LEARNING

Another way to engage a community in the learning experience is to organize them into teams that work together to discover solutions to real-life problems. As with the methods described above, **problem-based learning** encourages people to think in a critical way. Instead of just memorizing somebody's idea of "the right answer" to a problem, team members talk to and challenge each other to develop their own solutions. Examples of the types of problems that learners might address include (1) how to reduce and manage stress or (2) how to conduct outreach to link an underserved community with health care services.

In this model, there are no right answers as much as there are a range of possible answers that represent the experience, ideas, and values of the group. One significant benefit of this approach is that the group members get to know each other as individuals and learn how to work together as a team. This creates a sense of community, as well as building relationships across differences such as class, ethnicity, immigration status, language, and culture.

One challenge is that people can become accustomed to education or training that promotes "yes" and "no" or "right" and "wrong" ideas. It is sometimes uncomfortable, at first, for people to engage in learning that is less defined. People may look to you for guidance and judgment. In this case, problem-based learning may require additional explanation, and additional patience from you in your role as facilitator.

CHWs use participatory learning, popular education, problem-based learning, and other methods that actively involve community members in the process of learning. These methods respect the experience, knowledge, and wisdom of learners, and support them in using their knowledge to take action that will promote their health and well-being.

How might you apply these approaches to learning as you facilitate a training for CHWs on cultural humility?

20.4 Applying CHW Skills

Many essential CHW concepts and skills can be applied to the task of facilitating trainings.

CULTURAL HUMILITY

Cultural humility (see Chapter 7) guides you in respecting the cultural identities of the clients and communities you work with. It reminds us to acknowledge that all people are the experts in their own cultural identities, experiences, belief systems, and values. It cautions us about imposing our own cultural standards, beliefs, or assumptions onto others. Finally, cultural humility encourages us to transfer power away from ourselves and working to support the leadership and independence of clients and community members.

Let cultural humility guide your work as a trainer. Demonstrate respect for the cultural identities of all participants. Try to be aware of any moment when you may be imposing your own beliefs, assumptions, or biases. Sometimes participants will speak up to challenge you in these moments, and sometimes they will convey their discomfort or displeasure through body language, by leaving the training space or turning off their videoconferencing monitor. If this happens, try to re-engage the participants. Welcome their feedback. Ask them what they would like to add to the conversation.

STRENGTH-BASED PRACTICE

Strength-based practice is addressed in Chapters 6 and 9 and encourages CHWs to inquire about; acknowledge; and build upon a client's knowledge, skills, values, and accomplishments in their work together. Apply a strength-based approach to your work as a trainer by identifying, listening to, and validating the wisdom that participants bring to every training. If, for example, you are training people newly diagnosed with depression about their condition, start by asking participants to share what they have already learned about depression symptoms, challenges, and effective strategies for managing or treating depression.

BIG EYES, BIG EARS, SMALL MOUTH

Apply the concept of a CHW with Big Eyes, Big Ears, and a small mouth introduced in Chapter 9. Remember to listen carefully to participants. Observe the training space and the interactions, energy, and body language of participants. Are they engaging with each other and with trainers? Do they seem to be enjoying the experience? Do they look bored, upset, or offended? Have they stopped participating? Are you talking more than the participants in the training?

These clues can help you to assess the effectiveness of a training as it occurs and provides an opportunity for you to intervene or change things up. If you are working with a co-facilitator and you have questions about how the training is going, take a quick break and consult with them. Brainstorm strategies for working together to enhance the effectiveness of the training.

DEMONSTRATE PATIENCE AND EMPATHY

To be successful over time, CHWs must be able to authentically demonstrate patience and empathy with the clients and communities they work with. Not surprisingly, these qualities and skills are also important for your role as a trainer. To reflect on these issues, consider the following questions about the trainings you facilitate:

- Did you bring a sense of interpersonal warmth and regard to the training?
- Did you express interest in the experience, ideas, questions, and skills of participants?
- Were you patient when participants were struggling with particular concepts or training activities?
- Did you offer encouragement and motivation for learning?
- Did you provide positive feedback and acknowledge the meaningful contributions of participants?
- Did you demonstrate empathy and concern in moments when a participant may share that they are struggling or facing a challenge or crisis?

> **Joe Calderon:** I am always applying my CHW skills to my role as a trainer. As CHWs, we are trained to meet clients where they are at, and as a trainer, I try to do the same with participants. I try to bring my humility, just like when I am working with patients. I'm no bigger or better than anyone else. I use my Motivational Interviewing skills and ask Open-ended questions so that participants can share their knowledge and skills. I share Affirmations to let participants know that I value their contributions to the training. Even when I'm training, I'm always in CHW mode.

ACKNOWLEDGE YOUR MISTAKES

Chapter 9 introduces the concept of fallibility or the idea that all people are imperfect, and everyone makes mistakes. As a CHW and as a trainer, it is helpful to acknowledge your fallibility and the limits of your knowledge and skills. Modeling this also encourages the clients and training participants you work with to be more comfortable with their own fallibility and mistakes.

Here are some tips:

- Acknowledge when you have limited knowledge about a particular question or topic. Ask if others in the training have expertise or knowledge they would like to share. *"That's a great question, but not a topic that I know much about. Can anyone else here answer Marta's question?"*
- Acknowledge that some topics and questions are complex and may not have one simple or best answer. Encourage participants to brainstorm a number of ways of answering the question or approaching the task at hand.
- Be accountable when you make a mistake, large or small. *"Oh, I'm sorry, I totally skipped over a topic,"* or *"Norma, I said I'd answer your question and then I forgot to circle back to it. I'm sorry. Let's talk about it now."* When you do this authentically, it promotes a stronger connection with training participants.

CHW Profile

Silvia Ortega (she/her)

Community Health Worker and Trainer

Promotores Academy, San Manuel Gateway College, San Bernadino, CA

Doula, Doula Assistant Program, Riverside Health Foundation

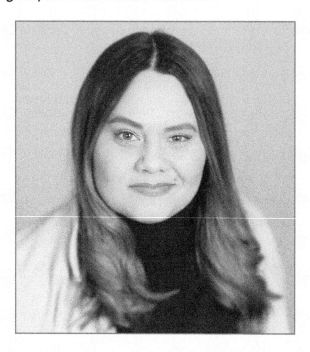

Becoming a CHW was a calling I had to answer. In college, I had some health issues. I took a leave of absence and began to do what I later found out was community health work. I wanted to live a healthier lifestyle, so I took a healthy cooking class, and started to change my lifestyle, little by little. After I graduated from college, I came back home and took a CHW training course.

I'm a CHW at San Manuel Gateway College, the same place I was a student 5 years ago. We work with low-income communities. The building we're in is like a one-stop shop. There are three floors with a clinic in the bottom, then behavioral health and dental care, and the top floor is the college. It is intentional to have a building for both education and health, so that the CHWs become part of an interdisciplinary team, working with doctors and residents.

I'm also a doula, working with low-income pregnant families and young mothers. I was the first CHW in the neonatal intensive care unit (NICU), following up with families through their stay in the NICU, then helping them transition back to their home.

One family that really impacted me was a family where the dad was disabled, and the mom had diabetes and almost had her foot amputated. When I met them in the NICU, the social workers were going to call CPS (Child Protective Services) because they didn't know who was going to take care of the baby. I told the social workers to give me two days to work with the family to see what we can do. We got them in the Ronald McDonald House, so they could visit the baby while I was working with them.

The dad was frustrated because he wasn't getting his SSI (Supplemental Security Income), so they couldn't pay rent. We got on the phone with his SSI worker that same day. Before the call I shared communication styles with him because he was very frustrated, very mad. I said, there's three basic communication styles: aggressive, passive-aggressive, and the one I use a lot is assertive. We agreed to use keywords, like expedite

(continues)

CHW Profile

(continued)

and critical, and to say that the family is in a very critical position right now with your baby in the NICU and your family really needs the money, so can they expedite your case. They got the SSI money the next week.

The dad felt supported, and they were able to rent a home. The mom went from being super depressed to having hope, being able to care for the baby in the NICU. The family says that because of me, their kids also communicate in an assertive way, where before they would scream at each other. And so, they all share their feelings, and the baby is very healthy.

Being a CHW has completely changed the way I see society. I think we are all put in this world to learn from each other. It has made me a more compassionate person. It taught me to have cultural humility. And I just fell in love with health. Without health, we really have nothing.

I tell CHWs starting their training to love what they do. It's a blessing, it's a calling. It's a responsibility to do the work that we do, but also think of the next generation. So, whatever I do, I don't just do it for me, or for my profession, but I do it thinking of how what I'm contributing can also impact the next generation's legacy. I call it the "love-acy," planting seeds for the future.

20.5 Training Methods

There are a wide variety of training methods that can be applied to both in-person and online trainings. We highlight a few common training methods here and encourage you to learn more by referring to the Additional Resources presented at the end of this chapter.

Short presentations/mini lecturettes: Short presentations or lectures are a valuable part of trainings, as long as they don't last too long and are balanced by using a variety of other methods that encourage more active participation. Try to keep any presentations short and focused. Share the stage and invite participants to present as well. Follow up any presentation with an opportunity for participatory and applied learning. Invite participants to discuss the presentation in small groups with a series of guiding questions. Ask them to share their questions and opinions about the topic. Provide them with a case study to analyze or a role play to practice the concepts or skills that have been shared.

Large and small group discussions: Use training methods that engage the entire group as well as opportunities for participants to work in smaller groups of two or more. Remember that some participants will feel more comfortable asking questions and sharing their experience and knowledge when speaking with a smaller group.

Applied learning: All trainings you facilitate will benefit from applied learning activities. If you are training people to learn or enhance any type of skill such as stress reduction, communication or advocacy skills, cultural humility, or chronic conditions management, think of an opportunity for participants to practice these skills in the training. Two classic types of applied training methods are *Case Studies* and *Role Plays*.

Case studies: Case studies present learners with a realistic scenario in which to apply the concepts and skills they are studying, and a series of questions to answer or tasks to complete. For example, trainers could use a case study about miscommunication between a provider and a patient to engage participants to talking about communication skills. Be sure to read the case study over with the large group to make sure that they understand the scenario and the questions or tasks you want them to complete. For examples of case study activities, see the *Foundations Training Guide* and other resources provided at the end of this chapter.

Role plays: Role plays are commonly used to train CHWs and other helping professionals, providing an opportunity to practice concepts and skills for working directly with clients. Role plays or skits can be used to address a wide variety of training topics and to engage learners with key content. You could use a role play to encourage participants to demonstrate stress reduction skills, advocacy skills, job interviewing skills, knowledge about reproductive health or safer sex, healthy nutrition, or other topics. Present learners with a clearly written and realistic role-play scenario and directions for what you want them to do. The role plays can be done in small groups or in front of a large group of learners. Ask participants to debrief and discuss the role play when it was done by asking a series of questions such as: "What did you observe in this role play?" "What questions or challenges did this role play highlight?" "How did the role play highlight or demonstrate the concepts and skills we have been learning?" For examples of role-play activities, see the *Foundations Training Guide* and other resources provided at the end of this chapter.

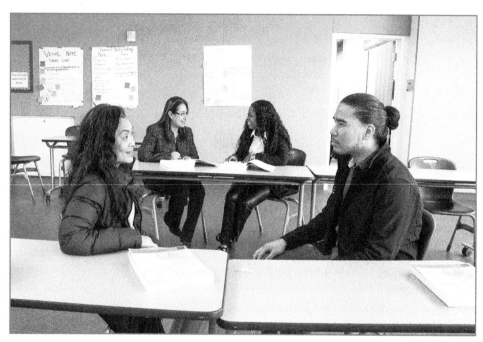

CHWs participating in role play practice.

Joe Calderon: In every training, I make sure that the participants have a chance to talk with each other in small groups. I use breakout groups on Zoom. In a smaller group, people connect more, things get more personal, they share more. The other technique that I always use is realistic case scenarios about situations that CHWs face in their clinics and communities. They need to apply their knowledge and skills to these scenarios because we're preparing CHWs to help communities that have been historically marginalized, stepped on, and left behind. These communities, the patients we work with, they need lifelines. CHWs are these lifelines. They are bridges across barriers and biases that our communities face, and good case scenarios prepare us to face these challenges.

Games: Games can be effective with participants of all ages and provide an opportunity for play, humor, and team-building. They can provide a great transition from one part of a training to another. You can find thousands of examples of icebreakers and other games online and in the Additional Resources provided at the end of this chapter. *What types of games or icebreakers have you played in trainings?*

Stress reduction activities: Learning should be fun and energizing. But it can also be stressful, particularly if the training is long or addresses challenging topics. Take a few minutes to facilitate a quick stress reduction activity or invite learners to share their own. This could be a two-minute deep breathing activity, such as the one highlighted in Chapter 12.

Plus/Delta analysis and feedback: A plus/delta (+/triangle image) discussion is a quick way to gather and categorize feedback. It can be applied to almost any training activity such as a video, a presentation, or a role-play demonstration. If you have a whiteboard or flip chart paper, draw two columns and label one with a Plus sign (+) and the other with a delta sign or triangle (Δ), a symbol that also represents change. If you are training online, you could use the chat box to help gather feedback. The plus side is for feedback about what went well or what participants liked or appreciated. The delta size is for what could be improved or done differently. It can also be used as a quick way to gather verbal feedback from all participants about a training. For example, trainers can ask participants questions such as:

Plus (+)

- What worked for you today?
- What supported your learning?
- What made you feel welcome and included?

Delta (Δ)

- What didn't work so well for you today?
- How could we make this training better?

Joe Calderon: I am always trying to read the room to see how the training is going. I can tell if it's going well by the level of participation. Are people speaking up? Are they asking questions? Are their cameras on? I observe their participation in small groups and how they debrief small group discussions or case scenarios. Do they seem engaged and energized by the material? Are they talking to each other, sharing stories and knowledge? Do they seem to be passionate about the topic? At the end of every training, I always ask the participants, "What are you taking away from today's training that you can see yourself using in the future?" Based on what they share, I can tell if the training was on point or not, if the topics we covered are relevant to their work.

20.6 Deciding If Training Is the Right Strategy

Training is often proposed as a strategy to address many community health issues. But training is not always the best way to address the challenge at hand. It may be more effective, for example, to conduct community health outreach, to facilitate a support group, to engage in community planning, or to facilitate community organizing and advocacy.

How do you figure out whether training is actually what a group needs?

The following questions are designed to guide you in deciding whether or not to conduct training:

- What does the group want to accomplish?
- What does the group want to learn to help them reach their goal?
- Are there other ways to accomplish these goals?
- What makes you think that training is the best way to accomplish it?
- Is there a better way to get the information to people?

In order to answer those questions, you will need to figure out:

- Who is your audience?
- Will participation in the training be voluntary or required?
- Would learning be better in a formal or informal setting?
- Is the group highly diverse (with different backgrounds, identities, and levels of knowledge about the training issues)?

- What are the possible barriers between you and your audience? Age, race, language, gender, sexual orientation, national origin, and literacy level are just a few of the walls that may stand between you and the people you are working with.
- Will the audience be expecting an "expert" as the teacher? What qualifies you to be the one to lead the session?
- Are you hoping to teach concepts or to teach skills?
- What will the cost of the training be? What is your budget? Is there a more cost-effective way to have your participants learn the material?

There is no simple formula to determine whether training is the right strategy use. Based on the answers to these questions, use your best judgment to decide whether training is the right approach for the challenge at hand.

20.7 How to Plan and Prepare Trainings

How will you prepare for the cultural humility training that you have been asked to facilitate (in the CHW Scenario presented at the beginning of this chapter)?

Your first task is to ask questions. You need to know what the audience or the person who contacted you wants to achieve, what the participants need, and what resources are available for this training.

The following list of general questions does not necessarily have to be answered in any particular order, but we recommend that you find out as much as you can about each one.

1. If you have been asked to conduct this training by someone else, *what are their primary goals*? In the case study presented at the beginning of the chapter, what are the supervisor's goals for the cultural humility training? What do they expect CHWs to learn in the workshop?

2. What do the participants *want to know*? What do the CHWs who will participate in the training most want to know about cultural humility and working with clients from a wide range of cultural identities and backgrounds? Have they experienced a lack of cultural humility in their own interactions with health care providers? Do they want to know specific strategies that demonstrate cultural humility with clients?

3. What do those who will participate in the training *already know*? For example, have the CHWs participated in workshops about cultural humility before? What do they currently do to ensure that their clients feel welcomed, respected, and understood?

CONDUCTING AN ASSESSMENT BEFORE DESIGNING A TRAINING

You will facilitate a better training if you understand what the participants already know and want to learn. If possible, conduct a *pre-assessment* to gather this information and prepare for the training. The assessment doesn't need to be complicated or lengthy; it just needs to provide you with some basic information. There are a number of options for how to gather the information, each with its own strengths and weaknesses.

Conduct Interviews Interviews with potential participants or another professional who works with the participants will provide useful information for planning your training. You might be able to visit an agency or group to talk with them in person about the proposed training or set up a conference call or Zoom meeting. Prepare a list of *open-ended questions,* being careful not to take too much time with the people you are interviewing (you don't want folks to think you are disrespecting the value of their time.) Decide how many people you are going to interview. Once you have conducted a few interviews, you can review your notes for common themes.

If you are able to speak with the CHWs who will participate in the cultural humility training, your questions might include:

- What is your level of interest in attending a training on cultural humility?
- What do you hope to get out of this training? What questions do you have that are related to the topic of cultural humility?
- Have you participated in prior trainings or classes on cultural humility? If so, what did these trainings cover?

- What do you already do to ensure that your clients are treated a culturally respectful manner?

- What topics do you not need me to cover in detail?

- What would you most like to learn about?

- What kind of trainings do you most enjoy? How do you best learn new information or skills?

  - *What other questions would you want to ask?*

ADMINISTER SURVEYS

Surveys are another resource for gathering information about future trainings. In general, surveys ask *closed-ended questions*. You need to decide on your goals before you design the survey and think about the type of answers that people may give to the questions you ask. You can conduct a survey by phone, Zoom, using a web-based survey instrument or by distributing paper copies, or with an in-person interview. Survey questions can be of many types, including multiple choice, yes/no, or *interval rating* (such as a Likert Scale, which asks people to rate their feeling or opinion on a 0–5, or 0–10 scale).

Learning to develop a good survey is an art that takes practice. It includes balancing the need for information against the likelihood that for the survey taker, time and patience may be limited. For more information about using surveys, please see the resources provided in Chapter 23 and at the end of this chapter.

CONDUCT A FOCUS GROUP

Focus Groups are an opportunity to bring together 6–12 members of a common group or community to facilitate a discussion about specific topics and record their responses. It is often used as part of a community diagnosis process, to develop new public health programs or educational materials or to evaluate programs, and it may be useful in designing your training as well. Focus groups take a lot of time to prepare for and, depending on the nature of your training, it may be a bigger project than the training itself merits. For more information on focus groups, see Chapter 23 and the additional resources presented at the end of this chapter.

CONDUCT ONLINE RESEARCH

No matter how much you already know about a training topic, we recommend that you conduct online research. Search for recent statistics, research studies, emerging standards or protocols, model programs, and other training models that you could adapt as you develop your own approach to the training topic.

Training CHWS on the Topic of Suicide Assessment: Joe Calderon

I was asked to develop a new training for CHWs who work with the Transitions Clinic Network (TCN). The TCN is a network of health clinics across the country that provide primary health care to patients returning home from prison. The focus of the training was on assessing patient risks for suicide.

To prepare for this training, I reflected on my own training and experience working with suicidal clients. I spoke with TCN health care providers and CHWs to identify their main priorities for the training. I spoke with several CHWs by phone and asked if they had prior training on suicide or suicide assessment and if they were aware of their clinic's protocols for assessing patients and completing mandatory reports for anyone found to be suicidal. I asked them what they most wanted to learn and practice during our training.

What I learned is that many of the CHWs didn't have prior training on assessing suicide, and many of them were anxious about having to talk with clients about the topic.

I also researched statistics on suicide, focusing on studies of people who are incarcerated or coming home after incarceration. I looked at suicide assessment protocols from organizations like the National Substance Abuse and Mental Health Services Administration (SAMHSA). I also asked TCN clinics to send me examples of their protocols for suicide assessment. What was interesting was that some of the clinics didn't have protocols. So that became another learning outcome for our training.

ARE YOU THE RIGHT PERSON TO FACILITATE THE TRAINING?

Once you have determined that training is an appropriate strategy to meet the needs of the community or organization, there are other questions to be answered. Are you the right person to deliver this training? Do you have the expertise and knowledge required? If your answer to that question is "no," you may be able to learn new information and skills that will prepare you to take the lead. Or you may want to identify someone who is more knowledgeable about the topic and ask that person to facilitate the training or to work with you as co-facilitator. Even if you are highly knowledgeable about the topic, you should still consider whether you are the right person to facilitate the training. In general, having a co-facilitator can improve your effectiveness as a trainer. With two trainers, there is more opportunity to notice a participant who needs extra support or adjust material if you hit a bump in the road.

Perhaps the most important issues to consider before deciding to do a training are the potential barriers that may exist between the training participants and trainer(s). While a facilitator does not necessarily need to resemble the people participating in the training, it is helpful if participants feel they can relate to the facilitator in some way. If trainers share things in common with participants, they may be able to establish a positive connection more quickly. If trainers don't share things in common with the group, you will want to consider whether differences in identity and experience are going to get in the way of the participants' learning experience.

Cultural identity and issues of class, ethnicity, immigration status, age, gender, and language are among the most obvious differences that may exist between you and the people you are hoping to train. Sometimes any or all of those differences can be such significant obstacles that you are not the right person to lead the training. Other times, by acknowledging the differences between you and the participants, by respecting and asking them to share their knowledge and experience during the training, and by doing plenty of homework to prepare ahead of time, you can serve as the trainer or co-trainer.

ESTABLISH GOALS AND LEARNING OUTCOMES

Once you have gathered information about training needs and expectations, it is time to establish the goals and learning outcomes or objectives for your training. (For the purpose of this chapter, we will use the terms *learning outcomes* and *objectives* interchangeably.) The feedback you received, whether from a survey, an interview, or a focus group, will be a critical part of determining what these goals and objectives will be.

What is the difference between a goal and a learning outcome? A goal is the broad statement that reflects a big idea about what we want to achieve. A **learning outcome** should be as specific as possible about what participants will know or know how to do as a result of the training. To learn more about developing goals and objectives, refer to the resources at the end of this chapter.

Here are the goals and two of the learning outcomes that were established for the Transitions Clinic Network training on Assessing Patient Risks for Suicide.

Training Goals

1. To increase awareness of the risks of suicide among the population served by the Transitions Clinic Network.
2. To enhance CHW knowledge and skills for assessing patient risks for suicide.
3. To prevent suicide among the TCN patient population.

Learning Outcomes

1. To explain guidelines for how and when to assess a patient's risk for suicide.
2. To discuss and demonstrate how to respond to patients who are and are not identified as being suicidal.
3. To discuss and understand organizational policies and procedures for reporting and responding to suicidal ideation

What are the possible goals and learning outcomes for the training on cultural humility that you have been asked to facilitate?

Goals:

Example: To enhance knowledge and skills for demonstrating cultural humility when engaging with clients and communities.

Learning Outcomes:

Example: Participants will demonstrate how to "transfer power" when working with a client to prioritize their knowledge, priorities, and skills

- *What are some other possible learning outcomes for the training on cultural humility?*

CREATE AN OUTLINE FOR YOUR TRAINING

After identifying your goals and learning outcomes, you are ready to develop a detailed outline of what you will do in the training. What information will you cover? What kinds of training methods are you going to use? Be specific about every step and topic you are going to cover. This will assist you in many ways, including allowing you to determine what you really have time to cover.

There are numerous ways to outline a training plan. Here is an excerpt from Joe Calderon's training on Assessing Risks for Suicide that he developed for the Transitions Clinic Network.

Sample Training Plan

JOE CALDERON, TRANSITIONS CLINIC NETWORK

Title of training: Assessing Patient Risks for Suicide.

Learning outcomes: By the end of the training, participants will be able to:

- Identify and discuss the prevalence of suicide in the United States, and among people with a history of incarceration
- Explain guidelines for how and when to assess a patient's risk for suicide
- Discuss and demonstrate how to respond to patients who are not suicidal
- Demonstrate how to respond to patients who are suicidal and how to implement guidelines for mandatory reporting
- Discuss TCN clinic policies and procedures for reporting and responding to suicidal ideation/emergencies
- Discuss the emotional challenge of working with clients who are suicidal and strategies for self-care
- Identify local, state, and national resources on suicide

Time required: Two Hours

Training methods:

- PowerPoint slides and presentation
- Small and large group discussions
- Testimony/stories
- Patient case scenario
- Role-play practice

Resources required:

- Current data on suicide rates and rates among incarcerated/formerly incarcerated communities
- First responder model for suicide assessment and 5150

(continues)

Sample Training Plan

(continued)

- ◦ Crisis response teams and other first responder agencies
- SAMHSA policies on suicide assessment
- TCN protocols for suicide assessment and mandated reporting
  - ◦ How do CHWs document and report a client who is suicidal? Who do they report this to? Who makes the report to a third party—police, crisis response team, etc.?

Trainer preparation:

- Research and identify suicide statistics and studies.
- Review SAMHSA guidelines on assessing for suicide.
- Summarize key information in a PowerPoint Slide.
- Decide what stories you to share with training participants to illustrate key concepts about suicide assessment
- Review TCN site policies and protocols re. suicide assessment and mandated reporting (identify a sample written policy to share during the training)
- Develop a step-by-step training plan with topics, methods, and estimated time for each activity

Learner preparation:

- Along with the training invitation and agenda, attach a copy of the SAMHSA suicide assessment guidelines and ask TCN CHWs to do the following in advance of the training date:
  - ◦ Review SAMHSA guidelines
  - ◦ Ask for and review clinic protocols for suicide assessment
  - ◦ Reflect on experience assessing and responding to patient risks for suicide

20.8 Tips for Facilitating a Participatory Training

With more experience as a trainer, you will continue to develop your own approaches and training methods. For now, here are some tips that we hope will be useful.

PREPARING THE TRAINING

For in-person trainings, make sure you have a safe, comfortable training space that is accessible to all participants: Will people be able to get to the training easily by bus, car, or on foot? If there are stairs, is there also a ramp or an elevator for those who are unable to use the stairs? Are there comfortable seats for everyone? Is there a source of fresh air (particularly important given COVID-19 concerns)?

Ask about the language needs of your participants: Do the trainers speak the same language as the participants? If you can't afford to pay for interpreters, are there community members who are willing to volunteer to play that role? Is there someone who requires sign-language interpretation? If so, make sure they have access to an interpreter and a comfortable place to sit where the participant can clearly see the interpreter and still be part of the group. Otherwise, you will need to let people know that the training is not accessible to all.

Assess child-care needs: If possible, try to arrange for child care, or have a plan for how to handle children if participants bring them. Your participants will appreciate knowing their children are safely occupied so that they can focus on the training. Inform participants in advance whether or not you are able to accommodate children or will provide child care.

Pack up your materials well ahead of time, including your training agenda, extra pens and paper, plenty of copies of any handouts, newsprint and an easel, markers, tape, and anything else you will be using. Make sure you haven't left anything out. We recommend making up a box with everything needed at least two days ahead.

Identify the need for technology: If you plan to show a video or PowerPoint presentation, make sure the appropriate technology (such as a laptop and LCD projector) will be available at the training site, or bring what you need with you. You do not want to waste valuable time at a training discovering that your systems aren't compatible or don't work at all.

Get to the training location at least thirty minutes in advance so that you have plenty of time to set up the room and to deal with any unexpected problems related to the space.

Double-Check and test all online materials: Before an online training, review your resources such as a posted online curriculum, slides, and videos to make sure that they are updated and that all web links are working. If you are using a videoconferencing resource like Zoom, make sure that the invitation and link are sent out to all participants. If you want to record the training, make sure that you have established this. As needed, practice using key features of the videoconferencing resources such as setting up breakout groups or using quizzes or polls.

- *What else would you want to do to prepare for the training session?*

FACILITATING A TRAINING SESSION

Setting the Stage

Set up the training space: Depending on the training topic and number of people expected, it can promote participation to set up chairs/tables either in a full circle or a u-shape. Make sure to set up chairs (and tables, if appropriate) ahead of time or request them to be set up as needed. If participants will be working a lot in small groups, you might want to set up tables with seats for four to five each throughout a room. What matters here is the comfort of the participants and the ability for everyone to see and hear each other.

Introduce yourself and welcome all participants: Review the topics that the training will address. Share the training goals and learning outcomes. Review the day's agenda so that participants know what to expect. Invite and respond to questions or concerns. Make sure participants know when breaks will occur, where the restrooms are, and any other logistical information they might need.

If you are training online via a videoconferencing resource, ask all participants to sign in to the group "chat" or discussion board with their name, and if appropriate, the agency they work for. Ask all participants to turn their video monitors on and to mute their microphones unless they are speaking.

Establish clear ground rules or learning agreements: Suggest some ground rules to the group and ask them if they would like to add to the list. Sample ground rules include: "No interruptions—let each person finish speaking before you begin," "Turn off cell phones," "Maintain confidentiality—don't share anyone's private or personal information with people outside of the training," and "Offer respect to all of the participants, even if you disagree with them." Ask everyone for their agreement in following the ground rules: this will be helpful if anything happens during the session that creates an unwelcome interruption or disturbance.

"Step Up, Step Back." Ask participants to monitor their own participation in the training. If they are someone who tends to speak a lot, encourage them to "step back" and allow other voices to be heard. If they are someone who tends to be quiet, encourage them to take risks and speak up so that others may benefit from their insight and experience.

Use icebreakers or opening activities to assist participants to relax and build trust. This will assist people in preparing for the work at hand and perhaps allow them to meet some or all of the people in the room. There are thousands of great ideas for icebreakers online. Be guided in your choices by how much time you want to spend on this activity. Take into consideration the degree to which the participants already know each other.

- *What else would you want to say or do at the beginning of a training?*

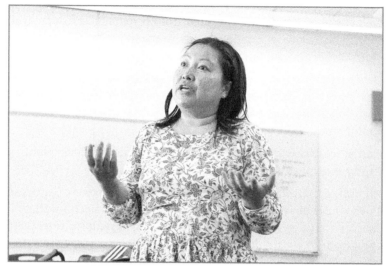

Darouny Somsanith facilitates a CHW training.

Organization and Logistics

Keep to the training schedule: You will break trust of the participants if you start a training late or don't finish on time. If for some reason you cannot begin on time, start no more than ten minutes after the session was scheduled to begin.

Schedule breaks during your session, particularly if you are working for more than an hour. People need time to stretch, use the bathroom, and return phone calls. They will be more capable of giving their full attention to the training if you let them know that they will be able to take care of these needs.

If possible, provide healthy refreshments for participants: Fruit, water, fresh vegetables, and dip are good things to provide, and also provide reassurance that you are concerned about the welfare of your participants.

Clarity

Connect your points together: Show how one idea leads to the next. Check-in regularly with participants to see if they understand what you are saying and doing. Ask them if they have any questions or concerns. Observe their body language. If you see looks of confusion on their faces, ask if you are communicating clearly enough.

Build on earlier lessons: They may be lessons learned at a different time entirely or lessons learned earlier during the same session. This aids in reinforcing learning.

Summarize your main points during the course of the session as a way to emphasize your message. Try asking participants to summarize key information. This is also a quick way to assess whether or not you have clearly conveyed essential concepts.

- *What else would you do to organize the training and to ensure that participants understand the information provided?*

Engaging Participants

Don't talk too much! Give people many opportunities to ask questions and to express their own knowledge and expertise. Don't allow your own anxiety or worry about silence to interfere with the learning process of the participants.

Ask questions: Acknowledge that everyone in the room has knowledge and experience to share. Your role is to facilitate learning, not to be the only source of information. Start a training by asking people to introduce themselves and answer a few questions. For example, you could ask, "How long have you worked here?" "What do you hope to learn today?" "What is one thing you would like to share with other people about your experience with this topic?"

Engage participants in problem-based learning instead of telling them what they need to know. For a workshop on cultural humility, you might assign participants to small teams, and ask each team to develop a proposal for what they and their agency can do differently to ensure that clients are treated respectfully.

Keep people moving: Sitting in one place throughout a training often makes it difficult for people to stay alert and to learn effectively. It can help to ask people to move around the room, meeting in different small groups, or writing down their ideas on large sheets of paper posted on the walls.

Use games and exercises: Once people are in small groups, they often enjoy an opportunity to compete in some way with the other groups. Teams might play a version of Jeopardy or another popular game show. Questions to be answered should reflect the material that you want the participants to learn.

Remember to break into small groups for discussions or applied learning activities.

Use participatory activities such as role plays, skits, or case studies.

Have teams teach each other a new skill: For example, in a workshop about managing hypertension or high blood pressure, you might give each group a handout about different components (such as healthy eating, active living, stress management, and medication management) of hypertension management. Each group is given enough time to understand and practice the method, and to make a plan for how to teach it to others. Each group then makes a presentation to the other participants about their assigned method for effective management of high blood pressure.

- *What else would you do to actively engage training participants?*

Tips for Facilitating Online Trainings

Increasingly, we participate in and facilitate trainings online using distance learning platforms and videoconferencing resources. Here are some tips that we have learned from facilitating online trainings:

- Practice and test the technology you are using. This will help to prevent glitches during the training and provide you with greater confidence so that you can focus on facilitating learning. You may need to spend some time upfront guiding participants in how to use the technology such as remembering to keep their video monitor on, to mute their microphone when they are not speaking, or how to post comments in a chat box.

- Online trainings can sometimes be more formal and passive than in-person alternatives. As a trainer, bring the energy you want participants to match. Speak with passion and convey your interest in the topics you are addressing.

- Don't lecture for too long! Remember to use a variety of training methods. You can adapt most training approaches and techniques—including the use of case studies, skits, and role plays—to the online environment.

- Use breakout groups to provide participants with opportunities to meet in smaller groups to discuss training topics or engage in applied learning activities.

- Monitor that chat to make sure that you track and respond to questions and comments posted by participants.

For multi-week or session trainings using an online learning platform.

- Use a blend of synchronous (live or in the moment learning opportunities such as a live videoconference meetings) and asynchronous activities such as posted videos, readings, and discussions that participants can engage in at their own pace.

- Quizzes can help participants to assess their progress in learning key concepts and skills.

- Discussion Forums. Some online learning platforms provide an opportunity for participants to engage in discussion with each other. This helps to foster connection among participants and creates an opportunity for them to share their knowledge, questions, and concerns about key topics. By reading the discussion forum, trainers can identify progress in meeting learning outcomes.

Joe Calderon: I train CHWs who are part of a national primary care network, so the only way to do this is online. One of the benefits of offering online trainings is being able to reach people who may not otherwise have an opportunity to participate. I think a lot of trainers get caught up in comparing in-person to online training or complain about conducting online trainings. But for me the job is the same, whether I'm with CHWs in-person in a classroom or talking to them over Zoom. To be effective, you need to prepare and bring your passion. Train from your experience, share from the heart, and create an atmosphere where community develops. Don't dominate or act like you have all the answers. Stay humble, share what you know, and make space for the participants to share what they know.

ENDING A TRAINING

Make sure you end on time: Even if you have not been able to cover all your material, respect people's time and end when you said that you would.

Acknowledge that people may still have questions and let them know where and how they can continue to learn about the topics addressed in the training. Give people a way to contact you if they don't already have that information.

Thank everyone for their participation.

Ask for feedback: You may want this in writing, as answers to a questionnaire, for instance, or you may ask students to discuss the "plusses and deltas" for a training. There is more information later in this chapter about some evaluation methods for a training.

Make sure that you leave the training space as you found it: This is particularly important if you are using space that was donated. Make sure your hosts want to invite you back.

20.9 Responding to Common Challenges

No matter how well you plan, something unexpected is sure to happen during a training. Mostly, this is a good thing (because extraordinary learning moments will spontaneously occur due to the contributions of participants), but sometimes it makes the work more challenging. Some of the training challenges that you are likely to experience are described below.

A PARTICIPANT WHO IS ARGUMENTATIVE OR DOMINATING

You may encounter a training participant who is argumentative, who has something to say about every statement you make, who is disrespectful to others, or in some other way makes it difficult to proceed smoothly with the training agenda. It is important to consider, however, how these behaviors may affect the other participants. As a facilitator, it is your responsibility to ensure a productive learning environment for everyone. There are a number of strategies that might work in this situation.

The ground rules established at the beginning of the training can be useful when challenges arise. If a person is openly disruptive, remind the group of the ground rules and why they are important for reaching your common goals. If a participant is dominating the discussion, you can make a point of calling on others to speak. You might begin to call on people who have not raised their hands or spoken up on their own. You might say, "Let's make sure we hear from everyone today." You can also speak directly to participants who are disrupting the training. Ask to speak with them privately, during a break, rather than doing so in front of other participants. Remember to be respectful and kind as you encourage them to support the mission and the established ground rules for the training.

Joe Calderon: One of the participants in a training I was facilitating was dominating the session. He wanted to answer almost every question and seemed to want everyone else to know that he was an expert about the training topic. I pulled him aside so we could speak privately. I said, "It is wonderful to have someone in the training who has so much experience and knowledge. But today I need to make sure that everyone has a chance to participate and share their ideas. I'd really appreciate your leadership in helping to make that happen." From that point on, the participant stepped back and let others speak up.

When you are working with a co-trainer, one of you can take responsibility for keeping their eye on the "room temperature," making sure that disruptions are handled quietly, perhaps even by asking the person to step out into the hallway to talk for a minute and asking them if they can agree to be present without being disruptive.

DOING OR SAYING SOMETHING THAT OFFENDS TRAINING PARTICIPANTS

As trainers, we fear saying or doing something that offends participants, undermining trust and perhaps the opportunity for future partnerships. We will all make mistakes from time to time and unintentionally do or say something that is hurtful or disrespectful to one or more of the training participants. Hopefully, when this occurs, it will be brought to your attention in some way. Ideally, participants will speak up to let you know that they are upset. If you don't learn about the problem, you won't have an opportunity to respond and to restore trust and collaboration.

Jill Tregor: When participants tell me that I have done something that they experienced as offensive, hurtful, or disrespectful, I need to give them my full attention. This is the most important time to be fully present in the training, to listen deeply, and not to respond defensively. What is most important is to honor the experience of the participant and try to restore a positive training relationship. I always offer an authentic apology and do my best not to repeat my mistake. If you have done a good and honest job at this, you may deepen or improve the quality of your relationship with participants by showing that you are a human being who makes mistakes, takes responsibility for them, and expresses your intention to build a respectful professional partnership.

20.10 Evaluation of Trainings

How will you measure what people learn during a training? For most trainings, you will want to keep the evaluation fairly simple. Determine what you want to know about the training. What information will allow you to do a better job next time you conduct a training? Do you want feedback about your training skills? Do you want to know how much people learned? Do you want to know what their favorite part of the training session was?

An evaluation can be as simple as asking participants to respond anonymously, in writing, to four questions: (1) What did you think of the training? (2) What did you learn? (3) What else did you want to learn? (4) What would you change about the training?

Or it can be a series of questions about each section of the training.

Here is a sample of a brief evaluation of the cultural humility training mentioned at the beginning of the chapter.

1. Name three things that you learned as a result of today's training.

2. How much has your knowledge of cultural humility increased as a result of this training?

   0 1 2 3 4 5 6 7 8 9 10

   Not at all   Neutral   A lot

3. What might you do differently now with a client as a result of this training on cultural humility?

4. Would you recommend this training to others (and please share why)?

5. What suggestions do you have for how to improve this training?

To learn more about evaluation, review the resources provided at the end of this chapter.

Chapter Review

PLAN YOUR OWN TRAINING

You have been asked to facilitate a 90-minute training on cultural humility for CHWs (the case study presented at the beginning of this chapter). You have a month to prepare for the training.

1. What steps will you take to plan this training?

2. What do you most want to know in order to prepare for the training?

3. How might you conduct a pre-assessment to prepare for the training? What questions might you ask?

4. What do you want the participants to come away with at the end of the training? What might be some of your goals and learning outcomes?

5. Explain what Paulo Freire called *conscientization*, or *critical consciousness*, and how this concept could be applied to the training you will facilitate.

6. What training methods will you use? How will you engage different types of learners?

7. Develop a specific training plan for at least one learning outcome and one training activity using the format provided in this chapter.

8. How will you evaluate this training?

Reference

Freire, P. (1970). *Pedagogy of the Oppressed*. New York. Seabury Press.

Additional Resources

American Evaluation Association. (2023). https://www.eval.org/.

American Friends Service Committee. (2023). Popular Education. https://www.afsc.org/resource/popular-education.

The California Academy of Sciences. (2023). Why do Icebreakers with Adult Learners? https://www.calacademy.org/educators/icebreakers-and-energizers.

Centers for Disease Control and Prevention. (2019). Understanding the Training of Trainers Model. https://www.cdc.gov/healthyschools/tths/train_trainers_model.htm (accessed 29 January 2023).

The Center for Innovative Teaching and Learning. (2023). Case Studies. Northern Illinois University. https://www.niu.edu/citl/resources/guides/instructional-guide/case-studies.shtml#:~:text=Case%20studies%20provide%20students%20with,safe%20and%20open%20learning%20environment.

The Center for Innovative Teaching and Learning. (2023) Role Playing. Northern Illinois University. https://www.niu.edu/citl/resources/guides/instructional-guide/role-playing.shtml.

Food and Agriculture Organization of the United Nations (FAO). (2023). Preparing for Training and Facilitating. https://www.fao.org/3/ad424e/ad424e02.htm (accessed 31 January 2023).

The Foundations for Community Health Workers Training Guide. (2016). Wiley. https://bcs.wiley.com/he-bcs/Books?action=index&itemId=1119060818&bcsId=10183 (accessed 30 January 2023).

Freire Institute. https://www.freire.org/.

The Hun School of Princeton. (2020). What is Problem-Based Learning? https://www.hunschool.org/resources/problem-based-learning.

International Labour Organization. (2020). Participatory Action-Oriented Training (PAOT). https://www.ilo.org/global/topics/safety-and-health-at-work/resources-library/training/WCMS_736031/lang--en/index.htm.

National Education Association. (2023). Project-based learning. https://www.neaclc.org/about-nea/our-approach/project-based-learning#:~:text=Project%2DBased%20Learning%20(PBL),world%20and%20personally%20meaningful%20projects.&text=Kindergarten%20learners%20hearing%20from%20an%20expert%20for%20the%20Community%20Helper%20Project. (accessed 31 January 2023).

Office of Population Affairs. (2020). Focus Group Tip Sheet. (2020). U.S. Department of Health and Human Services. https://opa.hhs.gov/sites/default/files/2021-08/focus-group-tip-sheet-april-2020.pdf.

Organization for Economic Co-operation and Development. (2020). The Potential of Online Learning for Adults. https://www.oecd.org/coronavirus/policy-responses/the-potential-of-online-learning-for-adults-early-lessons-from-the-covid-19-crisis-ee040002/.

Pew Research Center. (2023). Writing Survey Questions. https://www.pewresearch.org/our-methods/u-s-surveys/writing-survey-questions/.

QuizBreaker. (2022). The 10 Best Icebreakers for Adults (Tired & Tested). https://www.quizbreaker.com/icebreakers-for-adults.

Racial Equity Tools. (2023). Training and Popular Education. https://www.racialequitytools.org/resources/act/strategies/training-and-popular-education#:~:text=Training%20and%20popular%20education%20are,to%20act%20individually%20and%20collectively. (accessed 29 January 2023).

Rural Health Information Hub. (2023). Health Education. https://www.ruralhealthinfo.org/toolkits/health-promotion/2/strategies/health-education.

Science of People. (2023). 35 Fun Meeting Icebreakers to Warm Up Any Meeting. https://www.scienceofpeople.com/meeting-icebreakers/ (accessed 28 January 2023).

Schools for Future Youth. (2023). Participatory Learning Methods. https://sfyouth.eu/images/toolkit/global_citizenship_education/ParticipatoryLearningMethods.pdf (accessed 29 January 2023).

Substance Abuse and Mental Health Services Administration. (2023). SAMHSA Native Connections, Setting Goals and Developing Specific, Measurable, Achievable, Relevant, and Time-bound Objectives. Retrieved from https://www.samhsa.gov/sites/default/files/nc-smart-goals-fact-sheet.pdf.

Training for Change. (2023). https://www.trainingforchange.org/.

Transformative Learning in the Humanities. (2020). *What is Participatory Learning or Active Learning*. City University of New York (CUNY) Academic Commons. https://transform.commons.gc.cuny.edu/2020/12/21/what-is-participatory-or-active-learning/.

Group Facilitation

21

James Figueiredo

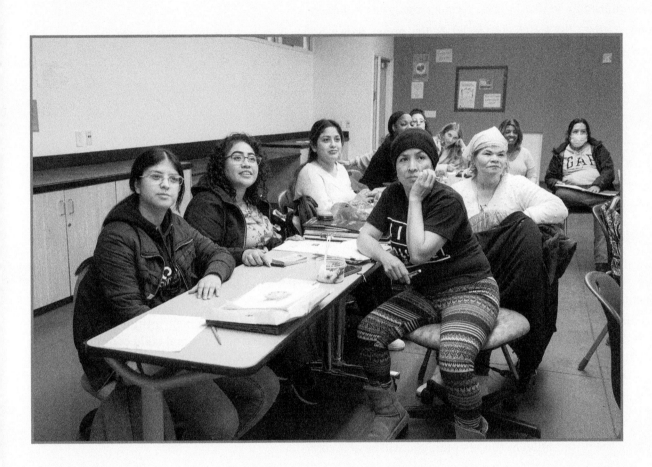

Foundations for Community Health Workers, Third Edition. Edited by Tim Berthold and Darouny Somsanith.
© 2024 John Wiley & Sons, Inc. Published 2024 by John Wiley & Sons, Inc.
Companion website: http://www.wiley.com/go/communityhealthworkers3E

CHW Scenario

You have been asked to start a group for older adults at a local senior center. The purpose of the group is to support participants in better managing and living with diabetes, and in preventing complications. The senior center members are at least 62 years old and diverse in terms of race, gender identity, ethnicity, socio-economic status, and immigration status.

The opportunity to facilitate this group feels both daunting and exciting. You realize the stakes are high and are determined to do what it takes to make the group a success.

If you were the CHW assigned to facilitate this group, how would you answer the following questions:

- What steps do you need to take to prepare to facilitate the group?
- What will be the main goals of the group?
- How will you establish group agreements?
- How will you help build a sense of trust among the participants?
- How will you make sure that everyone has a chance to participate?
- How will you handle disagreement and conflicts in the group?
- How will you know if the group is achieving the desired goals and outcomes?

Introduction

CHWs facilitate a variety of groups that bring people together to discuss common concerns and support each other in taking actions to enhance their health and well-being. This chapter provides an introduction to how to plan, facilitate, and evaluate groups.

Group facilitators promote discussions that positively impact people's thoughts, feelings, attitudes, behaviors, and actions. A healthy group dynamic has the power to foster new social connections and build community, which in itself supports and increases well-being.

The concepts and skills that guide your work with individual clients—such as healthy boundaries, cultural humility, motivational interviewing, and conflict resolution—can also guide your work as a group facilitator.

WHAT YOU WILL LEARN

By studying the information in this chapter, you will be able to:

- Identify and describe different types of groups
- Describe the unique benefits of group work
- Discuss the role of facilitators in shaping a group's culture and dynamic
- Discuss and apply group facilitation techniques
- Develop strategies designed to respond to common challenges of group work
- Explain key steps for preparing to facilitate a group by yourself or with a co-facilitator
- Use evaluation methods to measure success and continually improve the shared group experience

C3 Roles and Skills Addressed in Chapter 21

C3 Roles	C3 Project	C3 Skills
2. Providing Culturally Appropriate Health Education and Information	**C3 Project**	1. Communication Skills
6. Building Individual and Community Capacity	**Chapter 21**	6. Education and Facilitation Skills

Catharsis

Groupthink

21.1 Types of Groups

CHWs facilitate a wide variety of groups including educational, support, and social groups. Some groups contain a blend of these formats.

EDUCATIONAL GROUPS

Educational groups are generally the most time-limited type of group. They focus on providing health information and building skills that assist participants to improve their well-being. The group ends once the health information has been covered. People who attend educational groups may go on to join longer-term support groups or social groups to help them continue to support their goals.

Educational groups can be as short as a single session, such as Mental Health First Aid group in which participants learn how to respond appropriately to someone who may be experiencing a mental health challenge. Groups may last for several weeks or months, depending upon the goals and curriculum. For many people, educational groups are an opportunity to learn about their diagnosis with health conditions such as asthma, depression, HIV, bipolar disorder, asthma, or cancer.

Groups may be based on highly structured evidence-based curricula grounded in research demonstrating its success. A popular example of an evidence-based educational group is structured diabetes self-management groups. These educational have been shown to improve individual blood glucose levels and reduce the complications associated with diabetes (Centers for Disease Control and Prevention, 2023).

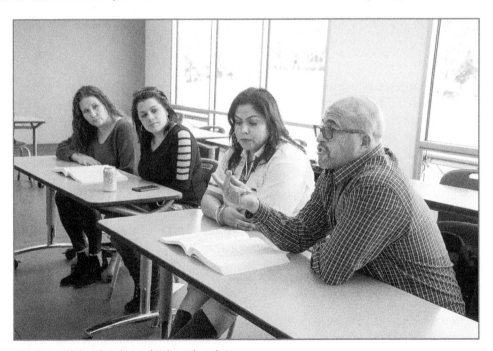

CHWs participating in and Educational Group

As a CHW, you may also be asked to develop or adapt existing health education content to meet the specific needs of a group. While a key purpose of an educational group may be to impart knowledge, simply being with people who share a common challenge or health condition can provide emotional benefits that are similar to those offered by support groups. For example, a group of people with diagnosed anxiety disorders learning new skills together helps to build community and contributes to the participants' sense of well-being. While educational groups led by CHWs require a baseline knowledge of the topic, they generally do not require a high level of academic or clinical knowledge. It does require understanding and being able to offer basic information as appropriate to your role.

An Educational Group for Older Adult Haitian Immigrants

The Villa Co-op is a large senior housing community located in Everett, Massachusetts. It is home to dozens of immigrants from Haiti aged 62 and over who meet income eligibility guidelines. Many of the residents have been diagnosed with diabetes, prediabetes, hypertension, heart disease, and/or high cholesterol levels. A Healthy Living education group was formed by two CHWs from Cambridge Health Alliance who were also Haitian immigrants living in the same neighborhood. The group focuses mainly on eating healthier food and increasing physical activity. The CHWs developed a curriculum with support from a physician and nutritionist. At times, a Haitian physician joined the group to answer questions that were beyond the scope of CHW practice.

Group members were able to identify their own long-established eating habits which may be harming their health. The education sessions emphasized the benefits of traditional foods, like black beans, which are both nutritious and affordable. The group also did experimental cooking together in the community kitchen, modifying typical Haitian recipes. Their experiments included frying plantains in healthier oils, reducing portion sizes, substituting white rice with a blend of white and brown rice, and substituting salt with spices, lemon, or vinegar. The members taste-tested the food and weighed in on what dietary changes they were willing and unwilling to modify.

During the time that the food was cooking or baking, the CHWs played traditional Haitian Kompa music to get people moving. Dancing to their oldies helped to increase the participants' level of physical activity. It led to a discussion on what types of physical activities they already enjoy and can continue to do after the course ends. This educational series went beyond being just linguistically accessible. Its success can largely be attributed to the CHWs' deep understanding of their community's strengths, health beliefs, and barriers.

- *How could educational groups benefit people in your community?*

What Do
YOU?
Think

SUPPORT GROUPS

Support groups place an emphasis on emotional support provided by peers. This type of group is widely used for people who have survived difficult experiences (e.g., sexual assault, domestic violence, and death of a loved one), are living with a specific health condition (e.g., HIV, breast cancer, substance use disorder, sickle cell anemia, and depression), or who face stigma and discrimination (e.g., LGBTQ+ youth, transgender women, and people who are or have been incarcerated). Support groups also exist to help caregivers who support people with chronic conditions (e.g., Alzheimer's disease, cancer, asthma, and bipolar disorder).

CHWs often co-facilitate support groups with a colleague, such as a nurse, social worker, or other professionally trained health care provider. While all CHWs and group facilitators should receive proper supervision from their employer, it is especially important for those running support groups. With the right training and supervision in place, CHWs leading groups often feel a great sense of reward as they assist others to face challenges that they themselves may have experienced.

Hugo Rengifo Ochoa: I observed my co-worker, a seasoned facilitator, and honestly felt that I'd never rise to their level. I was very intimidated at first, especially since I am not a native English speaker. When it was time for me to co-lead a group, I was unsure of my ability. I worried about how I would come across to people who are much older than me.

I was paired with a clinician to run my first group. I quickly noticed how well our skill sets combined. I was the expert in the community, and she used her clinical expertise. We both played off each other's strengths. It has been several years now. I still make mistakes but keep learning from them to improve my skillset and create positive experiences for all group members. I can now help newer CHWs the way that my colleague helped me.

SOCIAL GROUPS

Social groups are less formal than educational groups and support groups. In fact, some social groups exist without a group facilitator. Participants themselves may determine when and where they will meet, and what activities they will engage in. Organizing roles may belong to the members.

Many people already belong to social groups that do not involve CHWs. These groups may be run by faith-based organizations, senior centers, youth recreational programs, cultural centers, and neighborhood groups.

What all social groups have in common is that they involve people coming together, interacting, and gaining a sense of unity. Social groups can be highly effective in reducing social isolation. Effective social groups help people build relationships, establish a basis for trust, and gain a deeper sense of belonging.

Social groups vary widely. Examples include:

- A group of women diagnosed with debilitating mental health challenges operates a community garden in an urban area. The group is led jointly by a CHW and a clinical social worker. While the participants spend most of their time gardening together, there is a pre-meeting before they begin gardening with a check-in on how each member is doing. The harvest provides opportunities for the members to eat together, bring home healthy food, and donate vegetables to a nearby shelter for unhoused people. When needed, the social worker provides group members with support, while the CHW focuses on keeping the members engaged with their tasks and with each other.

- A social group for parents with transgender children. The host organization provides snacks and beverages one evening per month along with some informational brochures and a host, a transgender CHW who is available to answer questions and provide encouragement as people informally mingle.

- An older adult men's group that gathers regularly to watch sporting events together on a large screen television at a senior center. Rather than watch at home alone, they congregate not only to root for their teams, but also to spend several hours out of their homes and to participate in unstructured conversations with their peers. The CHW at the center primarily works to encourage more men to join the group and looks out for the members who may be experiencing a decline in their health.

- A group of gay men living with HIV who formed a bowling league and compete every Tuesday night. The CHW, also a person living with HIV, is primarily responsible for managing logistics, and recognizing and responding when a group member might be struggling and in need of extra attention outside of their time in the social group.

A Social Group for Older Adults

A social group aimed at reducing social isolation among older adults was launched in 2018 in collaboration between the Cambridge Health Alliance and the City of Everett Council on Aging. The idea for the group stemmed from a conversation that a CHW had with Mary A. Piorun, a 96-year-old CHW volunteering at the local senior center. Mary talked with the other CHW about her love of knitting hats and scarves, and how the cost of yarn made it a difficult hobby to afford on a fixed income. She added that she had garbage bags full of hats and scarves that she wanted to donate. The CHW arranged for the hats and scarves to be brought to the senior center and given away for free to all its members. This sparked interest among the members to learn how to knit. With funds from a local foundation, the CHW was able to provide free yarn and knitting needles. Rather than simply giving away the yarn, they decided to start a weekly knitting circle where members could gather, socialize, and knit together or learn this new skill from other members.

Mary successfully recruited 11 women who would gather in front of a large window to knit together. The members would chat, reminisce, tell stories, and informally offer each other emotional support. Mary recruited the participants and offered knitting lessons while the other CHW provided the supplies and briefly checked in with each member.

(continues)

A Social Group for Older Adults

(continued)

Over time, the group produced more hats than they were able to give away at the senior center. This prompted them to donate dozens of hats and scarves to the breast health center at a nearby hospital. The product of their collective labor was given to patients who lost their hair from their cancer treatment. Later, they donated their handiwork to the fire and police department for first responders to give to families who abruptly evacuated from house fires and youth who were under emergency removed from the care of their parents and guardians. At the city's Veterans Day parade, a group of younger CHWs helped set up a table along the parade route for the knitters to offer free hats and scarves to veterans and their families.

This group wound up achieving more than their main goal of reducing social isolation. There was the financial benefit of not having to pay for the yarn and the joy that came from being able to give back to others in their community. One member joyfully exclaimed, "before I was sitting down most of the day. This made me finally feel useful again!"

In Memoriam: Mary A. Piorun, 1921–1920

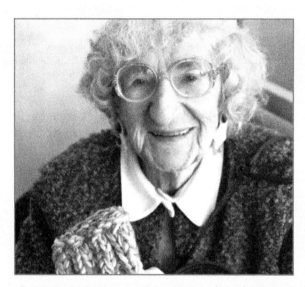

Mary Piorun, a volunteer CHW for the Cambridge Health Alliance (CHA), gave tirelessly to helping older adults in Everett, Massachusetts. She spent five days a week at the Edward G. Connolly Center, volunteering her time to CHA's Aging Wisely Everett Program. At the age of 96, she graduated from CHA's CHW Core Competency course, delivered over 12 weekends. She was a star student with perfect attendance and always ready to share her wisdom with her classmates.

In her 90s, Mary established a knitting group, recruited older adults to join chronic disease self-management groups, helped coordinate a gardening club, and was a panel presenter at the 2017 Massachusetts Department of Public Health's Suicide Prevention Conference on the topic of reducing social isolation among older adults.

A great loss was felt throughout the CHW world and local community when Mary died at the age of 99 from COVID-19 on April 22, 2022. She is a local legend who always exuded optimism and warmly welcomed everyone she encountered.

HYBRID GROUPS

Many groups combine elements from educational, social, or support group structures. For example, some groups may provide education about a specific health condition—such as HIV disease or breast cancer—and provide members with emotional support.

- *What types of groups have you participated in?*

- *What motivated you to participate in the group(s)?*

- *What was your experience like overall?*

- *What type of group would you be interested in facilitating, and why?*

21.2 Key Considerations Before You Start a Group

Before starting any group, there are several factors that are important to consider.

What Is the Focus Issue or Topic? This is a key early decision. Groups address a number of topics, such as parenting, recovery from drug use, mental health challenges, sexual assault, grief, and chronic health conditions. The list of possible topics is almost endless. Selecting a topic that is too wide or too narrow can present different challenges. Ideally, the group topic is one that community members have either proposed themselves or expressed an interest in addressing. The dynamics in the group will be shaped by the participants. Consider what might be the differences between a group generally focused on chronic conditions compared to one that is particularly focused on the topics of bipolar disorder, breast cancer, HIV, or asthma. The selected topic will also likely determine what level of knowledge you need to possess about the subject matter.

What Are the Goals and Purpose of the Group? Successful groups need a clear common purpose or goal. The group facilitator and participants should know at the outset what they are aiming to achieve. It becomes the facilitator's role to keep goals in mind. While some groups exist primarily to educate participants about a specific topic, other goals may include changing health-related behaviors, reducing stigma, building self-esteem and independence, maintaining recovery, and/or gaining a sense of belonging and acceptance.

What Are the Criteria for Joining the Group? Determining who can participate in a group can be a difficult decision. Setting clear eligibility criteria from the beginning will impact group dynamics. You will need to decide how broad or how narrow the eligibility criteria will be. Too narrow and you may have challenges with recruitment. If it is too broad, the group may lack a sense of shared identity or experience and find it more difficult to build connections. For example, imagine a diabetes group promoted as open to anyone living with diabetes compared to a group that is specifically to a particular linguistic, cultural, or age group. Members with shared identities will be able to understand each other in ways that a widely diverse group may not. A group of Haitian older adults would be more able to speak shorthand to each other because of their shared language, cultural norms, and practices. Opening the group to include adolescents with diabetes would almost certainly impact how its members choose to participate. Sometimes in trying to reach everybody we may design a group that doesn't benefit anyone. Having clearly defined membership criteria combined with a recruitment strategy that includes a simple application process and/or interview process can help contribute to achieving the stated goals of the group.

What Is the Size of the Group? The number of participants in groups varies considerably. Groups that are too small are more likely to lack a diversity of perspectives. Large groups can be unwieldy and frustrating for those wishing to actively contribute and be acknowledged. Right sizing a group is crucial to its continued success. You need to consider the impact on a group if some people stop attending. While five members may provide enough variety of perspectives for a group, the loss of just one or two members may be detrimental to the group's dynamic and effectiveness.

Is the Group Closed or Open? Closed groups include the same people who meet regularly over a specified period of time, while open or drop-in groups welcome new members at any time as long they meet the membership criteria. Both formats have advantages and disadvantages. Members in closed groups get to know each other very well. This makes it possible to form bonds and connections with other members that might be more difficult to achieve in open groups where new arrivals may feel like strangers and trust has to be re-established. A drawback of closed groups is when attrition occurs, the group may become too small to achieve the desired goals.

Open groups allow members to attend meetings as they wish. As with closed groups, members of open groups must also meet the criteria for membership. Alcoholics Anonymous (AA) is a well-known example of an open group. AA members attend when they wish and where they wish. Open groups take the pressure off the individual to attend and encourage people to join who may not have participated due to the time and commitment required of closed groups.

The dynamics of open and closed groups can differ considerably. Facilitators leading closed groups generally have an idea of what dynamics to expect as they become increasingly familiar with the members. Facilitators of open groups regularly welcome new members, which results in greater shifts in the group dynamic as established members and newcomers become acquainted with each other. The introduction of new people can re-energize a group or raise an unhealthy level of cautiousness among members. People who feel on guard will have difficulty deriving benefits from these gatherings. Imagine a 10-session support group where the members have opened up considerably by week 5. What might it look like if new people join in week 6 and again in week 7? While it may be a natural reaction to include new people, it is important to recognize how other members will be positively or negatively impacted by the change. In some cases, it will make most sense to offer people a spot when another group starts or identify other means of support for the people who cannot be immediately accommodated.

When Does the Group Meet? When scheduling group meetings, it is important to set times that maximize attendance. In some cases, the optimal time for a group to meet may be different from the CHW's regular working hours. For example, a diabetes education or support group for teenagers might not be optimal during school hours, while it may work well for many parents and older adults. If people are driving or taking a bus, will rush hour traffic impact their ability to join? Organizations may need to structure the work hours of group facilitators to accommodate the best meeting times for group members.

How Often Does the Group Meet? The frequency of meetings often influences people's decision to join groups. Groups that meet very frequently can be difficult for people to fit into their schedules, while groups that meet infrequently may struggle to develop close connections among participants. Understanding the purpose of the group and availability of members is helpful for striking a good balance. For example, a two-hour educational group on chronic disease self-management held over five consecutive weeks may be a good fit for those preferring to commit their time for a limited duration. In contrast, a support group for people living with chronic conditions with no scheduled end date that meets at least monthly for 90 minutes may prove more beneficial for members who will benefit from continued connection with others facing similar challenges.

What Is the Duration of Each Group Meeting? Determining how long each session will run requires knowledge about the community you wish to serve. Some people may decide not to join a group because it interferes with parenting or family responsibilities such as childcare and meal preparation.

When the duration of a meeting exceeds 90 minutes, it is helpful to build in break times. It is also important to adhere to each meeting's beginning and end time. Going beyond the scheduled ending time can be anxiety provoking for members who don't want to be perceived as rude for leaving but at the same time stressed about making it to their next obligation or missing a ride.

Where Does the Group Meet? There are a variety of factors to consider when selecting a location for a group. Is public transportation available? If so, how frequently does it run around the time of the meeting? Will people be commuting during rush hours? Will members be charged for parking? Will your organization validate parking? Is the space accessible for people with disabilities such as people who use wheelchairs or walkers? Are the restroom facilities appropriate? Is the meeting space pleasant? What physical safety concerns are in the neighborhood during the time the groups are held? What level of privacy will people have? What is the overall condition and appearance of the meeting room?

Anonymous: We found this beautiful meeting space with privacy, lots of natural light, and a beautiful garden area. It was a quarter-mile walk from a bus stop. We failed to consider how far that walk was for some people and how hard it would be during the winter. We wound up going back to our old space, even though it was not as pretty.

How Many Group Facilitators Are Needed? Most CHWs lead groups alone or with a co-facilitator. Two facilitators are optimal for larger groups and groups where challenging topics and emotions are likely to be expressed. While one facilitator leads a discussion or activity, their colleagues can observe group members, their level of participation, and keep an eye and an ear open for anyone who may be struggling or require additional support. Depending on the topic or nature of the group, it may prove beneficial for one of the facilitators to have a clinical background or strong subject matter expertise on the topic being covered.

CHW Profile

Pennie Jewell (She/Her)

Community Health Representative

Nottawaseppi Huron Band of the Potawatomi (NHBP) in Michigan

NHBP and other federally recognized tribal members

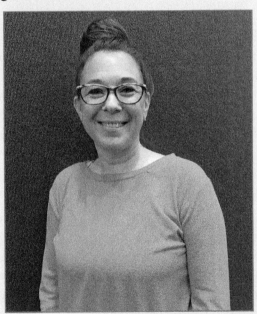

I have been a helper in my community for as long as I can remember whether it was helping my grandma or others. When I was nineteen, I became a certified nursing assistant (CNA) and started providing direct in-home care. I continued providing care in some form for the next twenty-five years until I heard about a job with the local tribe as a Community Health Representative (CHR). Transitioning to that position was fairly easy when I realized I had actually been performing community health worker roles my entire career.

My work varies, but I mainly work with the elders in the community. We have a full medical clinic including behavioral health and dental services. Chronic disease is a big issue in the community along with some members feeling isolated. I provide social support, capacity building, and case management services. My work is done both in the clinic and out in the community. However, most of my visits are at the client's home.

(continues)

CHW Profile

(continued)

As a Community Health Representative, I formed a group for adult community members with limited abilities called ELEVATE. We started out meeting every week but have since reduced the meetings to monthly. When the group started, I was facilitating it, coming up with activities and topics of conversation. But as time went by, the participants formed their own friendships and their own priorities and didn't need me as much. I've noticed these friendships continuing outside of the group. They've become their own community and claimed leadership of their group, which is very fulfilling for me.

I have effectively advocated for CHW/CHRs with the Nottawaseppi Huron Band of the Potawatomi and now for the CHW profession at the state and national levels. I am involved in many committees and conversations, giving feedback and input about the work of CHWs and the communities that we serve. I am a member of the Michigan CHW Association (MICHWA), the National Association of Community Health Workers (NACHW), and the leadership team for the CHW Common Indicators Project.

In 2020, I started a home care business to help with unmet needs in the greater community. We provide nonmedical services to clients in the area as well as serving the tribal community.

As a Community Health Representative, I help my community by first building a relationship and earning the participant's trust. This way, they feel comfortable reaching out to ask for assistance. The best reward is as simple as the smile on a person's face when you know you have helped meet a need, and it is appreciated.

There are a couple of things I would say to a CHW who is just starting out in their career. One is the idea of self-care and its importance. It is common for Community Health Workers to get wrapped up in their work and to take it home at night. That's natural because it is who we are. However, you must learn to take care of yourself first because as we all know, you won't be able to take care of your community if you are not taking care of yourself.

I also encourage Community Health Workers to use your voice. Sometimes people won't value our skills and our knowledge. Sometimes, our ideas and our input are overlooked. Don't let anyone else make you feel less important because you don't have letters behind your name or an academic degree. Your life experience is just as important. Just remember to trust your knowledge of the community and always make your opinion heard.

21.3 The Unique Advantages of Group Work

Dr. Irvin Yalom, author of The Theory and Practice of Group Psychotherapy, documented the unique benefits he observed among people in support groups (Yalom, 1995). While Yalom wrote specifically about the benefits of group psychotherapy led by a clinician, the benefits he identified are also present in groups led by CHWs. Some of the unique benefits of participating in groups include the following (adapted from Yalom's work):

Deeper connection: Being connected to others promotes our health and well-being. Social isolation and loneliness are public health challenges. While many people are more connected via the internet, they often lack authentic relationships. In groups, people have an opportunity to share their stories and listen to the stories of others. Some participants feel truly heard for the first time in their lives. Inevitably, this creates a sense of connection among group members.

Giving back: Groups not only provide participants with an opportunity to receive support, but they also provide an opportunity to offer meaningful encouragement and support to others. Offering support to others, particularly for people who are isolated or who have mostly been recipients of services, can help to build their confidence and self-esteem.

Self-Reflection: Groups encourage members to reflect on their own lives, knowledge, values, beliefs, and behaviors. This type of reflection promotes greater self-understanding. The more group members come to understand themselves, their past experiences and patterns of behavior, the better prepared they are to identify and take action to enhance their health and well-being.

Catharsis: The productive expression of strong emotions accompanied by new insight and knowledge.

Gaining information: In group settings, information is shared by facilitators and participants alike. Information about common challenges or health conditions is offered in the hope that it can support change and enhance well-being. For example, group members may share information about how they manage stress, grieve and heal from loss or trauma, take medications as prescribed, or eat healthier foods.

Building hope: A sense of hopelessness can prevent people from creating changes in their lives. Instilling hope is a strong motivator for people to begin a process of change. Hope is generated by witnessing others who have faced or are facing similar life challenges and sharing knowledge and strategies for enhancing health and wellness. Groups can help people to think and feel differently about their situation and to shift from despair to hopefulness.

Healing: Groups can support people to heal from difficult experiences such as war, incarceration, rape, the death of a loved one, and other forms of loss and trauma. Healing involves looking back at our pain and suffering, making sense of past experiences, and figuring out how to move forward. Participating in groups can support people to identify where they have been getting stuck in their journey of recovery or healing, and to develop new strategies for transforming their pain.

Building healthier relationships: Establishing positive connections with group members helps people have more harmonious personal and professional relationships outside the group. The established and agreed-upon norms of the group can teach members effective communication skills, how to address and negotiate disagreements or conflict, and how to offer meaningful support to others.

Developing social skills: Group members observe how others connect to and communicate with others. A healthy group supports members to learn new skills and to unlearn older patterns of behavior that have been holding them back in their lives.

Role modeling: The facilitator and the participants have opportunities to serve as positive role models for other group members. People in the room may observe others making life choices that they may want to incorporate into their own lives. The group setting is an opportunity to learn and emulate how others manage strong emotions, handle stressful situations, and adopt healthier behaviors.

> **Kayla Green:** I was facilitating a group at SSTAR in Fall River, Massachusetts. We had a single dad in recovery from drug addiction, who was very worried about the school year ending because of his inability to afford childcare for his seven-year-old son. He worried about his kid being exposed to violence and drugs, as he himself had experienced at a young age. Another single parent in the group had been in a similar situation and explained how she went to a childcare program and negotiated a large cost reduction for her daughter's care. At the next group meeting, we learned that this single dad was able to secure childcare there and that it was close to free. The whole group applauded him and the person who gave him this tip.

Please watch the following video ▶ interview with Alma Vasquez, a CHW working in San Francisco. Ms. Vasquez talks about her experience facilitating a support group for Latinas.

GROUP FACILITATION: (*Source:* Foundations for Community Health Workers/http://youtu.be/ 36IBED_1Nvk).

21.4 Roles and Abilities of Group Facilitators

Group facilitation is high-level work that requires the application of a variety of specialized skills in a relatively short and defined amount of time. As a group facilitator, you are tasked with setting a clear purpose, monitoring and promoting participation, maintaining safety of all group members, demonstrating professionalism, focusing on the process, and managing time. Luckily, many of the abilities required for successful work with individual clients, such as Cultural Humility and Motivational Interviewing, are transferable to your work in group settings.

ADMINISTRATIVE TASKS

Administrative tasks are required during every phase of group work. These tasks include developing and distributing promotional information about the group, interviewing and enrolling participants into group, documenting attendance, preparing handouts, scheduling guests to meet with the group, ordering supplies, audio/visual set up, developing evaluation forms, booking space, setting up the room, and following up with individual participants outside of group as needed.

As you plan a group, estimate the amount of time required to complete administrative tasks. This will depend on the level of support available at your organization. In some organizations, administrative tasks are solely the responsibility of the group facilitator, while other workplaces may delegate some of this work to colleagues. It is easy to underestimate the amount of administrative time needed to help ensure each meeting runs smoothly. Doing the upfront work will make for a better experience for group participants and support you in achieving the intended outcomes.

GROUP DYNAMICS AND STAGES

Facilitators play the lead role in shaping group dynamics. Dynamics are largely influenced by the ability to monitor and encourage participation, and to maintain a sense of safety among all members. As a facilitator, you will need to manage group dynamics while demonstrating your comfort in witnessing and responding to ambivalence, emotion, and conflict.

A basic understanding of what constitutes a healthy group dynamic will lead to more successful group outcomes. It is particularly helpful to understand that most groups move through a predictable set of stages to become an effective team. These stages were initially described by Bruce Tuckman, an American psychological researcher. Tuckman called these stages of group work forming, storming, norming, and performing, and later included a fifth stage, adjourning (Tuckman, 1965).

Understanding Tuckman's model can help facilitators identify what stage a group is in and what may be required to reach the next level. It may also benefit participants to become acquainted with these stages of group work and the common challenges and tasks they are likely to experience.

Forming: In this initial stage, participants are trying to understand the purpose of the group and getting to know each other. The tendency is for people to be polite and understanding, which is why this stage is sometimes referred to as "the honeymoon period." In this stage, the facilitator's role is to review the group's purpose and goals, set and ratify group agreements, assure inclusion of all members, and demonstrate qualities of respect, timeliness, honesty, humility, and kindness.

Storming: The storming stage involves greater conflict and a high degree of ambivalence (doubt or mixed thoughts and feelings) among group members. It is generally considered the most challenging stage to manage, when a group will either advance or fail to move forward productively. During the storming period, the facilitator's role becomes more prominent as members begin to talk directly about issues that motivated them to join the group, avoiding important topics and truths about themselves, and resisting the need to make changes. The facilitator's role is largely about facilitating agreement on the ways in which the group will work together to address common concerns and shared experiences.

Norming: This is the stage when group members begin to settle down. Progress occurs as the group is on board with the new norms and expectations for their interactions. During this stage, the group members' commitment to the group builds and they begin to trust each other even when they disagree. At this stage, the facilitator looks out for barriers to participation, makes adjustments to overcome them, and seeks ways to maintain and grow the group's momentum.

Performing: At this stage, the group is making progress in addressing key goals. Group members become more deeply committed to understanding themselves and others, express themselves with greater confidence, gain new insights, experience personal growth, and are more capable of identifying and expressing problems. There is less reliance on the facilitator to enforce group agreements or address conflict. However, it is important for the facilitator not to become complacent as the group can fall back to other stages.

Adjourning: This is the final stage when participants are preparing for the group to end. As the facilitator, your role is to guide participants to reflect upon and celebrate what they achieved and to say goodbye. While the tone of a final group meeting may be largely celebratory, facilitators should be prepared to support members to express sadness or other emotions that may accompany the ending of a highly valued experience.

MANAGE TIME

It is important to honor the commitment that participants have made to the group by beginning and ending each meeting at the scheduled time.

Some group discussions will run longer than planned, and others will not take nearly as long as anticipated. Develop a plan for responding to these circumstances. Being ahead or behind schedule is not necessarily counterproductive for meeting the group goals. Groups may run over the allotted time for discussions because participants are actively engaged. Nonetheless, facilitators are responsible for honoring the group's commitment to start and end on time. Going past the agreed-upon ending time may be a source of stress for participants who have other commitments but do not wish to appear impolite by leaving before others.

You may need to shift the allocation of time within a group meeting. For example, you may want to make more time for a discussion that is engaging participants and meeting a key goal. If you are co-facilitating the group, check in with your colleague. You can also transfer power to the group by asking them if they would like to spend more time on a specific discussion or activity (e.g., "What do you think is the best way to spend our time? We could stop and start a new discussion or give this discussion another 10–15 minutes and hold off some of the other topics until later."). Participants appreciate flexibility in the agenda, and the ability to voice their priorities. Involving the group in this decision is a way to demonstrate your person-centered approach.

Be aware that with some evidence-based programs (such as six-week diabetes management or another type of educational group), there may be a requirement to follow a pre-developed curriculum faithfully without skipping over or significantly shortening key topics or activities. In such cases, it is important to let the participants know from the beginning that some time constraints are mandated ("We are following a curriculum and have to make time to address each of the scheduled topics").

A large visible clock in the meeting room is a better resource for managing time than a wristwatch. Checking time on our watches or phones can make facilitators appear distracted or eager for a meeting to end. It is a common mistake not to allow enough time to wrap up or close a group session. Too often, facilitators notice that there are just a few minutes remaining and abruptly end the meeting. Give yourself and the participants breathing room at the end of each session to briefly summarize what was accomplished and allowing participants time to share their final thoughts. You might say something like, "Okay, we have just ten minutes left for our group. Let's wrap up this discussion and do our check-out. Who would like to begin?"

21.5 Establishing a Group Identity

An essential task for facilitators is to work with participants to establish a clear sense of identity for the group. A group identity is collectively created and is based on factors such as the purpose or goal of the group, the shared identities of the group members (what do they have in common?), group agreements, and the focus and tone of group discussions and interactions. Even if you facilitate ten groups with the same topics and goals, each group will have a slightly unique identity based on who participates, what they bring to the group, and how they connect with other members.

Group participants sometimes bring a painful history that may include experiences of stigma, prejudice, or discrimination. People who have been harmed by others in the past may be hesitant at first to connect with or trust new people. The shared group space cannot reflect the judgment and ugliness of the outside word. It must be a place of refuge that truly welcomes each and every participant and encourages them to share who they are, what they have experienced, and what they think and feel.

As the facilitator, you play a major part in setting the tone for the contributions of the participants. You can increase the odds of establishing a healthy group identity by modeling the behaviors you wish to observe in others. This includes asking questions to invite participants to share their stories, concerns and ideas, listening without interruption, and providing affirmations when someone shares something powerful or provides meaningful support to another group member. Your essential CHW skills—cultural humility, motivational interviewing, and conflict resolution—are foundational resources for establishing a strong, respectful, and dynamic group identity and process.

How you hold and demonstrate your authority as a facilitator is key to establishing a group that achieves its goals. There are times for you to lead the group process, such as in managing time and intervening to reinforce group agreements and protect the safety of group members. Most of the time, however, we encourage you to hold your authority lightly and to make room for group members to claim leadership of group discussions. As the facilitator, you should hold back from sharing your own ideas too frequently. Make space for group members to lead and carry discussions, to respond to the stories and questions that other participants share, and to offer support and share resources. Remember that a key value of group work is the opportunity for members to provide encouragement and support to others. If you dominate discussions and rush to validate or offer support to group members, you may prevent other members from doing so. In this way, a key component of your success as a group facilitator is to hold back and apply your Big Ears, Big Eyes, and small mouth.

When any new group forms, each person brings their own personality and cultural identity with them. Our cultural backgrounds influence how we communicate and connect with others, and our beliefs about group rules, roles, and boundaries. As a facilitator, you are responsible for establishing the group identity while demonstrating cultural humility (Chapter 7) and respect for the cultural identities of all group members. Balancing these responsibilities can be tricky.

As you work with participants to establish and maintain an inclusive and productive group identity, pay attention to how cultural identities and beliefs may impact the way that participants view the group and how they participate. Deeply held cultural beliefs mean that not every type of group setting is the right match for everyone. People may find the taboo nature of certain topics is not appropriate for group settings, no matter how much confidentiality is assured. For example, many people from Portuguese-speaking communities have often heard from their families "Não mete na praça" (Don't put it out in the Plaza), and there is the common saying in Spanish "La ropa sucia se lava en casa" (Dirty Laundry is washed at home). When such beliefs are deeply held by some community members, their participation in groups may be limited by the feeling that sharing vulnerabilities or secrets with "outsiders" is a form of betrayal to family and community. Culture is a powerful force, especially among people who come from societies that place a strong value on interdependence rather than autonomy or independence. The western biomedical model places a very high value on autonomy, which can be at odds with people who come from collectivistic cultures who are more likely to view themselves as part of a whole more than to asset their needs as individuals.

GROUP AGREEMENTS

Group agreements are sometimes referred to as ground rules or guidelines. They are a critical resource for creating a common identity for each group and for clarifying expectations for participation.

How group agreements are developed varies. Some facilitators introduce and explain a pre-developed list of group agreements and ask for additions to the list. Others ask the participants to develop the agreements together, adding suggestions as needed. The priority is for group members to understand and agree to follow the established group agreements.

It can be helpful to post the group agreements so they are visible during meetings and can serve as a reference when needed. The rules of the group may be very different from the rules the participants have at home or in their communities. It may take some time for people to adjust to these new expectations.

Safety is in part achieved through assuring confidentiality, inclusion of all members, and conveying humility and kindness toward each other. One of the most common group agreements is to demonstrate "Respect." Be sure that group members have an opportunity to discuss and clarify what they see as signs of respect and disrespect.

Group agreements serve to create a safe learning environment. A facilitator can name this by stating something like: "Our time together may not always feel comfortable, and that's okay because we can push through discomfort and grow from that experience. What's not okay is when people feel unsafe. Your safety is the top priority. Without it, these meetings hold little value."

Group agreements can also serve to keep participants on track by asserting the importance of timeliness for the beginning and end of each meeting, and when to return to the meeting space after breaks.

Once you have established group agreements, you may ask participants to ratify the guidelines with a show of hands. If there are any objections, make time to discuss them and to make any necessary adjustments. Some facilitators choose to go a step further with ratifying the agreements by having participants sign a document to indicate that they fully understand and commit to abiding by what has been agreed upon. You may also find it helpful to review and reinforce group agreements at the beginning of early group sessions for a closed group or at the beginning of every group meeting for an open or drop-in group.

Sample Group Agreements

Confidentiality: What is said in group stays in group. Participants must not tell people outside of the group who attend the group or reveal any personal information that they share. Breaking confidentiality breaks trust. This group agreement is so important that violation of it may result in dismissal from the group.

The only time when confidentiality may be broken is if facilitators are required by law to report potential harms such as suicide, child, or elder abuse.

Honor time: We will start every group session at _____ and end at _____. We kindly ask that everyone be on time, including after break(s).

Communicate your learning needs: As the facilitator of this group, my role is to help remove anything that might block your ability to engage. For example, you can ask us to speak more slowly or at a higher volume, request larger print handouts, or make us aware of something that you find distracting.

Engage: Give yourself permission to be fully present. Minimize distractions by turning off phones, not texting, and listening to what everyone has to say. Your participation is what brings this experience to life. Ask questions. We see this as an act of courage because if you are wondering about something and raise your hand, you are helping others who may be wondering the same thing.

Take space—make space: We understand that people participate in different ways. If you tend to be quiet and reserved in groups, we ask that you use this setting as an opportunity to share your voice, your experience, and your knowledge with us. If you are someone who eagerly participates and has lots to say, we ask that you hold on to that enthusiasm and at the same time make space for others to share their experiences and ideas.

Assume good intentions: Assume that everyone in the group has good intentions rather than assuming that they may be attempting to do or say something harmful or disrespectful. When a hurtful remark is made, we don't want to ignore it. There is an opportunity here for all of us to learn how to communicate and work with each other more effectively, and to take responsibility when we do or say something that is harmful to others.

Disagree agreeably: To put this simply, *"say what you mean, mean what you say, but don't say it mean."* We need a group where everyone can voice disagreement with each other in a kind and respectful way.

● *What other group agreements do you recommend?*

What Do
YOU?
Think

POSITIVE VERSUS NEGATIVE CONFLICT

As a group facilitator, it is important to understand the distinction between positive and negative conflict.

Negative conflict occurs when group members are unable to listen to each other calmly or to disagree respectfully. Participants may speak rudely to each other or attack each other's ideas or perspectives. When conflict is heated and unproductive, it can do irreparable harm to a group. Instead of learning new skills for communicating about differences or disagreements, group members may reenact negative patterns of conflict that they learned in the past. Negative conflict takes an emotional toll that often leaves people feeling worse off than when they first joined a group.

At the same time, the absence of conflict is not necessarily helpful for growth or learning. Group participants benefit from an environment where they can safely exchange their ideas productively, even while holding opposing views. A positive conflict dynamic supports group members to challenge each other's ideas and listen to and learn from new perspectives. As a group facilitator, you can model how to communicate in moments of disagreement or conflict by asking open-ended questions, listening calmly to what others say, and demonstrating respect for different points of view. In this way, groups offer an opportunity for participants to enhance their skills for negotiating conflict—essential communication skills for all types of interactions and relationships outside of the group.

Chapter 13 provides more detailed concepts and guidelines for conflict resolution.

BEWARE OF GROUPTHINK!

The term **groupthink** was first used in 1972 by social psychologist Irving L. Janus to describe a toxic form of group cohesion that occurs "when people get together and start to think collectively with one mind. This group becomes more concerned with maintaining unity than objectively evaluating situations, alternatives, and options" (Janus, 1982, p. 174). Often, group members and facilitators are unaware that groupthink is occurring because it may appear that the group has gained a sense of harmony and could be in the performing stage. Groupthink leads members to set aside their own beliefs and to adopt the accepted opinion of the rest of the group. Some members may hold back from sharing what they really think or feel just to keep the peace. Remember that group members benefit from the opportunity to navigate and manage challenges in a supportive and respectful environment.

Unchecked, a groupthink dynamic can lead members to express disapproval of participants who do not reflect the dominant shared beliefs. Facilitators must remain on high alert as this highly unhealthy dynamic can lead members to ignore or disrespect those who disagree with them, and to disregard new or different ideas and resources.

There are many actions group facilitators can take to prevent groupthink from becoming established. Encourage group members to think critically and let them know that you welcome new ideas and respectful challenges to what appears to be the dominant opinion of the group. Solicit new thinking by asking questions after someone expresses a particularly strong point of view. For example, you could ask, "What are some other ways of looking at this issue? Does anyone have a different perspective to share with the group?" Invite group members to reach out to you at any time if they are feeling hesitant or uncomfortable expressing themselves in the group. Facilitators can further encourage diversity of thinking by thanking people when they bring in a fresh point of view into the conversation. Making space for different ideas and opinions does not mean that facilitators agree with these ideas; it simply creates an opportunity for the group to consider and explore different perspectives. Sometimes the ideas expressed in group may be offensive to others, whether the speaker is aware of it or not. In an environment where trust and the group agreements have been firmly established, the group will be able to navigate these challenges without raising their voices or disrespecting one another. Again, this type of learning can be deeply beneficial for learning skills that can be applied in the group members' personal lives.

21.6 Facilitation Techniques for Support Groups

Skilled facilitators use a wide range of techniques to help group members to learn and build positive relationships with each other. Below is a partial list of key strategies you may want to apply as a group facilitator.

Calling people by their name: Be sure to ask each group participant what name they want to go by in the group. Hearing one's own name causes the brain to release the feel-good hormones dopamine and serotonin. The chemical reaction of hearing our names spoken sends unconscious signals of empathy, trust, and compassion. Use of name tags or tent cards where participants jot down their preferred names. Writing names on both sides of the tent cards serves to help the people sitting to their left and right to learn and remember each other's names.

Silence/Pauses: Pauses and silence during groups are natural, but we each have a different comfort level for silence (for more information about embracing silence, see Chapter 9). In groups, some people are ready to talk immediately after another participant finishes a sentence or asks a question, while others are pausing to reflect, translating what they want to express from their primary language to the dominant language, or simply demonstrating a different communication style. Pausing or taking time during a conversation also provides people who may have mental health or cognitive challenges with a greater opportunity to contribute to a conversation. In some cases, you may want to remind participants to leave room for reflection before responding to a question or statement. What's important is that you appear to be totally at ease with silence in the room, even if you are not.

Assessing participation: This is sometimes called "reading the room." Participation levels in groups naturally wax and wane. Scanning the room and noticing the participants' engagement level may help you determine when it is time to recommend a short break or quick stretch. As you get to know the participants, you may start to recognize when someone is preparing to speak. Some people communicate their readiness to speak via body language. A skilled facilitator is attuned to the group and able to maximize participation from people who are not raising their hands or immediately speaking up. Encourage participation, when appropriate, by saying something such as, "Is there anyone who hasn't had a chance to share tonight who would like to speak?"

Ask open-ended questions: Open ended questions (see Chapter 9) help to generate reflection and conversation and often start with When, How, What, or Why. In contrast, closed-ended questions can be answered with a one-word response such as "yes" or "no" and can provide useful information that can often be followed up with an open-ended question.

For example, "Have you ever felt depressed?" is a closed-ended question that participants can answer by nodding or shaking their head or by saying yes or no. It can provide some important information to the group. However, by asking an open-ended question such as, "How would you describe what depression is like for you?"—you can open up a conversation among group members and generate more information about their individual experiences.

Be careful about asking "why" questions, as they sometimes come across as judgmental. You can often substitute "why" questions by asking "what" questions. Rather than asking, "Why did you relapse (or return to prior behavior such as drinking alcohol)?" ask, "What was going on in your life around the time you relapsed?" The second example conveys a greater sense of concern and respect.

Asking "What have you heard?" is a particularly valuable open-ended question because there is no incorrect response. It is effective because it allows participants to share what they have heard, rather than putting them on the spot and asking them to share their own experience or beliefs. Consider the difference between asking "What do you know about depression?" versus "What have you heard about depression?" Starting this question with "What have you heard?" may make it easier for group members to speak up and share their knowledge.

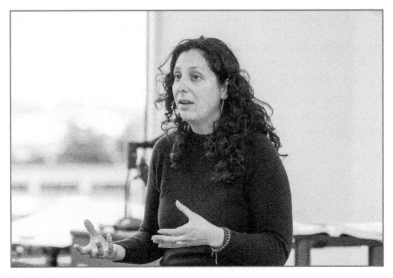

Facilitating a Group

Demonstrating support and encouragement: There are a wide range of actions you take to put people at ease and demonstrate that you care. This can include offering a person tissues, making time to listen to an important story, minimizing distractions in the room and outside the room, use of culturally appropriate room décor, body language that does not get misconstrued as disapproval, judgment, boredom, or impatience. While a facilitator may be crossing their arms to keep warm in a chilly room, it may be misinterpreted as demonstrating disapproval. Similarly, you may want to glance at your watch to keep track of time and have that action come across as if you are just hoping to get out of the room.

Bouncing back: This is when, instead of answering a question posed by a group member, the facilitator restates the question for that person or the group to answer. This gives the facilitator time to better formulate their own response and provides an opportunity for others to share their knowledge. For example, if a participant asks, "How can I find healthy food that I can afford?," rather than immediately answering the question, you could choose to bounce it back to the individual by asking, "What are some resources that you are already aware of?" and/or bouncing back the group by asking by asking "Does anyone have some ideas to share about how to find healthy and affordable food?"

Tact: Having tact requires addressing the group calmly and respectfully when you are called upon to intervene or interrupt a discussion or dynamic that is causing harm. It requires maintaining neutrality as emotions flare, and keeping calm when conflicts, disagreements or different points of view are being addressed by the group.

Humor: Humor and laughter also have a place in group settings. Even while the topics discussed in some sessions may be heavy, the tone does not always have to be somber or serious. Inclusion of lighter moments demonstrates how sorrow and joy can coexist. Humor can help the group bond when they laugh together.

Solicit opposing viewpoints: This strategy may be useful when it appears that the group is in full agreement, but you are concerned that different perspectives or viewpoints have not been expressed. Asking the group to contribute other ways of looking at the topic can highlight the diversity of opinions among participants. When the participants choose not to share alternate views, the facilitator may present other ideas for people to consider and discuss.

Shift the focus: If the discussion veers off-topic for more than a brief amount of time, a facilitator can simply remind participants that the conversation has moved away from the planned topic. You might say, "This new discussion is really interesting, but I'm going to put on my facilitator hat and ask that we get back to the topic of _____." In some circumstances, the new and unplanned discussion topic may be so compelling to the group that it may be more beneficial for the group to switch gears. In these relatively rare instances, the facilitator will want to seek permission from the group to move onto a new topic.

James Figueiredo: I was running a group in Boston around the time of the Patriot's Day bombing of the Boston Marathon. The participants were still reeling from what happened, and a couple Muslim participants were afraid that they or their kids would be victims of hate crimes. It just didn't feel right to keep to the agenda that was created before the bombing happened. I turned out to be a good call. People had a lot to say about what impact this had on their lives. If I had stuck with the original agenda, I don't think people would have been able to take in the information.

Third-Person perspective: This technique involves using the third-person point of view to express an idea or perspective in a less personal or challenging way. Sharing a different perspective in the third person (someone who is neither a group member nor a facilitator) can sometimes make it easier for people to consider. For example, a facilitator might say, "I know a colleague who thinks that . . ." or "I have heard some clients say . . ." This keeps the spotlight off the facilitator while making space for others to share about themselves more comfortably.

Third-personing can also be used to reduce a participant's embarrassment or shame for not having correct information. For instance, if you ask, "What have you heard about how mpox (previously monkeypox) is transmitted?" If a participant responds, "through getting a vaccine," you can kindly provide accurate information using third-personing by starting a sentence with "That's what a lot of people think," then adding health information (e.g., "What the latest research proves is that the vaccine saves lives and there have not been any cases of people getting mpox from being vaccinated." Using the third-person can help a group to talk more openly and with less anxiety about challenging topics.

EFFECTIVE APOLOGIES

It can be difficult for some people to apologize or say, "I'm sorry." As a group facilitator, we are bound to offend someone from time to time. While we all make mistakes, it is especially important for the facilitator to model or demonstrate how to provide an authentic apology (see the Art of Apology in Chapter 13).

When we hurt someone with our words or actions, an authentic apology serves to demonstrate humility and self-awareness, both qualities that we aim for every group member to demonstrate. Apologies are a sign of strength and an act of taking personal responsibility. Taking ownership of our actions can go a long way to repair relationships. The consequences of not apologizing can be harmful to the group process. It may lead members to feel uneasy around you and to limit what they share. It could also escalate to negative conflict among members.

How we apologize matters. Simply saying "I'm sorry" is not enough. It must be perceived by the person who was offended as genuine. The words we choose to offer are just as important as how we convey the message through our tone of voice, body language, and facial expressions.

Examples of effective apologies include:

- **Acknowledge and label your action**: Immediately say that you are sorry, own up to exactly what you did, and label the offending actions. "I'm sorry, my remark was rude/stigmatizing/disrespectful to you" or "I apologize for raising my voice at you. It was disrespectful of me to do that."

- **Tell them how you intend to repair the problem**: Communicate to the individual and the group that you care about not repeating the same mistake. "I'm going to be more thoughtful to avoid using those kinds of words again" or, "I'm going to commit to not raising my voice like that, even if we disagree."

- **Demonstrate change**: Even if the apology is immediately accepted and helps to heal the relationship, it is essential to demonstrate that we have learned from our mistakes by not repeating them. Repeatedly apologizing for the same type of offense will erode the group's trust in you. This merits a further reflection about why you continue to have strong reactions and an opportunity to develop a strategy for not allowing your feelings to disrupt the group process.

21.7 Responding to Facilitation Mistakes and Challenges

All helping professionals make mistakes (see Chapter 9 on fallibility). Here are some common errors that group facilitators make and some tips for how to avoid them.

A poor start: First impressions carry a lot of weight. Starting a group off poorly means you will need to work harder to correct a negative first impression. A strong start is especially important in setting the right tone for a new group and continues to be important at the beginning of each group meeting. Have a clear plan in place for how you want to welcome group members, introduce yourself, review the goals for the group, establish group agreements, and begin the first discussion or activity.

Appearing unprepared: CHWs have busy schedules. Facilitators sometimes find it difficult to allot the recommended two to three hours of preparation for every hour that a group meets. A facilitator's prep work may involve building one's knowledge base on the scheduled topic, identifying referral sources, setting the agenda, contacting participants, and preparing a list of questions to generate discussion. If necessary, talk with your supervisor to ask if it is possible to negotiate more designated work time to prepare for group sessions.

Appearing over-scripted: While preparation is necessary, sounding like we are reading from a script may come across as cold or inauthentic. Appearing robotic will get in the way of achieving a genuine sense of human connection. Speak as you normally do and be your authentic self. This will encourage group members to relax and be themselves as well.

Improper handling of questions: The way that questions are treated and answered by facilitators has a direct influence on the level of participation of group members. When a facilitator ignores or seems offended by a question, it inevitably leads participants to be more hesitant about asking questions. Another error that is easy to make is when a facilitator forgets to respond to questions that have been set aside to be answered later on. This is sometimes referred to as putting questions in the parking lot, often a visible list posted in the meeting room where topics and questions to be addressed in the future are written down. It can be easy for the facilitator to forget to go back and answer the question. This will leave group members feeling ignored and may lead them to ask fewer questions or to participate less in the future.

Lack of familiarity with certain topics: Facilitators should have a strong basic understanding of the key topics that the group will address. Knowledge may be based on previous training and work, provided by a detailed curriculum, or attained through a certification process. Imagine a facilitator leading a group for people living with HIV who do not understand the ways that the virus is transmitted or prevented. Lack of basic knowledge presents a credibility issue. In some instances, to meet the needs of the group, it may be necessary for the facilitator to be paired with someone with a clinical background and a deeper knowledge of the topic.

At the same time, none of us knows it all. It is always okay to acknowledge that we don't know something or are uncertain about how to answer a question. You might say, "I'm not sure. Let me research this and report back to you at our next meeting." You can also bounce the question back to the group. You might say, "Is anyone here knowledgeable about _____?"

Being behind schedule: When a facilitator responds to being behind schedule by rushing through content in order to fit it all in, it will overwhelm participants and reduce their input. Group members will generally be courteous as you zip through information but may not be following or understanding the information you present. Some participants may feel it would be rude to speak up and ask you to slow down. Conversely, participants can also sense it when you drag a discussion out in order to use the allotted time.

Adjust the schedule as necessary to take time for important content. Determine in advance what topics can be shortened—and how, if necessary, or postponed. Always have a few activities planned in case you end early and want to take advantage of additional time. This could be a great time to ask participants to evaluate their experience in the group so far (see the section below on Evaluation).

Taking on the expert role: Many participants assume that the group facilitator is the expert in the room. Don't fall into the expert trap, where you find yourself answering all the questions that come up. There are others in the room with expertise who would be happy to share their knowledge with others. Groups are not a class or a lecture, and you want to put on your Big Eyes, Big Ears, and small mouth (see Chapter 6) and encourage most of the contributions to come from group members themselves. Bounce the question back to the group, "Would someone like to share what you know about this topic?"

Dominating discussions: Remember that we are facilitating groups for a cause, not for applause. As a facilitator, our role is to encourage the group to connect with one another around their common experiences, to speak up, and to actively participate in discussions and activities. Once groups are established, facilitators may say very little during a session except to review the agenda and pose questions. When groups are well bonded, they can manage discussions on their own, making sure that everyone has an opportunity to participate. Once group sessions are over, reflect on your work on your own or with a co-facilitator. One question to ask is, "Who did most of the talking during the session?" If you find yourself talking a lot, reflect on why this is and what you can do to "transfer power" (see Chapter 7 on Cultural Humility) back to the group members.

Imposing personal values or beliefs: The concept of Cultural Humility cautions us against imposing our own cultural identities, values, and assumptions onto the clients and community members we work with. As the facilitator, your experience and your beliefs are less important than those of group members. Work in a way that privileges and emphasizes the identities, values, and wisdom of the participants. These are the resources group members most need to address life challenges and make lasting changes to enhance their health.

COMMON CHALLENGES

Just as you face challenges in your work with individual clients, you will also face challenges as a group facilitator. In these moments, strive to suspend judgment and to respond with patience, respect, and cultural humility. Remember that challenges are often opportunities to deepen and enhance the quality of your work with group members.

Common challenges for group work include a lack of energy and participation, one or more participants who dominate discussion, put-downs or disrespect, and bias or discrimination against some group members.

We encourage you to resist the temptation to make assumptions about why a participant is behaving in a way that may be disruptive or harmful to the group process or goals. Keep in mind that challenges sometimes arise because the group is doing good work, such as identifying important topics that are difficult to talk about or that generate strong emotions. Consider possible causes of the behavior, the impact of the behavior on the group, and how to respond effectively.

Group Facilitation Challenge: A Member Rarely or Never Speaks

Possible reasons for this behavior: Not everyone is comfortable speaking in front of groups, and some people participate by actively listening to others. A person who is quiet may be tired or preoccupied with personal problems. They may not feel safe or prepared to address the topic. They may not yet feel a sense of connection or trust with other group members or the facilitator, or they may lack confidence in their ability to express themselves in the dominant language of the group.

Potential impact on the group: Other group members may assume that the person who is silent is uncomfortable, disinterested, or not "pulling their weight." This challenge may result in a decline in participation from other group members or over-participation by some members who compensate for those who rarely speak.

Possible responses: Introduce activities that ask each group member to speak at least briefly. Facilitate smaller group activities such as asking participants to turn to the person on their left or right and share their thoughts about a particular topic or question. Facilitators may also approach the quiet person during a break or outside of group to kindly inquire about how to encourage them to share more with their peers. Ask the participant why they tend to be quieter in the group and consider offering the person other roles if appropriate (e.g., time-keeper and notetaking).

Challenge: The Conversation Veers Far Off Topic

Possible reasons for this behavior: Conversations may stray from the chosen topic for many reasons. Not everyone—or all cultures—places the same value on linear conversations and may be more accepting of side-stepping to address other topics. Some participants may find it difficult to stay attentive to a single topic for too long or may feel discomfort with the current topic and seek to switch the focus. And sometimes new topics arise spontaneously that are more important to address in the moment.

Potential impact on the group: The new focus of conversation may interrupt an important conversation and opportunity. Participants may feel annoyed or relieved by a sudden switch in focus. The new topic may represent an important question or topic and may be of greater interest to the group.

Possible responses: Address what is happening. You may wish to steer the group back to the selected topic. You can also ask the group if the selected topic has been sufficiently addressed and if they wish to switch to a new topic. You can ask if the topic that emerged spontaneously is one that they wish to discuss now or in a future group session.

Challenge: A Participant Often Challenges What Others Say

Possible reasons for this behavior: This may be a sign that group members are feeling comfortable with different points of view and navigating positive conflict. It could also be a sign that the participant is uncomfortable with the topic or other group members, feels threatened, or has learned elsewhere that this is an acceptable communication style.

Potential impact on the group: Being able to express different points of view is essential to the health of any group and fuels reflection, growth, and learning when handled with respect. When a participant challenges other people's perspective in an aggressive or highly critical manner, this can shut down conversation and harm group connection and cohesion. When a participant frequently challenges what others have to say, it can interrupt conversations and prevent other group members from sharing their experience and beliefs.

Possible responses: Validate moments when group members share or encourage different points of view in a respectful way. If a group member challenges other ideas in a rude, aggressive, or otherwise disrespectful manner, remind participants of the group agreements and the importance of welcoming all experiences and opinions.

In some cases, you may need to kindly but firmly interrupt the person who is repeatedly challenging others to make sure that the person who was originally speaking has an opportunity to finish sharing. You can also ask to hear from group members who haven't contributed recently.

You may need to speak to the person who is challenging others during a break or outside of group to draw their behavior to their intention and invite them to respond to different points of view with more sensitivity and respect. If a group member is unable to change the nature of their participation and continues to challenge others in ways that are disruptive and harmful to the group goals, you may need to ask the person to stop attending the group.

Challenge: Side Conversations

What are some possible reasons for this behavior? People may feel discomfort speaking in large groups, gossiping, boredom, and difficulty expressing themselves in the group's dominant language. A participant may only feel safe expressing disagreement with some members or helping the person next to them by explaining or interpreting what others in the room are saying.

Potential impact on the group: Shifts attention away from others who are respectfully speaking, encourages more side-conversations, resentment toward those causing the distraction and toward the facilitator for not intervening, as well as a loss of safety if members sense that the side talkers are gossiping about them or others in the group.

Possible responses: Refer to the group agreements, ask group members to listen to the large group and the person who is speaking at the moment, establish eye contact with the people holding the side conversation and walk toward them, and ask people to count off into small activity groups and to mix-up or change who people are seated next too.

Challenge: A Participant Stigmatizes or Makes Comments That Are Hurtful or perceived as offensive (e.g., misgendering, referring to people who use drugs as "addicts" or "junkies," stereotyping or using slurs based on the other member's race/ethnicity/gender identity/religion)

Possible reasons for this behavior: Early messages from childhood or influence from media, lack of understanding about how or why their comment hurt or offended others, a negative experience with a person or people belonging to a particular group which turns into an unfair generalization or stereotype of all others from a particular group, internalized oppression and identification with the community they are putting down or offending.

Potential impact on the group: Erosion of safety and trust. This is the ugliness of the outside world spilling into what should be a safe environment. Out of fear, participants may hide or lie about aspects of their identity to avoid being targeted. Negative conflict between and among members. Group members may stop participating and may not return to future meetings.

Possible responses: In these moments, the group is looking to the facilitator to interrupt harmful behavior and maintain group safety. You must speak up and let the person who made the remark—and the group as a whole—know that this type of behavior isn't acceptable.

Stay calm and be kind. Remind participants of the group agreements. Sometimes this will provide an opportunity for the participant to apologize for their remark, which may have been unintentional. This helps to model ways for the group members to make mistakes and be accountable.

If you are working with a co-facilitator, this can be a great opportunity for one of you to stay in the group while the other asks the person who made the disrespectful comment to talk privately in another space. The goal here is to see if the person who made the remark can identify what may have prompted their behavior and its impact on the group. Encourage the participant to return to group prepared to apologize for their remark and to participate in ways that build trust with others. Remind the participant that if they continue to stigmatize or disrespect others, they will be asked to leave the group.

- *What other types of challenges may you face as a group facilitator?*

21.8 Video-based Groups

Many groups have shifted from being delivered in-person to meeting by videoconferencing via Zoom or other videoconferencing platforms. This technology comes with advantages and challenges for group members and facilitators.

POTENTIAL BENEFITS OF VIDEO-BASED MEETINGS

- Less risk of exposure to infectious illnesses (cold, flu, COVID, etc.)
- Transportation issues are eliminated
- Cost savings related to travel (gas, parking, bus fare, and less loss of income from unpaid time off)
- Childcare coverage may be easier and/or less expensive
- Increased interest in attending groups for those apprehensive about in-person groups
- Spending less time away from family members and loved ones

POTENTIAL DRAWBACKS OF VIDEO-BASED MEETINGS

- Language barriers may become magnified
- Group members may not have access to the internet, smartphones, computers or tablets
- Group members may face challenges in accessing or using videoconferencing technology
- Home distractions and a lack of privacy at home
- Discomfort seeing oneself or been seen by others on screen
- A personal preference for in-person communication
- Privacy concerns
- Facilitators may miss identifying important health risks (e.g., smell of alcohol on breath, hygiene, anxiety, cuts, etc.)
- Limitations in responding to crisis situations
- Using videoconferencing technology can be exhausting and place strain on our eyes and stress on our bodies

Do's and Don'ts for Video-based Groups

DO:

- Position the camera at eye level and speak with your eyes looking at the screen
- Position yourself so the camera is seeing you from the chest up, instead of just seeing your head. This is more natural for the viewer. Afterall, in an in-person meeting you're usually seeing more of a person than just their face. This is especially beneficial if you tend to gesture with your hands.
- Silence personal devices and place yourself on "mute" when you are not speaking (this reduces feedback and makes it easier for others to listen).
- Monitor the "Chat Room" or comments and questions that group members may post during videoconferencing sessions.
- Set up your space beforehand.
- Follow your agency dress code.
- Notify people around you that you will be on a videoconference call.
- Support members in creating boundaries at home.
- Review how to use the technology you are using such as how to turn on video monitors, to mute speakers, and to post questions and ideas in a chat box or discussion forum.
- Notify and seek permission from members if recording.
- Consider requiring that all members be visible onscreen.
- Leave time for breaks and encourage member to step away from their screens.

DON'T:

- Work on other tasks while on a video call.
- Stare at yourself on the screen.
- Use a distracting background.
- Share images of anything that you don't feel comfortable with.
- Position yourself at a low angle.
- Get too close to the camera.
- Block the lighting in the room.

21.9 Co-Facilitation

CHWs may facilitate groups on their own or with a co-facilitator. It can be especially helpful for people who are new to group facilitation to be paired with a more experienced colleague. By working together, you will be able to observe, practice, and learn essential skills and techniques.

Co-facilitating a group has benefits and challenges that can generally be overcome with proper planning and effective communication between the facilitators. When you work alongside another facilitator, group members will be impacted by the whole group dynamic as well as how well the facilitators work and relate to each other. Both facilitators are responsible for working together in harmony to sustain a positive group process.

Co-facilitators usually have different speaking and facilitation styles. These differences can encourage increased participation and richer discussions. Disagreement expressed agreeably between the facilitators can be powerful in demonstrating how to collaborate and negotiate differences respectfully. Differences of opinion between facilitators that are not well managed can be detrimental to the group process. When there is noticeable disharmony between the facilitators, the members become like guests at a dinner party where the hosts are bickering at the table. It places participants in an awkward position and can contribute to a lack of unity or cohesion among the group, and they may choose to align with one facilitator over the other.

PREPARING WITH A CO-FACILITATOR

Preparation is essential when you are working with another facilitator.

Meet in advance: Before working together for the first time, set aside time to build a working relationship. Learn a bit about each other, your past experience and training, and what led you to this work. It is an opportunity to express what you want to achieve with the group, to review the established curriculum you are using, or to plan your own agenda for group sessions and establishing ground rules. These meetings also provide useful clues to both facilitators about each person's communication style.

Clarify the group goals: Discuss, clarify, and write down the goals for the group. Having clearly established goals will help you to evaluate your progress in meeting them.

Describe your facilitation style: Be frank about this. Are you someone who conveys a calming energy or are you more theatrical in your approach? Remember that your personal styles don't need to match. This is an opportunity to discuss how your different styles and skills can complement each other and help to keep the members engaged.

Identify opportunities for growth: All group facilitators have areas where they can continue to enhance their skills. Be open and honest about topics and challenges that you may be less knowledgeable about or confident addressing. Do you start to talk too fast when you are excited? Do you tend to go over the allotted time? Do you sometimes struggle to intervene or respond to conflict or other group challenges? Being honest with yourself and your co-facilitator helps to create a safe space for constructive feedback, growth, and professional development.

Discuss how to respond to common challenges: Make a plan for how you want to respond to common group challenges such as a lack of participation, a group member who dominates discussions, put-downs, conflict, or discriminatory behaviors. For the harmony and success of the group, it is important that you work together to address challenges and create opportunities for reflection and growth. If one facilitator freezes or is uncertain how to respond to a challenge, the other must be prepared to take action.

Establish how to interject: Ask each other how to respectfully speak up when the other person is leading a discussion or activity. What one person perceives as a helpful comment may be viewed as a rude interruption by another. Often, chiming in prematurely has to do with being excited about sharing something designed to benefit the group in the moment. As facilitators get to know each other better, they usually learn when their colleague has something they wish to add and can choose to invite them by asking if there is something they wish to contribute.

Establish how to provide assistance: As facilitators get to know each other, they typically learn to notice when their colleague needs assistance. It may be as simple as rephrasing something that may not have been clearly conveyed to the group or as complicated as responding to a particularly vulnerable or emotional contribution from a participant. Ask each other "How will I know if you need help?," "What type of assistance do you welcome?," and "What shouldn't I do?" The cue could be eye contact with a certain expression or simply asking for assistance in the moment ("_____ (co-facilitator's name), what are your thoughts about this?"). Co-facilitators helping each other is not a sign of weakness. It demonstrates collaboration and mutual support.

Determine how to use the break times: Some facilitators use scheduled breaks to take time for themselves. Others want to check-in with their co-facilitator to gauge participation and progress. A more balanced option is to quickly determine if there is a need or desire to check in during the break. If so, conduct a quick check in by asking questions such as, "How do you think it is going?" and "Do we need to make any changes to our plan for the rest of the session?" This allows for the facilitators to be mutually supportive of each other and make any last-minute course corrections.

Determine how to give and receive feedback: It is helpful to talk about how you and your co-facilitator wish to share and receive feedback. This includes the timing of when to offer feedback. While one person may want immediate feedback during a break session, others may find this overwhelming and feel better prepared to receive feedback after the group session has ended. Keep in mind that some people have had bad experiences with colleagues who provided more criticism than constructive feedback. Take your time to develop a collaborative approach to sharing feedback that heightens your connection and your ability to do effective work together. For more information about how to provide and receive feedback, please see Chapter 14.

Decide the divvy: A common misconception is that facilitators should each lead the group 50% of the time. There are a variety of reasons why one facilitator may be leading discussions significantly more or less than their colleague. A new facilitator may benefit from observing their more experienced partner. There will be times when a facilitator is facing a hardship or not feeling well, and their colleague needs to take the lead. As the discussion topics will vary from session to session, it is helpful to determine which facilitator may have more expertise or be better prepared to take the lead. This may be due to the nature of the topic or its potential for evoking strong emotional reactions. Rather than assuming that each facilitator will take the lead 50% of the time, be flexible and keep in mind that you are working together 100% of the time. When one facilitator is taking the lead for a discussion or activity, the other is carefully listening and observing the group and preparing, as necessary, to direct a question or comment to the group or their co-facilitator.

DEBRIEFING WITH YOUR CO-FACILITATOR

Make time to debrief each group session after it ends and immediately afterward if possible. While it is important to identity any challenges you experienced and opportunities to enhance your skills and improve the effectiveness of the group, it is just as important to identify and celebrate successes. Is the group making progress in achieving its goals? Are group members feeling more comfortable participating, addressing common challenges, and offering each other support and encouragement? Are they learning how to manage disagreements? Are group members demonstrating new insights, growth, and change? Identifying these markers of success provides motivation for your continued work together.

When done well, debriefing enhances the collaborative working relationship between facilitators. It may also reveal challenges that make it difficult to work together effectively. In such a case, it may be helpful to seek support from your supervisor. Ultimately, it is about meeting the needs of the group of people you are entrusted to serve.

A Framework for Debriefing with Your Co-facilitator

Take turns asking each other the following questions and listening with respect to what your colleague has to say:

- "What were the highlights of this group session?"
- "What were the challenges of this group session?"
- "How do you think we worked together?"
- "What did we do well?"
- "What could we have done better?"
- "How can we improve our work with the group?"

21.10 Ethics and Group Facilitation

As a group facilitator, you are likely to face ethical challenges (described in Chapter 5). Some of the most common ethical challenges include maintaining confidentiality, upholding professional boundaries, preventing discriminatory treatment, and promoting self-care.

Failing to protect a person's confidentiality or privacy is an ethical violation that is difficult for any group to recover from. For many CHWs, the requirement for maintaining confidentiality has been repeatedly reinforced by supervisors and human resource departments which seek to avoid costly liability issues resulting from HIPPA violations. These breaches of confidentiality have cost organizations millions of dollars and have resulted in termination of CHWs who have betrayed this trust.

While group facilitators have a legal and ethical duty to protect confidentiality, group members do not. Imagine a scenario in which a participant opens up to the group about their HIV-positive status and later learns that another group member disclosed this information to someone outside the group. This harms the individual, the group, the organization, and the community.

While there are no laws to prevent group members from gossiping, a facilitator can take steps to reduce the likelihood of such violations of privacy. CHWs can help minimize the risk of broken trust by establishing and reinforcing group agreements to protect the confidentiality of who participates in the group and any personal information they share. While you may feel like a broken record, reinforcing the ethical obligation to protect everyone's privacy serves to prevent serious problems. Facilitators can choose to underscore the importance of confidentiality by citing their organization's policies.

> **Hugo Rengifo Ochoa:** Whenever I notice a member share something that seems deeply personal or private, I make it a point to remind all of us that what was just shared must stay in the room.

Organizations that have successfully integrated CHWs into their programs provide professional supervision to support CHWs struggling with ethical dilemmas and the personal impact of the work. With supervision and support in place, CHWs can safely raise concerns and ask for guidance on how best to respond to the challenges they are facing. Just as the sense of safety members experience in the group is conducive to growth and learning, a healthy relationship between the CHW and their supervisor mirrors this dynamic.

21.11 Ending a Group

Ending or adjourning a group, like ending services with an individual client, is an opportunity to reflect upon and summarize key achievements and to anticipate next steps.

Recall the journey together: The facilitators can jog people's memories by asking them to summarize how the group started and how it ended. This walk down memory lane is an opportunity to review the achievements of the group as a whole and the contributions of each member. It is also an opportunity to acknowledge the challenges the group faced along the way and how they came together to achieve its goals. This is a good time to give space for members to share stories of personal experiences with being part of the group process.

> ## Think, Feel, Do. James Figueiredo
>
> I facilitated a 10-session group for people living with HIV/AIDS in South Africa who were learning to co-lead peer support groups. They taught me an activity for ending groups called *Think, Feel, Do.*
>
> We asked participants to draw an outline of a person. Next to the head, they documented something that the group experience made them *think*. Next to the heart, they documented how the time together made them *feel*. Finally, next to the feet, they documented something they planned *to do* as a result of their experience in the group. After giving people sufficient time to work on it alone, each participant shared their responses to the three questions with the entire group.

Acknowledge all members: The facilitators thank the group for its cooperation and support, and thank each member for something that they did that contributed to the group's success. This opens the door for participants to recognize the valuable contributions and achievement of other group members.

Certificates may be an appropriate form of acknowledgment for some groups, especially educational groups. Rather than providing one certificate per participant, you might award two identical copies. The first copy could be framed and handed to each person as part of a graduation ceremony. The second copy is for participants to jot down words of appreciation for other members of the group. Every member walked away with kind words from everyone in the group, including the facilitators.

Celebrate: How group members prefer to celebrate varies depending on cultural and individual preferences. Seeking input and ideas from the group will help you to shape an event that reflects their ideas. Celebrations may include providing food, festive décor, music, gifts, certificates, or some type of award. Beyond the festivities, the celebration should serve to reinforce the commitments that the participants have made to positive changes that will enhance their skills, health, and wellness.

> **Jaenia Fernandez:** On the second to last day of a 12-session group that I was facilitating for a dozen people in recovery from drug and alcohol addiction, we had the idea to ask each member to share the name and performer of their favorite song. We put all the songs onto a playlist. During the last group meeting, we listened to each other's music while we ate and socialized. In response to many of the group members, we wound up sending the playlist to the whole group. It was a parting gift that we had not planned.
>
> In another group that I facilitated, participants wanted a time set aside for two group members from Brazil who volunteered to give samba dancing lessons. I've learned that members have their own ideas, which I would not have come up with on my own. I have taken some of these new activities and used them successfully for other groups.

Expression of emotion: Some members may be feeling anxiety and sadness about the group ending. Make time for participants to share their thoughts and feelings about approaching the end of the group. While there is no one-size-fits-all approach to helping people move forward, your role is to demonstrate empathy and connect the struggling member to appropriate resources.

Next steps: Make time for participants to share how they will continue to practice or put into action the knowledge and skills they have learned in group. For example, how will they continue to manage their diabetes once the group has ended? What key resources are they bringing with them to promote their health and well-being?

21.12 Evaluation

There are several ways to evaluate the effectiveness of group work.

Many evidence-based programs such as Mental Health First Aid and the Stanford-Developed Chronic Disease Self-Management Program require the facilitator to administer a standardized evaluation form. These more robust data collection tools are generally survey forms which are available electronically or in hard copy. In many cases, these evaluations can be submitted anonymously.

Some groups conduct follow-up evaluations weeks or months after the last group session. This type of evaluation assesses the longer-term impact of the group by measuring each participant's ability to sustain changes and continued progress toward their stated wellness goals. The measures will vary depending on the nature of the group. A smoking cessation program will likely want to know how tobacco use has changed, while a diabetes self-management program will want to know if there were any sustainable changes related to diet, exercise, and medication adherence.

While a final evaluation during the adjournment stage of the group is valuable, you may also want to consider periodic evaluation throughout the group process. Ongoing feedback from the group members provides facilitators with essential information about how participants feel about the group, the role and performance of facilitators, and whether or not the group is meeting expectations. If you conduct an ongoing evaluation of a group, clearly explain that all input, positive or negative, is welcomed and will be carefully considered to enhance the management and effectiveness of the group. Continual evaluation can be regularly incorporated at the end of each group session by asking participants to share what they think went well and what could be changed to improve the group experience. Some group members may feel more comfortable providing their input anonymously. This could be done by handing out index cards and asking the participants to write down what they think is going well on one side of the card and what changes they propose on the other side.

Make time to carefully review the feedback that you receive from group members. If you work with a co-facilitator, review the feedback together. Focus on what you learn about the experience of participants, what seems to be working best for them, and what aspects of the group should be changed. With each group that you facilitate, you will learn new techniques, become more comfortable with your role, and learn how to incorporate feedback from participants to keep enhancing the quality of your practice.

For more information about program evaluation, please see Chapter 22.

Chapter Review

To test your understanding of the information provided in this chapter, answer the questions presented at the beginning of the chapter about facilitating a diabetes group for older adults, or answer the questions presented below about a group of your own design.

DESIGN YOUR OWN GROUP

Develop a plan for a group that you hope to facilitate in the future. Select a community to serve and a health issue to address that you are already familiar with.

1. Describe the community that will participate in the group.
2. What health issue or concern does the group have in common?
3. What will you call your group?
4. What are the key goals for this group?
5. What are the membership criteria for the group?
6. Where will you meet and how often?
7. How many times will the group meet?
8. Will the group be open or closed?
9. How will you start and end each session?
10. What group agreements will guide the work of the group? How will these be established?
11. What will you do to promote the participation of all group members?
12. How will you know if you have been successful in facilitating this group?

References

Centers for Disease Control and Prevention. (2023). Managing Diabetes. https://www.cdc.gov/learnmorefeelbetter/programs/diabetes.htm (accessed 2 June 2023).

Janus, I. L. (1982). *Group think: Psychological studies of policies, decisions and fiascos* (2nd ed.). Boston: Cengage Learning.

Tuckman, B. (1965). Developmental sequences in small groups. *Psychological Bulletin*, 63, 384–399.

Yalom, I. (1995). *Theory and practice of group psychotherapy*. New York, NY: Basic Books.

Additional Resources

Galla, S. (2023). *How to start & facilitate a support group in 6 steps.* Mensgroup. https://mensgroup.com/
start-support-group#:~:text=How%20to%20facilitate%20a%20support%20group%201%20
Welcome,no%20longer%20than%203-5%20minutes%20per%20person.%20 (accessed 28 March 2023).

The Harriet W. Sheridan Center for Teaching and Learning (2023). Tips on Facilitating Effective Group
Discussions. Brown University. https://www.brown.edu/sheridan/teaching-learning-resources/
teaching-resources/classroom-practices/learning-contexts/discussions/tips#:~:text=1%20Allow%20
participants%20to%20introduce%20themselves%20%E2%80%93%20you,Treat%20participants%20
with%20respect%20and%20consideration.%20More%20items (accessed 28 March 2023).

Mental Health America. Center for Peer Support. (2016). https://www.mhanational.org/sites/default/files/
MHA%20Support%20Group%20Facilitation%20Guide%202016.pdf (accessed 28 March 2023)

Psychology Today. (2023). Groupthink. https://www.psychologytoday.com/us/basics/groupthink
(accessed 28 March 2023).

Psychology Today. (2023). Groupthink: Ethics Defined. YouTube. https://www.youtube.com/watch?v=
ZOX79tmDox4 (accessed 28 March 2023).

Ryan, E. & Kelly, M. L. (2023). Do you use these words when you apologize? It's time to stop, researchers say.
NPR. https://www.npr.org/2023/01/25/1150972343/how-to-say-sorry-give-good-
apology#:~:text=They%20are%3A%201%20Say%20you%27re%20sorry.%20Not%20that,going%20to
%20pay%20for%20the%20dry%20cleaning.%20 (accessed 28 March 2023).

Research, Evaluation, and Dissemination of Findings

22

Lily K. Lee, Julie Ann St. John, J. Nell Brownstein, Pennie Jewell,
and Lisa Renee Holderby-Fox

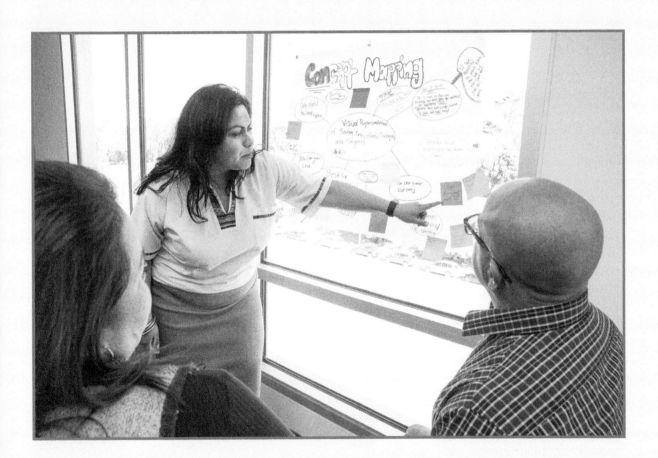

CHW Scenario: Evaluating a Physical Activity Intervention

You are a CHW working on a project to improve physical activity for members of a community. Your agency is working with a group of key partners (stakeholders) to evaluate the "outcome" and "impact" of the physical activity program (the intervention). As a member of the evaluation team, you are guiding the evaluators to use culturally appropriate evaluation methods and will share (disseminate) the findings with the community.

As the CHW in this scenario, how would you answer the following questions?

- What are your potential roles in the evaluation activities?
- How can you make sure the community is involved?
- How will you disseminate the findings with the community?
- How will you use the findings to improve the health of the community?

An Early Experience with Research and Evaluation

During my early career as a CHW, I was engaged in research and evaluation for a federally funded demonstration project and didn't even know it! I didn't understand what that meant. The terms "demonstration project" should have given me a clue. As I conducted home visits to high-risk pregnant women and teens, I was required to conduct ongoing assessments and surveys with program participants. I also accompanied participants to prenatal visits, arranged transportation, and connected them to community resources for basic needs such as food, housing, and health coverage. I was required to keep track of the number and length of home visits I conducted, and the number and type of all other activities I engaged in with program participants. Although I tracked all these numbers and filled out endless bubble forms, I didn't understand why.

One day our evaluator sat with the CHWs in the program and explained the need to capture the endless additional information. We were participating in the evaluation of our program to determine if CHWs could promote the health of participants by increasing prenatal visits, reducing high-risk deliveries and infant mortality in our county. She explained what the evaluation of our program could mean—more babies might be born healthier. She shared that if our program demonstrated that CHWs made a difference, our program and others could be funded to continue the important work we were doing in the communities we served. The evaluator's explanation made gathering the additional information a priority.

I didn't understand until years later that I had participated in a form of research and evaluation just like so many CHWs do every day. When CHWs participate in research or evaluation, it's helpful to recognize that our daily work is informing these processes and outcomes. Once we understand the connection, it broadens our knowledge and demystifies research and evaluation.

This is the experience of Lisa Renee Holderby-Fox, a CHW with over 20 years of CHW work experience. The program mentioned above was successful and continues in existence today with funding from various sources. The team of CHWs has grown and continues to impact pregnant and parenting families in the community.

Introduction

This chapter introduces basic definitions, concepts, and skills for research and evaluation. The knowledge gained through this chapter will also expand your leadership skills and ability to bridge partnerships with community members in both program evaluation and research efforts.

Research and evaluation are included in the list of CHW competencies identified by the Community Health Workers Core Consensus Project (C3) Project (Rosenthal, Menking, & St. John, 2018). The C3 Project is introduced in detail in Chapters 1 and 2.

WHAT YOU WILL LEARN

After studying this chapter, you will be able to:

- Define research and evaluation

- Describe types of research and evaluation framework and methods

- Develop tools for research and evaluation

- Discuss the role of CHWs in research and evaluation

- Share the interpretation of research and evaluation findings to the community

- Discuss trends in CHW research and evaluation

C3 Roles and Skills Addressed in Chapter 22

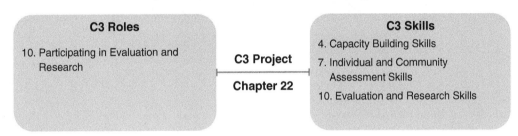

C3 Roles

10. Participating in Evaluation and Research

C3 Project

Chapter 22

C3 Skills

4. Capacity Building Skills

7. Individual and Community Assessment Skills

10. Evaluation and Research Skills

WORDS TO KNOW

Bias

Community Assessment

Community-based Participatory Research (CBPR)

Dissemination

Evaluation

Evaluation Framework

Institutional Review Board (IRB)

Logic Model

Research

Scientific Method

Qualitative Data

Quantitative Data

22.1 Defining Research and Evaluation

People define and use the terms research and evaluation differently. Some believe that research and evaluation overlap, while others believe evaluation is part of research. What is important is that the two share a common ground: the use of data to make or guide decisions (Wanzer, 2021).

DEFINITION OF RESEARCH

Research is a process to gain new knowledge and uses a systematic process called the **Scientific Method**. The scientific method guides the data collection for question(s) researchers intend to answer or prove. Researchers, now more than ever, need the help of CHWs to work in communities to identify problems that need to be solved such as high rates of infant mortality, incarceration, type two diabetes, or community members who are unhoused. They develop a prediction or explanation (called a hypothesis). They test the hypothesis using a study design (overall plan to address the research question) and a methodology, which is like a roadmap for carrying out the study and includes information about selecting subjects for the study, what will be measured, and how.

Researchers and CHWs then collect and analyze the data. The research team looks at these results and makes conclusions based on what they discover (the findings or evidence). Next, the research team shares the results with community members and key partners such as community organizations. This process can be visualized in Figure 22.1 and Table 22.1.

In **community-based participatory research** (CBPR), community assessments use methods and frameworks *designed and conducted by the community rather than by just researchers or outside experts*, although outsiders may be involved in the research or even sometimes start the research. Participatory research methods are also

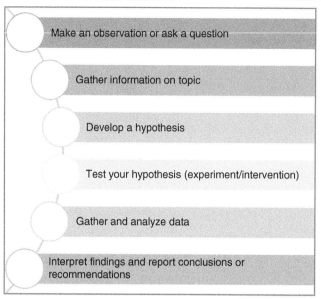

Figure 22.1 The Scientific Method

Table 22.1 Using the Scientific Method with a Physical Activity Example

STEPS IN SCIENTIFIC METHOD	CASE EXAMPLE—PHYSICAL ACTIVITY
Research question	How effective are CHWs in promoting a physical activity intervention program?
Gather information	• Root causes of why people are not physically active across the Social-Ecological Model. • Types of education, resources, and social support needed to increase physical activity • CHW's role in addressing root causes to support more physical activity
Hypothesis	CHWs can play an important role in improving physical activity in the community by educating members on access to and support to participate in physical activity opportunities.
Test hypothesis with an intervention (experiment)	**Control group**: CHW-led cancer screening **Experiment group**: CHW-led physical activity program at four levels across the Social Ecological Model to access and support participation in physical activities (Note: in a descriptive study, there will not be two groups. Researchers may conduct a survey to understand the *root causes* of why people have difficulty staying active in their communities or their attitudes about receiving CHW services—such as education or social support)
Gather and analyze data	**Qualitative data**: phone calls using motivational interview guide. Compare data on physical activity between control group and experiment group.
Interpret findings and report conclusions and recommendations	Interpret the results and draw conclusion on whether CHW education and social support were helpful to improve physical activity in the program compared to those in the control group. Researchers and CHWs then prepare a presentation, report, or an article to share (disseminate) the findings and recommendations for a plan of action. CHWs have an important role in applying cultural humility and knowledge about the community to select the best suitable method to share findings with the community.

clearly tied to a process of community organizing, advocacy, or action to transform or improve community conditions (see Chapter 23). After presenting the research findings or results, the research team (including CHWs), community members, and community partners work together to solve a community problem. They collaborate throughout all key steps of a project including a needs assessment, planning, developing the project or intervention, implementation, evaluation, and sharing results of the project (Samuel et al., 2018).

While the scientific method is the backbone of all research and evaluation, researchers may use different methods (tools) and methodologies (how to implement the plan or approach) to gather new knowledge. The three most common methodologies you may use are quantitative, qualitative, and mixed methods, which are talked about in more detail in Section 22.3.

TYPES OF RESEARCH STUDIES

There are many kinds of research studies. Most of them fall into two groups: descriptive and experimental.

In **descriptive studies**, researchers and CHWs may collect information from study participants at just one point in time.

In an **experimental study**, a treatment, procedure, or program is intentionally introduced, and data are collected to measure results or outcomes. Experimental studies or experiments generally include a control group (does not receive the treatment or program) and an intervention group (receives a treatment or program). Data from both groups are compared to gain knowledge about how well the treatment or program worked (effectiveness) or what difference the intervention made (impact).

Because of their unique connections to their communities, CHWs are often involved in community assessments (also known as community health assessment, community diagnosis or needs assessment). A **community assessment** gathers information about a community's current health status, needs, and the *root causes* of poor health (for more information about root causes, please see Chapters 3 and 4). For example, high rates of asthma, heart disease, cancer, and other health conditions are often symptoms of root causes, which may include discrimination and lack of access to essential resources caused or influenced by government and institutional practices and policies. Information gathered from the assessment can be used to develop a community health improvement plan for how and where resources should be used to best meet community needs (National Center for State, 2022). Although CHWs' roles in research have increased, more programs need to include CHWs in research and evaluation activities.

Root Causes

Root causes are the underlying reasons for poor health in a community (see Figure 22.2). The result (outcomes) of poor health—like high rates of depression, obesity, asthma, heart disease, and cancer—are often symptoms of root causes and health behaviors. Social determinants of health also play critical factors in differences in living conditions or opportunities that groups of people experience within the same community that are largely influenced by institutional practices and policies. The Health EquiTREE diagram below (Breen, 2022) shows how the elements underground (root causes, systemic culture, and narratives) and those above the ground (leaves, branches, and trunk) represent the components of health that are visible.

CASE STUDY: RESEARCH USING THE SCIENTIFIC METHOD

Consider the *problem* of the lack of physical activity in a community. Researchers in San Diego, California, studied a CHW-led the "Fe en Acción" (Faith in Action) program, a community-based program designed to increase moderate-to-vigorous physical activity among church-going Latinas (Arredondo et al., 2022) across the Social Ecological Model (Centers for Disease Control and Prevention, 2022b). Sixteen (16) Catholic churches were randomly assigned to either the physical activity intervention (*experiment group*) or the cancer screening intervention (*control group*), both CHW-led. Participants were followed from baseline (start) for 12 months and again for 24 months. The *hypothesis* of this research study was that CHWs play an effective role in improving physical activity in the community by educating members on access to and support to participate in physical activity opportunities.

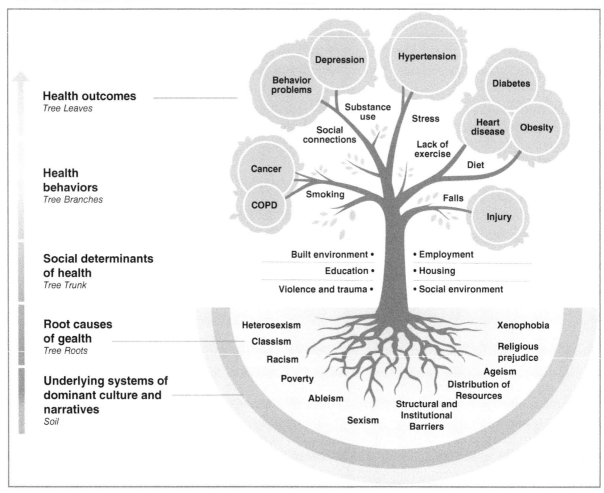

Figure 22.2 Health EquiTREE (Breen, 2022)

Let's apply the **scientific method** to this research case example:

Research studies like the physical activity case example clearly demonstrate that education and social support provided by CHWs do improve program outcomes (Haughton et al., 2015; Lee & Park, 2021). Other studies show CHW involvement in the intervention promotes health outcomes (Centers for Disease Control and Prevention, 2018a). See also Appendix A and B.

DEFINITION OF EVALUATION

Evaluation looks at whether a program or intervention results in anticipated improvements or changes. Evaluation is sometimes called evaluation research, applied research, or more commonly program evaluation.

An evaluation may be interested in assessing the impact of an intervention such as a new treatment method (high blood pressure medication) or innovations in services (high blood pressure self-management program for patients). Some program evaluations are designed to gather information about the program's performance or factors that affect behavior such as participation in physical activities (Centers for Medicare & Medicaid Services, 2020).

Some examples of evaluation questions are (Kosecoff & Fink, 1982):

- How well did the program achieve its goals, hopes, and expectations?
- Were the program's activities implemented as planned?
- For which groups was the program most or least successful?

Similar to the scientific method used in research, evaluations use a plan with rigorous processes for the collection and analysis of the data, which is referred to as **evaluation framework** or model. The Program Performance and Evaluation Office at the Centers for Disease Control and Prevention (2022c) provides steps in conducting an evaluation.

Steps in Evaluation Practice

1. **Engage key partners (stakeholders):** Engage those involved, those served or affected by the program, and primary users of the evaluation findings.

2. **Describe the program:** Describe the program, including the need, expected effects, activities, resources, context, and logic model (see Section 22.2).

3. **Focus on the evaluation design:** Select culturally appropriate approaches to focus on issues of greatest concern to key partners

4. **Gather credible evidence:** Gather information or data to analyze and interpret findings to make recommendations.

5. **Justify conclusions:** Interpret conclusions by linking them to the evidence gathered and relevant to the key partners

6. **Share lessons learned:** Share lessons learned with these components: program description, data-gathering methods, activities completed to carry out the evaluation, the findings, and plan for sharing with community (dissemination).

[Adapted from the (Centers for Disease Control and Prevention, 2022c)]

It is important to note that, although an evaluation design includes all the steps above, sometimes evaluators need to revisit previous steps (usually between steps 4 and 5) to ensure the data are capturing the whole picture of the conditions in the community or a specific population.

TYPES OF EVALUATION

The main types of evaluations are **formative, process, impact, outcome, and summative evaluations** (see Table 22.2). Generally, a comprehensive evaluation will include formative, process, impact, and outcome evaluations. The following table provides a quick guide to the different types of evaluations and sample questions they address.

In addition to the evaluation types presented above, you may come across *Summative Evaluation*. Summative Evaluation considers the entire program cycle and assists in decisions such as:

- Should the program be continued?
- If so, will the program be continued in its entirety?
- Is it possible to carry out the program in other settings?
- How sustainable is the program?
- What elements could have helped or hindered the program?
- What recommendations have evolved out of the program?

EVALUATION CASE EXAMPLE

In the Familias Sanas y Activas (Healthy and Active Families) study, researchers evaluated participants who took part in Promotora-led physical activity (PA) classes (Ayala and San Diego Prevention Research Center Team, 2011; Ayala et al., 2017). The evaluation measured physical improvements in participants and changes in their level of PA. Evaluation results found significant differences in self-reported moderate-to-vigorous PA at 12 months, but not at 24 months among the intervention participants (see Table 22.3).

Table 22.2 Description of Types of Evaluation

FORMATIVE EVALUATION	PROCESS EVALUATION
Identifies the problem, needs, or a risk to be evaluated. This is the *needs assessment* step.	Tracks or monitors the activities of the program, the quality of services provided, and the population served.
<ul><li>What is the main problem in the community or problem of interest?</li><li>Who is the target population?</li><li>What methods and tools should be used? How should they be adapted to be more culturally appropriate?</li><li>What questions or prompts should be addressed in a focus group?</li><li>Is training or pilot testing needed?</li><li>What are the goals and objectives?</li><li>What is the intervention?</li><li>What is the budget of the project or program?</li></ul>	<ul><li>Has the project reached the target group?</li><li>Are all project activities reaching all parts of the target group?</li><li>Are participants and other key partners satisfied with all aspects of the project?</li><li>Are all activities being carried out as intended? If not, why?</li><li>What changes (if any) have been made to intended activities?</li><li>Are all materials, information, and presentations suitable for the target audience?</li></ul>
IMPACT EVALUATION	**OUTCOME EVALUATION**
Measures the program effectiveness *immediately after* and *up to six months* after the completion of the program.	Concerned with the long-term effects of how well the program goal has been achieved, *at least six months after* the start of the program.
<ul><li>How well has the project achieved its objectives (and sub-objectives)?</li><li>How well have the desired short-term changes been achieved?</li><li>Are there changes in participants' attitude, self-esteem, confidence, or social connectedness, and other factors of program?</li><li>How much of the change was the result of the program (intervention)? How effective was the program?</li></ul>	<ul><li>Has the overall program goal been achieved?</li><li>What factors outside the program have contributed or hindered the desired change?</li><li>What unintended changes occurred because of the program?</li><li>Did the program help change overall mental and physical well-being, education and employment, or help-seeking behaviors? How or why not?</li></ul>

(*Source:* Adapted from "Evaluating Health Promotion: A Health Worker's Guide" Hawe, Degeling, Hall, & Brierley (1990).)

Table 22.3 Using the Evaluation Framework for a Case Example of a Promotora-led Physical Activity Program

STEPS IN EVALUATION FRAMEWORK	CASE EXAMPLE: PROMOTORA-LED PHYSICAL ACTIVITY PROGRAM IN SAN DIEGO, CA
Engage key partners	The San Diego Prevention Research Center Team, CHWs/Promotores, community members, community agencies.
Describe the program	The Familias Sanas y Activas study (Ayala, 2011) is a community-based program intended to increase moderate-to-vigorous physical activity among community Latinas in San Diego, California. Twenty-four community volunteers were trained as promotoras to lead group exercise classes. An optional, 11-session healthy lifestyle program was offered in addition to the regular exercise classes. Four hundred and forty-two Latinas took part in the classes. The classes were held at local schools, recreation centers, community centers, and public housing complexes.

(continues)

Table 22.3 (*continued*)

STEPS IN EVALUATION FRAMEWORK	CASE EXAMPLE: PROMOTORA-LED PHYSICAL ACTIVITY PROGRAM IN SAN DIEGO, CA
Evaluation design	Mixed methods (different kinds of methods): **Qualitative**: Observations by staff and self-reports from participants. **Quantitative**: Participant surveys and physical measurements.
Gather credible evidence	**Qualitative**: Research assistants noted observations of participants as they took part in physical measurements and asked them questions about their use of community resources. **Quantitative**: Records were kept of participants' blood pressure, weight, and waist circumference. Promotores kept attendance sheets at their classes. Participants filled-out questionnaires regarding their health and use of community recreational resources.
Justify conclusions	Promotores can promote physical activity in their community and achieve meaningful changes in the residents' health. At 6 and 12 months, measures of blood pressure, hamstring flexibility, waist circumference, aerobic fitness, heart rate recovery, improved mood, fewer barriers to being physically active, and social support improved significantly among participants.
Share lessons learned	The Promotora-led physical activity program was a success. Input from community members, trainings, and other support was helpful and necessary.

KEY DIFFERENCES BETWEEN RESEARCH AND EVALUATION

Institutional Review Boards (IRB)

An **Institutional Review Board** or IRB is a group of people who review an application for a research or evaluation project to make sure that the research is conducted in a way that protects the rights and safety of the participants involved in the research. In general, an IRB application is needed to conduct research involving people. Prior to beginning a research or evaluation project in a community, the research team should discuss and confirm if IRB approval is needed (U.S. Department of Health & Human Services National Institute of Health, 2022). IRBs are usually located in universities or other settings where research is a primary activity (including research centers, hospitals, labs, etc.).

Another type of IRB that is becoming more common is a *community-based IRB*. In a community-based IRB, communities establish ethics review processes for making decisions related to whether and how research is conducted in their communities (Puckett, 2017, Shore et al., 2011).

An alternative to an IRB application is a *quality improvement* application, which goes to a Quality Improvement Review Board (QIRB). A quality improvement project seeks to improve patient care and outcomes or results for participants/patients, health care systems, and organizations (Harrington, 2007). Projects whose focus is to improve some process in patient care can submit a proposal to a QIRB, who will review the proposed project and confirm whether a QIRB approval is sufficient or if the project is research and should be submitted to an IRB (Casarett, Karlawish, & Sugarman, 2000).

22.2 CHW Competencies and Framework for Research and Evaluation

In Section 22.1, we focused on the general definitions and methods with case examples of research and evaluation. In this section, you will learn about the set of core competencies, identified through the work of the C3 Project, that you can apply to research and evaluation programs. You will also learn about how these core competencies or skills relate to evaluation and research frameworks or models (see Table 22.4).

Table 22.4 Differences Between Research and Evaluation

	RESEARCH	EVALUATION
Purpose is to:	Test a theory and produce findings that apply to a population or community.	Look at (evaluate) how well a program did, based on what it said it would do. Did the program achieve expected results?
Questions start with:	A person in an academic or research setting with a particular expertise.	Key partners and those potentially affected by the findings/results.
Quality and Importance is judged by:	Peer review in a discipline such as public health, nursing, or medicine.	Those who will use the findings to make decisions and take actions.
Ultimate test of value is:	Contribution to knowledge.	Ability to improve programs for more efficiency or better results.

(*Source:* Adapted from "Evaluation versus Research" Patton (2017).)

Table 22.5 Framework for Program Evaluation in Public Health Mapped to CHW Competencies in Research and Evaluation

STEPS IN EVALUATION FRAMEWORK	CHW COMPETENCIES IN RESEARCH AND EVALUATION
Engage key partners/ stakeholders	a. Ability to identify important concerns and conduct evaluation and research to better understand root causes b. Ability to apply the practices of Community Based Participatory Research (CBPR)
Describe the program	c. Ability to participate in evaluation and research processes including: i. Identify priority issues and evaluation/research questions
Focus the evaluation design	ii. Develop evaluation/research design and methods
Gather credible evidence	iii. Data collection and interpretation
Justify conclusions	iv. Share results and findings
Ensure use and share lessons learned	v. Share results and findings vi. Engage stakeholders to take action on findings

CHW CORE COMPETENCIES IN RESEARCH AND EVALUATION

The CHW core competencies in research and evaluation identified by the C3 Project include (see Table 22.5):

1. Ability to identify important concerns and conduct evaluation and research to better understand root causes

2. Ability to apply the evidence-based practices of Community Based Participatory Research (CBPR)

3. Ability to participate in evaluation and research processes including:

   a. Identify priority issues and evaluation/research questions

   b. Develop evaluation/research design and methods

   c. Collect and interpret data

   d. Share results and findings

   e. Engage key partners to take action on findings

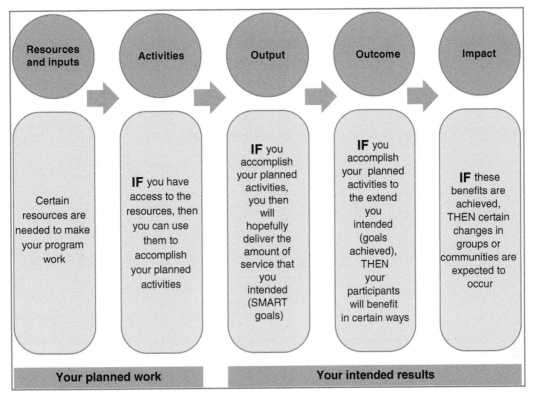

Figure 22.3 Logic Model: If ... Then Statements

FRAMEWORK FOR PROGRAM EVALUATION

Researchers and evaluators use frameworks or models to guide their work of gathering new knowledge. Learning about frameworks and models will help you understand the big picture of an evaluation project and the selected methodology. This understanding will help you identify areas where you can apply CHW competencies to lead or contribute to the project. The following section provides two frameworks mapped to the CHW competencies: Framework for program evaluation in public health and the Logic Model.

LOGIC MODELS

Some programs use a **logic model** (Figure 22.3) instead of evaluation framework to design a roadmap of how a program or intervention will produce results. Similar to the evaluation framework, a logic model shows the relationship between a program's resources and its proposed activities, outputs, outcomes, and impacts (Sharma & Petosa, 2014). Logic models differ widely in format and level of detail, and not all components are used in any given model. As a CHW, you may not be responsible for creating a logic model for a program but will benefit from understanding how the activities you will lead or participate come together and are measured or evaluated.

Key terms commonly used in logic models are presented here as *If/Then statements* (Centers for Disease Control and Prevention, 2020). A more detailed step-by-step guide to developing a logic model can be found on the Centers for Disease Control and Prevention Program Evaluation Framework webpage (2018b).

In addition to frameworks and models, in both research and evaluation, setting measurable goals and a clear timeline is critical—they determine the various components of the research design and serve to track the implementation of the activities and your intended results. Writing SMART goals is a critical skill you should learn as a CHW working in any research and evaluation work. In Chapters 9 and 10, you learned about developing and using *individual* SMART goals. The following worksheet, Table 22.6, with examples provides you a step-by-step guide to writing SMART goals *for research and evaluation projects*:

Table 22.6 Guide to Writing SMART Goals for Projects

LETTER	WORD	GUIDANCE (QUESTIONS TO CONSIDER)
S	**Specific**	**Who** needs to be involved to achieve the goal?
		What do we want to accomplish?
		When is the time frame?
		Where will the action occur?
		Which requirements, constraints, or obstacles need to be addressed?
		Why do we want to accomplish this goal?
M	**Measurable**	What metrics will we use to measure the goal?
		How will we measure progress?
		How will we know when the goal is accomplished?
A	**Achievable (attainable)**	How important is the goal to those involved?
		How can the goal be accomplished?
		What can you do to make the goal attainable?
		What are the logical steps we should take?
R	**Realistic/relevant**	Is this a worthwhile goal?
		Is this the right time?
		Do we have the necessary resources to accomplish this goal?
		Is this goal in line with our long-term objectives?
T	**Timely (time bound)**	How long will it take to accomplish this goal?
		When is the completion of this goal due?
		When are we going to work on this goal?

(*Source:* Adapted from "The Essential Guide to Writing SMART Goals" (Eby, 2019).)

In summary, understanding the roadmap for research and evaluation, whether it is using a framework or logic model, will help you piece together the various activities and tasks, and use your CHW competencies to contribute to telling the complete story of the community's needs, strengths, and opportunities to improve health and address social inequities.

CHW Profile

Mattie Clark, She/Her

Clinical Community Health Worker and Outreach Advocate

G.A. Carmichael Family Health Center, Belzoni, Mississippi

Underserved and Rural Communities

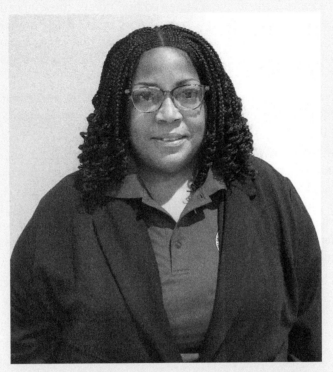

Growing up in Mississippi made me cognizant of the issues that arise when it comes to securing health care and other important needs in an underserved community. I know what it's like to struggle and to be around those who just need a helping hand to get back on their feet. I grew up in a small town, a farming community. There were times when my family struggled to keep the lights on and when the food didn't last. I started working in the fields when I was very young for two or three dollars a day. I was motivated to become a Clinical Community Health Worker because I want to help restore and give back to the community and because of my love for the people within it.

I provide services to rural communities and surrounding areas in person and via Telehealth. Some of the programs and services I provide are chronic disease self-management. I am a diabetes prevention lifestyle coach. I assist with HIV prevention and testing and counsel people about PrEP (antiretroviral medications to prevent infection with HIV). I do health fairs and COVID vaccinations. **I was part of a research team that demonstrated that CHWs can promote the health of community members with cardiovascular disease (see Chapter 16).**

I work with people living with chronic diseases who don't have transportation, are underinsured, or don't have health insurance. I set up participants with Medicaid or Medicare to get transportation assistance. I call three days in advance so they can get transportation to an appointment and back home. We also have volunteers that will drive people where they need to go. My motto is to meet people where they are.

(continues)

CHW Profile

(continued)

A participant was going through a rough patch after his home tragically burned down. He was staying on his land, living out of his car in the hot sun, with no water because it had been cut off. I contacted the Water Association and got him assistance with his bill. I also spoke with the USDA of Rural Development and secured a tiny home for the participant to live in. I helped him fill out the application. This gave him peace of mind, knowing he would have water and a tiny home set up on his property. I visit him every 30 days because he's a high-priority participant who needs extra help and follow-up. I make sure he understands his medications and is taking them properly. He's still waiting for the tiny home to be finished, but he's doing better.

My work has made me more confident because I'm a trusted figure in the community. While doing this work, I've been able to expand my knowledge, as well as my advocacy efforts. I've become closer with my community and really do my best to improve their lives any way I can.

Some tips I would share with new CHWs are to always lead with compassion, be your authentic self, and try your best not to get overwhelmed by the work. You really have to meet people where they are and try your best to help them. I don't stop until every resource is exhausted and I know that I've done everything I can do. I advocate. I send letters to our political representatives. I ask God for guidance, but no matter how hard we try, we can't win every battle. Don't beat yourself up if you're not able to help people with every problem that arises in their lives. Remember that we are a network. You are never alone. Reach out to your coworkers and your community and ask for help when you need it.

22.3 Selecting Research Tools and Methods

The next step after developing a road map for the research or evaluation project is to consider the most appropriate research tools and methods to use based on your understanding of the community. A research tool or method is used to gather information about the area of interest or focus. They assist you in gathering quantitative or qualitative data. Both are useful in understanding the problem that the community has identified.

Quantitative data let you know how many times something is happening, how many people share the same experience or opinion, or anything else that can be measured numerically or by counting. The tools and methods you will commonly use are surveys, mapping, counting, and public health data records. When you hear "quantitative," think of numbers.

Qualitative data give you an in-depth or deeper understanding of how people feel about or experience an issue. The tools and methods you will commonly use are interviews, focus groups, community forums, photovoice, or digital stories. When you hear "qualitative," think of words, stories, and pictures.

Mixed Methods research involves combining quantitative and qualitative methods for gathering data within the same study. Researchers can take advantage of the strength of both methods to explore and uncover relationships that may be presented on the research question or topic of interest. The choices of tools and methods are carefully decided based on the research topic, participants, and other cultural considerations.

An Example of Quantitative and Qualitative Data

The Question: How does smoking hurt our community?

Quantitative data: The number of people who report that their health has been harmed by smoking, the number of tobacco billboards or ads in a community, or data from the local health department on the number of people in the community who smoke and the number of people with chronic diseases that are caused by smoking such as emphysema, lung cancer, and heart disease.

Qualitative data: Real-life stories of how smoking hurts the community; the story of someone who died too young because they smoked; how a group of parents feels about tobacco advertising that targets their community; or how people feel about limiting smoking in public housing.

TYPES OF RESEARCH TOOLS AND METHODS

Both research and evaluation programs use a variety of research tools or methods to collect, measure, and analyze data. The key is to use tools wisely to ensure the outcomes achieved are measured appropriately. When designing and selecting research tools, keep cultural humility and literacy in mind. As a CHW, you can inform the team about tools that may be most acceptable and culturally appropriate for the communities you are working with (see Table 22.7).

Table 22.7 Uses of Specific Research Tools and Methods

TYPE OF TOOLS (T) AND METHODS (M)	DESCRIPTION	WHEN TO USE IT	WHEN NOT TO USE IT
Library (T)	Visit a local library and work with librarian and library computers to research your topic.	For access to local statistics, resources, and history that might not be available elsewhere.	If the information or data are available on the internet.
Internet (T)	Use search engines like "Google" or reputable health sites to get data or to network.	To do a quick initial search; a broad search; to access records or data unavailable locally.	If the information does not come from a reliable source
Existing policies, regulations (T)	Research at local, state, and federal levels whether there are existing policies relevant to your topic and whether they are being enforced.	This should be a standard part of your assessment!	This is always relevant!
Community forums (M)	Organize evening or weekend community meetings to gather community input, feedback, perceptions, and experiences.	When you want information from the community at large and want to raise awareness that an issue is being addressed.	If you do not have the resources available, as Community Forums are labor intensive

(continues)

Table 22.7 (*continued*)

TYPE OF TOOLS (T) AND METHODS (M)	DESCRIPTION	WHEN TO USE IT	WHEN NOT TO USE IT
Focus groups (M)	Strategically choose 6–12 people representing a variety of views on your issue. Facilitate a "group" discussion to get their perceptions and experiences.	When you want to get deep and in-depth qualitative information about your issue. This information complements information from community surveys. Focus groups also give people the opportunity to interact *with each other*, in addition to responding directly to a question. The conversation that participants have with each other is the richest part of any focus-group process.	If you want to be able to talk about what the community thinks "as a whole" about an issue, you may need to survey hundreds of people to get that broader view.
Key informant interview (M)	Strategically select individuals who play key roles in the community, related to the focus of the study. Using an interview guide, ask them questions to inform the needs and assets of the community on the topic of interest.	When you want more in-depth qualitative information about an issue from the perspective of a community member who is directly affected or involved in the focus of the study.	There is a potential bias if informants are not selected with care. The validity of the data can sometimes be difficult to prove.
Survey (M)	Decide on the number of people you will survey. Come up with a survey or questionnaire to use to ask those people what their opinions are on the issue you are concerned about.	When you want a representative sample of the communities' responses in an organized way. This information goes well with focus group information. Survey information can be counted, such as the number and percentage of those surveyed who share similar experiences, risks, or opinions.	May not provide you with the qualitative "stories" you are looking for.
Community mapping (T)	Take a large piece of paper and "map" a place such as a neighborhood, inside a store, etc. Plot important items you are looking for. "Google Maps" or other online tools can be used for digital mapping. Some cities and counties have websites with specific mapping tools (like GIS) for their community.	When you want a visual representation of a place. For example, to show how many liquor stores or parks are in your neighborhood. Also, when you want to compare the locations of two things—for example, traffic lights and car crashes.	When it is difficult to define the community geographically or the target involves multiple distant communities.

(continues)

Table 22.7 (continued)

TYPE OF TOOLS (T) AND METHODS (M)	DESCRIPTION	WHEN TO USE IT	WHEN NOT TO USE IT
Photovoice (traditionally done with still photographs, can also be done with video called Digital Stories (M)	Use cameras to document using pictures or videos of the issue you are working on. Usually, these pictures or videos are shared and discussed first among residents in a focus group, and then may be used later to tell the story to the public or a policymaker about the problem.	When sharing the story of the community as part of the community needs assessment. As a pathway for conversations to increase understanding and cultural respect. For healing and transformation; for behavioral change reflection and intentions. Digital stories can also be used to share (disseminate) findings and lessons learned.	When you don't have the resources.

Here are some examples of photovoice and digital stories for your reference:

Examples of photovoice:

- Using Photovoice to Describe the Assets and Barriers to Sexual and Reproductive Health among Latinos (Baquero, Goldman, Muqueeth, Eng, & Rhodes, 2014)
- Captivating views of CHWs (Cooper, 2022)

Examples of digital stories:

- National Center for Farmworker Health Digital Stories (National Center for Farmworker Health, 2022)
- National Indian Health Board Native Youth Summit Digital Story Films (National Indian Health Board, 2012)

A key aspect of using research tools and methods is the importance of consistency. Research or evaluation leaders must provide training to those who will collect data to ensure that the tool or methods are used correctly by all members of the data-collection team.

CHWs can also serve as liaisons to work with community members to identify research questions to ask and to recruit people to participate in surveys, focus groups, interviews, or forums. For example, you may want to convene an informational session or orientation for participants and community members to provide information on the purpose and steps involved in the activities planned for the study.

DEVELOPING RESEARCH TOOLS AND METHODS

Depending on your level of experience and team demands, you may be asked to develop or assist with the development of a research tool to ensure it is culturally appropriate. You may also be asked to use these tools to gather data for a project or program. In either case, the following are considerations to keep in mind when developing and understanding the application of some of the more common tools and methods used in research and evaluation.

Ethical Considerations When Doing Research and Evaluation

There are three key ethical principles to keep in mind when participating in research and evaluation (Quinn, 2015):

1. **Respect for persons**: This means people are treated as autonomous—they make the decisions that are best for him or herself. This also includes respect and protection for people who cannot make their own decisions.

2. **Beneficence**: This means respecting peoples' decisions, protecting people from harm, and keeping people safe (protecting their well-being). This principle means that research and evaluation should maximize possible benefits and minimize any potential harm.

(continues)

Ethical Considerations When Doing Research and Evaluation
(continued)

3. **Justice**: This means participants in research and evaluation are receive equal opportunity according to their need, effort, contributions to society, and merit.

These principles can help guide CHWs as part of the research or evaluation team in making decisions when working with people (human subjects is the common term used in IRB applications). These ethical considerations are especially important for certain groups of people who are considered "vulnerable populations." A vulnerable population refers to a group of people who have conditions that put them at greater risk of being placed in ethically inappropriate projects; this could mean that a person has difficulty providing voluntary, informed consent due to limitations in making decisions or situational circumstances or could also mean a person has a higher risk for being taken advantage of (Gordon, 2020). Common vulnerable populations acknowledged and protected by Institutional Review Boards (IRBs) include people who are incarcerated, pregnant women, fetuses, people with cognitive disabilities, and economically and educationally disadvantaged persons (Gordon, 2020).

CHWs have a unique opportunity to ensure that community members involved in research and or evaluation are treated ethically—with respect and not tricked or coerced into participating or doing something they do not really want to do. For example, a common ethical issue regarding research and evaluation is giving financial incentives for participating. On the one hand, people should be compensated for their time and not taken advantage of. For example, if $1000 is being offered to participate in a research study, a person with financial hardships may feel that they have to participate, though participating may not benefit them and could potentially harm them.

The principal investigator is responsible for protecting participants and that is also why researchers go through IRBs to get research and evaluation studies approved. Deciding whether something is ethical is *not* the sole responsibility of a CHW. Rather, as a CHW, you can be a champion for your community and help ensure their rights are protected by asking questions and getting additional information as needed.

METHODS USED FOR QUANTITATIVE DATA

The most commonly used quantitative research methods are surveys, polls, and questionnaires or forms. In the recent years, these methods have been distributed via email as a link, hyperlink, or QR code along with the informed consent, and participants have the option to complete them from their computers or mobile devices. These tools are created using online applications such as Survey Monkey or Qualtrics, Zoom polls, and other web-based platforms.

Surveys/Polls/Questionnaires

- **Identify the questions**: Start by working with community members to identify the type of information they want to gather and how that information will improve their understanding of the focus issue or concern (such as barriers to physical activity, how to improve blood pressure, or access to mental health services). Next, create a list of questions to include in the survey designed to gather this information. Narrow the questions down to no more than two pages. Use straightforward language, and do not use abbreviations. Finally, put your questions in a logical order, from the general to the more specific.

- **Organize the questions**: Start the survey with the questions that are the most interesting and least threatening. Save the more difficult questions for the end, and avoid leading questions (e.g., a question starting with "Don't you think that _____?").

- **Consider answer choices**: As much as possible, use closed-ended questions (yes or no answers) for surveys rather than open-ended ones (see Chapter 9). This will allow you to collect data and analyze your findings more easily. When including questions that ask people to compare or rate items, be sure to include options from both extremes. If you want to give respondents a list of answers or categories to choose from, try to keep it short (no more than five choices, for example, strongly agree, agree, neutral, disagree, and strongly disagree). Questions that ask people to remember things from the past should focus on the near past to document accurate information (e.g., "How many times in the last month have you. . . .").

- **Add an extra pair of eyes**: It is a good practice to involve someone with evaluation experience to review their survey tool and make suggestions.

- **Test the questions**: Once you have your survey in draft form, pilot the survey with a few community members who are representative of the group you want to survey. This will help to ensure that all the questions are clear and invite responses that are useful to the community assessment. Finally, come up with a brief memo called informed consent to attach to the survey describing who you are, why you are doing the survey, and how you will use the information gathered (see Ethical Considerations When Doing Research and Evaluation). The informed consent must be handed out to everyone whom you ask to participate in the survey.

METHODS USED FOR QUALITATIVE DATA

Several research tools are useful for finding out what the community is thinking or learning about their story. Community forums or meetings, key informant interviews, and focus groups are common, frequently used methods.

Focus Groups

- **Focus group size**: A focus group is essentially an interview conducted with a group of 5–8 people. Generally, you want to make sure there are enough people in the room to keep a good conversation going, but not so many that some participants won't have a chance to speak. In planning the number of participants, plan with the expectation that one or more individuals may not show up, so you may need to recruit 6–12 people. If everyone shows up, it would still be a manageable size for a focus group, and if fewer than 12 show up, you will still have enough people to keep the conversation flowing.

- **Diversity of perspective**: Often, having people who are similar in some way is useful—for example, having all the participants come from the same neighborhood, all be single parents, or all be of the same gender, age, or ethnicity. Other times, it's helpful to have more diversity. You might hold several focus groups on the same topic. Talk with your colleagues and community partners about what the right mix should be for the information you wish to learn.

- **Create the right environment to build rapport and trust**: Participants need reassurance that you and the other group members are trustworthy. Let people know what you are doing and why and follow through on any commitments you make to the group.

- **Ground rules**: Setting basic ground rules allows everyone to know what to expect. You might suggest some and then ask those in the group if they have any they want to add. Post them on flip-chart paper so everyone can keep them in mind.

- **Informed consent**: Participants should be provided with an *informed consent* detailing the purpose of the study, disclosing any risks to them for participating, rights to not participate or stop the interview, and contact information for any questions or concerns.

- **Confidentiality is important to discuss**. You need to assure participants that what they say will be treated confidentially by you, and they in turn need to agree to keep what they hear and say confidential. Let people know what you are going to do with the information they have provided.

- **Discussion guide**: Make sure that everyone has the chance to speak. Use a discussion guide (interview guide) of approximately 5–7 pre-formulated questions or prompts to facilitate the group discussion. These questions are developed based on research and knowledge of the community as well as the health and social issues in discussion.

- **Facilitation**: The best practice is to have two people facilitate the focus group—one to act as the moderator or facilitator, and another act as the recorder and to document what participants say.

- **Incentives for participation**: If you have a budget for this, small gift cards or other incentives such as refreshment table or individual snack or goodie bags will be appreciated by the participants and encourage them to show up for the focus group.

- **Length of time**: Focus groups are one to two hours.

- **After the focus group**: As soon after the session as possible, write down your thoughts and review your notes. Spend some time with your fellow facilitator and share your reflections. Identify strongly held views, major areas of agreement among participants, and surprising information.
- **Reaching saturation**: Saturation is defined as the point when the information or concepts of two consecutive focus groups reveal no additional "new" category of information (Hennink et al., 2019).

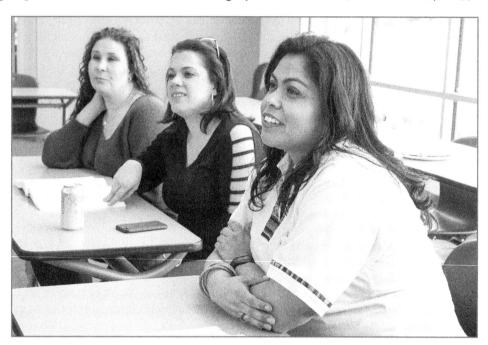

A focus group discussion about a community health concern.

Informed Consent or Release of Information

About the study: This focus group is part of a _____ study or evaluation program. The purpose is to _____. You have been invited to participate because you are a member of _____ community or have knowledge about _____ (topic or issue).

Benefits to participant: By participating in this focus group, you will have an opportunity to share your knowledge and perspectives on the _____ (topic or issue). You may choose to stop participating at any time during the interview. You will be provided with a _____ (incentive) in appreciation of your time and information.

Disclosures of *potential risk to participant*: There are _____ (e.g., minimal) risks to you for participating in this focus group. The focus group discussion will be recorded, and the information will be kept confidential and only used for the purpose of this study or evaluation. There will be no identifiers or names associated with your answers and comments.

If you have any questions about this study or evaluation, you may contact _____ (name of lead researcher or organization representative) at _____ (phone and email).

Consent:

I, _____, give _____ [name of interviewer] permission to use material from this interview for the purposes of the study or project.

Signed and dated:

_____

Note: If the person you are interviewing is less than 18 years old, a parent or guardian must give permission and sign the consent.

DEVELOPING AN INTERVIEW GUIDE

Focus groups and key informant interviews use interview guides, which are a set of pre-prepared questions based on the research and other information gathered about the topic of interest. Questions must be open-ended (not yes or no questions) and designed to inspire conversation. A question that is too open could leave participants confused or overwhelmed. It's smart to start with general, simple questions that are easier for people to understand and answer, then build the discussion with more complex or deeper questions. A sample set of questions might look like this:

1. What do you like about living in your neighborhood or community?
2. What are your concerns with physical activity in your community?
3. How do these concerns affect the community residents in staying physically active?
4. What needs to change to promote physical activity in your community?
5. What resources are available in your community to promote physical activity?

Managing Focus Group Challenges and Opportunities

A focus group was conducted with community members to talk with them about their thoughts, ideas, and opinions about physical activity and about potential barriers to not being physically active.

The focus group facilitator was aware that several women had younger children who were not yet in school. The facilitator also knew that different cultures and languages were present in the community.

To help with childcare, the facilitator arranged for licensed childcare providers to be in the same location where mothers could see their children and know they were safe while they participated in the group.

To address cultural and language factors, the facilitator developed questions with other CHWs who were from the community and had children. The facilitator then vetted the questions with local community nonprofit organizations who worked with similar priority population to make sure the questions were easy to understand and culturally appropriate, as well as to help translate the questions into appropriate languages.

A Word About Bias

It is possible to conduct research or evaluation so that you learn *only* what you want to hear. If you think that the community should start a campaign to turn an abandoned lot into a park, you can set up the study to increase the chances that this will be the outcome. After all, it's for a good cause, isn't it? But this type of manipulation contradicts the true purpose of the study, which is to gather information without prejudice and to let the community express their own concerns and their own ideas for change. This is called **bias**.

Common ways that bias can undermine a research or evaluation study include:

- **In participant selection**: Determining who participates in the community diagnosis—such as including only people who already agree with a certain position.
- **In discussion questions**: Asking *leading questions* or questions that lead people to the answers you want them to provide. For example, a leading question is: "Do you think that the empty lot by XYZ avenue should be converted into a community park?" Instead, an open-ended and unbiased question would be: "What do you think about the empty lot by XYZ avenue? How would you like this lot to be used in the community?"

(continues)

A Word About Bias

(continued)

- While you should avoid leading questions, it can be helpful to ask questions with a list of answers to choose among. These "multiple choice" questions may help people to think about the topic from different angles. They also make it easier to count the responses. An example would be, "Which of the following do you believe are possible options for the use of the empty lot? (a) residential housing, (b) community park, (c) recycling center, and (d) other." When you include the option of "other," you also decrease bias, since it allows the community members to add their own ideas. Make sure you give them the opportunity to state what they mean by "other." If all the options you list for a question are very similar, then that introduces bias because it guides people to think only one way.
- **In summary of responses:** Summarizing the discussion to highlight information that supports your position, while withholding data that do not, or presenting it in a confusing way.
- **In data analysis:** Guiding the analysis or trying to do the analysis for the community and telling them what the data say.
- **In action planning:** Guiding the development of the action plan, by calling on and supporting the voices of people who agree with you, or by asking questions that lead people to the type of action that you think is best.

It's important to be aware of your own biases. Allowing your own bias or that of your employer or organization to influence the results of a study is likely to undermine the community's trust in you and may also weaken and damage, rather than strengthen the community's own capacity.

DATA ANALYSIS

Quantitative data collected from surveys, questionnaires, or other tools can be analyzed by various methods and software applications. Usually, this is done by someone with specialized training, but it's helpful to understand and contribute to the interpretation of the results and findings.

There are different ways to analyze qualitative interviews. More commonly, interviews are transcribed word for word from a recording, then, identify key themes from one interview or common themes from more than one interview—this is called "content analysis." This will help you see common themes and what is important to people in the focus group.

For example, a qualitative focus group may reveal key factors (root causes) that influence physical activity in a local community. Analysis of the interview transcriptions (content analysis) might generate themes such as poorly maintained parks and recreational areas, lack of well-lit streets for walking or biking, the closing of a centralized community center, violence, or racism. In your summary and analysis of the interviews, do not only look for opinions and themes that were shared among the respondents, but also for particularly strong or powerful opinions. Write down insightful quotes to include in your analysis. To help visualize common themes, you can create a simple table (see Table 22.8) to identify the different themes mentioned and to count how many people mentioned them.

In a mixed-methods study, data from both a survey and a focus group are analyzed and reviewed to gain knowledge or understand the problem about a topic or issue. Whether qualitative, quantitative, or mixed methods, selecting the best set of methods and tools for information gathering (data collection) supports the efforts to understand the problem the community has identified. The analysis of the data then can provide new or supportive information to confirm, deny, or learn about the issues of interest.

Table 22.8 Example—Summary of Themes from the Physical Activity Qualitative Interviews

MAJOR THEMES	OUT OF 20 INTERVIEWS, THE NO. OF PEOPLE WHO MENTIONED THE THEME:
Poorly maintained parks and recreational areas	8
Lack of well-lit streets for walking and biking	12
Closing of the main community center	6
Violence and racism	15

22.4 Sharing Findings with the Community

After data analysis, a crucial next step in the process is to share the findings. This is called **dissemination**. Dissemination of findings helps community members identify a possible solution to their common concern and create opportunities to talk about actions that may force decision makers to do something about the issue. Yet, many research and evaluation efforts fail to invest sufficient time and resources to disseminate their findings. As a CHW, you can play an important role in connecting with the community and sharing relevant information, including lessons learned, benefits and risks of any intervention. You may use the following types of questions to assist in discussions:

- What does the information tell them about the issue they investigated?
- Who in the community is most affected by the problem?
- What percentage of people who participated in the research seem highly concerned about the problem?
- What does the community think about the causes and consequences of the problem?
- What are their proposed solutions?
- Do different parts of the community have different experiences or opinions—for example, do women express different opinions from men, and do youths express different opinions from elders? Are there any differences in opinion based on where people live in the community?

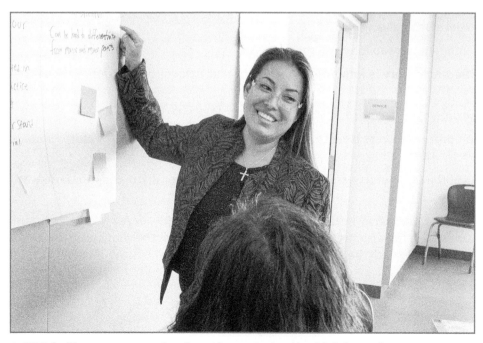

A CHW facilitates a community discussion to analyze health information.

As you prepare to share findings with the community consider the following additional points:

1. *Engage community members and partners early in the research and evaluation process.*

   - Find and engage community leaders, and other "gatekeepers," and introduce them to the research or evaluation team. These community members can be ambassadors and help with engage others throughout the project.

   - Include community members in decisions regarding plans to conduct research and best approach to disseminate findings.

2. *Promote the importance of sharing research and evaluation findings with the community.*

   - Discuss why and how the findings or results will be used.

   - Ask if there is a plan in place to share research findings with the community. Share your ideas with the researchers and evaluators.

   - Promote culturally appropriate ways to share information with the community. This may include social media, local newspapers and radio stations, a community forum or town hall, photo stories, or newsletters.

3. *Engage community members in the dissemination of the findings.*

   - Make sure community members who have taken part in the data gathering have access to the results or findings

   - As you gather data via surveys, interviews, or focus groups, ask people how they would like to hear about the findings.

   - Participants may want to assist in developing the plan for dissemination and to be actively involved in the dissemination of the findings. For example, a community member could co-present results with the research team.

4. *Know the communities you will be sharing information with.*

   - Be culturally aware to know how to break down information in simpler terms and ideas, what language(s) should the results be presented based on the community's primary languages.

   - Consider the people who will share information back to the community—are they a trusted source of information such as a well-known CHW or community leader?

5. *Don't take the data at face value.*

   - There are different ways to interpret the same data.

   - Showing the whole story is important! Information or data gathered cannot always tell the whole story.

6. *Provide soaking time.*

   - Allow community members time to absorb the information and react, before jumping to action ideas.

   - The results of the community assessment may be surprising or distressing to those who live in the community.

   - On the other hand, there may be important community strengths or aspects of community history that were not captured in the diagnosis—discussing the results with the community may provide an opportunity to add more detail to the picture.

Phuong An Doan-Billings: As someone who works as a CHW, you get trained to look at information in a certain way. But when you bring the information to the community, sometimes they close the door; they don't want to hear it. You have to figure out how they feel when you share bad news—like that nail salon chemicals can cause cancer. They don't think that's something they want to know. They'll think, you mean I harm myself, my customers, everyone who works here. And they will feel very, very sad. You assume that it's good information for people to know, but they don't feel that way. Someone might think, "It's not personal—it's a community issue," but that's an American way of thinking. The Vietnamese way is more indirect. You can't talk right into their face. What we do is, we find out what they don't like to hear, and then present that in a delicate way. It's a cultural difference—and that's why we are here as CHWs.

PREPARING YOUR FINDINGS IN A VISUALLY COMPELLING FORMAT

Once the community group has analyzed and interpreted the data and has a plan for dissemination, we recommend that you develop a clear way to present the results. You will want to share your key findings with members who will assist you to advocate for changes in the community and to policymakers. *How* you present the data often makes a difference in terms of whether people understand the findings and want to act on the results. More is not always better! It is important to identify key findings (usually three to five) from the results (data analysis). Consider the following points:

- What information is most compelling to the community?
- What are the community's concerns about the issue and what do they want done about it?
- What information will be useful in engaging policymakers to take action on the community's behalf?
- How is the community negatively affected by the issue compared with other communities?
- What policies or local solutions are already in place that address the issue?
- What presentation format (newsletter, social media post, video, community forum, and others) will be most helpful to use based on the audience? Consider potential access issues, such as internet for digital formats.

The presentation of the findings can vary. The expression "a picture is worth a thousand words" applies well here. Whether printed or digital, using tables, pie charts, bar or line graphs, photos or maps, case studies quotes, video or digital media, or infographics, are helpful ways to tell the story and promote discussions.

COMMUNITY-DRIVEN HEALTH EQUITY ACTION PLANS

Another important step is developing an *action plan* based on the analysis of research or evaluation findings. An action plan lays out the steps the community may take to make or advocate for change. It should be strategic, transformative, and practical (Data Center Research for Justice, 2022). It is similar to the action plans that CHWs support individual clients to develop (see Chapters 9 and 10). This process should be as inclusive as possible, providing an opportunity for all members of the community to participate if they choose. Getting this process right is more important than doing it quickly. If you rush and forget to include certain members of the community, you risk losing support for your action plan or creating a new conflict and problem in the community. Be as transparent, open, and honest as possible about this process; let everyone know how and when they can participate.

The National Academy of Medicine (NAM) Culture of Health Program developed a model for developing Community-Driven Health Equity Action Plans which has been piloted (tested the application) in five community teams (CA, OR & WA, NY, WV, and TX). These five community teams agreed to explore opportunities and barriers in advancing health equity at the community level while addressing health inequities locally through Community-Driven Health Equity Action Plans. Each community uniquely designed a plan for communities using the model with a seven-step guide: vision and goals, community context, research grounding, strategies and tactics, stakeholders, timeline, and sustainability (National Academy of Medicine, 2023).

Part of your action plan will be to identify potential allies who will assist in creating change. You will need allies at all levels—from the grassroots to City Hall or the State legislature. It's often helpful to identify a specific policymaker who might be sympathetic to your ideas and who has influence with other policymakers. This person could become a champion who helps facilitate the steps to attain your policy goals. Yet even champions sometimes need to be convinced or persuaded to achieve the results you want. For more information about Community Organizing and Advocacy, see Chapter 23.

CONSIDERATIONS WHEN RESEARCH IS NOT COMMUNITY DRIVEN

When research is not community driven, the problem identified, the plans, the analysis, the interpretation, and dissemination are not *in* the community nor *with* the community. As the member of the research or evaluation team with unique connections to the community intended to serve, your CHW voice FOR the community can ensure the project is community driven.

In addition to the considerations presented in earlier sections, here are some additional questions to determine whether a project is community driven or not:

- What issues or questions are the focus of this research? Are these topics and questions important to the community in which the research will be undertaken?

- To what extent will researchers involve local community members in the research process and project? Have community members been consulted about the research focus and methods? Will community members be hired to work on the study?

- How might the information gathered by research ultimately be used to promote the health and well-being of the community?

- How will the results of the study—including positive and negative results—be shared with the community and with the subjects of the research (the people who participate in surveys, questionnaires, and focus groups or who donate blood or other biological samples)?

- What is the past record of the lead researchers (sometimes called principal investigators)? Have they made efforts in the past to share research findings with the communities they studied? Has their research been used to promote the welfare of the communities they studied?

You can advocate and speak for your community when you come across research that is not community driven. Now that you have a greater understanding of the components of research and evaluation, and have acquired knowledge and ability to apply your CHW research and competency skills, you can contribute to all areas of the design, method selection, data collection, dissemination, and even action planning!

22.5 Trends in CHW Research and Evaluation

Research studies have demonstrated that CHWs contribute to improving the health and reducing health inequities of community members. CHWs engage in research in different ways. In some studies, CHWs are actively involved in the collection of data. In other projects, CHWs are actively engaged in leading and guiding the research and/or evaluation study. Both models highly engage CHWs, and there are several successes that have been published for both models.

Many studies have involved CHWs in research; some common roles of CHWs in research studies include participant recruitment and data collection (such as surveys, facilitating focus groups/interviews, etc.). Appendix A lists a few examples of studies that involved CHWs in research studies.

A growing trend in research is to actively engage CHWs as lead researchers within the research team. This includes CHWs as principal investigators and co-investigators in a research or evaluation study. Appendix B shows examples where CHWs are not only involved in doing the research (such as recruiting participants and collecting data), but they are also engaged in the design and carrying out the research—and have responsibilities such as making sure the IRB protocol is followed and that participants' rights are protected; provide leadership in proper collection of data and training project staff; participate in data analysis and reporting of the findings.

Evaluation of programs and services involving CHWs have grown in the past decade as well. But there are no national evaluation standards that can be used to compare evaluation results across different CHW programs. There is less documentation on CHW-led evaluation efforts and how CHWs are involved in leadership capacities. However, there's growing number of CHWs who have taken leadership roles in local, regional, and national evaluation programs and initiatives.

CHW led evaluation. An example of a CHW-led nation-wide effort is the CHW Common Indicators (CI) Project. The CI Project's purpose "is to contribute to the integrity, sustainability, and viability of CHW programs through the collaborative development and adoption of a set of common process and outcome constructs and indicators for CHW practice" (Rodela et al., 2021). Since its inception in 2015, the CI Project has sought to prioritize the knowledge, input, and leadership, including decision-making power, of CHWs at every stage of the project (Rodela et al., 2021).

CHWs have led the CI Project's workshops, videoconferences, and presentations using popular education techniques to balance power and the voices of key partners. This CHW-led initiative has resulted in the development of a list of a conceptual frame that brings attention to CHW processes and outcomes. This conceptual frame has served to evaluate CHW practices and programs and foster intentional collaborations between CHWs and the broader CHW evaluation communities.

CHW involved evaluation. The Centers for Disease Control and Prevention's (CDC) Community Health Workers for COVID Response and Resilient Communities—Evaluation and Technical Assistance CDC-RFA-DP21-2110 (CCR-ETA) grant has led to opportunities for CHWs to get involved in evaluation efforts at a national level CHWs serve in various groups (CHW council) to review and monitor data, and in the dissemination of evaluation results (Centers for Disease Control and Prevention, 2022a). Other CHWs work as program staff to coordinate national webinars and communities of practice, developing data-collection instruments, conducting data collections, and involved in other evaluation activities.

Recent trends have shown the value of CHW-driven evaluation frameworks, which are helping to shape stronger and more equitable health systems, improving public health, and helping wider publics understand what CHWs do and what they need to succeed. As a CHW, you can make a link to what you have already been doing on research and evaluation programs and understand the why and how to make your work acknowledged and recognized. You can also bridge knowledge gaps, educating researchers and evaluators on how to best involve CHWs to make the most contribution to the team and ultimately bring transforming solutions to improve health equity and social justice in communities.

Chapter Review

Assess your understanding of the key concepts and skills presented in Chapter 22. Review the CHW Scenario presented at the beginning of the chapter. How would you evaluate this Physical Activity Program? How could the information that you gather be used to influence and improve the health of the community?

Consider how to answer the following questions:

- What is the purpose of research and evaluation? How can research and evaluation contribute to promoting community health?
- What roles can CHWs play in research and evaluation?
- How does your understanding of frameworks and models help you identify areas where CHWs can contribute?
- What are some of the main differences between quantitative and qualitative data?
- What are some of the different tools and methods that can be used in research and evaluation?
- Why do you think it is important for CHWs to exercise leadership in research and evaluation?
- Why is it important for research and evaluation efforts to collaborate closely with the communities in which research and evaluation are being undertaken?
- How can you bridge the gaps in disseminating research and evaluation findings with your community?

References

Arredondo, E. M., Haughton, J., Ayala, G. X., Slymen, D., Sallis, J. F., Perez, L. G., . . . Lopez, N. V. (2022). Two-year outcomes of Faith in Action/Fe en Acción: a randomized controlled trial of physical activity promotion in Latinas. *International Journal of Behavioral Nutrition and Physical Activity*, 19, 1–10.

Ayala, G. X., Molina, M., Madanat, H., Nichols, J. F., Mckenzie, T. L., Ji, M., . . . Labarca, C. (2017). Intervention effects on Latinas' physical activity and other health indicators. *American Journal of Preventive Medicine*, 52, S279–S283.

Ayala, G. X. & San Diego Prevention Research Center Team. (2011). Effects of a promotor-based intervention to promote physical activity: Familias Sanas y Activas. *American Journal of Public Health*, 101, 2261–2268.

Baquero, B., Goldman, S. N., Muqueeth, S., Eng, E. & Rhodes, S. D. (2014). Mi Cuerpo, Nuestro Responsabilidad: Using Photovoice to Describe the Assets and Barriers to Sexual and Reproductive Health among Latinos.

Breen, E. (2022). The Health Tree Metaphor and the Importance of Shared Language. Health Resource in Action. https://hria.org/2022/04/03/healthequitree/ (accessed 6 May 2022).

Casarett, D., Karlawish, J. H. & Sugarman, J. (2000). Determining when quality improvement initiatives should be considered research: proposed criteria and potential implications. *JAMA*, 283, 2275–2280.

Centers for Disease Control and Prevention. (2018a). Pasos Adelante Program. https://www.cdc.gov/prc/study-findings/research-briefs/pasos-adelantes.htm (accessed 6 May 2022).

Centers for Disease Control and Prevention. (2018b). Program Evaluation Framework Checklist for Step 2: Describe the Program. https://www.cdc.gov/evaluation/steps/step2/index.htm (accessed 6 May 2022).

Centers for Disease Control and Prevention. (2020). Developing a Logic Model. https://www.cdc.gov/tb/programs/evaluation/Logic_Model.html (accessed 6 May 2022).

Centers for Disease Control and Prevention. (2022a). Community Health Workers for COVID Response and Resilient Communities—Evaluation and Technical Assistance CDC-RFA-DP21-2110 (CCR-ETA). National Center for Chronic Disease Prevention and Health Promotion (NCCDPHP). https://www.cdc.gov/chronicdisease/programs-impact/nofo/covid-response-assistance.htm (accessed 6 May 2022).

Centers for Disease Control and Prevention. (2022b). The Social-Ecological Model: A Framework for Prevention. https://www.cdc.gov/violenceprevention/about/social-ecologicalmodel.html (accessed 6 May 2022).

Centers for Disease Control and Prevention. (2022c). Program Evaluation. Office of Policy, Performance, and Evaluation. https://www.cdc.gov/evaluation/index.htm (accessed 6 May 2022).

Centers for Medicare & Medicaid Services. (2020). Intro to Evaluation: Guidance for Community Officials and Organizations on Introduction Steps to Evaluate Community Needs and Capacity for a LTSS Program. https://www.hhs.gov/guidance/document/intro-evaluation (accessed 6 May 2022).

Cooper, L. (2022). Captivating Views. of Community Health Workers. Johns Hopkinds University. https://hub.jhu.edu/2022/10/21/lisa-cooper-latoya-ruby-frazier-more-than-conquerors/ (accessed 6 May 2022).

Data Center Research for Justice. (2022). Research for Community Power. https://www.datacenter.org/services-offered/#:~:text=Community%2Ddriven%20research%20engages%20communities,investment%20in%20fighting%20for%20solutions. (accessed 6 May 2022).

Eby, K. (2019). The Essential Guide to Writing Smart Goals. Luettavissa. https://www.smartsheet.com/blog/essential-guide-writing-smart-goals (accessed 6 May 2022).

Gordon, B. G. (2020). Vulnerability in research: basic ethical concepts and general approach to review. *The Ochsner Journal*, 20, 34–38.

Harrington, L. (2007). Quality improvement, research, and the institutional review board. *Journal for Healthcare Quality*, 29, 4–9.

Haughton, J., Ayala, G. X., Burke, K. H., Elder, J. P., Montañez, J. & Arredondo, E. M. (2015). Community health workers promoting physical activity: targeting multiple levels of the social ecological model. *The Journal of Ambulatory Care Management*, 38, 309–320.

Hawe, P., Degeling, D., Hall, J. & Brierley, A. (1990). *Evaluating health promotion: a health worker's guide*, MacLennan & Petty Sydney.

Hennink, M. M., Kaiser, B. N. & Weber, M. B. (2019). What influences saturation? estimating sample sizes in focus group research. *Qualitative Health Research*, 29, 1483–1496.

Kosecoff, J. & Fink, A. (1982). *Evaluation basics: A practitioner's manual*, SAGE Publications, Incorporated.

Lee, Y. & Park, S. (2021). Understanding of physical activity in social ecological perspective: application of multilevel model. *Frontiers in Psychology*, 12, 622929.

National Academy of Medicine. (2023). Culture of Health: Community-Driven Heath Equity Action Plans. https://nam.edu/programs/culture-of-health/community-driven-health-equity-action-plans/ (accessed 6 May 2022).

National Center for Farmworker Health. (2022). Digital Stories. http://www.ncfh.org/digital-stories.html (accessed 6 May 2022).

National Center for State, T., Local, & Territorial Public Health Infrastructure and Workforce. (2022). Community Health Assessments & Health Improvement Plans. Centers for Disease Control and Prevention. https://www.cdc.gov/publichealthgateway/cha/plan.html#print (accessed 6 May 2022).

National Indian Health Board. (2012). 2012 National Indian Health Board Native Youth Summit Digital Story Films. https://www.nihb.org/communications/2012_nyt_films.php (accessed May 6 2022).

Patton, M. Q. (2017). Evaluation Flash Cards: Embedding Evaluative Thinking in Organizational Culture. Otto Bremer Trust. https://ottobremer.org/wp-content/uploads/2017/12/OBT_flashcards_201712.pdf.

Puckett, Y. (2017). Bringing the IRB into the community: a new framework for the ethical regulation of CBPR. *MOJ Public Health*, 5, 183–188.

Quinn, C. R. (2015). General considerations for research with vulnerable populations: ten lessons for success. *Health & Justice*, 3, 1–7.

Rodela, K., Wiggins, N., Maes, K., Campos-Dominguez, T., Adewumi, V., Jewell, P. & Mayfield-Johnson, S. (2021). The Community Health Worker (CHW) common indicators project: engaging CHWs in measurement to sustain the profession. *Frontiers in Public Health*, 9, 674858.

Rosenthal, E., Menking, P. & . St John, J. (2018). *The community health worker core consensus (C3) project: A report of the C3 project: phase 1 and 2, together leaning toward the sky. a national project to inform CHW policy and practice.* El Paso, Texas.

Samuel, C. A., Lightfoot, A. F., Schaal, J., Yongue, C., Black, K., Ellis, K., . . . Eng, E. (2018). Establishing new community-based participatory research partnerships using the community-based participatory research charrette model: lessons from the cancer health accountability for managing pain and symptoms study. *Progress in Community Health Partnerships*, 12, 89–99.

Sharma, M. & Petosa, R. L. (2014). *Measurement and evaluation for health educators*, Jones & Bartlett Publishers.

Shore, N., Brazauskas, R., Drew, E., Wong, K. A., Moy, L., Baden, A. C., . . . Seifer, S. D. (2011). Understanding community-based processes for research ethics review: a national study. *American Journal of Public Health*, 101, S359–S364.

U.S. Department of Health & Human Services National Institute of Health. (2022). NIH Clinical Research Trial and You: The Basics. https://www.nih.gov/health-information/nih-clinical-research-trials-you/basics (accessed 6 May 2022).

Wanzer, D. L. (2021). What is evaluation?: perspectives of how evaluation differs (or not) from research. *American Journal of Evaluation*, 42, 28–46.

Appendix A: Examples of CHW Roles in Research in Published Studies (*mapped to C3 Project CHW Core roles)

Facilitation of assessment activities (focus groups, interviews, etc.) ***C3 Project roles:** #8 Implementing individual and community assessments #10 Participating in evaluation and research	Health disparities	Shah, V. O., Ghahate, D. M., Bobelu, J., Sandy, P., Newman, S., Helitzer, D. L., … & Zager, P. (2014). Identifying barriers to health care to reduce health disparity in Zuni Indians using focus group conducted by community health workers. *Clinical and Translational Science*, 7(1), 6–11.
	Behavioral health services	Ingram, M., Murrietta, L., de Zapien, J. G., Herman, P. M., & Carvajal, S. C. (2015). Community health workers as focus group facilitators: A participatory action research method to improve behavioral health services for farmworkers in a primary care setting. *Action Research*, 13(1), 48–64.
Identification and recruitment of participants ***C3 Project roles:** #1 Providing culturally appropriate HE and information #3 Care coord., CM, and Sys, navigation #5 Advocating for Indiv. And communities #10 Participating in evaluation and research	Recruit and match participants for different research studies	Varma, D. S., Strelnick, A. H., Bennett, N., Piechowski, P., Aguilar-Gaxiola, S., & Cottler, L. B. (2020). Improving community participation in clinical and translational research: CTSA Sentinel Network proof of concept study. *Journal of Clinical Translational Science*, 4(4), 322–330. doi:10.1017/cts.2020.21.
	Health disparities	Brown, L. D, Vasquez, D., Salinas, J. J., Tang, X., & Balcázar, H. (2018). Evaluation of healthy fit: a community health worker model to address Hispanic health disparities. *Preventing Chronic Disease*, 15, E49. doi:10.5888/pcd15.170347.
	Physical activity	Vidoni, M. L., Lee, M., Mitchell-Bennett, L., & Reininger, B. M. (2019). Home visit intervention promotes lifestyle changes: results of an RCT in Mexican Americans. *American Journal of Preventive Medicine*, 57(5), 611–620. doi:10.1016/j.amepre.2019.06.020.
Health outreach and education ***C3 Project roles:** #1 Providing culturally appropriate HE and information #2 Providing Culturally Appropriate HEd and Information #9 Conducting outreach #10 Participating in evaluation and research	Medical home intervention	Rogers, E. A., Manser, S. T., Cleary, J., Joseph, A. M., Harwood, E. M., & Call, K. T. (2018). Integrating community health workers into medical homes. *Annals of Family Medicine*, 16(1), 14–20. doi:10.1370/afm.2171.
	Breast, cervical, and colorectal cancer intervention	Krok-Schoen, J. L., Weier, R. C., Hohl, S. D., Thompson, B., & Paskett, E. D. (2016). Involving community health workers in the centers for population health and health disparities research projects: benefits and challenges. *Journal Health Care Poor Underserved*, 27(3), 1252–1266. doi:10.1353/hpu.2016.0145.
Variety of research activities ***C3 Project roles:** #10 Participating in evaluation and research	Review of several studies involving CHWs in research	Coulter, K., Ingram, M., McClelland, D. J., & Lohr, A. (2020). Positionality of community health workers on health intervention research teams: a scoping review. *Frontiers in Public Health*, 8, 208. doi:10.3389/fpubh.2020.00208.

Appendix B: Examples of CHWs as Researchers in Published Studies

RESEARCH FOCUS	STUDY TEAM/CITATION
Access to parks/ environmental changes	Arredondo, E., Mueller, K., Mejia, E., Rovira-Oswalder, T., Richardson, D., & Hoos, T. (2013). Advocating for environmental changes to increase access to parks: engaging promotoras and youth leaders. *Health Promotion Practice*, 14, 759–766. doi: 10.1177/1524839912473303.
CHW Common Indicators	Rodela, K., Wiggins, N., Maes, K., Campos-Dominguez, T., Adewumi, V., Jewell, P, & Mayfield-Johnson, S. (2021). The community health worker (CHW) common indicators project: Engaging CHWs in measurement to sustain the profession. *Frontiers in Public Health*, 9, 674858. doi: 10.3389/fpubh.2021.674858.
Food security and access	St John, J. A., Johnson, C. M., Sharkey, J. R., Dean, W. R., & Arandia, G. (2013). Empowerment of promotoras as promotora-researchers in the Comidas Saludables & Gente Sana en las Colonias del Sur de Tejas (Healthy Food and Healthy People in South Texas Colonias) program. *Journal of Primary Prevention*, 34(1–2), 41–57. doi:10.1007/s10935-013-0296-1.
Health disparities	Johnson, C. M., Sharkey, J. R., Dean, W. R., St John, J. A., & Castillo, M. (2013). Promotoras as research partners to engage health disparity communities. *Journal of the Academy of Nutrition and Dietetics*, 113(5), 638–642. doi:10.1016/j.jand.2012.11.014.

Community Organizing

Rama Ali Kased, Larry Salomon, and Savita Malik

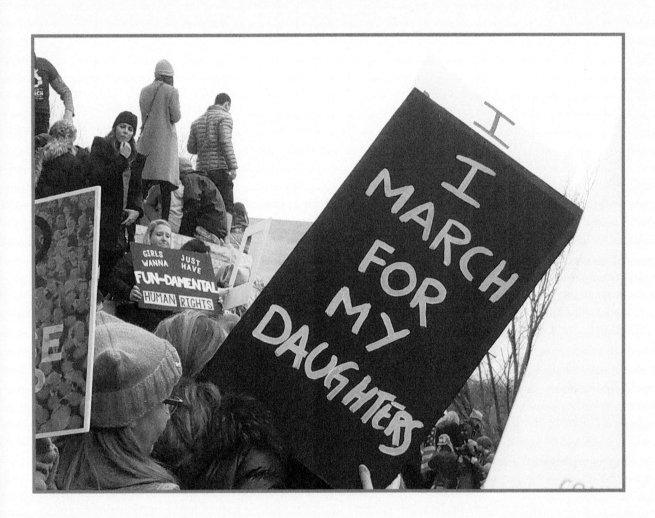

Foundations for Community Health Workers, Third Edition. Edited by Tim Berthold and Darouny Somsanith.
© 2024 John Wiley & Sons, Inc. Published 2024 by John Wiley & Sons, Inc.
Companion website: http://www.wiley.com/go/communityhealthworkers3E

"You didn't see me on television, you didn't see news stories about me. The kind of role that I tried to play was to pick up pieces or put together pieces out of which I hoped organization might come. My theory is, strong people don't need strong leaders."

—Ella Baker (Fraser, 1986).

Introduction

What do you think of when the words "civil rights movement" come to mind? If you're like most people, chances are you imagine Dr. Martin Luther King, Jr. You can probably even hear part of his famous "I Have a Dream" speech. Maybe you envision some moving images—in black-and-white of course—of people gathered in massive numbers, holding signs that read "FREEDOM NOW" or "WE DEMAND VOTING RIGHTS!" or "WE SHALL OVERCOME."

This is only one part of one movement building and community organizing, but for many of us, this is what sticks out in our memories. We've gotten used to hearing inspiring speeches from great leaders, who command the attention of thousands of people gathered together. And the people all look serious in our mind's eye. With their fists in the air, they respond to the speaker's appeal to march—and off they go. That's how the people fight for power. That's how people make change. That's how the movement happens.

But not really.

These inspiring moments are not really how movements are built or sustained. The truth is more complicated. The reality is that social movements and social change mostly happen away from the spotlight. As Mrs. Baker said above, it almost always happens far away from the television cameras.

CHWs are often ideally situated to facilitate community organizing efforts. CHWs are also skilled at connecting community members to information and resources that can assist them in finding solutions to their identified problems or concerns. CHWs honor people's cultural identities, knowledge and skills, and support their autonomy and leadership. Like Mrs. Baker's work, CHW's work is often not recognized by television cameras but is nevertheless important and vital work to bring about change in communities.

- *Can you think of other examples of successful community organizing campaigns and movements in the United States or elsewhere in the world?*

- *Have you or your family and close friends ever participated in community organizing efforts?*

23.1 Overview

Typically, a chapter about community organizing emphasizes the role of individual activists. Often, they will feature an introductory quote famous leaders like Martin Luther King, Jr. or Cesar Chavez or Malcolm X. But have you ever wondered why it's always just a few of the same names and why maybe so many other deserving names from our past seem consigned to forever living in the shadows?

Let's go back to that quote from Ella Baker at the beginning of this chapter. If Ella Baker were alive today, she would probably not mind that she wasn't as famous as some other leaders. While she thought that some of those leaders took too much of the credit for the work being done by countless others, she might tell us that it makes sense that many people don't know her name. After all, what she did in the movement was done behind the scenes, away from the spotlight of the cameras and microphones.

That's because Ella Baker was an organizer. Ella Baker got other people involved. Ella Baker trained people to become fellow organizers. Ella Baker made sure those organizers stayed committed to the goal of creating strong organizations made up of grassroots leaders. Leaders who came from the community, but whose work would likely not land them on the cover of magazines or speaking in front of 250,000 people at a massive march and rally.

Maybe this is a problem of our larger culture. We love a story about an individual hero. Maybe a lawyer or politician who turned down fame and fortune to do the right thing. Those stories sure fill us with hope. But perhaps instead of looking for hope in the latest political superstar, we should take a peek behind the scenes. We just might find the organizers, like CHWs, working with regular, everyday kinds of people, trying to find ways to build power among those who desperately need it.

WHAT YOU WILL LEARN

By studying this information in this chapter, you will be able to:

- Discuss how people in the community come together to make change.

- Define and discuss community organizing.

- Explain the difference between community organizing, advocacy, mobilizing, activism, and direct services.

- Discuss the CHW's roles and responsibilities in the community organizing process, and put them into practice

- Define popular education and understand as an approach to community organizing.

C3 Roles and Skills Addressed in Chapter 23

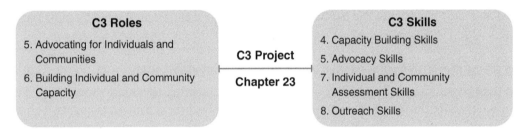

C3 Roles		**C3 Skills**
5. Advocating for Individuals and Communities	**C3 Project**	4. Capacity Building Skills
		5. Advocacy Skills
6. Building Individual and Community Capacity	**Chapter 23**	7. Individual and Community Assessment Skills
		8. Outreach Skills

WORDS TO KNOW

Activism

Community Organizing

Critical Consciousness

Solidarity

23.2 What Is Organizing? What Does an Organizer Do?

Organizing is a process in which regular people get together to address their common problems. The goal is to involve lots of people to take on roles in a strong collective group, also known as an organization. The larger goal is for the organization, made up of the *people most affected by a particular issue*, to become large and strong enough to demand and create change.

Notice the description emphasizes regular, everyday people who are most negatively impacted by social problems. This is also commonly referred to as *grassroots* organizing because the work requires the people to take on leadership responsibilities and to move the agenda. The people at the grassroots. Not the lawyers. Not the politicians. Not even the advocates, which is just a fancy word for those who speak on behalf of others. In organizing, the people speak and act and lead and inspire and sometimes even win—all on their own behalf.

Floribella Redondo-Martinez: Not all CHWs will be tasked with the role of community organizing, but when they are, they have a very special task at hand. The role of CHWs in organizing is to help communities find the gaps and the common problems that impact their health and well-being, and then to support community members to create lasting changes to fill in those gaps.

Organizing is a constantly evolving process which, at its best, "builds a culture of solidarity, community, and a deep sense of belonging *while* sharpening a vision for alternative ways to structure systems and society. It's a dynamic process, largely influenced by cultural practices and traditions of the base" (Calpotura, work in preparation). The "base" is a reference to the members of an organization. In community organizing, the people who get involved are asked to join up and become members. Not just volunteers. Not just occasional activists. But members which means the organization belongs to them in both formal and informal ways.

Community organizing identifies and supports leadership from within the community and increases their capacity and skills to work together and take effective action for social change. In this way, the balance of power and resources shifts toward the community.

Community organizing is a strategy for promoting social justice and health equity and can be used to advocate for a wide variety of issues that impact the health of local communities such as access to safe and affordable housing, food equity or access to affordable and nutritious food, access to health care and mental health service, voting rights and other civil rights, police violence, gun violence, minimum wage and universal income, decriminalization of drug use, and many other issues. Community organizing:

- Mobilizes the community to do for themselves, to advocate on their own behalf.
- It is usually led by "grassroots" leaders, sometimes with the support of professionals like Community Health Workers.
- Helps to build and shift power into the hands of the people who are most impacted by injustices.
- Develops capacity and leadership skills of community members to take effective actions for social change.

ALL ORGANIZERS ARE ACTIVISTS. NOT ALL ACTIVISTS ARE ORGANIZERS

Many of us find time to volunteer, to speak out at a school board meeting, to donate money, or even to attend a rally and march. All of those things make us activists. We get involved from time to time. Maybe we're involved often. But we're often involved as individuals, not as members of a group. And our involvement, though fulfilling and hopefully impactful, is nevertheless not the same as what organizers do.

What makes an organizer different is that they are trying to get others involved. They are trying to bring others from isolation into community. And not just for a moment, or for a rally, or for a donation. They are working to build an organization of the people, from the ground up. They spend lots of time talking with people in the community and asking them to join an organization made up of others like them. They try to build and sustain people's involvement. All the people involved in this kind of effort are activists because they too decided to get off the sidelines and into the fight. But what they are involved with is the work of constantly building something that lasts beyond the rally or the march. That's part of what makes organizing different from activism.

ORGANIZING IS NOT ABOUT SPEAKING ON BEHALF OF OTHERS

Organizing is also different from advocacy in this similar regard: Organizers are concerned with getting other people involved and developing their leadership. Lara Kiswani is the director of a San Francisco grassroots organization called the Arab Resource and Organizing Center (AROC, 2023). While AROC provides some services to the community, especially legal advice, Kiswani cautions against allowing direct services to overwhelm the agenda of an organization devoted to developing the power of regular people who get involved in AROC's work.

One of the programs AROC sponsors is called Arab Youth Organizing (AYO), essentially a committee made up of middle and high school–aged students within the larger organization. AYO's young people learn how to recruit other youth, to identify issues that affect their families and communities, and they grow to understand how to run issue-based campaigns to win more rights and benefits. Recently, AYO pushed an agenda within AROC to have the entire organization conduct a campaign to get the San Francisco Unified School District to include Arabic as one of the district's language pathways for students. The Arabic language campaign was won, and the district currently provides resources in Arabic language courses. Because of this grassroots leadership and the way it was cultivated by AROC's organizing staff, the youth developed not only their own leadership, but an organizing agenda as well. This is an example of how organizing differs from advocacy. The organizers made sure the bases were involved in the work, in a conversation with Lara Kiswani, she said, "we don't speak for others ... we work to help amplify their voices."

THE DIFFERENCE BETWEEN MOBILIZING AND ORGANIZING

During the summer of 2020, there were more rallies and demonstrations than at any other moment in U.S. history. Enraged by the police murder of George Floyd in Minneapolis, people all over the country took to the streets demanding justice—both in Minnesota and in their own communities. It was an extended expression of anger that saw millions of people participated in thousands of protests in hundreds of cities during the weeks that followed. Calls to "Defund the Police!" and "End White Supremacy!" were loud and constant.

Activists put out the call for mass mobilization and so many people who had never before been to a protest suddenly found outlets to make their feelings of righteous fury known. Seeing all those unified people was inspiring beyond words. But it's also fair to conclude that it didn't result in changes to many policies. Calls to defund police departments went unheeded, for the most part. That's because the vast majority of those powerful demonstrations were temporary expressions of discontent. These were protests, not targeted campaigns with specific demands on specific targets.

Where changes did occur was in places where grassroots organizations, the ones made up of members from communities most affected by police racism and violence, stayed on the case well after the demonstrations came to an end. They stayed on the case because they engaged in base building long before the mobilizations and ran *issue-based campaigns* that, in some cases, took years to bear fruit.

23.3 A Story of Grassroots Organizing in Oakland, California

Let's consider the example of the Black Organizing Project (BOP), a 10-year-old organization in Oakland, California, that used that moment of rage to increase their pressure for a campaign to eliminate the official police presence in Oakland public schools (BOP, 2023). For years, the Oakland Unified School District had deployed its own police force. After a neighborhood man named Raheim Brown was shot and killed by one of these officers, there were protests, but local organizers knew they would be insufficient because those in power could just wait them out. The anger and energy would go away at some point. What happened instead was that local organizers decided it was time to build a strong community organization and fight back.

In a conversation, Jackie Byers, a BOP organizer said, "we told his mother that we would work to change the system." Byers said, "we would work not just to get justice for Raheim, but for all sons of mothers who have to cry and wonder what happened to their children."

The Black Organizing Project did not immediately call for a mass mobilization demanding justice. Like Byers, these seasoned organizers knew that the Oakland mayor, city council, and school board could just patiently wait them out. What they needed instead of a rally was an organization. But they also knew that they had to build it slowly and carefully.

BOP organizers decided to meet with as many community members as they could. Invitations went out to people in the community to come to listening sessions to testify about what they wanted to see change in their neighborhoods and in their lives. This was the point Ella Baker insisted upon all those years earlier: Strong people don't need strong leaders. The very best experts and leaders are already in the community. And many of them came forward to explain what they and their families experienced at the grassroots level.

The job of the BOP organizer was to listen and take notes in order to best understand people's issues and interests. The notes recognized those who seemed to have natural leadership skills. The good organizer is always looking to see who is going to step up, and if they would be willing to take on an important role in this new organization.

All of this occurred before any protest. Taking time and energy for mobilization would defeat the purpose of building a genuine organization led by the people themselves. From the beginning, BOP took building its membership seriously. Organizers met with each new prospective member in one-on-one meetings and then vetted them to see if they were a good match with what was fast becoming the organizational culture and mission. BOP did what big rallies and marches can't do: build relationships with everyday people in the community. With members young and old and in between, BOP organizers worked to create something that would last.

Organizing requires thoughtful and careful deliberation. There is almost nothing spontaneous about the work that organizers do. So, when BOP organizers were conducting their listening sessions and taking careful note of what people wanted to do, they considered a range of options before launching what would later be known as the Bettering Our School System (BOSS) campaign. They had to be intentional in this process and, with every step, involve their growing membership in planning and decision-making.

First, they had to identify the issue. That seemed pretty straightforward, given all the testimony at the listening sessions. They also used surveys to gather data about the top problems that needed to be challenged. This is why organizers make a distinction between problems and issues. The problem, in this case, was oppressive and racist policing. But how to turn that big of a problem into an issue the community could campaign against? Maybe it was smart not to broadly take on all of the policing in the East Bay, but the specific issue of OUSD cops in the schools.

Following a tried-and-true methodology in organizing practice, BOP had to consider several dimensions of a possible campaign. According to Rinku Sen's book Stir it Up: Lessons in Community Organizing and Advocacy (Sen, 2003), there are key principles that any good organization should think through:

- Is the campaign issue winnable?
- Does this campaign have a clear target?
- Will this campaign provide an opportunity to build grassroots leadership among the members?
- Is this issue deeply felt among the base?
- Will this campaign give the community a sense of its strength and potential?
- Fundamentally, will it challenge power?

Sen writes, "Campaigns indicate sustained intervention on a specific issue; they have clear short- and long term goals, a timeline, creative incremental demands, targets who can meet those demands, and an organizing plan to build a constituency and build internal capacity" (Sen, 2003, pp. 81).

BOP has engaged in protests for over ten years, but they have always been targeted and strategic, designed to keep pressure on those in power. As an organization in the middle of a campaign, it doesn't always make sense to just do marches and rallies. One key to longevity is that you pay attention to your base. BOP has constantly developed their membership and have made it clear they are in it together for the long haul.

BOP has lasted for over a decade and continues to grow strong. After Raheim Brown was killed, and after months of consulting community members and building an organization, BOP launched a campaign against the Oakland Unified School District. Their demands centered around the dismantling of the OUSD School Police Force. They engaged in occasional protest actions to keep public pressure on city and school district leaders; they showed up to every Board of Education meeting, having their members make public comment, always letting officials know they were from the Black Organizing Project. They recruited allied organizations and other community members to become part of their growing campaign. But mostly, they continued to grow and develop their membership. When the opportunity arose to increase pressure, they did.

In the summer of 2020, amidst national mobilizations and mainstream attention being paid to the issue, BOP turned the volume all the way up. Their demands now took on an added urgency. At Board of Education meeting, they introduced the George Floyd Resolution, which would eliminate the Oakland School Police Department. They put the pressure on by filling the board meetings regularly. And in 2020, BOP won. The George Floyd Resolution was historic, as it marked the first time any school district's internal police department had been dismantled.

This was a "defund the police" effort that made headlines because it actually succeeded. It succeeded because a group made up of real people, conducted a pressure campaign with a serious set of demands. They located the right target for this campaign, and they won.

- *What steps did the Black Organizing Project take to build a successful community organizing campaign?*
- *Can you think of examples of successful community organizing campaigns that took place—or are occurring now—in the communities where you live and work?*

What Do YOU? Think !

CHW Profile

Floribella Redondo-Martinez

CHW/Promotora, Co-founder and CEO, Arizona CHW Association

APHA CHW Section Chair

Co-founder National Association of Community Health Workers

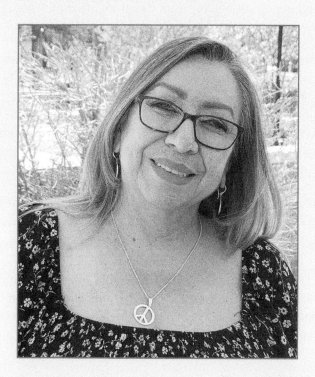

I started as a Promotora more than thirty years ago. The Farmworker Justice Fund, a group from Washington DC, came to Yuma, Arizona to start a promotores project. I was working in the fields and was recruited to be a Promotora de Salud addressing HIV among my peers. I participated in trainings, started to work, and realized I had something of value to offer. I could connect with my community; we spoke the same language- what we call the "campesino" (farmworker) language. I soon realized I was already a Promotora/CHW because when I wasn't working in the field, I was helping people by interpreting, writing letters, and telling them about resources in the community. As an HIV outreach Promotora, I am particularly proud of my work with women because they were the most vulnerable and uninformed about the risks of HIV.

I began talking with other Promotores about why we were so disconnected from other CHWs in our own states. We started planning how to connect with our peers. We established the Arizona CHWs Association (AzCHOW). I got a little funding and started unifying the voices of CHWs, Community Health Representatives and promotores de salud around the state. Through storytelling and shared experiences via focus groups we were able to gather the voices of the workforce. Using this documented voice, we put together recommendations that became the basis for the legislation that created Voluntary CHW Certification in Arizona. It took many years and a lot of sacrifices to get to this point. Now we have a unified CHW workforce that comes together in unity and equity to advocate together in one voice for the Arizona CHWs.

Now, after many years, I direct AzCHOW with a mission to build a strong unified CHW workforce in Arizona. We advocate for policy and systems change in our state as we build capacity by providing training on topics such as chronic conditions, advocacy, equity, SDOH, and mental health. We were the first to respond to the

(continues)

CHW Profile

(continued)

mental health needs of the CHW workforce during COVID-19 pandemic. We started doing webinars in English and Spanish the first week the pandemic was declared. CHWs were on the frontlines and were feeling anxious and stressed. There was a need and we responded to it.

As a CHW, I learned that anything is possible. My work has given me confidence in the knowledge that I have. I can look at a challenge, analyze it from all sides, and find a door for an opportunity to create a response. When I was working with farmworkers and knocking on doors talking with men and women about HIV, it made me a stronger and more confident woman. Being a CHW has allowed me to recognize that I have valued life experience, and my voice has an impact that can help lift other CHWs in the field.

CHWs just starting out probably enter the workforce on a specific project. This is just the door, the first step in your career, but you should never stop at just one step—there's a full ladder in front of you. Learn every single thing that you can. Ask your supervisor for opportunities to connect with other CHWs, and to attend meetings/conferences. Every situation and conversation bring an opportunity to keep growing in your profession. One important thing—don't forget to pause along the way to reflect on who you are; never lose your essence. Remember that it is okay if sometimes we have to regroup and reconnect with our knowledge and compassion, our love for the community, and our passion for service; this is what makes us who we are.

Floribella Redondo-Martinez is a Community Health Worker and a community organizer. She built relationships with other CHWs and Promotores de Salud in Arizona. She gathered CHWs together to voice their concerns and priorities. Flor knew that change would only come about through a unity of purpose and effort among CHWs. She knew early on that successful actions would not happen with just one person demanding for changes, but with many *regular people* who struggled from the same issues demanding change.

ORGANIZING HAS A RICH HISTORY

Saul Alinksy is an influential figure in the history of organizing. As a frustrated social worker, he came to an early realization that people only needed to recognize the potential of their own power. Poor people don't have money, but they have numbers, he reasoned. And if those communities could become organized, they could win almost any demand.

The basic gospel of "Alinskyism" included building power locally through the deliberate and strategic organization of poor people, developing local leadership who would be best equipped to articulate community interests, and, most importantly, being certain that any and all efforts came about "organically out of the needs of local communities" (Fisher, 1994).

During the Great Depression, Alinsky's "Back-of-the-Yards" organization in Chicago focused on organizing poor people through the establishment of what the historian Robert Fisher termed neighborhood "organizations of organizations" that brought together local labor unions, social service groups, neighborhood clubs, and churches.

Alinsky's organizing theory and practice centered around the belief that local, geographically distinct communities could build power bases that could influence the decisions of local governments regarding the distribution of resources.

In the Alinsky model, victories—over slum lords, police departments, unscrupulous neighborhood lenders, and various departments of city hall, etc.—are essential, not only because they help people get what they have demanded, but also because they contribute to the continued building of the organization.

Alinsky's community organizing model "was extended by Fred Ross, who helped develop the Community Service Organization (CSO) in the 1940s to organize Latinos in the southwest. Ross, who recruited and later worked alongside Cesar Chavez in various organizing efforts, is credited with instituting an organizing approach based on issues—which was distinct from the Alinsky model of organizing local institutions—and developing innovative organizing structures." Ross is also remembered for training new organizers with the tactic of the "house meeting" (Fisher, 1994).

Gilbert Padilla, one of the co-founders of the United Farm Workers, emphasizes the importance of the house meeting:

> *These gatherings create comfortable and brave spaces for people to gather and form genuine relationships. This is especially important at the early stages of organizations when maybe we did not have a space of our own. It is also a way of bringing in new members, and members who may have children or other family they take care of. With house meetings you make the meetings personal. One member brings the pan dulce and the other brings champurado. This creates more than just organizers working together, but a sense of community at a personal level. (Padilla, 2017)*

Despite the work of these early community organizing pioneers, it was not until the advent of the political and cultural ferment of the 1950s and 1960s that community organizing emerged as a "full-scale movement."

Organizing has a long tradition. In fact, there are many activities that qualify under the definition of organizing, even if the people engaged in that work so many years ago would not have labeled themselves with that language. The Underground Railroad, which relied on a sophisticated network of people who were trained to play specific roles and develop others to do the same. Or consider the efforts of Filipino and Mexican farm workers to not only engage fellow workers, but their families and communities as well. These and countless other examples existed outside of the influence of Saul Alinsky.

The most well-known example of organizing people comes from the civil rights movement. We began this chapter drawing a contrast between Ella Baker and Dr. King, mainly to emphasize how their approaches to fighting white supremacy differed. In the Ella Baker model, people take leadership at the grassroots. They work in organizations designed to showcase their power. Their voices are the ones that matter most in getting others involved. Ella Baker was a sharp critic of "the traditional paradigm of leadership, that stemmed mostly from the Black church: charismatic masculine leadership based on oratory and exhibitionism" (Wilkson, 2020).

One of the most unsung aspects of the struggle for civil rights is the role of the organizer. News accounts of the tumultuous era highlighted the marches, speeches, and sometimes-violent pitched battles in the streets. Popular historical accounts largely have done the same. Most veterans of American movements, large and small, will be quick to point out that none of those "big moments" could have happened without the grinding, laborious efforts of actual organizers.

- *What is are the histories of organizing in the communities that you belong to or work with?*

- *What issues have these communities sought to influence and change through organizing?*

What Do YOU? Think

ORGANIZING IS ABOUT BUILDING RELATIONSHIPS

One of the many dramatic moments of the early civil rights movement came when young students at some of the Historically Black Colleges and Universities in the South decided to test racial segregation by conducting "sit-ins" at dining establishments. Months into this series of actions, the students decided to gather at a conference to discuss where this emerging energy would go next. Ella Baker, by then a seasoned organizer and trainer, strongly advised the students not to get influenced by the ministers and the lawyers. Instead, she cautioned, stay independent, but if you want to make a lasting impact, devote yourselves not just to student activism, but to organizing at the grassroots, in communities throughout the Deep South, where segregation was all-powerful.

The lesson the student organizers learned was that *strong people don't need strong leaders.* The point was to develop the leadership of regular, everyday kinds of people, not just inspire them with great speeches and big marches. The students named their organization the Student Nonviolent Coordinating Committee (SNCC, pronounced "SNICK"). Out of all the many organizations in the history of the civil rights movement, SNCC was the one most dedicated to the strategy of grassroots organizing.

Mrs. Baker knew that the only way to truly contend for power and have the effort last over time was to build local organizations, made up of leaders who came from those communities. Her influence was felt among the students, and so many others who were attracted to this form of grassroots democracy in action. One of those people was a young teacher from New York, who decided to accept Mrs. Baker's challenge and devote his life to developing other people's potential. His name was Bob Moses, and he became one of the most effective organizers in the entire civil rights movement. Until recently, most people who have studied the movement, didn't really know who he was, since the best organizer remains in the background, recruiting, involving, guiding, developing, and cultivating the leadership of others.

Bob Moses was once asked how you organize a town (Larson, 2021, p. 56):

"By bouncing a ball," he answered quietly.

"What?"

"You stand on a street and bounce a ball. Soon all the children come around. You keep on bouncing the ball. Before long, it runs under someone's porch and then you meet the adults."

The point is that organizing starts with natural conversations. These are key to building lasting relationships. The person you meet on the street, or at their doorstep, or at their workplace might end up being one of the greatest local leaders. But if all that person ever gets is to listen to some big speech, it is not very likely they will get involved or stay involved in the fight for their own liberation.

Historian Charles Payne concluded about what happens when we don't understand the role of organizing in the history of movements: "Overemphasizing the movement's more dramatic features," he wrote, "we undervalue the patient and sustained effort, the slow, respectful work, that made the dramatic moments possible" (Payne, 1995, pp. 183).

A DIFFERENT KIND OF LEADERSHIP

The practice of organizing has evolved over these many decades since SNCC organizers were busy in the Mississippi Delta. But perhaps their greatest legacy is the commitment they made to something organizers call "leadership development." We've already discussed several examples of grassroots leadership, from the youth at Arab Youth Organizing to the community members in the Black Organizing Project to the everyday people who lived in Jim Crow Mississippi but found an organization that allowed them to assert themselves.

This is one of the defining features of grassroots organizing: *you can't claim "people power" if others are always making decisions for the people.* Members of grassroots organizations are the reason they exist. As Rinku Sen (2003) explains in her organizing textbook Stir it Up, the genuine organizer is always planning for the regeneration of leadership. Members are not just seen as props to make the organization look inclusive at a press conference, or on the home page of an organization's website; instead, they are actively developed and ideally transitioned into organizers themselves.

This means that organizing has to be about the business of developing members and recruiting new people. "If we see the same three faces at every event," Sen writes, "then perhaps enough new recruitment is not happening. If an organization has had one executive director for twenty-five years while a string of short-term staff people pass through, perhaps founder's syndrome is preventing the organization from new challenges" (Sen, 2003, pp. 97).

Community organizers have to be honest about the internal dynamics and organizational culture that can sometimes feel exclusive and elitist. Sen writes, "[The traditional approach to identifying grassroots leaders] does not take seriously enough the fact that existing leadership is often based on existing power structures. Certain characteristics are more readily given the stamp of leadership, such as connections to money, maleness, being formally college-educated, having English language skills, etc." (Sen, 2003, pp. 99)

State and national CHW Associations are constantly working to recruit new members and train them to help develop new leadership (see Chapter 2). New members are encouraged to participate in organizing and advocacy efforts to change policies and secure outcomes such as formal recognition of the profession, CHW-determined training standards, hiring of community members with lived experience, opportunities for professional advancement, living wages, and benefits.

ORGANIZING IS INTENTIONAL AND DYNAMIC

What all effective grassroots organizing practices have in common is their reliance on personal relationships with people who are accountable to each other in ways that passing along an online petition or liking something on your social media account can never be. Organizations that are built from the ground up usually last because everyone in the organization—from directors to full-time staff organizers to active leaders in the membership—cares about building people's power. They care about changing the conditions that have too much control over their lives. And they know that only through intentional organizing, can the base expand and a liberatory vision and strategy be put into effect.

It's important to emphasize the word intentional here. None of this happens naturally. Organizations collapse all the time. Members who don't feel connected to the work, stop showing up. Leaders who are ignored in favor of professional staff, get discouraged and stop showing up. There are internal tensions in organizations, just like there are in our families. And organizations that take on the ambitious work of building a multi-generational, multi-racial constituency, understand that this process can be delicate.

Celi Tamayo-Lee, an organizer with the group SF Rising, argues that we can't simply assume natural solidarity among diverse groups of people in multi-racial organizations. "You still have to put in the work to bring communities together around common concerns. Often, that just requires doing some very intentional political education" (Tamayo-Lee, 2022). In this sense, political education is about the process of developing consciousness; in other words, understanding how the world works, our place in it, and the lessons to be learned from past struggles. In this sense, ideology is really just an understanding of our place in the world and our role in shaping it.

Most good organizers recognize the importance of not imposing ideology or some official line, but rather "meeting people where they are." Phillip Agnew, an organizer with Black Men Build, makes the same point while talking about the problem of dismissing people's potential if they don't immediately ascribe to a particular set of ideas. Here's how Agnew describes the approach of his organization: "Come as you are, grow as you go. That's not cancel culture, that's movement culture." (Yamhatta-Taylor, 2021).

In her review of Black Lives Matter co-founder Alicia Garza's book, Keeanga Yamahtta-Taylor quotes the longtime Bay Area organizer:

> We can't be afraid to establish a base that is larger than the people we feel comfortable with. Movements and bases cannot be cliques of people who already know each other. We have to reach beyond the choir and take seriously the task of organizing the unorganized—the people who don't already speak the same language, the people who don't eat, sleep and breathe social justice, the people who have everything at stake and are looking to be less isolated." Widely co-credited with coining the generational movement phrase Black Lives Matter, Garza nevertheless concludes that, "Hashtags don't build movements. people do. (Yamhatta-Taylor, 2021)

ORGANIZING WILL NOT WAIT FOR INDIVIDUAL SAVIORS

Longtime organizer and teacher Marshall Ganz (2018) explained what he thought was most important to understand about what makes organizing different from other approaches to social change:

> This is what the craft of organizing is all about: Organizers recruit, train, and develop leadership; build a constituency with that leadership; and enable this constituency to turn its own resources—time, energy, imagination, money—into the power it needs to effectively pursue its goals. The test of effective leadership, in turn, is not in how many hats one can wear but in how many others one can get to wear hats. This is how you get to scale. (Ganz, 2018)

The "scale" that Ganz references is not just one organizational base, but a collection of them. That is how you get to be a movement. But it doesn't begin with a march. It begins with the intentional process of building an organization, from the grassroots. Alinksy was known to say, "Look, you don't have to put up with all this shit. But to accomplish anything you've got to have power and you'll only get it through organization." Fifty years later, in her interview with Yahmatta-Taylor, Black Lives Matter founder Garza echoes the same theme: "What we should learn from the latest iteration of the movement is that we need more organization, not less, and that we need clearer points of entry into such organizations for those who wish to do more than just demonstrate" (Yamhatta-Taylor, 2021).

We began this chapter with Ella Baker's critique of how we view social movements. Instead of always emphasizing the charismatic speaker who inspires all those people at a mass demonstration, we would be smart to understand movement building through the practice of organizing one person at a time.

Historian Robin D.G. Kelley (2013) makes this point in his critique of the famous 1963 March on Washington:

> I simply want to suggest that we stay mindful of the lessons of 1963. Big glitzy marches do not make a movement; the organizations and activists who came to Washington, D. C., will continue to do their work, fight their fights, and make connections between disparate struggles, no matter what happens in the limelight. The moral and political arc of movements for social justice is also very, very long. And this is why it is important to think beyond the march, "the speech," the spectacle. To understand August 28, 1963 is to understand the entire era. It requires following those movements that fall outside the spotlight, the movements organized and led by the very women who were excluded from the mic on that incredibly hot and humid Washington afternoon. The work of social movements is not always sexy, nor is it necessarily inspiring. But they are the engines for change and the incubators of new dreams. (Kelley, 2013)

23.4 Health Is Always Political

Health is a political issue since it impacts all factors of life and community, including where people live, learn, play, and work. Public health and the well-being of communities is impacted by the political systems, local and national governments, and even international governments. Promoting health and well-being includes engaging with the state and local political systems in some way. Organizing and advocating for better health conditions could include engaging in various political debates and struggles, including but limited to funding, land use, health care access, and environmental justice. It may include community members engaging different bodies of government including school boards and city councils. As CHWs, your role is to support community members to engage in the political processes and ensure their concerns are heard.

Jason Gee: Prioritizing the well-being of communities should be a top priority for all governing bodies. If systems shifted their focus to invest in people, we'd have a healthier, happier population who would be less likely to develop diseases and illnesses, less likely to participate in violence, crime, and other anti-social behaviors. Governing bodies and systems should be responsible for its population's health, and if they are not, then we need to organize and demand that they are.

We all want to live in healthy communities. Yet many communities lack access to the basic resources necessary for health such as clean water and air, safety, housing, food, education, employment, health care, and civil rights. They face a wide range of other public health problems such as high rates of infant mortality, heart disease, HIV/AIDS, drug use, incarceration, police brutality, or homelessness. They may live close to an oil refinery or waste incinerator. These health inequities are almost always tied back to historical and/or contemporary political forces making decisions that did not center on the well-being of these communities. It is because they face these challenges that communities come together and organize for social change. They want a better life for themselves and their children.

INSTITUTIONAL POWER VERSUS PEOPLE POWER

There are two types of power that function in our society. One is institutional power, and this power is usually held by institutions like the media, corporations, and governments. This type of power is usually held by a smaller quantity of people who make decisions that impact a much wider amount of people. The other type of power is *people power* or *power of the people*. This type of power is exercised when a larger number of people come together, organize themselves, and demand changes. One goal of community organizing is to exercise people power and usually against institutional power.

Unions are a good example of people power: Think about a corporation and unions; there's a CEO who holds institutional power, who oversees all the decisions of the corporation including wages, working conditions, and benefits. The CEO is usually one person, but the corporation usually includes a larger number of workers. When workers are unionized, and exercise their people power, they can demand changes to working conditions. They can demand higher wages, better working conditions, and better benefits. If their demands are not met, they can practice their power by going on strike until their demands are met.

23.5 Organizing for Health and Social Justice

The health inequities that exist in marginalized communities can be changed. Community Health Workers can play a significant role in organizing for changes that promote social justice and health equity. This begins by honoring the resources, wisdom, skills, and leadership present in all communities.

> **Floribella Redondo-Martinez:** CHWs' role in organizing efforts should include bringing as many people as possible to the table and helping create **one** powerful voice of many impacted by health inequities, a voice that is heard far and wide.

Community organizing is vital for the struggle for health equity and social justice. It is one of the most effective strategies for creating lasting social changes that will improve the lives and health status of large groups of people. For example, community organizing efforts significantly expanded the rights of disabled people for access to basic resources such as transportation, education, housing, and employment. In the first decades of the AIDS epidemic, community organizing by groups like ACT UP and the AIDS Treatment Action Group significantly expanded the rights of people living with HIV disease and their access to medical treatments and other basic resources. Community organizing captures the attention of the media and the public and puts pressure on policy makers to do something about such diverse concerns as accountable policing, environmental health, reproductive justice, and international trade agreements.

- *What changes are needed to promote the health of the communities you belong to and work with?*

23.6 Popular Education

One way to engage in community organizing is by using a popular education approach. Popular education (also addressed in Chapter 20) was introduced by Paulo Freire as an approach to engage marginalized communities to take action to change the inequities of their lives. Popular education means that everyone, including CHWs, is engaged in learning from one another. This process begins with acknowledging everyone's experience as valuable information and building upon those experiences to identify needs and create change. The role of the CHW is to facilitate a space where community members' experiences and voices are heard and centered in the conversations.

CRITICAL CONSCIOUSNESS

The goal of popular education is to develop critical consciousness or what Freire refers to as "conscientization." Critical consciousness is a tool for community members to understand the world around them, and to be able to use their knowledge, experience, and power to create change in their communities. This process helps community members to analyze the social injustices around them and realize their own power to create change. Freire defines critical consciousness in three steps (Freire, 1970):

Critical reflection: This step helps community members to reflect and question the social injustices they see in their communities. This step engages community members to develop an analysis of the issues in their communities. This step could include studying data and understanding the collective issues their communities face.

Critical motivation: This step involves dialogue among community members and creating relationships and commitment to making changes. This step could include regular meetings and creating relationships.

Critical action: This step includes developing a plan and taking action to create the change they want to see in their communities.

EMPOWERMENT

A goal of popular education and critical consciousness is to empower community members to lead efforts for social change. This is a strength-based approach that focuses not only on what communities lack and need, but also on the resources they already have. By developing connections within and among communities, these approaches often emphasize self-help and collaboration.

Empowerment is an essential component of community organizing (Wallerstein, 2006). Empowerment comes about through the broad participation of people, organizations, and communities, overcoming barriers to increase access to vital resources through engaging with and influencing political structures. Empowerment is achieved through the development of critical consciousness and confidence among community members, as well as through concrete actions that increase community control and improve community conditions.

POLICY DEVELOPMENT

Within the field of public health, community organizing often takes a more collaborative focus to build bridges among allies and to persuade policy makers. In order to establish new policies that promote health, we need to learn how to influence the decisions of policy makers. A policy is a principle or protocol that guides actions and decisions, often by establishing incentives or penalties. Policies include state and Federal laws (legislation), regulations that explain how these laws or decisions are to be carried out; local ordinances (municipal decisions); codes of ethics such as those created by professional organizations; and institutional rules and practices. An example of a national policy is the 2010 Affordable Care Act that requires every U.S. citizen (with some exceptions) to have health insurance. The law details who must have insurance and how insurance will be made available, among other things.

Policies are made by the U.S. Congress, state legislatures, municipal governments (city, town, village, or borough), school boards, Tribal governments, professional associations, and other organizations and institutions. We refer to them as policy makers or decision makers because they set the rules and policies that influence our health. As CHWs involved in organizing or advocacy, your job is to help ensure that the voices of the community are heard and their concerns resolved through policy changes.

Community organizing and efforts to change or introduce new policies are often reliant on building **solidarity** or collaborative alliances with other communities and organizations with common interests or goals.

As highlighted in her CHW Profile, Floribella Redondo-Martinez brought CHWs and Promotores de Salud together to organize their profession in Arizona. They crossed the state to build a network of CHWs, to listen to their experiences and needs, and to develop a unified proposal for legislation that would finally recognize their profession and its contributions to promoting health and social justice in Arizona.

- *Have you participated in efforts to change policies in your city, county, or state? What did you learn about the process of working with others to change policies?*

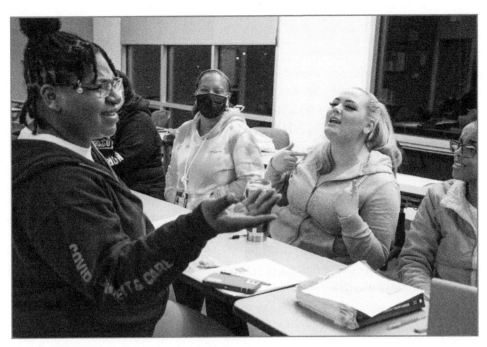

A community discussion about priority concerns.

GRASSROOTS RESEARCH

As illustrated above, the Black Organizing Project's months of "listening sessions" and careful use of surveys and one-on-one conversations helped not only shape their membership but also define their campaign. An effective campaign comes from deep conversations with community members and careful planning. It also relies on effective research, often conducted by and otherwise involving the very people for whom the campaign is built.

Jessie Fernandez, an organizer with the San Francisco-based group PODER, explained the importance of how training members in research—often through the use of surveys—can help define which issues the organization will tackle. "If we involve the community in researching issues and designing the solutions, we are more likely to be able to sustain longer and more ambitious struggles." (Fernandez, 2022).

A good survey offers many benefits to a grassroots organizer. For one, it can form the rationale to start a conversation. And if a person engages in that conversation, the organizer can collect information about their interests and desires, but also they can acquire contact information which can be used to follow up with that person. The organizer isn't out in the community to make speeches or to provide services; the organizer wants to develop relationships. Surveys can establish data to be used in a future campaign, but they can also help in the building of the membership base.

For more information about surveys and other resources for gathering information with and about communities, see Chapter 22 on Research and Evaluation.

23.7 Education Equity Campaign Case Study

Coleman Advocates for Children and Youth is a San Francisco community-based organization that has led many campaigns to improve the lives of Families of Color in the City (Coleman Advocates, 2023). Over 50 years old, the organization has been involved in various community organizing campaigns including struggles for affordable housing, living wage jobs, and education equity. One of their most successful and student-led efforts was the A-G campaign, which helped more students of color gain access to college preparatory courses. As a result of this campaign, a policy in San Francisco was passed making A-G coursework the curriculum for all and the high school requirement for graduation.

Before this policy was passed, students were graduating high school without the proper A-G courses to apply and be admitted to public four-year universities, such as the University of California (UC) and California State Universities (CSU). A-G coursework is the minimum admissions requirement for public universities like the UC and CSUs. At the time of this campaign, Coleman's organizing model included paid youth organizers who were placed at three San Francisco high schools. These high schools had some of the highest enrollment of students of color and were part of the base they were building. The organizers were building relationships with students, school staff, and faculty. They meet with students weekly to discuss concerns and issues they were facing in their schools that impeded their success.

While working with students on college applications, a Coleman organizer realized that a senior student did not have the proper courses to apply for any CSU or UCs. This began a conversation between other Coleman organizers and after speaking to more students, they found this was a common problem. Having access to public universities is important for historically marginalized communities for many different reasons including that public universities are more affordable than private ones. Also, research has indicated that people who obtain a college degree are more likely to live longer and healthier lives. Obtaining a college degree can lead to lower rates of unemployment, higher wages, and more social mobility. This fit into Coleman's overall work around supporting families of color and jumped on the chance to make change around this issue.

The steps below were taken to win the A-G campaign:

STEP 1: IDENTIFY A PROBLEM

Work with the community by fostering conversations and asking questions to find common problems that can be changed.

Coleman leaders realized after meeting and building with students, that many of them were interested in applying and attending four-year public colleges, like UCs and CSUs, but were not on track to graduate with the appropriate A-G classes to apply and be admitted to those universities. Coleman organizers soon learned that the San Francisco high school graduation requirements did not align with A-G coursework. In other words, students were graduating high school without the appropriate completed courses to apply and be admitted to UC and CSUs.

STEP 2: RESEARCH THE PROBLEM

Data helps in determining and pinpointing the problem.

Coleman leaders began a data-collection process soon after they witnessed a number of students with the same problem. They collected data on graduation rates of students of color and their A-G completion rates. They found a large number of students of color were graduating without the A-G requirements. They also collected first-hand stories from students and their families.

STEP 3: EDUCATE ABOUT THE PROBLEM

Educate as many as possible about the issue, especially those who are most impacted.

After they collected the data, Coleman leaders began meeting with families, students, and community leaders to inform them of their findings. They also met with teachers, staff, and other administrators and educational leaders to ask questions about this problem. Their goal was to inform those who may have not known about this program and to build momentum around it. They found that many did not know this problem even existed.

STEP 4: BUILD A BASE

We are more powerful when we are working with a large number of people.

As part of the education process, they also started building a broader base around the problem. They collected signatures and contact information of those who were impacted by the problem and interested in making a difference. They held regular meetings at school sites and in the community. They developed presentations and handouts about the issues.

STEP 5: CREATE CLEAR DEMANDS

Develop clear asks of change-makers and those in power.

After conducting research and educating others, Coleman leaders held listening sessions about what changes needed to be made. They explored different options to resolve the problem, including hiring more high school counselors, hiring more teachers, and making classes more available. However, they realized to make the most impact, they wanted to push for a policy change that would impact as many students of color as possible. Members of Coleman decided they wanted to change the entire process of the high school graduation requirements and make A–G as part of those requirements.

STEP 6: POWER MAP

Identify who has the power to make the changes.

Once they had their base in place, and decided the change they wanted to make, Coleman conducted a power map. They begin by drawing out who has the power to make the possible changes. They assessed all elected bodies, including the Mayor and the City Council. After power mapping, they learned the elected School Board had the power to pass and implement the policy. They also identified other organizations to work with including the teacher unions, leaders from local universities, and other student organizations.

They used the power mapping process to identify at least one elected school member who can support and stand behind the campaign. They met with this school board member, and she agreed to support the policy. She introduced the policy proposal to the rest of the school board when the campaign launched.

STEP 7: DEVELOP EFFECTIVE COMMUNICATION

Create language and slogans that everyone can understand and most people would support.

"College for All" was the slogan for this campaign. The slogan is easy to understand, and a large number of people can support it. They made t-shirts and buttons that were worn by students, their families, and other supporters. They made posters to hang in various places including the windows of homes of Coleman families. This helped gain attention to the campaign and garner more supporters.

STEP 8: LAUNCH THE CAMPAIGN

Go public with your campaign.

While there are different ways to launch your campaign, Coleman held a press conference in front of the school board building as the first part of launching their campaign. They invited students, media, community members, and educational leaders. This press conference gained attention in the local media. They also held teach-ins at school sites and community centers. They sent out mailers, e-mails, and used social media. They also called and texted families in their bases to update them regularly on the campaign and inform them of the next steps.

STEP 9: ENACT TACTICS

Enact the activity and action that will get you closer to your campaign goal.

The first tactic was for Coleman leaders and members to meet one-on-one with school board members. These meetings included students and families. They shared their own experiences with the school systems and their hopes and desires to attend college. They also shared the data they collected and introduced the proposal policy. The goal was to assess whether they had the support of the school board members.

The second tactic was to bring the base to the school board meetings and to provide public testimony about the problem. They wore their t-shirts and packed the board meetings.

Surprisingly, Coleman leaders and members were met with opposition. They were met with resistance from leaders who did not want to change the status quo. The opposition were claiming the policy will shift the high school curriculum too much and that they lacked the capacity to do so.

As result, Coleman leaders and members escalated their action and their third tactic was to protest in front of the school building. They held peaceful protests in front of the building each time before the board meetings for close to six months. They wanted disrupt business as usual to ensure their voices were amplified.

After a year of working on the campaign, the school board voted on the new policy, and it was passed.

STEP 10: IMPLEMENTATION

Follow up to be sure the policy is enacted.

Many times campaigns are won and promises are made, but the changes are not implemented or not fully implemented. As part of this campaign, Coleman asked to be part of the implementation team. They received regular updates and attended meetings on the district level to ensure implementation. After a year of the launch of the campaign, the policy was fully implemented at the district level and the requirements for graduation changed.

Each step of this campaign was important for its success. In every process of the campaign, community members were involved. They had input in every step of the way.

- *How may the success of Coleman Advocates' A-G campaign improve the lives of students of color and their families?*

23.8 The Role of CHWs

Community Health Workers have knowledge, skills, and values to support community organizing including:

- A commitment to social justice
- The ability to develop and maintain trusting relationships with diverse clients and communities
- Cultural humility
- The ability to listen to the concerns, experiences, and ideas of others with compassion and without judgment
- Information about resources that may be beneficial to the community
- Strong communication skills
- Group facilitation and teamwork skills
- Respect for the experience, wisdom, and skills of others
- Flexibility and the ability to adapt to changing circumstances
- A person- and community-centered approach to their work and a commitment to supporting the self-determination of individuals and communities

The same concepts and skills that you apply when working with individual clients can be applied to community organizing efforts. For example, CHWs apply person-centered concepts and skills to support the autonomy or independence of individual clients. You demonstrate cultural humility and recognize that clients are the only true experts regarding their own experience, knowledge, and health goals. You use a strength-based approach to focus on the resources that clients can draw upon as they work to promote their own health. These same skills can be applied to community-centered practice. Demonstrate cultural humility. Learn about and validate the strengths that reside in all communities—resources, leadership, wisdom, skills, and accomplishments. Work in a way that shifts power away from yourself to support the autonomy and leadership of community members. Just as any action plan to promote individual health should come from the individual themselves, the vision for social change must come from the community itself.

- *What other CHW knowledge and skills can be applied to community organizing efforts?*

> **Abdul Hafeedh Bin Abdullah:** There is power in the community. As CHWs, we build real relationships with the people we serve on a day-to-day basis. We are willing to advocate, and to serve and provide basic needs. We create space for healing and connection. This is all part of the process as a sustainable strategy for better health outcomes for all. All of this is part of a CHW's identity and profession. And, through organizing, we are able to leverage more impact and our impact is more sustained for health equity.

Community organizing may take place with or without the participation of a CHW, and the CHW may or may not belong to the community in question. Regardless of whether you are a member of the community, we hope you keep the following suggestions in mind. When participating in community organizing efforts, **we hope that CHWs** *will not*:

- **Assume that they know or understand the problems that most affect the community**: Only by listening to the community can you come to understand these problems.

- **Be the leader**: The role of the CHW is to facilitate the leadership of others rather than to assume it themselves.

- **Decide who participates**: All members of the affected community should be invited to take a place at the table and to contribute their knowledge and skills to the community organizing effort.

- **Prioritize tasks and activities or make key decisions**: The community must decide which issues or problems to work on and what actions they will take.

- **Do all the work**: Remember that your role is to assist people in acquiring new skills so that they can take ownership of their own community organizing efforts.

WE HOPE THAT CHWS *WILL*

- **Listen to the community**: Your most important job is to listen deeply to the concerns, ideas, aspirations, fears, and accomplishments of the community. You can facilitate this by creating opportunities for people to meet together and by asking simple open-ended questions that encourage people to speak up and share their knowledge. Use your motivational interviewing skills!

- **Learn local history**: Take time to learn about the history of the community, including past community organizing efforts and accomplishments, and any previous attempts to address the same problem or concern.

- **Recruit and honor the participation of diverse members of the community**: Drawing upon your existing connections in the community, reach out and invite all members to participate.

- **Provide training to community members**: You may have a role to play in supporting community members in enhancing their skills in areas such as the social determinants of health, group facilitation, planning, using surveys, or conducting a focus group. As always, you need to take direction from the community about which areas, if any, they would like to learn more about. You may provide the training yourself or identify others who can facilitate workshops for the community.

- **Mentor key people**: Often CHWs play a key role in mentoring community participants and leaders, assisting them to learn new skills and to gain confidence in their own ability to contribute to and to lead a community organizing effort.

- **Assist in the critical thinking process**: CHWs often support the development of critical consciousness by facilitating meetings and posing open-ended questions designed to provide community members with an opportunity to "speak their word" and arrive at a deeper understanding of the problems they face. As people begin to gain a common understanding of the problems affecting their communities, they will come up with possible actions and strategies to address these problems.

- **Assist the community to build on their strengths**: By supporting community members in conducting a community diagnosis, you can help them identify existing resources (experience, knowledge, skills, institutions, and leaders).

- **Support communities in shaping strategy**: By facilitating meeting and discussions (or teaching others to do this), you can help communities identify the policies they want to change and the decision makers or policy makers they want to reach. By sharing information and facilitating discussion of strategies and tactics, you can help communities find creative ways to win support for their proposals.

- **Facilitate the implementation process**: Once an action plan has been developed, CHWs can help the community to implement it. Again, you may facilitate group discussions or mentor others to facilitate this process. The community will have a lot of decisions to make: What activities will we undertake? Who will do which activities? How much money do we need? How will we raise these funds? Whom do we need to reach to participate in our efforts? What potential allies do we need to talk with? What additional training and resources do we need?

  - *What else can CHWs do to support community organizing efforts?*

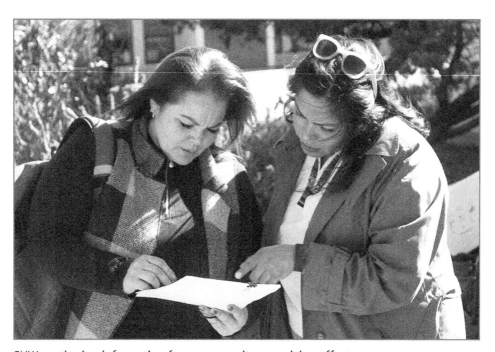

CHWs gathering information for a community organizing effort.

A CHECKLIST FOR CHWS ENGAGED IN COMMUNITY ORGANIZING

We have adapted the following checklist from a number of sources (Blackwell & Colmenar, 2012; Community Toolbox, 2023; Sen, 2003). As you participate in or develop community organizing and advocacy campaigns, use this checklist to reflect on how your efforts might be made more community-centered and effective.

PROMISING PRACTICE	WHAT DOES IT LOOK LIKE?	FILL IN HERE: HOW CAN YOU USE THIS PRACTICE?
Plan with people, not for them	• Listen to community members. • Involve them from the start • Ask questions and let ideas emerge	

(continues)

(continued)

PROMISING PRACTICE	WHAT DOES IT LOOK LIKE?	FILL IN HERE: HOW CAN YOU USE THIS PRACTICE?
Clarify the focus of your project and its goals	• Facilitate the identification of a clear purpose or goal for the campaign or program • State it concisely in a few sentences • Use plain language and ensure everyone is on board	
Assess strengths as well as needs	• Identify and celebrate community strengths • Listen for community issues or concerns • Find ways to use the strengths in addressing the needs	
Build local capacity for problem-solving	• Develop leaders through capacity building and developing knowledge and skills together • Foster connections between the community and local institutions, agencies, and government	
Deal explicitly with health inequities and discriminatory social conditions such as those associated with race, ethnicity, gender, etc.	• Recognize that community issues often have different impacts on different groups • Develop policies and proposals that consider the needs of various populations in the community	
Ensure language access	• Work with interpreters and translators as needed • Partner with bilingual and bicultural (or multilingual and multicultural) CHWs and community residents	
Connect the community to relevant resources and expertise	• Share contact information • Help form bridges between the community and other resources	
Build partnerships	• Identify other communities and organizations to partner with • Develop both short-term coalitions and long-term collaborations • Foster the sharing of information and resources	
Develop strategies and an action plan	• Select an overall action or goal that is attainable and significant • Analyze the policy makers who can act on that goal, their interests or influences • Develop activities or tactics to urge policy makers to take the desired action	
Use the media	• Use social media to develop and mobilize networks • Arrange for a media advocacy training	
Build in mechanisms for accountability to the community	• Feedback loops that link community and policy makers • Include community standards and measures of success in the long-term monitoring of the policy implementation	

(continues)

(continued)

PROMISING PRACTICE	WHAT DOES IT LOOK LIKE?	FILL IN HERE: HOW CAN YOU USE THIS PRACTICE?
Stay grounded in the community	• Regularly reach out to new community members to listen to their concerns	
Strengthen commitment—in yourself and in others	• Recognize that making change often takes time • Speak to the deeper motivations for action • Find fun and creative approaches that energize	
Take care of yourself as you take care of others	• Celebrate victories, large and small • Build in self-care to prevent burnout over time	

Chapter Review

To review your understanding of community organizing concepts, please do your best to answer the following questions:

- How would you define or explain community organizing to a new CHW colleague?
- What did Ella Baker mean when she said: "Strong people don't need strong leaders?"
- Why is the leadership of community members essential for effective community organizing?
- What steps led to the success of the Black Organizing Project in Oakland, California? What did they achieve, and how?
- What was the community that Floribella Redondo-Martinez helped to organize? What types of changes did they create?
- What types of policy changes do Community Health Workers and Promotores de Salud want to achieve in the state where you live and work?
- What roles might a CHW play in community organizing efforts? What types of actions or roles are not recommended for CHWs?
- Which core CHW concepts and skills can be applied to support community organizing efforts?
- How might you use principles of popular education? Specifically, what would you do?

What steps lead to the success of the A–G campaign? What steps stood out for you most?

References

The Arab Resource and Organizing Center. (2023). https://aroc.herokuapp.com/ (accessed 16 March 2023).

The Black Organizing Project. (2023). https://blackorganizingproject.org/ (accessed 16 March 2023).

Blackwell, A. G. & Colmenar, R. A. (2012). Principles of community organizing. In: M. Minkler (Ed.), *Community organizing and community building for health and welfare* (p. 423). New Brunswick, N.J.: Rutgers University Press.

Coleman Advocates. (2023). https://colemanadvocates.org/ (accessed 26 April 2023).

Community Tool Box. (2023). Chapter 1: Our Model for Community Change and Improvement. https://ctb.ku.edu/en/table-of-contents/overview/model-for-community-change-and-improvement (accessed 27 April 2023).

Fernandez, J. (2022). Guest Lecturer in Grassroots Organizing in Communities of Color. San Francisco State University. February 18, 2002.

Fisher, R. (1994). *Let the people decide: Neighborhood organizing in America*. New York: Twayne.

Fraser, C. Gerald. (1986) Ella Baker, Organizer for Groups in Civil Rights Movement in the South. *New York Times*. December 17, 1986.

Freire, P. (1970). *Pedagogy of the oppressed*. New York: Continuum.

Ganz, M. (2018). How to Organize to Win. *The Nation*. March 16.

Kelley, R. D. G. (2013). Big, Glitzy Marches are not Movements. *Boston Review*. August 28.

Larson, K. C. (2021). *Walk with me: a biography of Fannie Lou Hamer*. New York, N.Y: Oxford University Press.

Padilla, G. (2017). Guest Lecture: Grassroots Organizing in Communities of Color. San Francisco State University. April 25, 2017.

Payne, C. (1995). *I've got the light of freedom: The organizing tradition and the Mississippi freedom struggle*. University of California Press.

Sen, R. (2003). *Stir it up. Lessons of community organizing and advocacy*. Jossey-Bass.

Tamayo-Lee, C. (2022). Guest Lecture: Grassroots Organizing in Communities of Color. San Francisco State University. March 10, 2022.

Wallerstein, N. (2006). What is the Evidence on Effectiveness of Empowerment to Improve Health? Copenhagen, Denmark: WHO Regional Office for Europe. Retrieved from http://www.euro.who.int/Document/E88086.pdf.

Wilkinson, A. (2020). Biden Called Ella Baker a Giant of the Civil Rights Movement. Her Life Was Extraordinary. *Vox*. August 21.

Yamahtta-Taylor, K. (2021) A Black Lives Matter Founder on Building Modern Movements. *The New Yorker*. January 18.

Additional Resources

Mann, E. (2011). *Playbook for progressives: 16 qualities of the successful organizer*. Boston: Beacon Press.

Moberg, D. (1999) Alinsky for the Ages. Chicago

Wallerstein, N. (1992). Powerlessness, empowerment, and health: Implications for health promotion programs. *American Journal of Health Promotion*, 6, 197–205.

Walter, C. L. & Hyde, C. A. (2012). Community building practice: An expanded conceptual framework. In M. Minkler (Ed.), *Community organizing and community building for health and welfare* (3rd ed., pp. 78–90). New Brunswick, NJ: Rutgers.

C3 Project CHW Roles and Competencies Review Checklist

Use the following checklists to assess how CHW's role and skills linked to CHW trainings, practices, and/or policies align with the Community Health Worker Core Consensus Project.

ROLES

Table C3.1 Community Health Worker Roles/Scope of Practice

☐ Checklist for personal, programmatic, and policy review	**Community Health Worker Core Consensus Project** Roles/Scope of Practice
Role: Functions that CHWs serve in communities and the health care system. For example, CHWs provide health education.	
Scope of Practice: An all-inclusive list of roles and tasks which an occupation includes in its scope of work. The exact mix of these roles and tasks for any one individual will vary based on the needs of those served and host organizations.	

ROLE	SUB-ROLES
☐ 1. **Cultural Mediation Among Individuals, Communities, and Health and Social Service Systems**	a. Educating individuals and communities about how to use health and social service systems (including understanding how systems operate) b. Educating systems about community perspectives and cultural norms (including supporting implementation of Culturally and Linguistically Appropriate Services [CLAS] standards) c. Building health literacy and cross-cultural communication
☐ 2. **Providing Culturally Appropriate Health Education and Information**	a. Conducting health promotion and disease prevention education in a manner that matches linguistic and cultural needs of participants or community b. Providing necessary information to understand and prevent diseases and to help people manage health conditions (including chronic disease)

(continues)

Foundations for Community Health Workers, Third Edition. Edited by Tim Berthold and Darouny Somsanith.
© 2024 John Wiley & Sons, Inc. Published 2024 by John Wiley & Sons, Inc.
Companion website: http://www.wiley.com/go/communityhealthworkers3E

☐ 3. **Care Coordination, Case Management, and System Navigation**	a. Participating in care coordination and/or case management b. Making referrals and providing follow-up c. Facilitating transportation to services and helping address barriers to services d. Documenting and tracking individual and population-level data e. Informing people and systems about community assets and challenges
☐ 4. **Providing Coaching and Social Support**	a. Providing individual support and coaching b. Motivating and encouraging people to obtain care and other services c. Supporting self-management of disease prevention and management of health conditions (including chronic disease) d. Planning and/or leading support groups
☐ 5. **Advocating for Individuals and Communities**	a. Advocating for the needs and perspectives of communities b. Connecting to resources and advocating for basic needs (e.g., food and housing) c. Conducting policy advocacy
☐ 6. **Building Individual and Community Capacity**	a. Building individual capacity b. Building community capacity c. Training and building individual capacity with peers and among CHW groups
☐ 7. **Providing Direct Service**	a. Providing basic screening tests (e.g., height, weight, and blood pressure) b. Providing basic services (e.g., first aid and diabetic foot checks) c. Meeting basic needs (e.g., direct provision of food and other resources)
☐ 8. **Implementing Individual and Community Assessments***	a. Participating in design, implementation, and interpretation of individual-level assessments (e.g., home environmental assessment) b. Participating in design, implementation, and interpretation of community-level assessments (e.g., windshield survey of community assets and challenges, and community asset mapping)
☐ 9. **Conducting Outreach***	a. Case-finding/recruitment of individuals, families, and community groups to services and systems b. Follow-up on health and social service encounters with individuals, families, and community groups c. Home visiting to provide education, assessment, and social support d. Presenting at local agencies and community events

(continues)

Table C3.1 *(continued)*

☐ 10. **Participating in Evaluation and Research***	a. Engaging in evaluating CHW services and programs
	b. Identifying and engaging community members as research partners, including community consent processes
	c. Participating in evaluation and research:
	   i. Identification of priority issues and evaluation/ research questions
	   ii. Development of evaluation/research design and methods
	   iii. Data collection and interpretation
	   iv. Sharing results and findings
	   v. Engaging stakeholders to take action on findings

C3 Project, 2018|www.C3Project.org	

* *Asterisks denote new roles from 1998 to 2016; several subroles have been expanded.*

Table C3.2 Community Health Worker Competencies: Skills

☐ Checklist for personal, programmatic, and policy review	**Community Health Worker Core Consensus Project** Skills
Skill: The ability, coming from one's knowledge, practice, and aptitude, to do something well. A core role or a task that must be performed may be supported by multiple skills.	
SKILLS	**SUB–SKILL/DESCRIPTION**
☐ 1. **Communication Skills**	a. Ability to use language confidently b. Ability to use language in ways that engage and motivate c. Ability to communicate using plain and clear language d. Ability to communicate with empathy e. Ability to listen actively f. Ability to prepare written communication including electronic communication (e.g., email, telecommunication device for the deaf) g. Ability to document work h. Ability to communicate with the community served (may not be fluent in language of all communities served)
☐ 2. **Interpersonal and Relationship-Building Skills**	a. Ability to provide coaching and social support b. Ability to conduct self-management coaching c. Ability to use interviewing techniques (e.g., motivational interviewing) d. Ability to work as a team member e. Ability to manage conflict f. Ability to practice cultural humility

(continues)

☐ 3. **Service Coordination and Navigation Skills**	a. Ability to coordinate care (including identifying and accessing resources and overcoming barriers) b. Ability to make appropriate referrals c. Ability to facilitate development of an individual and/or group action plan and goal attainment d. Ability to coordinate CHW activities with clinical and other community services e. Ability to follow-up and track care and referral outcomes
☐ 4. **Capacity Building Skills**	a. Ability to help others identify goals and develop to their fullest potential b. Ability to work in ways that increase individual and community empowerment c. Ability to network, build community connections, and build coalitions d. Ability to teach self-advocacy skills e. Ability to conduct community organizing
☐ 5. **Advocacy Skills**	a. Ability to contribute to policy development b. Ability to advocate for policy change c. Ability to speak up for individuals and communities
☐ 6. **Education and Facilitation Skills**	a. Ability to use empowering and learner-centered teaching strategies b. Ability to use a range of appropriate and effective educational techniques c. Ability to facilitate group discussions and decision-making d. Ability to plan and conduct classes and presentations for a variety of groups e. Ability to seek out appropriate information and respond to questions about pertinent topics f. Ability to find and share requested information g. Ability to collaborate with other educators h. Ability to collect and use information from and with community members
☐ 7. **Individual and Community Assessment Skills***	a. Ability to participate in individual assessment through observation and active inquiry b. Ability to participate in community assessment through observation and active inquiry
☐ 8. **Outreach Skills***	a. Ability to conduct case-finding, recruitment, and follow-up b. Ability to prepare and disseminate materials c. Ability to build and maintain a current resource inventory
☐ 9. **Professional Skills and Conduct**	a. Ability to set goals and to develop and follow a work plan b. Ability to balance priorities and to manage time c. Ability to apply critical thinking techniques and problem solving d. Ability to use pertinent technology e. Ability to pursue continuing education and life-long learning opportunities f. Ability to maximize personal safety while working in community and/or clinical settings

(continues)

Table C3.2 *(continued)*

	g. Ability to observe ethical and legal standards (e.g., CHW Code of Ethics, Americans with Disabilities Act [ADA], Health Insurance Portability and Accountability Act [HIPAA]) h. Ability to identify situations calling for mandatory reporting and carry out mandatory reporting requirements i. Ability to participate in professional development of peer CHWs and in networking among CHW groups j. Ability to set boundaries and practice self-care

☐ 10. **Evaluation and Research Skills***	a. Ability to identify important concerns and conduct evaluation and research to better understand root causes
	b. Ability to apply the evidence-based practices of Community Based Participatory Research (CBPR) and Participatory Action Research (PAR)
	c. Ability to participate in evaluation and research processes including:
	   i. Identifying priority issues and evaluation/research questions
	   ii. Developing evaluation/research design and methods
	   iii. Data collection and interpretation
	   iv. Sharing results and findings
	   v. Engaging stakeholders to take action on findings

☐ 11. **Knowledge Base**	a. Knowledge about social determinants of health and related disparities b. Knowledge about pertinent health issues c. Knowledge about healthy lifestyles and self-care d. Knowledge about mental/behavioral health issues and their connection to physical health e. Knowledge about health behavior theories f. Knowledge of basic public health principles g. Knowledge about the community served h. Knowledge about United States health and social service systems
C3 Project, 2018|www.C3Project.org	

* *Asterisks denote new skills from 1998 to 2016; several subskills have been expanded.*

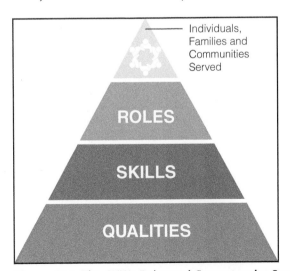

Figure C3.1 The CHWs Roles and Competencies Support Pyramid

C3 Roles and Skills Checklist

C3 CHW Competencies and Professional Development Which of these Core CHW Roles are you trained to provide?		
C3. Core CHW Roles	**My level of training or experience** A. No training/experience B. Some training/experience C. Extensive training/experience	
1. Cultural Mediation Among Individuals, Communities, and Health and Social Service Systems		
2. Providing Culturally Appropriate Health Education and Information		
3. Care Coordination, Case Management and Systems Navigation		
4. Providing Coaching and Social Support		
5. Advocating for Individuals and Communities		
6. Building Individual and Community Capacity		
7. Providing Direct Services		
8. Implementing Individual and Community Assessments		
9. Conducting Outreach		
10. Participating in Evaluation and Research		

Foundations for Community Health Workers, Third Edition. Edited by Tim Berthold and Darouny Somsanith.
© 2024 John Wiley & Sons, Inc. Published 2024 by John Wiley & Sons, Inc.
Companion website: http://www.wiley.com/go/communityhealthworkers3E

Which of these Core CHW Skills are you trained to provide?		
C3. Core CHW Skills		**My level of training and skill** A. No Training B. Some Training C. Extensive Training
1. Communication Skills		
2. Interpersonal and Relationship –Building Skills		
3. Service Coordination and Navigation Skills		
4. Capacity Building Skills		
5. Advocacy Skills		
6. Education and Facilitation Skills		
7. Individual and Community Assessment Skills		
8. Outreach Skills		
9. Professional Skills and Conduct		
10. Evaluation and Research Skills		
11. Knowledge Base		

Video Index

All videos are posted to the Foundations for CHWs YouTube Channel:
https://www.youtube.com/@foundationsforcommunityhea6889/search

CHAPTER	TITLE	DESCRIPTION	URL	QR CODE
Introduction	CHW Digital Story Robert's Story	How Robert Scott became a CHW.	http://youtu.be/Acaf7cKFGy0	
	CHW Digital Story Luciana's Story	How Luciana Padia became a CHW.	http://youtu.be/FS9leOmwACk	
PART 1: Community Health Work: The Big Picture				
Chapter 1: The Role of CHWs	Becoming a CHW CHW Interview	Two working CHWs share what they value about their profession.	http://youtu.be/BASkvuq1epw	
PART 2: Core Competencies for Providing Direct Services				
Chapter 5: Guiding Principles	Setting Boundaries with Clients: Role Play, Counter	A CHW has difficulty setting professional boundaries with a client.	http://youtu.be/kziHCHrwtzo	
	Setting Boundaries with Clients: Role Play, Demo	A CHW sets a professional boundary with a client.	http://youtu.be/pX9x_w8ME9s	
	Setting Professional Boundaries: Faculty Interview	The challenges of communicating, establishing, and maintaining boundaries with clients.	http://youtu.be/WXn-tvVILbY	

CHAPTER	TITLE	DESCRIPTION	URL	QR CODE
	Self-Disclosure Role Play, Counter	A CHW over-discloses personal information.	http://youtu.be/7CpFvjXO-rs	
	Self-Disclosure Role Play, Demo	A CHW demonstrates a limited self-disclosure.	http://youtu.be/12s4zgUUJFs	
	Self-Disclosure: Faculty Interview	The challenges and potential benefits of self-disclosure.	http://youtu.be/ihcr6GvBAAg	
Chapter 6: Behavior Change	Giving Advice: Role Play, Counter	A CHW makes the mistake of giving advice	https://youtu.be/Our62-cD0gk	
	Giving Advice: Role Play, Demo	A CHW uses client-centered skills rather than giving advice.	https://youtu.be/J8Jn__okskAM	
	Big Eyes, Big Ears, Small Mouth: Faculty Interview	The value for CHWs of speaking less and observing and listening more.	http://youtu.be/jE9uNHRhLA4	
	Talking Too Much Role Play, Counter	A CHW who talks too much rather than listening.	http://youtu.be/VhDFNaF0w6c	
	Strength-based Practice: Faculty Interview	The advantages of working with clients using a "strength-based" approach.	http://youtu.be/Cq4PX89tlZE	
	Your Approach to Client-Centered Counseling: Faculty Interview	Key aspects for developing your own approach to client-centered counseling.	http://youtu.be/yHIf0qqkxJI	

CHAPTER	TITLE	DESCRIPTION	URL	QR CODE
Chapter 7: Cultural Humility	Cultural Humility Faculty Interview	Instructor Abby Rincon describes the importance of cultural humility for CHW success with clients.	http://youtu.be/yV3DxgK5pn4	
	Nutrition and Culture Role Play, Counter	A CHW misses an opportunity to demonstrate cultural humility.	http://youtu.be/2Ck3V4johPM	
	Depression, Religion and Cultural Humility: Role Play, Counter	A CHW misses an opportunity to demonstrate cultural humility.	http://youtu.be/y6d-GdXi8go	
	Depression, Religion and Cultural Humility: Role Play, Demo	A CHW demonstrates cultural humility in working with a client.	http://youtu.be/Bgr6TXWknQQ	
Chapter 8: Initial Assessments	Welcoming a Client: Faculty Interview	How a warm welcome helps to build rapport with a new client.	http://youtu.be/iQrlmzhjAls	
	Communicating with Body Language, Role Play, Counter	How negative body language can undermine a relationship with a client.	http://youtu.be/DbsgG-LObPE	
	Communicating with Body Language, Role Play, Demo	A CHW who incorporates effective body language as they work with a client.	http://youtu.be/WDV2OPRzfYo	
	Taking Notes: Role Play, Demo	A CHW demonstrates how to talk with a client about taking notes.	http://youtu.be/yZ6FiTr3O4o	
Chapter 9: Counseling	Relapse Prevention: Role Play, Demo	A CHW talks with a client about preventing a relapse to prior risk behaviors.	http://youtu.be/g7UiLRJ-QkE	

CHAPTER	TITLE	DESCRIPTION	URL	QR CODE
	Relapse Prevention: Role Play, Debrief Faculty Interview	Concepts and skills for relapse prevention, and a discussion of the role play demonstration, "Relapse Prevention".	http://youtu.be/EaXhsT6B8y8	
	Providing an Affirmation: Role Play, Demo	A CHW provides an affirmation to a client.	http://youtu.be/FrggzUE7Z_I	
	Safer Sex & Using a Motivation Scale: Role Play, Demo	A CHW uses motivational interviewing and a motivation scale to support a client with behavior change.	http://youtu.be/h9MP3W4vFFE	
	Rolling with Resistance: Role Play, Counter	A CHW struggles to respond to a client's ambivalence about behavior change.	http://youtu.be/x_hyIMRMy7A	
	Rolling with Resistance: Role Play, Demo	A CHW demonstrates how to roll with resistance when a client is ambivalent about behavior change.	http://youtu.be/rgqrusY2MJI	
	Rolling with Resistance: Faculty Interview	The value of rolling with resistance when a client is ambivalent about behavior change.	http://youtu.be/9vNeWuNUflo	
	The Use of Silence: Role Play, Counter	A CHW who is uncomfortable with silence during a meeting with a client.	http://youtu.be/e98j0ohaQwU	
	The Use of Silence: Role Play, Demo	A CHW who is comfortable with silence during a meeting with client.	http://youtu.be/N5NyZ7OLcMA	
	The Use of Silence: Faculty Interview	Accepting silence as a natural part of conversations with clients.	http://youtu.be/DZNOeVxZfIs	

CHAPTER	TITLE	DESCRIPTION	URL	QR CODE
	Developing Your Client-Centered Practice: Faculty Interview	Key aspects for developing your own client-centered practice.	http://youtu.be/A71MPjMuYh8	
Chapter 10: Case Management	Establishing Client Priorities: Faculty Interview	The importance of supporting a client to establish their own priorities.	http://youtu.be/isOQoAF4kAA	
	Providing a Client-Centered Referral Role Play, Counter	A CHW does not provide a client-centered referral.	http://youtu.be/SzYoL5tA4DU	
	Providing a Client-Centered Referral Role Play, Demo	A CHW demonstrates one way of providing a client-centered referral.	http://youtu.be/2Gol8gJGSZg	
	Developing a List of Referrals CHW Interview	A CHW describes how to develop a list of reliable and culturally relevant referral resources.	http://youtu.be/xKJQo6HExq4	
Chapter 11: Home Visits	Conducting Home Visits: CHW Interview	A CHW shares strategies for conducting successful home visits.	http://youtu.be/BSgqpdyvZ5w	
PART 3: Enhancing Professional Skills				
PART 3				
Chapter 12: Stress	Action Planning and Stress Management: Role Play, Demo	A CHW supports a client with stress management.	http://youtu.be/H_62Cbm5W_c	
	Stress Management: Faculty Interview	The value of stress management for clients and CHWs.	http://youtu.be/YH2na2xuuuo	

CHAPTER	TITLE	DESCRIPTION	URL	QR CODE
Chapter 13: Conflict	Conflict between Two CHWs: Role Play	A conflict between two CHW co-workers.	http://youtu.be/8wHwNAnhC1Y	
	Responding to Anger: Role Play, Counter	A CHW does not respond well to a client's anger.	http://youtu.be/kOZWxisLm5s	
	Responding to Anger: Role Play, Demo	A CHW responds effectively to a client's anger.	http://youtu.be/IMxXFufpHFc	
	The Art of Apology: Faculty Interview	The value of learning when and how to offer a sincere apology to the clients you work with.	http://youtu.be/obtQn3fdGOY	
Chapter 14: Professional Skills	Providing & Receiving Constructive Feedback: Faculty Interview	The importance of learning how to provide and receive constructive feedback in a professional manner.	http://youtu.be/7NqVU0-foEw	
PART 4				
Chapter 15: Incarceration	Listening to a Client's Priorities, Role Play, Counter	A CHW does not do a good job of listening to the client's priorities.	http://youtu.be/n96TZKnnhec	
	Incarceration as a Public Health Issue, Faculty Interview	Donna Willmott, a teacher at CCSF, talks about why understanding people's incarceration histories is part of promoting their health.	http://youtu.be/o7AdDUAyu54	
	First Meeting between a Patient and a CHW, Interview	A client with a history of incarceration speaks about her first impressions of her CHW and the difficulty of trusting a stranger to help her.	http://youtu.be/OrfXKN8IgxA	

CHAPTER	TITLE	DESCRIPTION	URL	QR CODE
	A CHW with a History of Incarceration, CHW Interview	A CHW with a history of incarceration talks about the value of his experiences in building relationships with his clients.	http://youtu.be/PfBJ9GCvkKk	
	CHW Digital Story Ron's Story: A Grandmother's Love	CHW Ron Sanders tells his story.	http://youtu.be/ePDOB5OtjzM	
	CHW Digital Story Juanita's Story: Everyone Has Purpose in Life	CHW Juanita Alvarado tells her story.	http://youtu.be/_AfVE1DCEVc	
	CHW Digital Story Tracy's Story: From Deliverance to Recovery	CHW Tracy Reed tells her story.	http://youtu.be/KEVRnTTGQlw	
	CHW Digital Story Ernest's Story	CHW Certificate Program Graduate Ernest tells his story.	http://youtu.be/2HVB_ZDRs1s	
	CHW Digital Story Lee's Story: Change	Freeman, a patient with the Transitions Clinic in Richmond, CA, tells his story.	http://youtu.be/VEIbOb7BkmQ	
Chapter 16: Chronic Conditions	Action Planning, Revising an Action Plan: Role Play, Counter	A CHW has difficulty addressing a client's challenges in implementing her Action Plan.	http://youtu.be/g6l5omhDSHU	
	Action Planning, Revising an Action Plan: Role Play, Demo	A CHW supports a client to revise their Action Plan.	http://youtu.be/Clr5pcdzo74	
	Action Planning, Revising an Action Plan: Faculty Interview	How to support a client to revise an action plan.	http://youtu.be/JUtog9cd29Q	

CHAPTER	TITLE	DESCRIPTION	URL	QR CODE
	Self-Management: Finding Reasons to Live Interview	A health coach discusses his approach to supporting clients to uncover their motivation for making changes in their life.	http://youtu.be/nRChT90HOMM	
	Action Planning: Faculty Interview	Strategies for supporting a client to develop an Action Plan.	http://youtu.be/51J58BJeQak	
	Medications Management, Part 1: Role Play, Demo	A CHW supports a client with medications management, Part 1 of 4.	http://youtu.be/gleMEwoN72k	
	Medications Management, Part 2: Role Play, Demo	A CHW supports a client with medications management, Part 2 of 4.	http://youtu.be/eLRe6wVkLuw	
	Medications Management, Part 3: Role Play, Demo	A CHW supports a client with medications management, Part 3 of 4.	http://youtu.be/F2Mndwvfu-c	
	Medications Management, Part 4: Role Play, Demo	A CHW supports a client with medications management, Part 4 of 4.	http://youtu.be/SVWbGyEKblk	
Chapter 17: HEAL	Talking about Weight and Health Role Play, Counter	A CHW does not do an effective job of talking with a client about weight.	http://youtu.be/FLpx7QHjMRY	
	Talking about Weight and Health Role Play, Demo	A CHW talks with a client about weight and health.	http://youtu.be/83EeBQuXOXo	

CHAPTER	TITLE	DESCRIPTION	URL	QR CODE
	Action Planning and Exercise: Role Play, Demo	A CHW supports a client to develop an Action Plan to manage chronic health conditions.	http://youtu.be/x9kt4EusdwA	
	Client-Centered Counseling and Nutrition Role Play, Demo	A CHW supports a client to make changes to her diet.	http://youtu.be/73-ebSBGQUo	
	The Value of Taking Small Steps Interview	A health coach discusses how he supports clients to initiate realistic but meaningful change in their life.	http://youtu.be/4ILopSTH7lk	
	Hypertension and Healthy Eating, Part 1 Role Play, Demo	A CHW provides health education about nutrition to a client with high blood pressure.	http://youtu.be/aGuViTC42G4	
	Hypertension and Healthy Eating, Part 2 Role Play, Demo	A CHW provides health education about nutrition to a client with high blood pressure.	http://youtu.be/271pMgUIuNg	
	Hypertension and Healthy Eating, Part 3 Role Play, Demo	A CHW provides health education about nutrition to a client with high blood pressure.	http://youtu.be/gVIV_8iM_HA	
PART 5: Working with Groups and Communities				
Chapter 21: Group Facilitation	Group Facilitation CHW Interview	A CHW describes her work facilitating a support group for Latinas.	http://youtu.be/36IBED_1Nvk	

Index

Note: Page numbers followed by *f* indicate a figure; followed by *t* indicate a table.

Foundations for Community Health Workers, Third Edition. Edited by Tim Berthold and Darouny Somsanith.
© 2024 John Wiley & Sons, Inc. Published 2024 by John Wiley & Sons, Inc.
Companion website: http://www.wiley.com/go/communityhealthworkers3E

American Heart Association, 454
American Public Health Association
    (APHA), 38
anger
  conflict resolution, 365–367
  home visit clients, 326
  person-centered counseling, 250
Annie E. Casey Foundation, 45
anti-discrimination, 125
anti-trans legislation, population
    health, 99
APHA CHW Section, 52
apologies, conflict resolution, 370
applications, jobs, 384–385
applied learning, 611
apprenticeships, 42–43
arthritis, 444, 447
Asians, health inequities, 103
assertive communication, conflict
    resolution, 365
assessments, 189–216, 207f
  beginning, 192–200
  body language, 198–199
  case management plan, 269
  clarification, 211
  client focus, 200–201
  client resources, 202–203
  closed-ended questions, 191, 203
  confidentiality polity, 197–198
  connection, building, 194
  contact information, 214
  demographic information, 202
  documenting, 214–216
  elements of, 193
  ending phase, 192–193, 213–214
  explaining, 196
  forms, 214–216
  Health Insurance Portability and
      Accountability Act (HIPAA), 197
  home visits, 316–317
  individual and community
      assessment skills, 191
  informed consent, 198
  initial, 191–193
  interview space, 194
  key health issues, 205
  language, accessibility, 201
  language of service, 195–196
  middle phase, 192, 200–213
  open-ended questions, 191, 203–204
  pace, 204–205
  person-centered counseling, 221
  providing direct service, 191

  public health, 77–78
  rapport, 194
  referrals, 214
  review, 213
  right to privacy, 202
  scope of practice, 130, 192
  skills, 66, 191
  strength-based approach, 202–203
  summarize, 212
  telehealth, 195, 198
  thanking client, 214
  time management, 202, 213
  tone of voice, 198–199
  training, 614–615
  Vital Signs Life Assessment and
      Rating form, 207f–210f
  wellness issues, 205
assurance, 77–78
asthma, 444, 446–447
ASTHO (Association of State and
    Territorial Health Officials), 51
attire
  home visits, 311
  job interviews, 389
  professional, 391–392
auditory learners, 602, 605
avoidance, conflict resolution, 361

B

Because Black Is Still Beautiful, 433–434
behavior change, 149–156
  accountability, addressing, 155–156
  advice, giving mistake, 153–154
  client blaming, 154–155
  community factors, 150t, 151–152
  criminal justice, 152
  discrimination, 151
  ecological approach, 150–152
  economics, 150t, 152
  family factors, 150t, 151
  friend factors, 150t, 151
  individual factors, 150t, 151
  information reliance mistake, 153
  media, 150t, 152
  mistakes, facilitation, 152–156
  natural events, 152
  neighborhood factors, 150t, 151
  politics, 150t, 151
  prejudice, 151
  societal factors, 150t, 151–152
behavioral responses
  stress, 340
  trauma, 534

beliefs, 118
bias, 659, 672t, 677–678
Big Eyes, Big Ears, and small mouth,
    159f, 369, 465, 609
birthing parent mortality, 92, 100, 102t
Black Organizing Project (BOP),
    693–694
Black Panther Party, 38
Black people, health inequities,
    102, 102t
blame versus contribution, conflict
    resolution, 368–369
blood pressure, 47–48
body language, 198–199, 392–395
body mass index (BMI), 490, 494
Body Positive, 512
boundary crossing, 117, 134–135
Bubble Chart, 246–247, 247f
building capacity, cultural humility,
    176–179
building individual and community
    capacity, 9t, 12, 31, 66, 92, 117,
    148, 184, 221, 333, 357, 378, 409,
    489, 525, 628, 691
bullying, conflict resolution, 359
burnout, 333, 341–342

C

C3 Project, xiv–xvi, 9, 33
Cambridge Health Alliance (CHA), 632
cancer, 46, 70, 444, 447
capacity-building skills, 15f, 17, 41, 409
  community organization, 691
  cultural humility, 176–179
  person-centered counseling, 221
  research and evaluation, 659
cardiovascular diseases, 443, 445, 447
care coordination, case management,
    and system navigation, 9t, 11,
    261, 301, 443
career readiness, 381–391
  action words, 386
  applications, jobs, 384–385
  attire, job interviews, 389
  closing interviews, 390
  communications, 381
  cover letters, 385
  critical thinking, 381
  equity, 381
  experience, 386
  inclusion, 381
  interviewing, 388–391
  job description, 384

chronic conditions (*Continued*)
  harm reduction, 465
  Harvard School of Public Health, 455
  health data, 444
  health education, 465
  health goals, 468
  health inequities, 447
  health-related behaviors, 451
  healthy living, 505
  Hepatitis C, 444
  high blood pressure, 453–454
  HIV Disease, 444, 447
  holistic therapies, 451
  hypertension, 453–454
  integrative therapies, 451
  kidney disease, 444
  management models, 455
  management, 444–447, 455,
      467–471
  Mayo Clinic, 455
  medical equipment, 451
  medical interventions, 451
  medication labels, 473–474
  medication management, 443, 468,
      471–476
  medications, 451, 471–473
  medicine and public health models
      integration, 455–456
  mental health, 444, 451
  motivation, 470–471
  motivational interviewing (MI), 465
  multiple sclerosis, 444
  muscular dystrophy, 444, 447
  National Cancer Institute, 454
  National Institute of Mental Health,
      454
  National Institutes of Health, 454
  National Library of Medicine, 454
  nutrition, 448
  person-centered, 459–460, 464–465
  physical activity, 448
  physical assistance, 451
  population health management, 443,
      458–459, 462
  post-traumatic stress, 444, 449
  relapse, 477–478
  respiratory diseases, 444
  schizophrenia, 444
  scope of practice, 461–462
  second-hand smoke, 448
  self-determination, 464
  self-management, 459–461
  services, ending, 480–481

social change movements, 457
  societal factors, 448–449
  strength-based approach, 465
  stress, 449
  teamwork, 141, 457–458
  therapy, 451
  tobacco use, 448
  treatment, 451–454
  tuberculosis, 444
  US Centers for Disease Control and
      Prevention, 454
  World Health Organization, 455
chronic obstructive pulmonary disease
      (COPD), 444
chronic stress, 333, 336, 340–341, 344
CHW Common Indicators (CI) Project,
      see CI Project
CHWs
  characteristics, 4
  chronic conditions, 444–445
  community organization, 706–710,
      708t–710t
  competencies, 9t, 9–10, 16–18,
      33–34, 665–668
  conferences, 51
  defined, 4–5, 32–33
  health-care team, 141–142
  histories, 30–31
  models of care, 8
  multilingual, 21–22
  networks, 51–54
  number in U.S., 7
  public health, 8
  qualities, 4, 14t, 14–16
  roles, 4f, 4–6, 9t, 9–10, 20–22, 31,
      33–34, 66, 92, 141–142, 426–431
  skills, 4f, 9t, 9, 31, 66, 92
  titles, 6t, 6–7
  trauma survivors, 549–558
    action planning, 556–557
    do's and don'ts, 549–551
    listening, 550
    meeting, ending, 555–556
    referrals, 554
    responding, trauma stories, 551–552
    safety, 555
    self-care, 551
    services, 555
  workforce, 34–35, 48–51
  workforce policy, 48–51
CI Project, 18–19
cisgender, 92, 97, 104
client blaming, 154–155

client conflicts, conflict resolution,
      359–360
client consent, 265
client files, 289–290, 306, 308–309
client focus, assessments, 200–201
client relationships, 125
client resources, 202–203
client support, 130
client's time, home visits, 310
climate change, 40
clinical teams, 139–141
closed groups, 633–634
closed-ended questions, 191, 203
closing interviews, 390
clutter, home visits, 325
Code of Ethics, 123–126
  advocacy for change in law and
      policy, 125
  advocacy for the profession, 126
  anti-discrimination, 125
  client relationships, 125
  conduct, 125
  confidentiality, 124
  continuing education, 125
  cooperation, 125
  cultural humility, 124
  enhancing community capacity, 125
  honesty, 123
  interactions with other service
      providers, 125
  legal obligations, 124
  loyalty to the profession, 126
  maintaining community trust, 124
  professional rights and
      responsibilities, 125–126
  promotion of equitable relationships,
      124–125
  quality of care, 124
  recognition of others, 126
  referral to appropriate services, 124
  respect for human rights, 124
  responsibility in the delivery of care,
      123–124
  scope of ability, 124
  self-presentation, 125
  training, 124
  wellness and safety, 126
code switching, 378–380
co-facilitating social/support groups,
      scope of practice, 132, 650–652
cognitive responses
  stress, 339–340
  trauma, 534–535

social gradient, 92, 101
social groups
    group facilitation, 631–632
    trauma survivors, 542
social justice, 4–5, 8, 15f, 22–23,
        83–86, 105–109
    advocacy for, 108
    community organization, 701
    economic justice, 108–109
    targeted universalism, 105–106
social marketing, community outreach,
        575, 583–585
social media, community outreach,
        584–585
social skills, 637
social workers, 46
society
    behavior change, 150t, 151–152
    ecological model, 79–80
solidarity, 691–692, 699, 702
somatic therapies, 525, 543
sources of conflict, 358–359
speaking clarity, home visits, 311–312
spectrum of prevention, 66, 80–81,
        81t, 87t
spirit, MI, 236
spiritual responses
    stress, 340
    trauma, 536–537, 543
spirituality, self-care, 347–348
stages, case management, 266
stages of change model, 221, 232–234,
        233t
status, trauma survivors, 538–540
stigma, incarceration, 409–410, 416,
        421–422, 424–426, 429, 432
Stockton Economic Empowerment
        Demonstration (SEED), 109
strength-based approach, 148, 160–162
    chronic conditions, 465
    assessments, 202–203
strength-based practice, 608
strengths, client, 269
stress, 331–352
    allostatic load, 333, 340
    associations, 344
    behavioral responses, 340
    burnout, 333, 341–342
    chronic conditions, 449
    chronic stress, 333, 336,
        340–341, 344
    cognitive responses, 339–340

deep breathing, self-care, 347
defined, 333–334
discrimination, 335–336
emotional responses, 339
external resources, 333, 337–338
faith, self-care, 347–348
healthy eating, self-care, 349
internal resources, 333, 337–338
managing, 343–346
meditation, self-care, 348–349
mindfulness, self-care, 348
networks, 344
peer support, self-care, 350
physical activity, self-care,
        346–347
physical responses, 339
post-traumatic stress, 333, 341–342
prayer, self-care, 347–348
Professional Quality of Life Scale
        (ProQOL), 342
professional services, 349–350
reduction activities, 612
relaxing, 345–346
resources, 343–344
responses, 339–340
risk assessment, 342
root causes, 344
secondary resilience, 333
secondary trauma, 333, 341
self-assessment, 342
self-care, 346–350
self-reflection, 342
spiritual responses, 340
spirituality, self-care, 347–348
stress reduction, 350–351
stressors, 333–335
supportive supervision, 333, 343
vicarious trauma, 341
weathering, 333, 340
wellness, CHW, 343
stress reduction, 350–351
stressors, 333–335
stroke, 70
structural discrimination, cultural
        diversity, 167
structural racism, cultural
        diversity, 167
suburban settings, home visits, 302
suicide assessments, 558–560, 615
summarize
    assessments, 212
    MI, 242

supervision
    case management, 265, 294–295
    community outreach, 598–599
    conflict resolution, 358
    person-centered counseling, 251
supervisors, 120, 397–398
support
    professional development, 400
    trauma survivors, 543
support groups, 542, 630
supportive and corrective feedback,
        378–379, 395–397
supportive supervision, stress, 333, 343
surveys, training, 615
survivor's guilt, 533

T
targeted universalism, 92, 105–106
task conflict, 358
team-based care, 140–141
team meetings, case management,
        293–294
teamwork, multidisciplinary, 138–143
    case management, person-centered,
        141, 266
    case management plan, 275
    challenges, 142–143
    chronic conditions, 141, 457–458
    CHW role, health-care team,
        141–142
    clinical teams, 139–141
    communication, 140–141
    community outreach, 594
    culture of unity, 141
    growth opportunities, 141
    hierarchies, 142
    home visits, 142
    medication management, 141
    mission, shared, 140
    outcomes, measurable, 141
    outreach, 141
    patient education, 141
    role clarity, 140
    strategies, 143
    team-based care benefits, 140
    team-based care characteristics,
        140–141
    vision, shared, 140
    workload equity, 142
teamwork
    person-centered counseling, 251
    professional development, 381